Assessment of Dynamic Lung Functions: Essential Pulmonology

Assessment of Dynamic Lung Functions: Essential Pulmonology

Editor: Louie Foster

AMERICAN
MEDICAL PUBLISHERS
www.americanmedicalpublishers.com

AMERICAN
MEDICAL PUBLISHERS
www.americanmedicalpublishers.com

Cataloging-in-Publication Data

Assessment of dynamic lung functions : essential pulmonology / edited by Louie Foster.
p. cm.
Includes bibliographical references and index.
ISBN 979-8-88740-573-5
1. Lungs--Diseases. 2. Respiratory organs--Diseases. 3. Pulmonary circulation.
4. Pulmonary function tests. I. Foster, Louie.
RC756 .A87 2023
616.24--dc23

American Medical Publishers,
41 Flatbush Avenue,
1st Floor, New York,
NY 11217, USA

ISBN 979-8-88740-573-5 (Hardback)

Contents

Preface

The lungs are vital organs situated on both sides of the chest. They have a variety of functions. However, their primary function is gas exchange between the blood and lung. Lungs are also integral to the maintenance of homeostasis and blood pressure. They can be affected by various diseases and disorders which are studied and treated under the discipline of pulmonology. This area of medicine is involved in the management of various respiratory diseases, including asthma, emphysema, tuberculosis and pneumonia. There are several clinical procedures that can be used for the diagnosis of pulmonary diseases, which include blood tests, arterial blood gas tests, pulmonary function testing, bronchoscopy, CT scan, chest X-rays, and positron emission therapy. This book provides comprehensive insights on dynamic lung functions. It presents researches and studies performed by experts across the globe. The book is appropriate for medical students and professionals seeking detailed information in this area of pulmonology.

After months of intensive research and writing, this book is the end result of all who devoted their time and efforts in the initiation and progress of this book. It will surely be a source of reference in enhancing the required knowledge of the new developments in the area. During the course of developing this book, certain measures such as accuracy, authenticity and research focused analytical studies were given preference in order to produce a comprehensive book in the area of study.

This book would not have been possible without the efforts of the authors and the publisher. I extend my sincere thanks to them. Secondly, I express my gratitude to my family and well-wishers. And most importantly, I thank my students for constantly expressing their willingness and curiosity in enhancing their knowledge in the field, which encourages me to take up further research projects for the advancement of the area.

Editor

1

Ventilation and Perfusion at the Alveolar Level: Insights from Lung Intravital Microscopy

Jasmin Matuszak[1], *Arata Tabuchi*[2] *and Wolfgang M. Kuebler*[1,3]*

[1] *Institute of Physiology, Charité – Universitätsmedizin Berlin, Corporate Member of Freie Universität Berlin, Humboldt-Universität zu Berlin, and Berlin Institute of Health, Berlin, Germany,* [2] *The Keenan Research Centre for Biomedical Science at St. Michael's, Toronto, ON, Canada,* [3] *Departments of Surgery and Physiology, University of Toronto, Toronto, ON, Canada*

Correspondence:
Wolfgang M. Kuebler
wolfgang.kuebler@charite.de

Intravital microscopy (IVM) offers unique possibilities for the observation of biological processes and disease related mechanisms *in vivo*. Especially for anatomically complex and dynamic organs such as the lung and its main functional unit, the alveolus, IVM provides exclusive advantages in terms of spatial and temporal resolution. By the use of lung windows, which have advanced and improved over time, direct access to the lung surface is provided. In this review we will discuss two main topics, namely alveolar dynamics and perfusion from the perspective of IVM-based studies. Of special interest are unanswered questions regarding alveolar dynamics such as: What are physiologic alveolar dynamics? How do these dynamics change under pathologic conditions and how do those changes contribute to ventilator-induced lung injury? How can alveolar dynamics be targeted in a beneficial way? With respect to alveolar perfusion IVM has propelled our understanding of the pulmonary microcirculation and its perfusion, as well as pulmonary vasoreactivity, permeability and immunological aspects. Whereas the general mechanism behind these processes are understood, we still lack a proper understanding of the complex, multidimensional interplay between alveolar ventilation and microvascular perfusion, capillary recruitment, or vascular immune responses under physiologic and pathologic conditions. These are only part of the unanswered questions and problems, which we still have to overcome. IVM as the tool of choice might allow us to answer part of these questions within the next years or decades. As every method, IVM has advantages as well as limitations, which have to be taken into account for data analysis and interpretation, which will be addressed in this review.

Keywords: intravital microscopy, alveolar dynamics, alveolar perfusion, pulmonary microcirculation, acute lung injury, lung video microscopy

INTRODUCTION

Intravital microscopy (IVM) is a two-dimensional imaging technique that allows for visualization of biological processes *in vivo*. It is highly versatile as it can be adjusted to various tissues and can be combined with high quality state-of-the-art microscopy enabling high resolution of tissue and single cells in the natural and complex environment of a multicellular organism (**Figure 1**). Some tissues in experimental animals are easily accessible, such as the vessels of the ear or can be easily exteriorized in mice for vascular IVM studies such as the mesentery or the cremaster muscle. For internal organs and/or chronic observation, the implantation of imaging windows is typically required, and widely used as abdominal, cranial and thoracic windows, as well as dorsal skin fold chambers. Depending on the desired penetration depth, the spatial resolution and the temporal resolution, different microscopic methods can be applied, ranging from widefield, laser scanning confocal, spinning disk, multi-photon microscopy or others. The use of fluorescent dyes and transgenic animals expressing fluorescent markers opens seemingly endless possibilities for the visualization of *in vivo* biological processes down to the subcellular level.

Albeit generations of excellent scientists have advanced our understanding of respiratory physiology to the current stage (Rahn et al., 1946; Suki and Bates, 2011), one of the most basic physiological principles, i.e., alveolar dynamics, is still surprisingly poorly understood. Our insight into the dynamic processes has been hampered by the limited accessibility of alveoli for dynamic studies at the microscale *in vivo* (Grune et al., 2019). Due to the lung's complex structure, direct visualization by IVM is only possible for structures close to the lungs surface, such as subpleural alveoli. *In vitro*, as well as *ex vivo* or *in situ* models can only partially reflect the complex physiologic situation at the level of the alveolus and its surrounding capillary network in health and disease. Standard clinical and experimental imaging approaches including X-ray, computer tomography (CT), magnet resonance imaging (MRI), positron emission tomography (PET) and single photon emission computed tomography (SPECT) are able to image the whole lung and thus, provide important insight into disease state and general mechanisms, but are unsuitable to detect structures and processes at the microscale alveolar level. At the moment no non-invasive imaging technique is available that would enable the imaging of the alveolar or capillary microarchitecture *in vivo* at single-cell or subcellular resolution. The same applies to dynamic phenomena, such as alveolar dynamics, defined here as changes in alveolar size and morphology over the time course of the respiratory cycle in consideration of the underlying biophysical forces, or capillary microhemodynamics, i.e., microvascular flow characteristics and their determining factors in alveolar capillaries. Due to its anatomical complexity (Schneider et al., 2019) and dynamic behavior both at the level of ventilation and perfusion, direct imaging can provide unique insights into our understanding of lung physiology, perfusion and immunology, especially at the alveolar level. Yet, IVM of the lung simultaneously poses a series of unique problems, such as the restricted accessibility of the organ within an anatomical cavity at physiologically subatmospheric pressures. The three-dimensional structure of the alveolo-capillary unit comprises abundant air-liquid interfaces which prevent exploitation of e.g., multiphoton imaging for deep tissue penetration. The dynamic behavior of the lung tissue poses unique problems in terms of motion control. And finally its immunoprivileged status predilects the lung for immune reactions in response to surgical trauma or mechanical ventilation. Although IVM has been successfully used to study pulmonary microvascular responses as well as alveolar mechanics in real-time, the emerging understanding of alveolar physiology and pathophysiology are both still far from complete. Importantly, these limitations in our understanding are only in part attributable to a relatively small number of studies due to the complexity of such analyses. Adding to such limitations are controversial interpretations of the observations obtained from IVM. Such differences in interpretation relate in part to the above-mentioned methodological limitations of IVM, but also to the question how alveolar dynamics should be described, and what constitutes normal vs. pathological behavior, as will be discussed later in this review.

The key function of the pulmonary system is gas exchange, which is predominantly localized in the highly specialized respiratory zone, the alveoli. Interestingly, alveolarization and maturation of the microvasculature are the only developmental processes of the lung that continue after birth, up to 21 years (Schittny, 2017), emphasizing the importance and intricacy of the alveolar system. Alveoli are the dead-end of the respiratory tree and enable the uptake of oxygen and the removal of carbon dioxide at the alveolar membrane. To this end, the total alveolo-capillary membrane, comprised of the alveolar epithelial wall facing the gas side, the endothelial wall at the blood side, and a single fused basement membrane between the two, is extremely thin (at some places <100 nm thick). Almost 90% of the lung acts as a functional respiratory zone (parenchyma) with 300 million alveoli and an incredible surface area of 143 m^2 (Gehr et al., 1978). The quality of gas exchange of the lung is directly dependent on the number of functional alveoli, the thickness of the alveolo-capillary membrane, alveolar vascularization and perfusion. In various lung diseases, this delicate alveolar design can be compromised leading to injured and dysfunctional alveoli and impaired gas exchange which in some cases will require supplemental oxygen or even mechanical ventilation. A prime example for such an acute scenario is the acute respiratory distress syndrome (ARDS), an acute failure of the respiratory system with an in-hospital death rate of approximately 30% (Petrucci and Iacovelli, 2007). ARDS is a multifactorial disease with various underlying causes, but is usually characterized by a rapid onset, an extensive inflammation of the lungs, and clinical characteristics such as failure of the alveolo-capillary barrier resulting in severely impaired gas exchange and abnormal low blood oxygenation (hypoxemia). In the absence of effective pharmacological treatments, mechanical ventilation is presently the mainstay of therapy to warrant oxygenation in ARDS. Yet, mechanical ventilation is a double-edged sword and has to be used with caution. On the one hand mechanical ventilation is essential for the patients' survival, but on the other hand it can inflict permanent damage to the lung referred to as ventilator-induced lung injury (VILI) or ventilator-associated lung injury (VALI) (Amato et al., 1998), which negatively impacts both survival and post-survival life-quality. In already injured alveoli mechanical ventilation can impose further damage to the alveolar wall by physical and biological stresses, such as volutrauma, biotrauma or ergotrauma (which will be discussed in greater detail in the section: intravital microscopy for analysis of alveolar dynamics), although there is no consensus with respect to the main mechanism of injury.

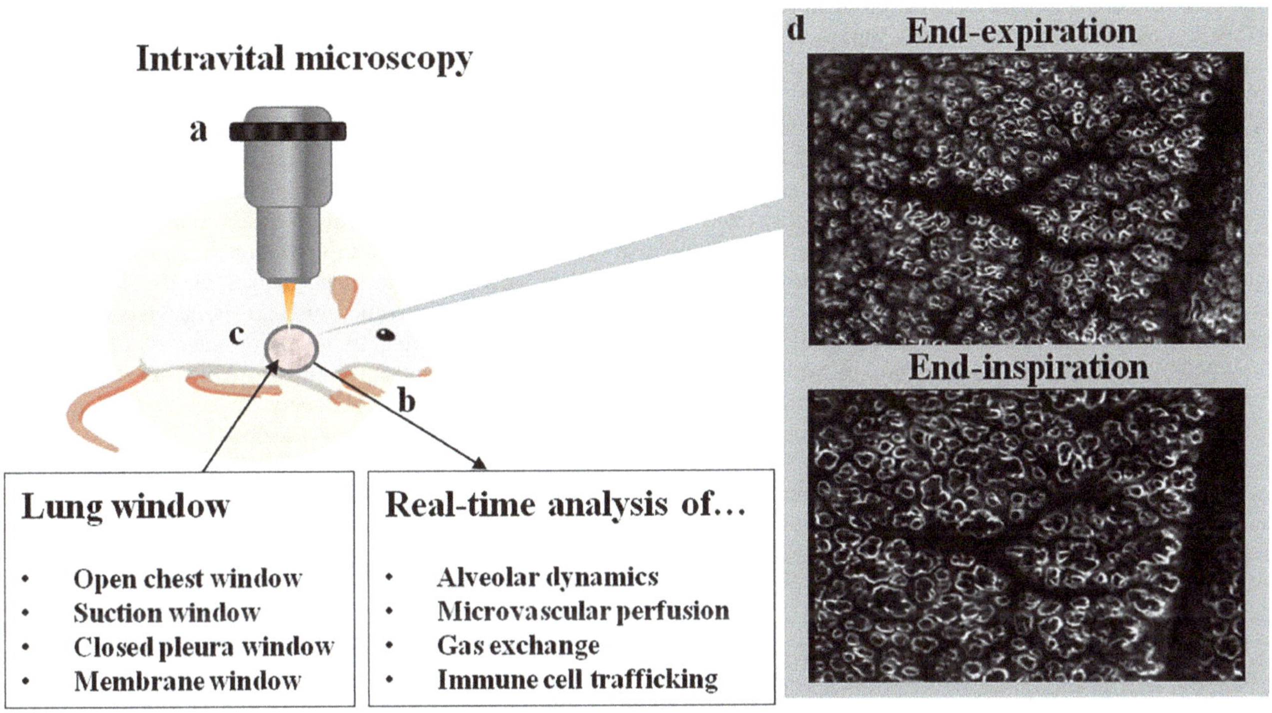

FIGURE 1 | Schematic overview of a lung window and IVM. Intravital microscopy **(a)** is typically performed in mechanically ventilated animals (**b**; e.g., mouse, rat, swine, dog). Access to the lung is gained via excision of a surgical window **(c)** from the thoracic wall, with different types of windows currently in use. Imaging can be performed with several light microscopic applications ranging from widefield microscopy to multiphoton microscopy. In **(d)** two representative images of subpleural alveoli imaged by darkfield illumination at end-inspiration and end-expiration are shown. In the center of the image, a vascular tree can be seen with its terminal branches, surrounded by alveoli which distend during inspiration. On the right side of the image, the rim of the lung lobe can be seen. Ethical approval for the animal experiment was obtained from the Animal Care Committee of St. Michael's Hospital Toronto. The figure was designed using resources from Freepik.com.

Although – as will be discussed later – important limitations exist, IVM is currently the gold standard for visualization of alveoli *in vivo* and offers a broad potential to provide new insight into alveolar dynamics. In this review we will draw attention to the opportunities but also to the challenges and limitations of IVM in this context. We will discuss the use of IVM in different fields of lung research and provide a perspective for future areas of research. First, we will begin with a brief background on the development of IVM in lung research.

INTRAVITAL MICROSCOPY OF THE LUNG – FROM EARLY BEGINNINGS TO CURRENT STATE-OF-THE-ART

Although IVM of the lung will be considered by many as a very modern or recent technique, it was in fact applied as early as in 1661 by Marcello Malpighi. Malpighi observed the pulmonary microvasculature of the frog lung with a microscope and described for the first time alveoli and the surrounding alveolar capillaries (Young, 1929). More than 250 years later in 1925, Harry Hall visualized the pulmonary microcirculation in cats and rabbits by transilluminating the lung lobes outside of the chest (Hall and Chapman, 1925). Taking into account the importance of the natural physiologic environment of the lung, Hall's approach to open up the chest and remove the lung for examination was successively replaced by a more elegant method, the thoracic window technique. The first attempt to create a thoracic window was accomplished by the removal of muscle from the rib cage with the parietal pleura being left intact (Wearn et al., 1934). The lung of the paralyzed animals was then transilluminated with a beam of light entering from a second window in the diaphragm. With this technique, Wearn et al. (1934) were able to describe the basis of capillary recruitment in the lung. The analysis of subpleural alveoli under closed thorax/chest condition was established in 1935 by Terry by implantation of a hollow metal cylinder centered by a cover glass (Terry, 1939). This revealed, however, a new problem of intravital imaging, namely the cyclic respiratory movements of the lung leading to motion artifacts. Wagner (1969) solved this problem in a canine model by a suction device which fixed the lung surface to a coverglass via negative pressure that was applied through a series of bore holes. This suction manifold was able to markedly reduce respiratory motion within the window of observation. Almost 50 years later, an improved lung window for stabilized imaging in mice was established by Looney et al. (2011) enabling live-imaging and in particular single cell tracking by two-photon imaging in an area of observation that is immobilized by a suction device. Vacuum suction stabilized lung windows are now widely used to analyze the pulmonary immune system (Looney et al.,

2011). This includes neutrophil margination (Kuebler et al., 1994, 1997; Park et al., 2019) or immune cell – tumor cell interactions (Hanna et al., 2016), as well as infections of the lung (Sewald, 2018; Ueki et al., 2018).

Yet, although suction devices can effectively reduce or even eliminate motion artifacts in IVM, mechanical stabilization of the lung surface generates a non-physiological situation that prevents adequate assessment of alveolar dynamics and the effects of ventilation on microvascular perfusion. In addition, suction of the lung surface to a glass window for observation may potentially injure the sensible lung surface and stimulate inflammatory responses. To overcome these limitations, Tabuchi et al. (2008) developed a thoracic window without suction in which the lung is allowed to move freely within a closed chest cavity, thus mimicking physiological situations at the expense of image stabilization. In this approach, a thoracic window of 7 mm in diameter is generated by removal of chest muscles and ribs, and a transparent membrane is glued to the thoracic wall to re-create a closed-chest situation. With the help of a transdiaphragmal catheter the pleural air is removed and negative pleural pressure re-established, lifting the lung surface to the membrane-sealed lung window for microscopic observation. Although movements from respiratory and cardiac cycles persist in this model, identical areas will return into the microscopic focus plane during the inspiratory or expiratory plateau phase, allowing for ventilation-triggered imaging acquisition during these periods. By use of this approach Tabuchi and colleagues studied blood oxygenation (Tabuchi et al., 2013) and alveolar dynamics in healthy and diseased lungs (Mertens et al., 2009; Nickles et al., 2014; Tabuchi et al., 2016).

Similar to the "pleural window" by Wearn et al. (1934), Mazzuca et al. (2014) created an "intact pleural window" (size 0.5 cm^2) by removing tissue down to the transparent parietal pleura allowing for direct visualization under closed-chest conditions without the implantation of a "artificial" lung window. This technique combines the advantages of the "physiological" free-moving lung in the Tabuchi model with a reduced surgical trauma at the expense of a smaller area of observation (i.e., one intercostal space). Other researchers adjusted their lung window by placing it in a small chamber at 37°C to exclude temperature-related adverse effects on the tissue directly located under the window surface (Kreisel et al., 2010).

All of the abovementioned lung windows are typically used for short-time imaging that does not exceed several hours. Only a few lung windows have been reported that may allow for long-term observations in dogs, rabbits (De Alva and Rainer, 1963), rats (Fingar et al., 1994) or mice (Kimura et al., 2010), albeit without stabilization and at low spatial resolution. Recently, however, Entenberg and colleagues developed an impressive model of a permanently implanted lung window in mice, which is minimally invasive, allowing the mouse to awake from the surgical intervention and breathe independently. For this approach the authors used an inert and corrosion-resistant steel window for high-resolution imaging of the lung (WHRIL) that allows for long term observation of the different stages of lung metastasis (Entenberg et al., 2018). According to this initial report, the window offers similar high-quality images as classic suction-fixed lung windows, with the possibility to visualize the same lung area repeatedly over several weeks by use of an established technique for microcartography (Entenberg et al., 2018). If this approach should be replicable in other labs and allow for longitudinal observations, it would open multiple new opportunities to monitor the progression of lung diseases. This would include changes in alveolar dynamics, microhemodynamics, microvascular tone regulation, and immune cell trafficking in animal models of different lung diseases including but not limited to ARDS/acute lung injury, lung fibrosis, COPD, pulmonary hypertension, and other parenchymal and vascular lung diseases.

Beside their "classic" use for intravital imaging, lung windows have also been effectively used to measure alveolar pressures in a closed-chest model in dogs (Bates et al., 1989), illustrating the versatility of the lung window approach. To this end, a small incision was made into the parietal pleura, and visceral and parietal pleura were glued together in this area. Next, a small plastic capsule was glued to the surface of the lung with a piezoresistive pressure transducer puncturing the visceral pleura for alveolar pressure measurement.

Despite the successful application of lung windows over several decades, some key limitations have to be taken into consideration for the study of alveolar dynamics. These restrictions relate in particular to four points, which will be discussed in greater detail in the chapter "Limitations of IVM": First, IVM limitation to two-dimensional imaging, preventing three-dimensional analysis of alveolar dynamics. Second, IVM is presently restricted to structures at or close to the organ surface such as subpleural alveoli, while deeper lung compartments cannot be accessed. Third, IVM can only image and analyze a small percentage of the total number of alveoli. Fourth, the specific location at which IVM is performed may impact the findings, e.g., due to its position within the hydrostatic gradient of the lung (pulmonary bases vs. apex).

INTRAVITAL MICROSCOPY FOR ANALYSIS OF ALVEOLAR DYNAMICS

Breathing is a complex process, in which air flows into the lung via the airways along a pressure gradient created by the contraction of the diaphragm and the external intercostal muscles. When external intercostal muscles and the diaphragm relax, lung elastic fibers and alveolar surface tension will cause a decrease in lung volume and thus, exhalation of carbon dioxide rich gas. Although the anatomical and physiological changes during the respiratory cycle at the level of the whole lung are well understood, there is presently no consensus on the corresponding tissue dynamics at the alveolar levels. Rather, different and in part mutually exclusive concepts and theories have been proposed how alveoli may behave during the physiological respiratory cycle, and in particular in diseased lungs, which will be described in more detail in the following paragraphs.

Alveolar Dynamics in Healthy Lungs

In 1929 the physiologist Charles Clifford Macklin was one of the first to study the mechanics of the distal airspaces during the respiratory cycle. He assumed that the main volume change in the respiratory area during breathing occurs in the alveolar ducts and not the alveoli itself. This concept was based on the notion that alveoli experience almost no stretch, except for the border area between alveolar duct and alveoli. Rather, ventilation would be controlled by a continuous muscle system running form the larynx to the alveoli (Macklin, 1929). Approximately 40 years later this theory was questioned by experiments in feline (Storey and Staub, 1962) and guinea pig lungs (Forrest, 1970) where a rapid-freeze method was applied to analyze lungs at different volumes of inflation. Morphometric methods were applied to quantify the impact of lung volume change on alveolar and alveolar duct dimensions. These studies revealed an increase in alveolar volume (2×) and surface area (70%) when lung volume increased from functional residual capacity to 75–80% of total lung capacity (Storey and Staub, 1962) suggesting isotropic "balloon-like" distension of the alveoli. Subsequent studies by Gil and Weibel using electron microscopy of fixed rabbit lungs similarly suggested a change of alveolar volume as a function of total lung volume and explained it with an unfolding of alveolar septal pleats and folds and uncrumpling of the alveolar surface (Gil and Weibel, 1972; Gil et al., 1979). Notably, the notion of septal unfolding and uncrumpling – albeit providing an intuitive concept for the extraordinary capacity of the lung to accommodate considerable volume changes within the normal breathing range with relatively minor pressure increase – has at large been neglected over the past decade in the discussion of alveolar dynamics. While generations of scientists have studied the effects of mechanical stretch on alveolar epithelial cells using various commercially available or custom-designed stretch devices it is important to note that alveolar epithelial stretch – at least within the confines of normal tidal volumes – may be minimal if alveolar distension and contraction are primarily the result of surface folding/crumpling and unfolding/uncrumpling. Beside unfolding of alveolar septa and isotropic "balloon-like" changes of alveolar size, two other mechanism have been proposed as theoretically possible causes for the change of lung volume during inflation, namely a sequential recruitment of previously collapsed alveolar units or simultaneous changes in alveolar shape and size (i.e., non-isotropic distension) (Gil et al., 1979).

Importantly, the above reported findings were unanimously derived from morphological examinations and stereological analyses of excised and fixed lungs, prevented the analysis of the effects of different inflation levels within the same lung. More importantly, *post mortem* findings can only reflect static conditions yet not the dynamic behavior of alveoli over the respiratory cycle. Just as static and dynamic lung compliance diverge considerably; extrapolations from static end-point measurements of alveolar mechanics may lead to potentially erroneous interpretations regarding the dynamic behavior of alveoli in the intact lung. Important insights on such dynamic relationships was initially derived from theoretical models, notably the landmark paper by Jere Mead, who demonstrated the role lung distension and its relevance for the uniform expansion of air spaces (Mead et al., 1970). Other important topics addressed by theoretical models were stress-strain relationships (Fung, 1975), the dynamics of single vs. multiple alveoli (Schirrmann et al., 2010), as well as more complex alveolar regions (Tsuda et al., 2008; Sznitman et al., 2009).

Moreci and Norman (1973) performed the first *in vivo* observations of alveolar dynamics in a rat open chest preparation using incident light photomicrography. In this study, the authors observed a marked change in the size of the alveolar duct, whereas the alveolar volume only showed minor changes over the respiratory cycle. These findings were confirmed in a subsequent study from the same group (Daly et al., 1975) and would suggest the alveolar duct rather than the individual alveolus as the main site for airspace volume change. The group of Gary Nieman and colleagues, however, who performed an extensive series of IVM studies on alveolar dynamics in healthy and diseased lungs came to very different conclusions. At the end of the 1990s they proposed the concept of alveolar recruitment and derecruitment (R/D) in healthy dog lungs as the main mechanism for lung volume increase (Carney et al., 1999). Specifically, they proposed the recruitment (opening) of new (previously collapsed) alveoli when lung volume was increased from functional residual capacity (FRC) to 80% of total lung capacity (TLC). By IVM of dog lungs in an open chest approach via a glass coverslip that was carefully lowered onto the lung surface, the authors observed a small extent of isotropic alveolar distention during lung inflation, yet only up to 20% of TLC, with no detectable change in alveolar volume with further increases in lung volume. From these data and the observation that the number of alveoli per area of observation increased with higher lung volume, the authors concluded that changes in alveolar number due to recruitment rather than isotropic distension of alveoli (or alveolar ducts) must constitute the primary mechanism of physiological lung volume changes (Carney et al., 1999). In support of this notion, Hajari et al. (2012) calculated a linear increase in the number of alveoli with increasing total gas volume based on measurements by hyperpolarized ^{3}He diffusion and MRI in healthy human subjects.

The concept of R/D as primary mechanism of lung volume change during the physiological respiratory cycle contrasts, however, with previous findings of alveolar distension and contraction as the predominant mechanism of volume change in healthy lungs (Storey and Staub, 1962; Forrest, 1970). Analogous to these latter reports, IVM studies of the mechanically unimpaired lung by use of the thoracic window technique developed by Tabuchi et al. (2008) identified alveolar clusters to expand gradually with increasing inspiratory pressure in ventilated mice. The resulting pressure-volume relationship for the individual alveolus followed a sigmoid curve (Mertens et al., 2009) that is largely reminiscent of the classic pressure-volume curve for the entire lung (Rahn et al., 1946). In contrast, the total number of alveoli per area of interest remained unchanged, indicating alveolar distension and contraction rather than R/D as the main mechanism of lung volume change in this study (Mertens et al., 2009). As IVM is always hampered by the extrapolation of two-dimensional observations to the three-dimensional stage, the latter study was further validated by parallel optical coherence tomography (OCT) which confirmed alveolar distension and contraction at the three-dimensional level (Gaertner et al., 2012).

While IVM in intact, live animals - ideally under minimally invasive, closed chest conditions or even under spontaneous ventilation - is the gold standard for the visualization of alveolar dynamics, a common alternative - albeit less physiological - model used to analyze alveolar dynamics that allows for optimal control of ventilation and perfusion are excised, mechanically ventilated and constantly perfused lungs. By this approach, Namati et al. (2008) observed alveolar distension during lung inflation, yet at the end of inspiration the number of alveoli increased while alveolar volume decreased. The authors interpreted this finding as evidence for R/D and developed the concept of secondary daughter alveoli that get recruited by the primary (mother) alveoli via the pores of Kohn, i.e., hole-like interfaces between neighboring alveoli, rather than the conducting airways (Namati et al., 2008). In subsequent studies the same group switched from isolated lungs to *in vivo* optical frequency domain imaging (OFDI) in swine. Remarkably, in these studies alveolar dynamics were best fitted by uniform alveolar distension, although a heterogeneous component of airspace distension was observed as well (Namati et al., 2013), yet no R/D. These two studies from the same group highlight exemplarily the impact of the chosen experimental model on the results generated. Accordingly, one crucial factor for discordant results in the field of alveolar dynamics might be based on the use of different experimental models and methods, which are further complicated by species differences.

Although in the past 50 years several different groups tried to shed light on alveolar dynamics with different models and methods, no overall consent has been developed and as such, the topic remains controversial. A recent editorial by Nieman (2012) discussing Hajari et al.'s (2012) analysis of alveolar dynamics by MRI-based ^{3}He lung morphometry *in vivo* ensued a subsequent debate (Mitzner and Smaldone, 2012; Smaldone and Mitzner, 2012; Weibel et al., 2012) which summed up the different viewpoints and potential problems. As mentioned before Hajari et al. (2012) suggested that alveoli are regularly recruited and derecruited during inflation and expiration with no change of the inner surface area. Smaldone and Mitzner pointed out that these results, albeit showing parallels to their own work, critically depend on adjusting the parameters of a model to a single alveolar duct, thereby simplifying physiologic conditions (Smaldone and Mitzner, 2012). In the same discussion, Weibel highlighted that alveoli are often regarded as a unique structure itself, but that this is a misjudgment and the surrounding tissue and its interactions such as fiber tension and surface forces "make" alveoli. Schittny proposed that alveolar folding can be a proper explanation for recruitment in adult lungs and that R/D may be based on surfactant and surface tensions (Weibel et al., 2012). These different opinions highlight the current state of uncertainty with respect to alveolar dynamics, as - in the words of Smaldone and Mitzner - "what happens to lung acinar structure with lung inflation in a pathologic or even in a normal healthy lung remains unresolved" (Smaldone and Mitzner, 2012).

Alveolar Dynamics in Diseased Lungs

The present lack of a consensus regarding normal alveolar dynamics constitutes one of the major obstacles for our understanding of pathological alveolar dynamics in various lung diseases. This is particularly relevant as an appropriate understanding of alveolar dynamics in the diseased lung is likely crucial for the development of optimized or personalized ventilation regimes and for the development of novel therapeutic strategies. The only current consensus on alveolar dynamics in diseased lungs is that they differ from normal alveolar dynamics and that this differential behavior will likely contribute to or aggravate VILI. The situation under pathologic conditions is further complicated by the expected heterogeneity of pathological alveolar dynamics. Alveolar mechanics under physiological conditions can be expected to be essentially uniform over time and even between species. In contrast, alveolar dynamics in injured lungs can be expected to be more heterogeneous at the regional or even local level (i.e., between neighboring alveoli), and may further differ depending on the etiology of ARDS (e.g., direct vs. indirect lung injury), its severity and time course, as well as the presence or absence of additional disease-related comorbidities.

The most popular concept for alveolar dynamics in the acutely injured lung postulates that alveoli become unstable, leading to collapse and reopening during spontaneous respiration and - in particular - mechanical ventilation. Several groups using a diverse set of methods have provided evidence in support of this concept. Taskar and colleagues ventilated rabbits with either healthy lungs (Taskar et al., 1995) or with lungs in which surfactant function had been impaired by inhalation of dioctyl sodium sulfosuccinate (DOSS) (Taskar et al., 1997) in an open chest setting. In both scenarios, ventilation with negative end-expiratory pressure (NEEP) caused R/D. In healthy lungs R/D as a consequence of NEEP ventilation caused a transient yet reversible decrease in arterial oxygenation and lung compliance, but no overt direct injury of the lung tissue on histological examination (Taskar et al., 1995). In contrast, in lungs with impaired surfactant function simulating an acutely injured lung, NEEP caused persistent severe tissue damage with impaired lung mechanics and gas exchange (Taskar et al., 1997). These effects were prevented by ventilation with positive end-expiratory airway pressure, suggesting that R/D may aggravate VILI in pre-injured but not necessarily in healthy lung. In line with these findings, Seah et al. (2011) showed in that a combination of high tidal volume and zero end-expiratory pressure (ZEEP) causes VILI due to R/D in a murine model, which was not the case when mice were ventilated with either high tidal volume or ZEEP. Based on these findings the authors postulated a "map" of "safe" and "unsafe" ventilation settings, highlighting that the "unsafe" area can dramatically widen in injured lungs. A time- and pressure-dependent effect on R/D was observed in saline-lavaged rat lungs following recruitment maneuvers (Albert et al., 2009). While rapid inflation occurred within 1–2 s, recruitment was notably delayed in that it was absent for the first seconds and then continued to progress over the entire measured time-frame of 40 s. This delayed recruitment response may be clinically relevant, as inspiratory time in the clinical setting is commonly in the range of 0.5–1.5 s, thus potentially preventing R/D in the clinical context.

In a different study, Neumann et al. (1998) tested three different injury models for their impact on alveolar dynamics as assessed by CT. After induction of lung injury by oleic acid, endotoxin, or lung lavage in six ventilated pigs, the authors measured lung density and observed a quick onset of R/D in all experimental models. The notion that R/D is a frequent form of impaired alveolar dynamics in injured lungs was further supported by a substantial number of IVM studies from the group of Gary Nieman. In one of their initial studies Nieman et al. (1981) demonstrated the importance of the surfactant stabilizing effect on alveoli in a canine model of surfactant deactivation by pulmonary lavage with Tween 20 or saline (as control), respectively. Surfactant deactivation by Tween lead to distinct changes in alveolar size, with total collapse at end-expiration, later defined as R/D. Within the 4 h of the experimental protocol, alveolar stability was restored. In subsequent studies with Tween-mediated surfactant deactivation in pigs the authors observed heterogeneous lung injury (Schiller et al., 2001) and progressive alveolar instability – notably defined as change in alveolar shape and size, see below – when tidal volume was increased from 6 to 12 and 15 mL/kg bw (Steinberg et al., 2002). A positive end-expiratory–pressure (PEEP) level of 10 cmH_2O was able to stabilize alveoli, while lower PEEP levels resulted in R/D (Halter et al., 2003). In rats over-ventilated with an inspiratory peak pressure (IPP) of 45 cm H_2O the authors observed alveolar instability or R/D after 45 min, which persisted for 90 min until the end of the study, yet contrary to what could be expected, gross damage to the alveolar epithelium was not observed. As such, the latter findings argue against a decisive role for R/D in the pathogenesis of VILI (Pavone et al., 2007). This notion is also supported by a series of preclinical and clinical studies suggesting that VILI is less pronounced in areas of cyclic R/D or atelectasis as compared to areas of high stretch and overventilation (Tsuchida et al., 2006; Bellani et al., 2011; Wakabayashi et al., 2014).

In a model of surfactant depletion by Tween instillation Andrews et al. (2015) tested the possibility that R/D may be masked by a proper oxygenation rate, although alveolar dynamics are impaired. The group observed R/D, yet no decline in oxygenation, suggesting that the partial pressure of oxygen (PaO_2) is not a parameter to identify impairment of alveolar dynamics, such as R/D. This important claim was subsequently validated by Allen et al. (2005) in a rat model of overinflation injury analyzed by pulmonary impedance measurements and *in vivo* imaging. They showed in their study that injurious mechanical ventilation leads to alveolar instability, but already before imbalances in the gas exchange are measurable. It is important to note, however, that the interpretation of these findings critically depends upon the underlying concept of what constitutes physiological vs. pathophysiological alveolar dynamics – and hence, upon a matter of considerable controversy (**Figure 2**). In the work by Andrews et al. (2015), R/D was defined as increase in alveolar size from expiration to inspiration – a behavior that many other studies would consider as physiological alveolar dynamics. Specifically, whereas some define distension of alveoli as a pathologic phenomenon, others interpret the distension from expiration to inspiration as the normal physiologic situation and no change in size as a sign for abnormalities. Conversely, as in the studies by Nieman cited above, a lack of change in alveolar size or shape is considered by some as physiological scenario and accordingly termed "alveolar stability", whereas "alveolar instability" is used in these instances to describe any change in alveolar size or volume during the respiratory cycle. In contrast, other studies interpret alveoli with no volume change as pathological, and alveoli which distend and contract over the respiratory cycle [and would hence be considered as "instable" by Nieman et al. (1981), or as R/D according to Andrews et al. (2015)] as "normal" (Tabuchi et al., 2016). It goes without saying that these critical differences in terminology and interpretation have greatly contributed to the present lack of consensus on alveolar dynamics, and instead have added a substantial degree of confusion to the field. To limit the resulting ambiguity, we suggest here an unbiased terminology which categorizes alveolar dynamics into either "static" (i.e., no volume change), "aligned" (i.e., volume change in accordance with the parallel transpulmonary pressure changes), "paradoxical" (i.e., volume change that is not in accordance with the parallel transpulmonary pressure changes), and "opening-and-collapse" (R/D) (**Figure 2**). Notably, we refrain from a classification of these terms into physiological vs. pathological dynamics due to the ongoing controversy in this field. We hope that such a unifying terminology may ease comparability between future studies with the aim to ultimately allow for the development of a consensual concept.

In part, but not solely as a result of these ambiguities in terminology, the concept of R/D as postulated by the previously described studies has been opposed by a series of IVM studies that failed to observe any R/D under both physiological and pathological conditions (Mertens et al., 2009; Tabuchi et al., 2016). In a murine model of acid-induced lung injury a reduction of alveolar compliance was observed by dark field IVM that was especially pronounced in small alveolar clusters, thus causing a shift of alveolar ventilation to larger alveoli. Such a mechanism would amplify the heterogeneity of alveolar ventilation and thereby, promote alveolar overdistension (Mertens et al., 2009). Additionally, although no R/D was observed, several other "dyskinesias" such as pendelluft, alveolar stunning or reversed ventilation of alveoli were reported in different models of lung injury (**Figure 2**) including hydrochloric acid aspiration, Tween instillation for surfactant depletion and antibody mediated transfusion-related lung injury (Tabuchi et al., 2016). In all three models, the inflicted lung injury resulted in asynchronous alveolar ventilation, manifesting as alveolar pendelluft, as well as impaired gas exchange that was detected as local impairment of blood oxygenation. Notably, individual sighs of 10 s length were identified as an effective measure to reconstitute physiologic alveolar dynamics in some (acid-induced lung injury) but not all (Tween-injury) models of lung injury.

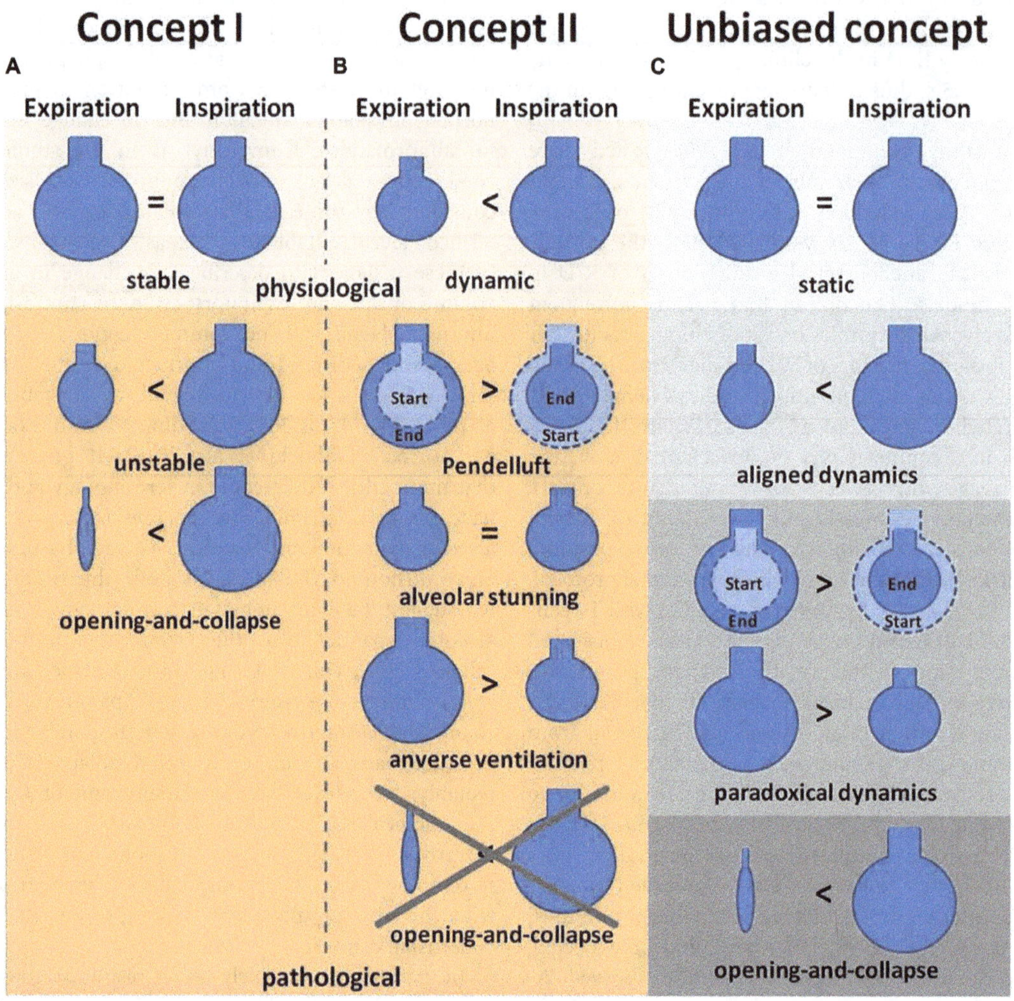

FIGURE 2 | Concepts of alveolar dynamics. **(A)** Concept I describes alveoli under physiologic conditions as stable (i.e., with no change in volume) during expiration and inspiration, whereas pathological situations lead to alveolar instability (defined as size and/or volume change) or even opening-and-collapse of alveoli (Carney et al., 1999). **(B)** Concept II describes alveoli under physiologic conditions as alveoli that increase in volume during inspiration and contract during expiration, whereas pathological conditions are associated with an arrest of alveolar dynamics (alveolar stunning) or paradoxical motions, such as Pendelluft or inverse ventilation (Mertens et al., 2009; Tabuchi et al., 2016). **(C)** The proposed third concept is an unbiased terminology to describe alveolar dynamics. In this concept alveoli are classified as being either static (i.e., with no change in volume during ex- or inspiration), or showing aligned (volume increase during inspiration, decrease during expiration) or paradoxical (volume increase during expiration, decrease during inspiration) dynamics, or opening-and-collapse (i.e., complete volume loss during expiration). Notably this concept refrains from a classification into physiological vs. pathological dynamics.

As such, considerable controversy exists regarding the characteristics and relevance of impaired alveolar mechanics in injured lungs in general, and the role of R/D in particular. Part of this controversy is attributable to different opinions on what constitutes "normal" alveolar dynamics and resulting differences in terminologies, definitions and interpretations. Methodological differences between analytical techniques (IVM vs. static) as well as specifics and limitations of the IVM technique itself (observation confined to subpleural alveoli, differences between hypostatic and apical lung zones, effects of alveolar edema) may contribute to seemingly opposing findings, while differences between species or models of acute lung injury are probably less likely to underlie these divergent findings.

INTRAVITAL MICROSCOPY FOR ANALYSIS OF ALVEOLAR PERFUSION, GAS EXCHANGE, AND IMMUNE CELL TRAFFICKING

Alveoli are the functional units of the lung with the overall task to warrant gas exchange, i.e., oxygen supply and carbon dioxide removal from the body. Besides alveolar ventilation, alveolar gas exchange is critically dependent on microvascular capillary network architecture and perfusion. Accordingly, capillary perfusion and its regulation have been a key interest for IVM studies in the past. In the late 1960s, Wagner (1969) developed a lung window with a suction device for dogs and applied it to analyze the pulmonary capillary transit time in local lung regions (Wagner et al., 1982). This development was a major advance, as before it had only been possible to measure the transit time for the entire lung which does not adequately reflect transit times in individual capillary beds. The measurement of pulmonary capillary transit time in dog lungs was realized by the injection of fluorescein isothiocyanate (FITC) labeled dextran into the corresponding lobe artery and subsequent microscopic observation of its passage through the pulmonary microvasculature. Notably, the mean capillary transit time was much longer than expected, namely 12.7 ± 3.2 (mean ± standard error) seconds in comparison to the 0.75 s for the whole lung capillary transit as measured by indirect methods. Wagner et al. (1982) concluded that this difference likely reflects the hydrostatic pressure gradient in the lung causing a similar vertical gradient of transit times.

Using a similar approach as Wagner, Fingar et al. (1994) implanted a transparent window chamber over the right lung lobe of Sprague Dawley rats to observe vessel permeability and edema formation in arterioles, capillaries and postcapillary venules. Pulmonary edema was induced by either oleic acid or compound 48/80 and measured by FITC-albumin leakage from the vessels into the alveolar space. Vascular leak was progressive over the observed time interval of 90 min and peaked after 30 min, with no measurable leak in control animals. Capillary leak from lung capillaries was similarly visualized by IVM as increase in alveolar septal thickness in a rabbit model of lung injury following complement activation by cobra venom factor (Kuhnle et al., 1999). The development of edema is a characteristic finding in ARDS that contributes critically to the propagation of VILI by diluting and inhibiting alveolar protective surfactant (Kobayashi et al., 1991), by reducing the fraction of aerated lung tissue that will consequently receive higher tidal volumes ("baby lung concept") (Gattinoni and Pesenti, 2005), and by the development of transient liquid bridges which exert excessive shear stress to airway epithelial cells (Bilek et al., 2003; Huh et al., 2007).

In addition to the detection of edema formation, IVM has also been used extensively to characterize the processes of capillary recruitment and derecruitment (not to be confused with alveolar R/D discussed above). IVM studies in mechanically ventilated rabbits or dogs or isolated rat lungs have demonstrated the considerable potential for capillary recruitment in the pulmonary vasculature at high perfusion rates or pressures (Wagner, 1988; Hanson et al., 1989; Kuhnle et al., 1995; Baumgartner et al., 2003), respectively. Importantly, this topic has recently gained considerable translational attention since several clinical studies of pulmonary hemodynamics at rest and during exercise in healthy resting supine subjects suggest that most of the pulmonary microvasculature is already recruited at baseline. Specifically, these studies show that even a three- to fourfold increase in pulmonary flow results only in a small decrease in pulmonary vascular resistance (Argiento et al., 2012; Kovacs et al., 2012; Wolsk et al., 2017). As a consequence, the evidence for capillary recruitment in healthy, spontaneously breathing subjects remains inconsistent, and comparative studies using IVM (or similar techniques) under conditions of both mechanical ventilation and spontaneous breathing would be important to clarify this hallmark of classic lung physiology.

In addition to changes in capillary density, pulmonary vasoreactivity has been a subject of lung IVM studies, in particular focusing on the site and mechanism of hypoxic pulmonary vasoconstriction. Although IVM is limited to the visualization of blood vessels close to the lung surface, such as smaller arterioles and venules, it offers a versatile tool for the analysis of pulmonary vasoreactivity with unmatched temporal and spatial resolution in an intact anatomical and morphological context (McCormack et al., 2000). By use of the murine lung window technique Tabuchi and colleagues were able to monitor and quantify the vasoreactive response of pulmonary arterioles and venules as small as 20–30 μm in diameter to hypoxia (11% O_2) or the thromboxane analog U-46619 in real-time (Tabuchi et al., 2008; Mertens et al., 2009). The typical vasoconstrictive response was predominantly located to arterioles with a diameter of 30–50 μm, less prominent in arterioles smaller than 30 μm and largely absent in venules. Hypoxic pulmonary vasoconstriction was similarly evident in pulmonary arterioles of the non-ventilated lung in rabbits undergoing one-lung ventilation (Groh et al., 1992).

In the early 2000's, the group of Axel Pries developed a novel IVM technique to directly visualize microvascular oxygen saturation in individual vessel segments *in vivo* (Styp-Rekowska et al., 2007). To this end they utilized multispectral oximetry, i.e., the recording of entire absorption spectra over the wavelength range from 480–630 nm from the surface of a vascular network, subsequent pixel-based matching of the recorded spectra to the known absorption spectra of oxy- and deoxyhemoglobin, and vascular segmentation to ultimately generate oxygenation maps of intact microvascular networks. In combination with Tabuchi's murine window technique, this approach allowed for the first direct visualization of the blood oxygenation process in the intact lung, an approach that surprisingly revealed that 50% of the total oxygen uptake at rest occurs in the precapillary arterioles before the blood enters the capillary network proper (Tabuchi et al., 2013). Combination of multispectral oximetry with IVM of alveolar dynamics and/or capillary perfusion as well as microhemodynamics yields a complex but versatile tool (**Figure 3**) that can provide unique insights into the process of alveolo-capillary gas exchange in the healthy and diseased lung (Tabuchi et al., 2016).

Leukocytes play key roles in inflammatory and immune responses of the lung. By use of IVM, the alveolar capillary bed has been identified as the main site of leukocyte retention during their passage through the lung (Lien et al., 1991; Kuebler et al., 1994), where they accumulate to form the so-called "marginated pool" (Kuebler and Goetz, 2002). This accumulation is attributable to the fact that the passing of leukocytes through the narrow capillary segments of the pulmonary microvasculature requires considerable neutrophil deformation, a process that has been termed neutrophil margination or sequestration (Doerschuk, 2001). Mechanical hindrance during the passage through the alveolar capillary network (Gebb et al., 1995; Kuebler et al., 1999) and the contribution of endothelial adhesion molecules and their interaction with

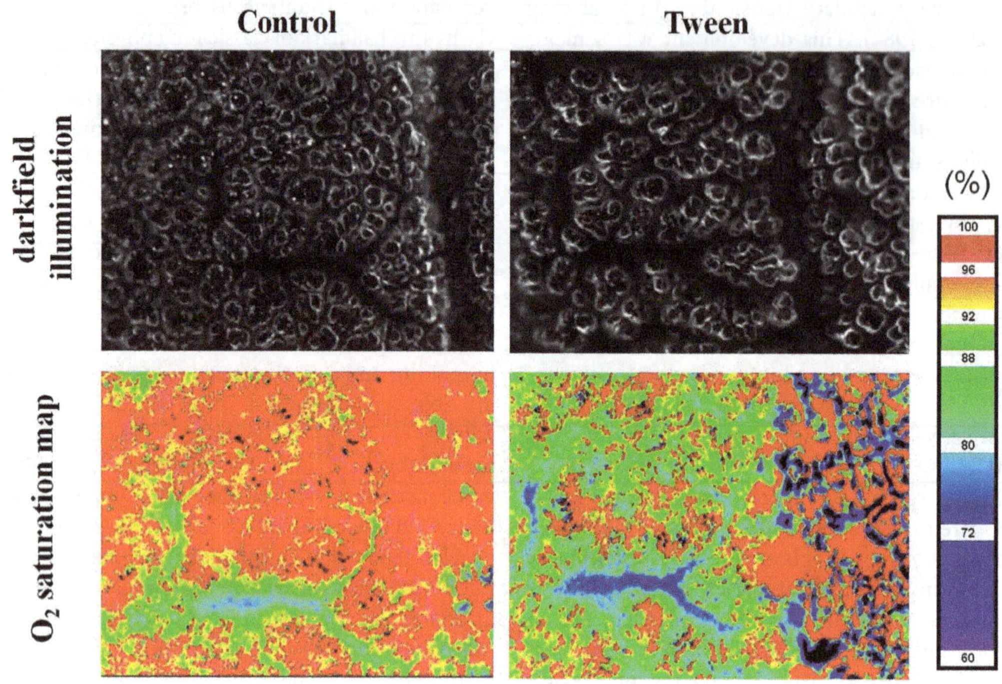

FIGURE 3 | Oxygen saturation map. Representative images of a pulmonary arteriolar vessel tree in a ventilated mouse with the surrounding alveolar capillary network under control conditions and after treatment with tween imaged by darkfield microscopy (top) and multi-spectral oximetry resulting in the generation of a corresponding oxygen saturation map (bottom). Note impaired alveolar structure and oxygenation in the Tween model of acute lung injury. Ethical approval for the animal experiment was obtained from the Animal Care Committee of St. Michael's Hospital Toronto.

leukocytes (Kuebler et al., 1997) constitute the predominant mechanisms that determine leukocyte sequestration and – upon appropriate chemotactic gradients – emigration into the alveolar space. Lien et al. (1991) suggested that leukocytes accumulate as a result of a misbalance between neutrophil delivery to the lung and divergent transit times along the capillaries. Kuebler and Kuhnle used IVM in a series of studies to identify the site of leukocyte sequestration (Kuebler et al., 1994), the effects of microvascular blood flow on leukocyte trafficking (Kuhnle et al., 1995), and the role of selectins in leukocyte margination (Kuebler et al., 1997). In addition to the dyes used for leukocyte labeling *in vivo* or *ex vivo*, these analyses were frequently combined with the use of other fluorescent dyes for concomitant analysis of edema formation by the assessment of vascular permeability, or for visualization and quantification of blood flow with plasma markers or labeled red blood cells. E.g., studies by Kuebler et al. (1994, 1997) and Kuhnle et al. (1995) in rabbits used FITC-labeled erythrocytes which were injected intravenously (i.v.) for quantification of blood flow velocity, red cell flux, and microhematocrit and i.v. administered rhodamine6G (**Figure 4**) as a marker for leukocytes with subsequent detailed analysis by IVM. Early on, the role of neutrophils within the pool of marginated and emigrating leukocytes has been of specific interest given their critical role in acute lung injury, pneumonia, and ARDS. Neutrophils not only play a critical role in the defense against pathogens, but also promote host tissue damage by the release of reactive oxygen species (ROS) (Simon et al., 1986; Smedly et al., 1986) thus aggravating edema formation and worsening outcome in ARDS patients (Steinberg et al., 1994). However, in early IVM studies the lack of specific dyes precluded a differentiation between different leukocyte subsets (Kuebler et al., 1994, 2000). In recent years, this limitation has been overcome by e.g., combinations of fluorescent dyes and antibodies to differentiate leukocyte subsets. To address the role of neutrophils in a model of sepsis-induced lung injury, Park et al. (2019) labeled erythrocytes *ex vivo* with DiD and reinfused them via a catheter. Concomitantly, vessels were visualized with FITC and Tetramethylrhodamine (TMR) conjugated dextran and neutrophils were specifically labeled *in vivo* with an anti-Ly6G$^+$ monoclonal antibody tagged with a fluorophore. In this study, the authors confirmed the previously described retention of neutrophils within the pulmonary microvascular system (Doerschuk et al., 1987; Lien et al., 1987, 1991; Kuebler et al., 1994), but in addition could link it to an increase in dead space ventilation due to microvascular injury by ROS, ultimately causing impaired oxygenation and hypoxemia. Mark Looney and his group, which had revitalized the study of immune cells in the lung by their development of a stabilized murine lung window (Looney et al., 2011), performed a series of studies in which they addressed the kinetics of neutrophils in the lung. In a recent paper from 2018 they showed that the reduction of neutrophil extracellular trap (NET), a form of innate defense mechanism, by pharmacological or genetic tools resulted in less lung injury and improved outcome in a model of pneumonia induced by methicillin-resistant *staphylococcus aureus* (MRSA) infection. Conversely, in patients with ARDS high levels of NET

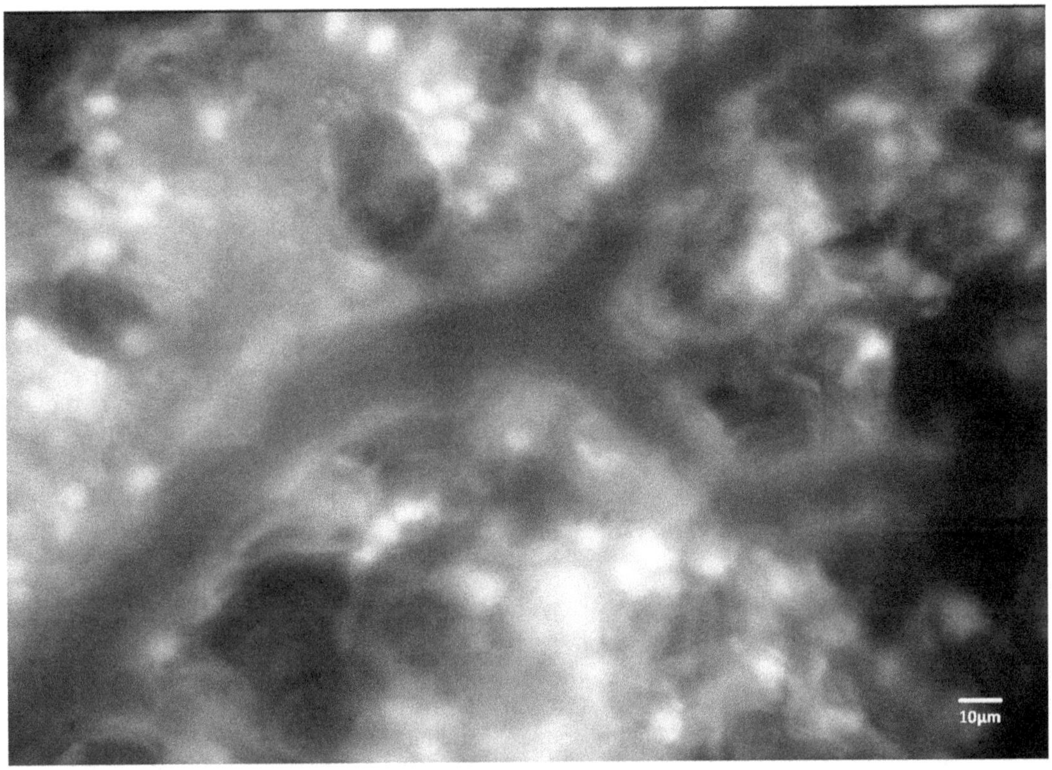

FIGURE 4 | Fluorescence imaging of immune cells in the mouse lung. Representative image of a pulmonary microvessel after i.v. injection of rhodamine 6G. Note the accumulation of stained leukocytes in the alveolar networks outside of the larger pulmonary microvessel in the image center. Ethical approval for the animal experiment was obtained from the Animal Care Committee of St. Michael's Hospital Toronto.

formation were associated with increased mortality (Lefrancais et al., 2018). Studies by Yipp et al. (2017) identified a defense niche for neutrophils during infection with *Escherichia coli*, in that neutrophils can respond almost instantaneously via TLR4-MyD88 and abl tyrosine kinase signaling to gram-negative pathogens and endotoxins. These findings highlight the potential of IVM to unravel novel mechanisms of lung immunosurveillance and the roles of innate and adaptive immune cells in lung health and disease.

LIMITATIONS OF IVM

Intravital microscopy is a versatile tool that offers multiple possibilities to analyze biological processes in a realistic anatomical and physiological multicellular environment. IVM can be applied to a large variety of different organs, often in combination with other imaging modalities such as optical coherence tomography (Mertens et al., 2009; Gaertner et al., 2012). In case of internal organs or structures window techniques are commonly applied to provide visual access to the organ of interest such as the skeletal muscle. The lung, however, is an especially complex organ and difficult to image due to its inherent respiratory movements, the propagation of cardiac motion artifacts to the lung surface, as well as to the lung's vulnerability to mechanical stress. Accordingly, preparation of lung windows without irritation of the lung surface and with maintenance of physiologic cardiovascular body functions (heart rate, arterial blood pressure, oxygenation, and cardiac output) throughout the experimental protocol with ongoing anesthesia and mechanical ventilation is challenging. Some lung windows are constructed to stabilize the lung surface for improved imaging with reduced motion artifacts. While this technique has proven highly efficient for tracking of immune cells, it will impair assessment of basic physiological phenomena, specifically alveolar dynamics and ventilation-dependent effects on lung perfusion due to the artificial removal of respiratory movements in the area of observation. In some studies IVM has been applied in open lung approaches by simply removing part of the thoracic wall and observation of the lung through this opening in the absence of a window. These approaches not only bear the risk of rapid drying of the area of observation and/or its exposure to artificial surfaces (such as cover slips) or environmental pathogens. It should also be considered that the mechanics of the thoracic wall and the interplay between intrapleural and transpulmonary pressures are fundamental factors of respiratory physiology. The disregard of these factors will have significant consequences on alveolar dynamics as well as microvascular perfusion and may contribute to the differential results obtained in studies of alveolar dynamics and the subsequent controversies.

In a pioneering study the group of Gary Nieman proposed that the volume change in healthy lungs is primarily based on the opening (recruitment) and collapse (derecruitment) of individual alveoli rather than the distension and contraction of alveoli (Carney et al., 1999). In this study which used an open chest technique the authors refrained from suction stabilization of the lung surface. Instead, a coverslip connected to the microscope objective was lowered onto the lung surface to generate a horizontal optical plane. While care was taken not to impact the underlying tissue, it seems difficult to conceive that this procedure would not lead to compression of the underlying alveolar structures. Other studies which used closed chest models in mice without suction applied to the lung surface, thus allowing for free movement of the lung, did not observe any R/D under physiologic conditions (Mertens et al., 2009), but instead described alveolar distension as the predominant mechanism of lung volume change.

While these discordant findings highlight how seemingly minor differences in experimental models and approaches may result in rather opposing results and interpretations, some general limitations that apply to all IVM models should not go unmentioned.

First, in many IVM models the lung surface is exposed to varying temperatures or room temperature, which will affect temperature-sensitive processes. Such processes are e.g., the activation of ion channels critical for the regulation of endothelial barrier function and neutrophil activation in ARDS (Goldenberg et al., 2015; Ahl et al., 2019). This can be avoided by the use of warmed lung window chambers (Kreisel et al., 2010) or simply by use of water immersion microscopy and continuous superfusion of the window with a pre-warmed solution (Kuhnle et al., 1993; Kuebler et al., 1994). Second, IVM of the lung is currently limited to the observation of subpleural alveoli, due to the restricted penetration depth of conventional fluorescence (approximately 30–50 μm), confocal (approximately 50–60 μm), and even two-photon microscopy (approximately 100 μm), therefore excluding deeper structures from analysis (Looney et al., 2011). Second, traction forces exerted by surrounding alveoli will differ between subpleural alveoli and deeper lung regions. Subpleural alveoli are on one side attached to the visceral pleura whereas in deeper lung regions alveoli are surrounded on all sides by other alveoli. Next, it should be considered that different regions of the lung differ in terms of ventilation and perfusion due to the vertical gravitational gradient. Consequentially, IVM observations, which are always restricted to a specific location, may differ considerably between lung base and apex. Both considerations (i.e., the problem of subpleural alveoli and the problem of different lung regions) relate to a more general limitation of IVM, namely the fact that the number of visualized (and analyzed) alveoli is commonly only a small fraction of the total alveoli in the lung and thus, not necessarily representative. Third, the limitation of IVM in terms of longitudinal studies should be considered. The majority of lung windows is too invasive to allow for long-term studies. The recently developed permanent lung window by Entenberg et al. (2018) is a notable exception, and may present a promising tool for future long-term observations. Fourth, albeit still the gold standard in terms of temporal and spatial resolution, IVM is a two-dimensional imaging method, giving only limited information about three-dimensional alveolar dynamics. While walls and outer diameter of the alveoli are commonly visible as bright reflections, it should be noted that these reflections can also result from capillaries or collagen in the pleura, making interpretations about the real alveolar dimension difficult. In healthy lungs air-filled alveoli appear as white ring structures in dark-field images; however, these rings are in fact the result of specific reflection processes, such as partial reflection and total internal reflection between neighboring alveoli. As a consequence, IVM dark-field images may result in an overestimation of actual alveolar size by a factor as big as $\sim$1.6 (Gaertner et al., 2015).

Optical coherence tomography, as a three-dimensional imaging modality albeit with a lesser temporal and spatial resolution as compared to IVM, avoids the above problem (Meissner et al., 2010) and further reveals another disadvantage of IVM, namely the inability to differentiate between collapsed or liquid filled alveoli (Gaertner et al., 2015). In ARDS the development of alveolar edema is a critical factor for impaired lung function and gas exchange, respectively, but its effect on alveolar dynamics is only partly understood. Edema fluid entering the alveolar space as a result of increased permeability of the alveolar wall accumulates in and ultimately floods entire alveoli. Alveolar flooding in turn impairs gas exchange and affects alveolar stability by diluting and inactivating surfactant, which functions as alveolar stabilizer by decreasing surface tension. In studies of alveolar micromechanics under pathologic conditions (such as instillation of the lung with liquid for mimicking edema, surfactant deactivation, or models of lung infection) cyclic disappearance and re-appearance of alveoli in IVM are commonly interpreted as R/D (Nieman et al., 1981; Schiller et al., 2001; Steinberg et al., 2002; Halter et al., 2003). In fact, however, this observation may similarly reflect fluid-filled alveoli becoming cyclically aerated and deaerated over the respiratory cycle. This was elegantly demonstrated by Gaertner et al. (2015) in a study directly comparing IVM and OCT imaging in fluid-filled lungs. Whereas in OCT the alveolar walls remained clearly visible (and showed open, yet fluid-filled alveoli), alveolar walls had seemingly disappeared in IVM images given the false impression of alveolar collapse.

CONCLUSION

While IVM remains a key technology for the assessment of alveolar dynamics and perfusion, its inherent limitations necessitate validation by and combination with additional three- or even four-dimensional imaging techniques such as e.g., OCT. Only a combination of different imaging modalities, measurements of lung mechanics (e.g., by forced oscillations), and theoretical models can be expected to ultimately clarify the ongoing controversies in the field. Such a joint, interdisciplinary approach may not advance our understanding of respiratory physiology, but may promote the development of optimized and personalized ventilation modes based on a better understanding of alveolar dynamics and their impact on alveolar perfusion and gas exchange in healthy and diseased lungs.

AUTHOR CONTRIBUTIONS

WK, JM and AT contributed to the conception and design of the manuscript and wrote the sections of the manuscript. JM wrote the first draft of the manuscript. All authors contributed to the manuscript revision, and read and approved the submitted version.

ACKNOWLEDGMENTS

We acknowledge support by the German Research Foundation (DFG) and the Open Access Publication Fund of Charité – Universitätsmedizin Berlin. **Figure 1** has been designed using resources from Freepik.com.

REFERENCES

Ahl, D., Eriksson, O., Sedin, J., Seignez, C., Schwan, E., Kreuger, J., et al. (2019). Turning up the heat: local temperature control during *in vivo* imaging of immune cells. *Front. Immunol.* 10:2036. doi: 10.3389/fimmu.2019.02036

Albert, S. P., DiRocco, J., Allen, G. B., Bates, J. H., Lafollette, R., Kubiak, B. D., et al. (2009). The role of time and pressure on alveolar recruitment. *J. Appl. Physiol.* 106, 757–765. doi: 10.1152/japplphysiol.90735.2008

Allen, G. B., Pavone, L. A., DiRocco, J. D., Bates, J. H., and Nieman, G. F. (2005). Pulmonary impedance and alveolar instability during injurious ventilation in rats. *J. Appl. Physiol.* 99, 723–730. doi: 10.1152/japplphysiol.01339.2004

Amato, M. B., Barbas, C. S., Medeiros, D. M., Magaldi, R. B., Schettino, G. P., Lorenzi-Filho, G., et al. (1998). Effect of a protective-ventilation strategy on mortality in the acute respiratory distress syndrome. *N. Engl. J. Med.* 338, 347–354. doi: 10.1056/NEJM199802053380602

Andrews, P. L., Sadowitz, B., Kollisch-Singule, M., Satalin, J., Roy, S., Snyder, K., et al. (2015). Alveolar instability (atelectrauma) is not identified by arterial oxygenation predisposing the development of an occult ventilator-induced lung injury. *Intensive Care Med. Exp.* 3:16. doi: 10.1186/s40635-015-0054-1

Argiento, P., Vanderpool, R. R., Mule, M., Russo, M. G., D'Alto, M., Bossone, E., et al. (2012). Exercise stress echocardiography of the pulmonary circulation: limits of normal and sex differences. *Chest* 142, 1158–1165. doi: 10.1378/chest.12-0071

Bates, J. H., Abe, T., Romero, P. V., and Sato, J. (1989). Measurement of alveolar pressure in closed-chest dogs during flow interruption. *J. Appl. Physiol.* 67, 488–492. doi: 10.1152/jappl.1989.67.1.488

Baumgartner, W. A. Jr., Jaryszak, E. M., Peterson, A. J., Presson, R. G. Jr., and Wagner, W. W. Jr. (2003). Heterogeneous capillary recruitment among adjoining alveoli. *J. Appl. Physiol.* 95, 469–476. doi: 10.1152/japplphysiol.01115.2002

Bellani, G., Guerra, L., Musch, G., Zanella, A., Patroniti, N., Mauri, T., et al. (2011). Lung regional metabolic activity and gas volume changes induced by tidal ventilation in patients with acute lung injury. *Am. J. Respir. Crit. Care Med.* 183, 1193–1199. doi: 10.1164/rccm.201008-1318OC

Bilek, A. M., Dee, K. C., and Gaver, D. P. III (2003). Mechanisms of surface-tension-induced epithelial cell damage in a model of pulmonary airway reopening. *J. Appl. Physiol.* 94, 770–783. doi: 10.1152/japplphysiol.00764.2002

Carney, D. E., Bredenberg, C. E., Schiller, H. J., Picone, A. L., McCann, U. G., Gatto, L. A., et al. (1999). The mechanism of lung volume change during mechanical ventilation. *Am. J. Respir. Crit. Care Med.* 160(5 Pt 1), 1697–1702.

Daly, B. D., Parks, G. E., Edmonds, C. H., Hibbs, C. W., and Norman, J. C. (1975). Dynamic alveolar mechanics as studied by videomicroscopy. *Respir. Physiol.* 24, 217–232. doi: 10.1016/0034-5687(75)90115-2

De Alva, W. E., and Rainer, W. G. (1963). A method of high speed *in vivo* pulmonary microcinematography under physiologic conditions. *Angiology* 14, 160–164. doi: 10.1177/000331976301400402

Doerschuk, C. M. (2001). Mechanisms of leukocyte sequestration in inflamed lungs. *Microcirculation* 8, 71–88. doi: 10.1111/j.1549-8719.2001.tb00159.x

Doerschuk, C. M., Allard, M. F., Martin, B. A., MacKenzie, A., Autor, A. P., and Hogg, J. C. (1987). Marginated pool of neutrophils in rabbit lungs. *J. Appl. Physiol.* 63, 1806–1815. doi: 10.1152/jappl.1987.63.5.1806

Entenberg, D., Voiculescu, S., Guo, P., Borriello, L., Wang, Y., Karagiannis, G. S., et al. (2018). A permanent window for the murine lung enables high-resolution imaging of cancer metastasis. *Nat. Methods* 15, 73–80. doi: 10.1038/nmeth.4511

Fingar, V. H., Taber, S. W., and Wieman, T. J. (1994). A new model for the study of pulmonary microcirculation: determination of pulmonary edema in rats. *J. Surg. Res.* 57, 385–393. doi: 10.1006/jsre.1994.1159

Forrest, J. B. (1970). The effect of changes in lung volume on the size and shape of alveoli. *J. Physiol.* 210, 533–547. doi: 10.1113/jphysiol.1970.sp009225

Fung, Y. C. (1975). Stress, deformation, and atelectasis of the lung. *Circ. Res.* 37, 481–496. doi: 10.1161/01.res.37.4.481

Gaertner, M., Cimalla, P., Meissner, S., Kuebler, W. M., and Koch, E. (2012). Three-dimensional simultaneous optical coherence tomography and confocal fluorescence microscopy for investigation of lung tissue. *J. Biomed. Opt.* 17:071310. doi: 10.1117/1.JBO.17.7.071310

Gaertner, M., Schirrmann, K., Schnabel, C., Meissner, S., Kertzscher, U., Kirsten, L., et al. (2015). Toward a comprehensive interpretation of intravital microscopy images in studies of lung tissue dynamics. *J. Biomed. Opt.* 20:066009. doi: 10.1117/1.JBO.20.6.066009

Gattinoni, L., and Pesenti, A. (2005). The concept of "baby lung". *Intensive Care Med.* 31, 776–784. doi: 10.1007/s00134-005-2627-z

Gebb, S. A., Graham, J. A., Hanger, C. C., Godbey, P. S., Capen, R. L., Doerschuk, C. M., et al. (1995). Sites of leukocyte sequestration in the pulmonary microcirculation. *J. Appl. Physiol.* 79, 493–497. doi: 10.1152/jappl.1995.79.2.493

Gehr, P., Bachofen, M., and Weibel, E. R. (1978). The normal human lung: ultrastructure and morphometric estimation of diffusion capacity. *Respir. Physiol.* 32, 121–140. doi: 10.1016/0034-5687(78)90104-4

Gil, J., Bachofen, H., Gehr, P., and Weibel, E. R. (1979). Alveolar volume-surface area relation in air- and saline-filled lungs fixed by vascular perfusion. *J. Appl. Physiol. Respir Environ. Exerc. Physiol.* 47, 990–1001. doi: 10.1152/jappl.1979.47.5.990

Gil, J., and Weibel, E. R. (1972). Morphological study of pressure-volume hysteresis in rat lungs fixed by vascular perfusion. *Respir. Physiol.* 15, 190–213. doi: 10.1016/0034-5687(72)90098-9

Goldenberg, N. M., Ravindran, K., and Kuebler, W. M. (2015). TRPV4: physiological role and therapeutic potential in respiratory diseases. *Naunyn. Schmiedebergs. Arch. Pharmacol.* 388, 421–436. doi: 10.1007/s00210-014-1058-1

Groh, J., Kuhnle, G. E., Kuebler, W. M., and Goetz, A. E. (1992). An experimental model for simultaneous quantitative analysis of pulmonary micro- and macrocirculation during unilateral hypoxia *in vivo*. *Res. Exp. Med.* 192, 431–441. doi: 10.1007/bf02576301

Grune, J., Tabuchi, A., and Kuebler, W. M. (2019). Alveolar dynamics during mechanical ventilation in the healthy and injured lung. *Intensive Care Med. Exp.* 7(Suppl. 1):34. doi: 10.1186/s40635-019-0226-5

Hajari, A. J., Yablonskiy, D. A., Sukstanskii, A. L., Quirk, J. D., Conradi, M. S., and Woods, J. C. (2012). Morphometric changes in the human pulmonary acinus during inflation. *J. Appl. Physiol.* 112, 937–943. doi: 10.1152/japplphysiol.00768.2011

Hall, R. J., and Chapman, A. W. (1925). A study of the efficiency of sterilization of dressings. *Br. Med. J.* 1, 1119–1120. doi: 10.1136/bmj.1.3364.1119

Halter, J. M., Steinberg, J. M., Schiller, H. J., DaSilva, M., Gatto, L. A., Landas, S., et al. (2003). Positive end-expiratory pressure after a recruitment maneuver prevents both alveolar collapse and recruitment/derecruitment. *Am. J. Respir. Crit. Care Med.* 167, 1620–1626. doi: 10.1164/rccm.200205-435OC

Hanna, R. N., Chodaczek, G., and Hedrick, C. C. (2016). *In vivo* imaging of tumor and immune cell interactions in the lung. *Bio Protoc.* 6:e1973. doi: 10.21769/BioProtoc.1973

Hanson, W. L., Emhardt, J. D., Bartek, J. P., Latham, L. P., Checkley, L. L., Capen, R. L., et al. (1989). Site of recruitment in the pulmonary microcirculation. *J. Appl. Physiol.* 66, 2079–2083. doi: 10.1152/jappl.1989.66.5.2079

Huh, D., Fujioka, H., Tung, Y. C., Futai, N., Paine, R. III, Grotberg, J. B., et al. (2007). Acoustically detectable cellular-level lung injury induced by fluid mechanical stresses in microfluidic airway systems. *Proc. Natl. Acad. Sci. U.S.A.* 104, 18886–18891. doi: 10.1073/pnas.0610868104

Kimura, H., Hayashi, K., Yamauchi, K., Yamamoto, N., Tsuchiya, H., Tomita, K., et al. (2010). Real-time imaging of single cancer-cell dynamics of lung metastasis. *J. Cell. Biochem.* 109, 58–64. doi: 10.1002/jcb.22379

Kobayashi, T., Nitta, K., Ganzuka, M., Inui, S., Grossmann, G., and Robertson, B. (1991). Inactivation of exogenous surfactant by pulmonary edema fluid. *Pediatr. Res.* 29(4 Pt 1), 353–356. doi: 10.1203/00006450-199104000-00005

Kovacs, G., Olschewski, A., Berghold, A., and Olschewski, H. (2012). Pulmonary vascular resistances during exercise in normal subjects: a systematic review. *Eur. Respir. J.* 39, 319–328. doi: 10.1183/09031936.00008611

Kreisel, D., Nava, R. G., Li, W., Zinselmeyer, B. H., Wang, B., Lai, J., et al. (2010). *In vivo* two-photon imaging reveals monocyte-dependent neutrophil extravasation during pulmonary inflammation. *Proc. Natl. Acad. Sci. U.S.A.* 107, 18073–18078. doi: 10.1073/pnas.1008737107

Kuebler, W. M., Borges, J., Sckell, A., Kuhnle, G. E., Bergh, K., Messmer, K., et al. (2000). Role of L-selectin in leukocyte sequestration in lung capillaries in a rabbit model of endotoxemia. *Am. J. Respir. Crit. Care Med.* 161, 36–43. doi: 10.1164/ajrccm.161.1.9901039

Kuebler, W. M., and Goetz, A. E. (2002). The marginated pool. *Eur. Surg. Res.* 34, 92–100. doi: 10.1159/000048894

Kuebler, W. M., Kuhnle, G. E., and Goetz, A. E. (1999). Leukocyte margination in alveolar capillaries: interrelationship with functional capillary geometry and microhemodynamics. *J. Vasc. Res.* 36, 282–288. doi: 10.1159/000025656

Kuebler, W. M., Kuhnle, G. E., Groh, J., and Goetz, A. E. (1994). Leukocyte kinetics in pulmonary microcirculation: intravital fluorescence microscopic study. *J. Appl. Physiol.* 76, 65–71. doi: 10.1152/jappl.1994.76.1.65

Kuebler, W. M., Kuhnle, G. E., Groh, J., and Goetz, A. E. (1997). Contribution of selectins to leucocyte sequestration in pulmonary microvessels by intravital microscopy in rabbits. *J. Physiol.* 501(Pt 2), 375–386. doi: 10.1111/j.1469-7793.1997.375bn.x

Kuhnle, G. E., Kiefmann, R., Sckell, A., Kuebler, W. M., Groh, J., and Goetz, A. E. (1999). Leukocyte sequestration in pulmonary microvessels and lung injury following systemic complement activation in rabbits. *J. Vasc. Res.* 36, 289–298. doi: 10.1159/000025657

Kuhnle, G. E., Kuebler, W. M., Groh, J., and Goetz, A. E. (1995). Effect of blood flow on the leukocyte-endothelium interaction in pulmonary microvessels. *Am. J. Respir. Crit. Care Med.* 152(4 Pt 1), 1221–1228. doi: 10.1164/ajrccm.152.4.7551374

Kuhnle, G. E., Leipfinger, F. H., and Goetz, A. E. (1993). Measurement of microhemodynamics in the ventilated rabbit lung by intravital fluorescence microscopy. *J. Appl. Physiol.* 74, 1462–1471. doi: 10.1152/jappl.1993.74.3.1462

Lefrancais, E., Mallavia, B., Zhuo, H., Calfee, C. S., and Looney, M. R. (2018). Maladaptive role of neutrophil extracellular traps in pathogen-induced lung injury. *JCI Insight* 3:e98178. doi: 10.1172/jci.insight.98178

Lien, D. C., Henson, P. M., Capen, R. L., Henson, J. E., Hanson, W. L., Wagner, W. W., et al. (1991). Neutrophil kinetics in the pulmonary microcirculation during acute inflammation. *Lab. Invest.* 65, 145–159.

Lien, D. C., Wagner, W. W. Jr., Capen, R. L., Haslett, C., Hanson, W. L., Hofmeister, S. E., et al. (1987). Physiological neutrophil sequestration in the lung: visual evidence for localization in capillaries. *J. Appl. Physiol.* 62, 1236–1243. doi: 10.1152/jappl.1987.62.3.1236

Looney, M. R., Thornton, E. E., Sen, D., Lamm, W. J., Glenny, R. W., and Krummel, M. F. (2011). Stabilized imaging of immune surveillance in the mouse lung. *Nat. Methods* 8, 91–96. doi: 10.1038/nmeth.1543

Macklin, C. C. (1929). The musculature of the bronchi and lungs: a retrospect. *Can. Med. Assoc. J.* 20:404.

Mazzuca, E., Salito, C., Rivolta, I., Aliverti, A., and Miserocchi, G. (2014). From morphological heterogeneity at alveolar level to the overall mechanical lung behavior: an *in vivo* microscopic imaging study. *Physiol. Rep.* 2:e00221. doi: 10.1002/phy2.221

McCormack, D. G., Mehta, S., Tyml, K., Scott, J. A., Potter, R., and Rohan, M. (2000). Pulmonary microvascular changes during sepsis: evaluation using intravital videomicroscopy. *Microvasc. Res.* 60, 131–140. doi: 10.1006/mvre.2000.2261

Mead, J., Takishima, T., and Leith, D. (1970). Stress distribution in lungs: a model of pulmonary elasticity. *J. Appl. Physiol.* 28, 596–608. doi: 10.1152/jappl.1970.28.5.596

Meissner, S., Tabuchi, A., Mertens, M., Kuebler, W. M., and Koch, E. (2010). Virtual four-dimensional imaging of lung parenchyma by optical coherence tomography in mice. *J. Biomed. Opt.* 15:036016. doi: 10.1117/1.3425654

Mertens, M., Tabuchi, A., Meissner, S., Krueger, A., Schirrmann, K., Kertzscher, U., et al. (2009). Alveolar dynamics in acute lung injury: heterogeneous distension rather than cyclic opening and collapse. *Crit. Care Med.* 37, 2604–2611. doi: 10.1097/CCM.0b013e3181a5544d

Mitzner, W., and Smaldone, G. (2012). Last word on viewpoint: unresolved mysteries. *J. Appl. Physiol.* 113:1950. doi: 10.1152/japplphysiol.01224.2012

Moreci, A. P., and Norman, J. C. (1973). Measurements of alveolar sac diameters by incident-light photomicrography. Effects of positive-pressure respiration. *Ann. Thorac. Surg.* 15, 179–186. doi: 10.1016/s0003-4975(10)64951-x

Namati, E., Thiesse, J., de Ryk, J., and McLennan, G. (2008). Alveolar dynamics during respiration: are the pores of Kohn a pathway to recruitment? *Am. J. Respir. Cell Mol. Biol.* 38, 572–578. doi: 10.1165/rcmb.2007-0120OC

Namati, E., Warger, W. C. II, Unglert, C. I., Eckert, J. E., Hostens, J., Bouma, B. E., et al. (2013). Four-dimensional visualization of subpleural alveolar dynamics *in vivo* during uninterrupted mechanical ventilation of living swine. *Biomed. Opt. Express* 4, 2492–2506. doi: 10.1364/BOE.4.002492

Neumann, P., Berglund, J. E., Fernandez Mondejar, E., Magnusson, A., and Hedenstierna, G. (1998). Dynamics of lung collapse and recruitment during prolonged breathing in porcine lung injury. *J. Appl. Physiol.* 85, 1533–1543. doi: 10.1152/jappl.1998.85.4.1533

Nickles, H. T., Sumkauskaite, M., Wang, X., Wegner, I., Puderbach, M., and Kuebler, W. M. (2014). Mechanical ventilation causes airway distension with proinflammatory sequelae in mice. *Am. J. Physiol. Lung Cell Mol. Physiol.* 307, L27–L37. doi: 10.1152/ajplung.00288.2013

Nieman, G. F. (2012). Amelia Earhart, alveolar mechanics, and other great mysteries. *J. Appl. Physiol.* 112, 935–936. doi: 10.1152/japplphysiol.01482.2011

Nieman, G. F., Bredenberg, C. E., Clark, W. R., and West, N. R. (1981). Alveolar function following surfactant deactivation. *J. Appl. Physiol. Respir. Environ. Exerc. Physiol.* 51, 895–904. doi: 10.1152/jappl.1981.51.4.895

Park, I., Kim, M., Choe, K., Song, E., Seo, H., Hwang, Y., et al. (2019). Neutrophils disturb pulmonary microcirculation in sepsis-induced acute lung injury. *Eur. Respir. J.* 53:1800786. doi: 10.1183/13993003.00786-2018

Pavone, L. A., Dirocco, J. D., Carney, D. E., Gatto, L. A., McBride, N. T., Norton, J. A., et al. (2007). Absence of alveolar tears in rat lungs with significant alveolar instability. *Respiration* 74, 439–446. doi: 10.1159/000101476

Petrucci, N., and Iacovelli, W. (2007). Lung protective ventilation strategy for the acute respiratory distress syndrome. *Cochrane Database Syst. Rev.* 2013:CD003844. doi: 10.1002/14651858.CD003844.pub3

Rahn, H., Otis, A. B., Chadwick, L. E., and Fenn, W. O. (1946). The pressure-volume diagram of the thorax and lung. *Am. J. Physiol.* 146, 161–178. doi: 10.1152/ajplegacy.1946.146.2.161

Schiller, H. J., McCann, U. G. II, Carney, D. E., Gatto, L. A., Steinberg, J. M., and Nieman, G. F. (2001). Altered alveolar mechanics in the acutely injured lung. *Crit. Care Med.* 29, 1049–1055. doi: 10.1097/00003246-200105000-00036

Schirrmann, K., Mertens, M., Kertzscher, U., Kuebler, W. M., and Affeld, K. (2010). Theoretical modeling of the interaction between alveoli during inflation and deflation in normal and diseased lungs. *J. Biomech.* 43, 1202–1207. doi: 10.1016/j.jbiomech.2009.11.025

Schittny, J. C. (2017). Development of the lung. *Cell Tissue Res.* 367, 427–444. doi: 10.1007/s00441-016-2545-0

Schneider, J. P., Wrede, C., Hegermann, J., Weibel, E. R., Muhlfeld, C., and Ochs, M. (2019). On the topological complexity of human alveolar epithelial type 1 cells. *Am. J. Respir. Crit. Care Med.* 199, 1153–1156. doi: 10.1164/rccm.201810-1866LE

Seah, A. S., Grant, K. A., Aliyeva, M., Allen, G. B., and Bates, J. H. (2011). Quantifying the roles of tidal volume and PEEP in the pathogenesis of ventilator-induced lung injury. *Ann. Biomed. Eng.* 39, 1505–1516. doi: 10.1007/s10439-010-0237-6

Sewald, X. (2018). Visualizing viral infection *in vivo* by multi-photon intravital microscopy. *Viruses* 10:E337. doi: 10.3390/v10060337

Simon, R. H., DeHart, P. D., and Todd, R. F. III (1986). Neutrophil-induced injury of rat pulmonary alveolar epithelial cells. *J. Clin. Invest.* 78, 1375–1386. doi: 10.1172/JCI112724

Smaldone, G. C., and Mitzner, W. (2012). Viewpoint: unresolved mysteries. *J. Appl. Physiol.* 113, 1945–1947. doi: 10.1152/japplphysiol.00545.2012

Smedly, L. A., Tonnesen, M. G., Sandhaus, R. A., Haslett, C., Guthrie, L. A., Johnston, R. B., et al. (1986). Neutrophil-mediated injury to endothelial cells. Enhancement by endotoxin and essential role of neutrophil elastase. *J. Clin. Invest.* 77, 1233–1243. doi: 10.1172/JCI112426

Steinberg, J., Schiller, H. J., Halter, J. M., Gatto, L. A., Dasilva, M., Amato, M., et al. (2002). Tidal volume increases do not affect alveolar mechanics in normal lung but cause alveolar overdistension and exacerbate alveolar instability after surfactant deactivation. *Crit. Care Med.* 30, 2675–2683. doi: 10.1097/00003246-200212000-00011

Steinberg, K. P., Milberg, J. A., Martin, T. R., Maunder, R. J., Cockrill, B. A., and Hudson, L. D. (1994). Evolution of bronchoalveolar cell populations in the adult respiratory distress syndrome. *Am. J. Respir. Crit. Care Med.* 150, 113–122. doi: 10.1164/ajrccm.150.1.8025736

Storey, W. F., and Staub, N. C. (1962). Ventilation of terminal air units. *J. Appl. Physiol.* 17, 391–397. doi: 10.1152/jappl.1962.17.3.391

Styp-Rekowska, B., Disassa, N. M., Reglin, B., Ulm, L., Kuppe, H., Secomb, T. W., et al. (2007). An imaging spectroscopy approach for measurement of oxygen saturation and hematocrit during intravital microscopy. *Microcirculation* 14, 207–221. doi: 10.1080/10739680601139302

Suki, B., and Bates, J. H. (2011). Lung tissue mechanics as an emergent phenomenon. *J. Appl. Physiol.* 110, 1111–1118. doi: 10.1152/japplphysiol.01244.2010

Sznitman, J., Heimsch, T., Wildhaber, J. H., Tsuda, A., and Rosgen, T. (2009). Respiratory flow phenomena and gravitational deposition in a three-dimensional space-filling model of the pulmonary acinar tree. *J. Biomech. Eng.* 131:031010. doi: 10.1115/1.3049481

Tabuchi, A., Mertens, M., Kuppe, H., Pries, A. R., and Kuebler, W. M. (2008). Intravital microscopy of the murine pulmonary microcirculation. *J. Appl. Physiol.* 104, 338–346. doi: 10.1152/japplphysiol.00348.2007

Tabuchi, A., Nickles, H. T., Kim, M., Semple, J. W., Koch, E., Brochard, L., et al. (2016). Acute lung injury causes asynchronous alveolar ventilation that can be corrected by individual sighs. *Am. J. Respir. Crit. Care Med.* 193, 396–406. doi: 10.1164/rccm.201505-0901OC

Tabuchi, A., Styp-Rekowska, B., Slutsky, A. S., Wagner, P. D., Pries, A. R., and Kuebler, W. M. (2013). Precapillary oxygenation contributes relevantly to gas exchange in the intact lung. *Am. J. Respir. Crit. Care Med.* 188, 474–481. doi: 10.1164/rccm.201212-2177OC

Taskar, V., John, J., Evander, E., Robertson, B., and Jonson, B. (1997). Surfactant dysfunction makes lungs vulnerable to repetitive collapse and reexpansion. *Am. J. Respir. Crit. Care Med.* 155, 313–320. doi: 10.1164/ajrccm.155.1.9001330

Taskar, V., John, J., Evander, E., Wollmer, P., Robertson, B., and Jonson, B. (1995). Healthy lungs tolerate repetitive collapse and reopening during short periods of mechanical ventilation. *Acta Anaesthesiol. Scand.* 39, 370–376. doi: 10.1111/j.1399-6576.1995.tb04080.x

Terry, R. J. (1939). A thoracic window for observation of the lung in a living animal. *Science* 90, 43–44. doi: 10.1126/science.90.2324.43

Tsuchida, S., Engelberts, D., Peltekova, V., Hopkins, N., Frndova, H., Babyn, P., et al. (2006). Atelectasis causes alveolar injury in nonatelectatic lung regions. *Am. J. Respir. Crit. Care Med.* 174, 279–289. doi: 10.1164/rccm.200506-1006OC

Tsuda, A., Henry, F. S., and Butler, J. P. (2008). Gas and aerosol mixing in the acinus. *Respir. Physiol. Neurobiol.* 163, 139–149. doi: 10.1016/j.resp.2008.02.010

Ueki, H., Wang, I. H., Fukuyama, S., Katsura, H., da Silva Lopes, T. J., Neumann, G., et al. (2018). *In vivo* imaging of the pathophysiological changes and neutrophil dynamics in influenza virus-infected mouse lungs. *Proc. Natl. Acad. Sci. U.S.A.* 115, E6622–E6629. doi: 10.1073/pnas.1806265115

Wagner, W. W. Jr. (1969). Pulmonary microcirculatory observations *in vivo* under physiological conditions. *J. Appl. Physiol.* 26, 375–377. doi: 10.1152/jappl.1969.26.3.375

Wagner, W. W. Jr. (1988). Capillary recruitment in the pulmonary microcirculation. *Chest* 93(3 Suppl.), 85S–88S. doi: 10.1378/chest.93.3_supplement.85s

Wagner, W. W. Jr., Latham, L. P., Gillespie, M. N., Guenther, J. P., and Capen, R. L. (1982). Direct measurement of pulmonary capillary transit times. *Science* 218, 379–381. doi: 10.1126/science.7123237

Wakabayashi, K., Wilson, M. R., Tatham, K. C., O'Dea, K. P., and Takata, M. (2014). Volutrauma, but not atelectrauma, induces systemic cytokine production by lung-marginated monocytes. *Crit. Care Med.* 42, e49–e57. doi: 10.1097/CCM.0b013e31829a822a

Wearn, J. T., Ernstene, A. C., Bromer, A. W., Barr, J. S., German, W. J., and Zschiesche, L. J. (1934). The normal behavior of the pulmonary blood vessels with observations on the intermittence of the flow of blood in the arterioles. *Am. J. Physiol. Leg. Content* 109, 236–256. doi: 10.1152/ajplegacy.1934.109.2.236

Weibel, E. R., Nieman, G. F., Gatto, L. A., Frazer, D. G., Schittny, J. C., Woods, J. C., et al. (2012). Commentaries on viewpoint: unresolved mysteries. *J. Appl. Physiol.* 113, 1948–1949. doi: 10.1152/japplphysiol.01203.2012

Wolsk, E., Bakkestrom, R., Thomsen, J. H., Balling, L., Andersen, M. J., Dahl, J. S., et al. (2017). The influence of age on hemodynamic parameters during rest and exercise in healthy individuals. *JACC Heart Fail.* 5, 337–346. doi: 10.1016/j.jchf.2016.10.012

Yipp, B. G., Kim, J. H., Lima, R., Zbytnuik, L. D., Petri, B., Swanlund, N., et al. (2017). The lung is a host defense niche for immediate neutrophil-mediated vascular protection. *Sci. Immunol.* 2:eaam8929. doi: 10.1126/sciimmunol.aam8929

Young, J. (1929). Malpighi's "De Pulmonibus". *Proc. R. Soc. Med.* 23, 1–11. doi: 10.1177/003591572902300101

2

An Analytical Model for Estimating Alveolar Wall Elastic Moduli from Lung Tissue Uniaxial Stress-Strain Curves

Samer Bou Jawde[1]*, Ayuko Takahashi*[1]*, Jason H. T. Bates*[2] *and Béla Suki*[1*]

[1] *Biomedical Engineering, Boston University, Boston, MA, United States,* [2] *Department of Medicine, Larner College of Medicine, University of Vermont, Burlington, VT, United States*

***Correspondence:**
Béla Suki
bsuki@bu.edu

The non-linear stress-strain behavior of uniaxially-stretched lung parenchyma is thought to be an emergent phenomenon arising from the ensemble behavior of its microscopic constituents. Such behavior includes the alignment and elongation of randomly oriented alveolar walls with initially flaccid fibers in the direction of strain. To account for the link between microscopic wall behavior and the macroscopic stress-strain curve, we developed an analytical model that represents both alignment and elongation of alveolar walls during uniaxial stretching. The model includes the kinetics and mechanical behavior of randomly oriented elastic alveolar walls that have a bending stiffness at their intersections. The alignment and stretch of the walls following incremental stretch of the tissue were determined based on energy minimization, and the total stress was obtained by differentiating the total energy density with respect to strain. The stress-strain curves predicted by the model were comparable to curves generated by a previously published numerical alveolar network model. The model was also fit to experimentally measured stress-strain curves in parenchymal strips obtained from mice with decreased lung collagen content, and from young and aged mice. This yielded estimates for the elastic modulus of an alveolar wall, which increased with age from 4.4 to 5.9 kPa ($p = 0.043$), and for the elastic modulus of fibers within the wall, which increased with age from 311 to 620 kPa ($p = 0.001$). This demonstrates the possibility of estimating alveolar wall mechanical properties in biological soft tissue from its macroscopic behavior given appropriate assumptions about tissue structure.

Keywords: multiscale, alignment, tensile modulus, bond-bending modulus, aging

INTRODUCTION

The macroscopic mechanical behavior of a biological tissue such as the lung parenchyma arises from the ensemble behavior of its microscopic constituents (Suki and Bates, 2011). This macroscopic behavior is usually very different from the behaviors of the constituents themselves. Furthermore, while macroscopic behavior determines physiological phenotype, disease processes and pharmacotherapies invariably act at the microscale level. It is thus crucial to understand macroscopic mechanical behavior of tissue as an emergent consequence of structure and function at the microscale. In particular, the strain-stiffening behavior of biological soft tissues has been primarily attributed to the way in which load-bearing fibers are recruited via alignment and/or straightening within the extracellular matrix (ECM) (Wuyts et al., 1995; Suki et al., 2005; Suki and Bates, 2011). The progressive recruitment of collagen fibers with increasing strain has been modeled specifically for lung parenchymal tissue (Maksym and Bates, 1997), human vein, fascia, tympanic membrane, rabbit papillary muscle (Decraemer et al., 1980), and ligament (Liao and Belkoff, 1999). Both recruitment and fiber reorientation were simultaneously taken into account by Lanir (1979). Nevertheless, the stress-strain behavior of the individual tissue constituents themselves must also be taken into account for a complete understanding of tissue mechanics. Determining this behavior experimentally is challenging because of the tiny length scales involved, but Sacks was able to determine fiber orientation using small-angle light scattering and numerically solved the constitutive equations to estimate the stress-strain behavior of individual collagen fibers (Sacks, 2003). Furthermore, these fibers do not act in isolation. They interact with each other and with other components of the ECM through electrostatic forces arising, for example, from negatively charged proteoglycans (PGs) that exert repulsive forces on each other (Cavalcante et al., 2005; Ritter et al., 2009).

These models, however, all fail to capture the foam-like structure of lung parenchyma comprised of alveoli and alveolar ducts. Models based on 3-dimensional alveolar geometry have been proposed (Denny and Schroter, 2006; Parameswaran et al., 2011; Pidaparti et al., 2013), but these all assume constitutive properties for the alveolar wall and predict tissue behavior on this basis. Here we seek to do the reverse, namely to infer alveolar wall properties from the macroscopic mechanical behavior of lung parenchyma. Most models of lung tissue that have been proposed to date are limited in this regard because they are numerical (Maksym et al., 1998; Cavalcante et al., 2005; Takahashi et al., 2014), and are thus computationally expensive. Also, the insights provided by numerical models are limited to the particular parameter sets used to calculate examples of model behavior. Analytical models, in contrast, have the potential to provide general insight that is not bound by particular exemplars. Analytical models can also usually be solved much more quickly than numerical models, which makes them more suited to the present inverse modeling application, although they invariably require significant simplifying assumptions in order to be tractable.

Accordingly, the goal of this study was to develop an analytical multi-scale model that links the elastic stiffness and the alignment mechanism of the alveolar walls to the macroscopic mechanical stress-strain behavior of the lung tissue itself. We test the predictions of this model by comparing its macroscopic stress-strain curves to those made by a previously developed numerical model. We also tested model predictions against experimental data obtained in parenchymal tissue strips under uniaxial stretching. These conditions modulate fiber stretching and alignment without being confounded by other phenomena operative in the 3-dimensional expansion of lungs *in situ* such as volumetric expansion, shear, and surface tension (Wilson and Bachofen, 1982; Bachofen and Schürch, 2001; Denny and Schroter, 2006). This enabled us to focus exclusively on the mechanical properties of the tissue fibers and how they change with age, the latter being known to principally affect the fibers (Kohn et al., 2015; Panwar et al., 2015).

METHODS

Model Development

We assume that a 2-dimensional strip of lung tissue with length L and width W is held in place at one end and stretched uniaxially from the other in a sequence of equal increments. The tissue strip is modeled as a network of hexagonal alveoli. Each of the N alveolar walls in the strip (**Figure 1A**) has a tensile Young's modulus Y_a, while adjacent walls are bonded together at intersections that have bond-bending modulus Y_b that resists changes in angle between neighboring walls. The volume fraction of the tissue comprised of alveolar walls is $\delta_{V,w}$, so the effective tensile and bond-bending moduli of the tissue are $Y_{ae} = Y_a\,\delta_{V,w}$ and $Y_{be} = Y_b\,\delta_{V,w}$, respectively (assuming that whatever fills the alveolar lumen makes no contribution to either). At incremental stretch step $s-1$, the nth alveolar wall has length $l_{n,s-1}$ and strain $\varepsilon_{n,s-1}$ and is oriented at an angle $\theta_{n,s-1}$ with respect to the direction of tissue stretch (**Figure 1B**).

An incremental displacement x of the right-hand end of the alveolar wall in the direction of tissue stretch will, in general, cause the wall itself to undergo some combination of alignment and elongation (**Figure 1C**). Elongation of the wall increases its elastic energy, while alignment alters the elastic energy stored within its wall-wall bonds (**Figure 1D**). The configuration of the various walls within the tissue at any time step s will be that which minimizes the sum of all these energies. The stress within the tissue is then the derivative of the energy density of the system with respect to macroscopic strain. To establish the global stress-strain equation for the tissue, we further assume

- constant tensile and wall-bending moduli,
- affine tissue deformation characterized by the microscopic incremental tissue strain ($d\epsilon_x$) due to the microscopic incremental displacement x being equal to the macroscopic incremental strain ($d\epsilon_X$) due to the macroscopic incremental displacement X $\left(d\epsilon_x = d\epsilon_X\right)$,
- extension and alignment of the alveolar wall bear a linear relationship to each other when strained incrementally,
- boundary effects are minimal (i.e., $L \gg l_{s-1}$ and $W \gg l_{s-1}$).

These assumptions lead to the following equation relating macroscopic tissue stress σ_T at the current stretch step s to the alveolar wall constitutive properties, the current strains, angles, and initial angles $\theta_{n,o}$ for all walls ($n = 1,\ldots,N$), and the incremental tissue strain (see **Appendix A** for a detailed derivation):

$$\sigma_T(s) = Y_{ae}\frac{1}{N}\sum_{n=1}^{N}\frac{d\epsilon_X + \varepsilon_{n,s-1} + \left(1+\varepsilon_{n,s-1}\right)\left(\theta_{n,0}-\theta_{n,s-1}\right)\tan(\theta_{n,s-1})}{1+\frac{Y_{ae}}{Y_{be}}\left(1+\varepsilon_{n,s-1}\right)^2\tan^2\left(\theta_{n,s-1}\right)} \tag{1}$$

In the limit of large macroscopic stretch, all the alveolar walls become aligned, the denominator of the above equation tends to 1, and the last term of the numerator tends to 0. At this point, the equation reduces to the description of an arbitrary number of

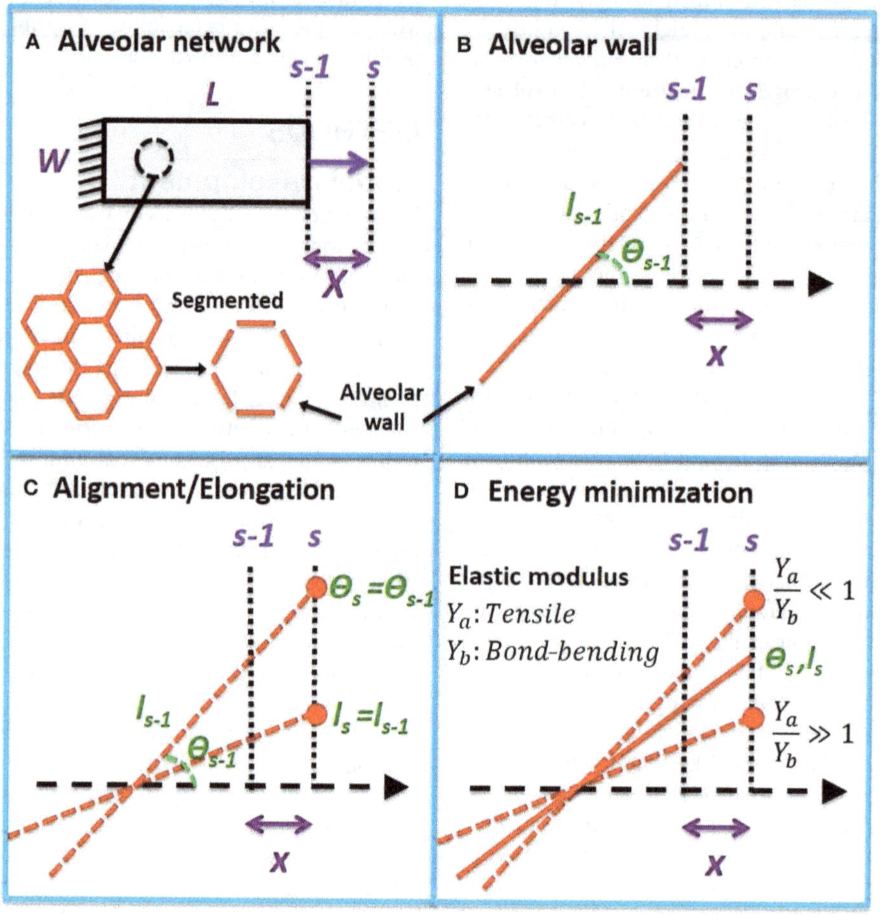

FIGURE 1 | Uniaxial model development. **(A)** Uniaxial stretching of a tissue strip from step $s - 1$ to s with an incremental macroscopic displacement X. The tissue is composed of a hexagonal network which can be partitioned into alveolar wall segments. **(B)** A single wall segment with length l_{s-1} and angle θ_{s-1} with respect to the direction of stretch at step $s - 1$. A microscopic displacement x will cause the wall to align by rotation and stretch. **(C)** The alveolar wall will follow the microscopic displacement between two extremes of pure elongation and pure rotation. **(D)** When the tensile modulus of the wall is much larger than its bond-bending modulus ($Y_a > Y_b$), it will rotate, and when its bond-bending modulus is much larger ($Y_b >> Y_a$), it will elongate in order to minimize energy. The new angle (θ_s) and length (l_s) at step s will lie between these two extremes at a location that minimizes the total elastic energy.

linearly elastic walls in parallel thus:

$$\sigma_T = Y_{ae}(d\epsilon_X + \bar{\varepsilon}_{s-1}) \tag{2}$$

where $\bar{\varepsilon}_{s-1}$ is the mean wall strain. The slope of this stress-strain relationship is independent of angle because, at full alignment, the bond-bending energy remains constant. The asymptotically linear portion of the stress-strain curve at high strain thus depends only on Y_{ae}. In general, however, the macroscopic stress-strain relationship expressed by Equation 1 involves the two elastic moduli Y_{ae} and Y_{be}, which can be estimated by fitting Equation 1 to experimental measurements of σ_T and ϵ_X. Finally, if the average fiber volume fraction ($\delta_{V,f}$) within the alveolar wall is known, and assuming that the fibers are the major contributors to the wall tensile modulus, then the average elastic modulus of a single fiber (Y_f) can be estimated as.

$$Y_f \cong \frac{Y_a}{\delta_{V,f}} \cong \frac{Y_{ae}}{\delta_{V,w}\delta_{V,f}} \tag{3}$$

Computational Model Validation

We compared the predictions of the above model to stress-strain relationships generated by a previously described numerical model. The numerical model, introduced by Cavalcante et al. (2005), consists of a hexagonal cell network representing a strip of lung parenchyma, where each hexagonal cell represents an alveolus in cross-section and each hexagonal segment represents an alveolar wall. (**Figure 9A** in **Appendix B**). Each wall is modeled as a spring with spring constant k in units of [N/m]. The relative rotation of two alveolar walls about their point of intersection is hindered by a bond-bending spring with an elastic constant b in units of [Nm/rad^2]. When b is zero, the hexagonal structure is unstable and collapses upon shear or uniaxial stretch, while when b is very high the symmetric configuration of the hexagon strongly resists a change in shape. In any case, the walls each align and elongate in such a way that the total energy of the network is minimized at each strain step. In this way, the model of Cavalcante et al. (2005) takes into consideration the deformation energy stored within all the individual alveolar walls and all the bonds between their respective neighboring walls in a network.

In contrast, the analytical model developed above considers the tensile and bending energies of alveolar walls in isolation (i.e., it does not take into account how the presence of neighboring walls might affect a given wall's configuration). Both models, however, should predict the same total elastic energy in the tissue strip at each tissue strain. When their respective expressions for total energy are equated (see **Appendix B** for details), we find that

$$Y_{ae} = u\frac{9}{4}l_o^2 k \quad (4)$$

$$Y_{be} = u18b \quad (5)$$

where l_o is the mean initial length of the walls in the numerical model, and u is a unity constant that ensures both sides of Equations 4 and 5 have the same dimensions.

Experimental Model Validation

We tested the predictions of the analytical model against three different sets of experimental data. The first set comprised the stress-strain measurements made in excised rat lung slices ($n = 5$ per group) published by Cavalcante et al. (2005). Measurements were made while the strips were bathed in normal, hypertonic, and hypotonic saline in order to modulate the charge densities on the proteoglycans in the tissue, which affects tissue stiffness due to altered repulsive forces acting on alveolar walls. Because the surface charges on elastin and collagen are significantly lower than those on proteoglycans (Maroudas and Bannon, 1981; Chalmers et al., 1999), altering saline tonicity is expected to mainly affect Y_{be} with relatively little influence on Y_{ae}.

The second test data set was comprised of quasi-static stress-strain curves measured in mice published by Shiwen et al. (2015). We used data from both wild-type mice (WT, $n = 6$) and from age-matched mice in which myocardin-related transcription factor-A (MRTF-A) had been knocked out (KO, $n = 6$). MRTF-A is known to lead to a reduction in type I collagen deposition, leading to tissue softening, and indeed these investigators showed that KO had reduced tissue stresses compared to WT. The reduction in stress was attributed to both a decrease in collagen content and a decrease in fibril diameter from 97 ± 24 nm in WT to 58 ± 9 nm in KO. It is thus expected that both Y_f and Y_{ae} should be reduced in the KO mice, with minimal alterations to Y_{be}.

The third data set was collected in our laboratory in a study approved by the Institutional Animal Care and Use Committee of Boston University. We investigated the effects of aging on alveolar wall tensile and bond-bending moduli by fitting lung tissue stress-strain curves obtained in young ($n = 5$; 5 months) and old ($n = 6$; 19, and 24 months) mice. The young mice were obtained from Charles River Laboratories (Boston, MA). The mice were anesthetized by intraperitoneal injection of pentobarbital sodium (80 mg/kg), tracheostomized and cannulated with an 18-guage steel needle in the supine position followed by median abdominal incision and sternotomy under deep anesthesia. Euthanasia was obtained during exsanguination by cutting the abdominal aorta and inferior vena cava while the pulmonary artery was flushed with phosphate buffered saline (PBS). For the aged mice, isolated lungs were obtained from Brigham and Women's Hospital, Harvard Medical School. The left lung in each group was cut into strips with dimensions of 5 × 2 × 1 mm, and used to obtain tissue strip mechanics. Uniaxial quasi-static stress-strain curves were obtained as previously described (Cavalcante et al., 2005). Briefly, the system consists of a computer-controlled lever arm (Aurora Scientific, Ontario, Canada) and a sensitive force transducer (model 300B; Aurora Scientific, Ontario, Canada) both attached to an acrylic base housing a 24 mL tissue bath maintained at a temperature of 37°C. Small metal plates were glued to each end of the strip with cyanoacrylate. The plates were attached to the force transducer and lever-arm via steel wires and the strip was submerged in the tissue bath containing PBS. The strips were preconditioned by applying three consecutive triangular displacement signals peaking at 60% uniaxial macroscopic strain at a rate of 2 %/s. After a 5-min equilibration period, force-displacement data were collected. Stress and strain were calculated as the force divided by the initial cross-sectional area and the displacement divided by the initial length of the strip, respectively.

Model Fitting and Statistical Analysis

Data simulation and curve fitting were performed using either MATLAB R2015a or R2018b (MathWorks, CA), while statistical tests were performed using SigmaPlot 11.0 (Systat Software, CA). A paired t-test was applied for the rat tissue slices bathed in different tonicities, while a t-test was used for the collagen knockout and aging study. Statistical significance was accepted at $p < 0.05$.

The *nlinfit* function in MATLAB was used to fit the model to data. The *nlinfit* solver was provided with initial guesses for Y_{ae} and Y_{be} and an initial uniform distribution of 5,000 alveolar wall angles between 0 and $\pi/2$ was assumed. The initial alveolar strains were set to zero. Since the model predictions (Equation 1) are based on the assumption of small incremental strains, while in most cases the experimental strain steps were large, we iteratively calculated the alveolar wall strains and angles as well as the total tissue stress for strains ranging from zero up to the maximum experimental strain, in strain steps of 0.001. The predicted model tissue stress was then compared to the experimental stress values at the experimental strains, the predicted values of Y_{ae} and Y_{be} were updated, and the process was repeated. Further investigations with the model indicated that at least 2,000 alveolar walls and an incremental strain of <0.01 are required for the model to converge—see **Appendix C**.

RESULTS

Model Behavior

Figure 2 plots the normalized stress-strain curves for five different Y_{ae}/Y_{be} ratios (**Figure 2A**) as well as the means and standard deviations of the alveolar angles and strains for ratios of 0.1, 1, and 10 (**Figures 2B,C**, respectively). The normalized stress-strain relationship for a ratio of 0.01 is essentially linear (**Figure 2A**) while the mean wall angle of $\pi/4$

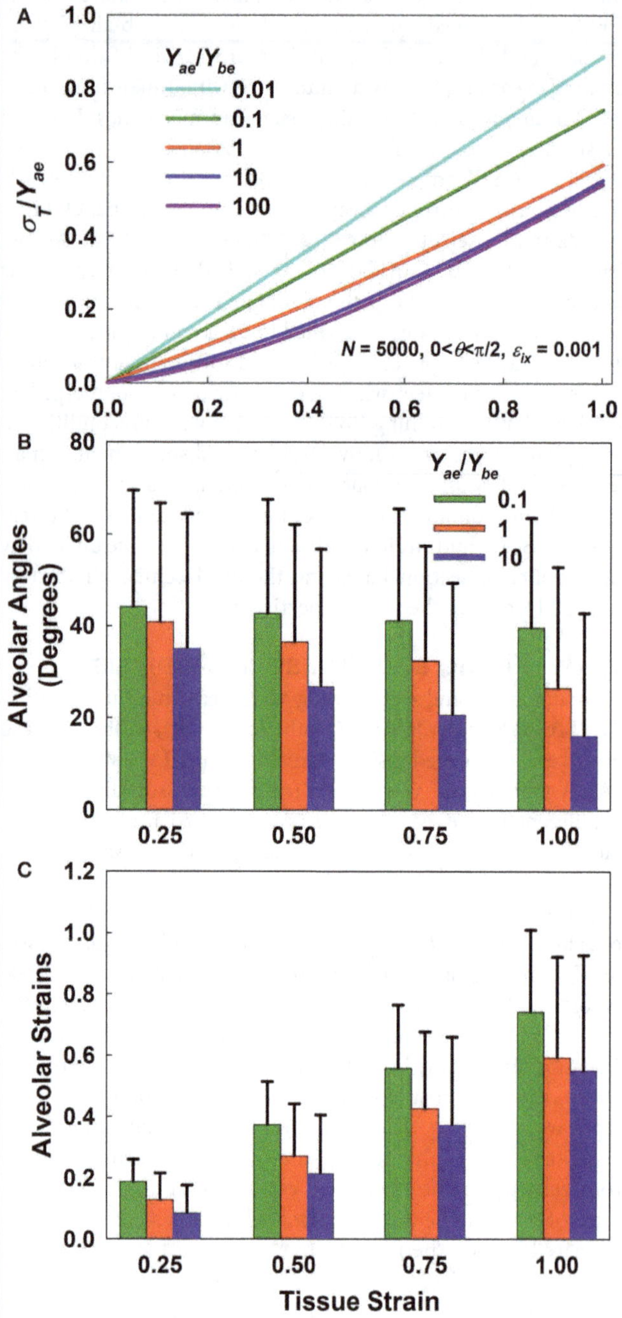

FIGURE 2 | Forward simulation results. **(A)** Normalized stress-strain curves for different Y_{ae}/Y_{be} ratios. **(B,C)** Mean and standard deviation of alveolar angles and strains, respectively, as a function of macroscopic tissue strain for Y_{ae}/Y_{be} ratios of 0.1, 1, and 10. Alveolar angles at a strain of zero were uniformly distributed between 0 and $\pi/2$ while alveolar strains were set to zero.

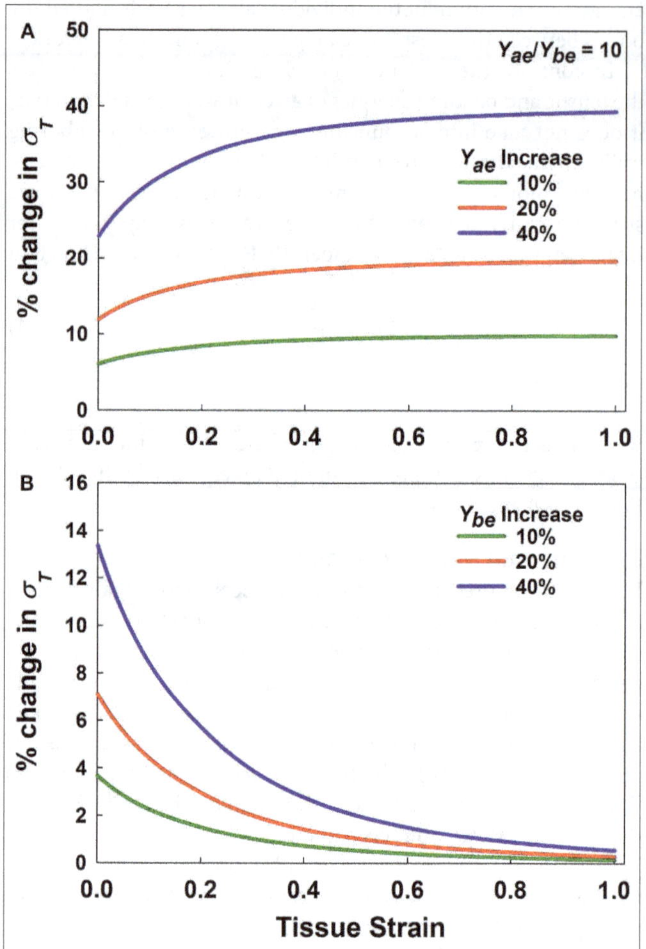

FIGURE 3 | Sensitivity analysis. **(A,B)** % change in stress for increasing Y_{ae} and Y_{be}, respectively by 10, 20, and 40% for $Y_{ae}/Y_{be} = 10$.

shows that alignment was minimal, demonstrating that strain was accommodated almost entirely through wall elongation. As Y_{ae}/Y_{be} increases, however, the stress-strain relationships (**Figure 2A**) become progressively more non-linear and thus similar to the experimentally observed stress-strain curves, while the mean wall angles depart increasingly from $\pi/4$, indicative of an increasing degree of wall alignment with macroscopic stretch. Above a Y_{ae}/Y_{be} ratio of 100 the macroscopic stretch of the tissue was accommodated almost entirely by wall alignment. Additional investigations of the effects of alveolar number and incremental strain are presented in **Appendix C**.

Figure 3 presents a sensitivity analysis of the effects of variations in Y_{ae} and Y_{be} on model stress for a Y_{ae}/Y_{be} ratio of 10. The effects of these two parameters are opposite; increasing Y_{ae} causes stress to increase (**Figure 3A**), while increasing Y_{be} causes stress to decrease (**Figure 3B**) with strain. Furthermore, variations in Y_{ae} have a stronger impact at high strains, while the opposite is true for Y_{be}. Clearly, once strain is high enough to bring the alveolar walls into alignment, Y_{be} has no further effect on the stress-strain curve, so with further strain there is a linear relationship between Y_{ae} and stress. In contrast, a linear relationship between Y_{be} and stress is not possible. **Figure 3** also shows that the rate of change of stress with either Y_{ae} or Y_{be} is greatest at low stress. This indicates that fitting the stress-strain relationship predicted by the model to experimental data over a range of strains from 0 to 30% should be sufficient to reliably estimate both elastic moduli.

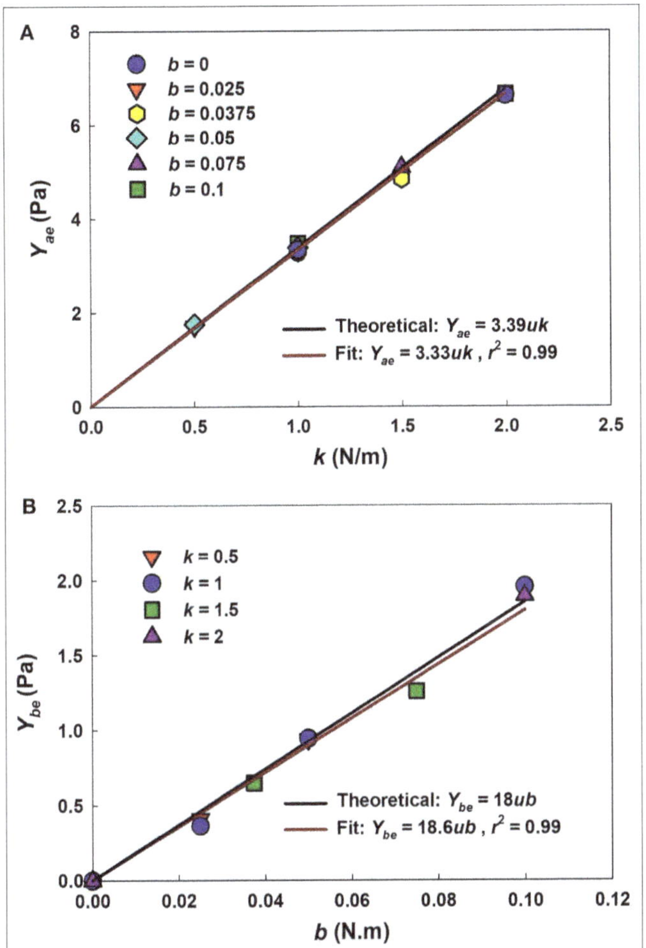

FIGURE 4 | Uniaxial model-based estimates of network parameters. **(A)** Y_{ae} vs. k for different b values. **(B)** Y_{be} vs. b for different k values. Solid black lines represent the theoretical relationships between network and model parameters. Solid dark red lines represent the fits with the r^2 as the adjusted coefficient of determination for the linear fit.

Model Validation

Figure 4 shows that estimates of Y_{ae} and Y_{be} from the analytical model (Equations 4 and 5, respectively) agree closely with those used in the numerical network model over a range of parameter values, with r^2 values of 0.99. This supports the utility of the analytical model as a computationally much faster alternative to the numerical model.

The distributions of alveolar wall angle and wall strain at four different tissue strains for the analytical and numerical models are compared in **Figure 5**. There is generally good agreement between the two models in terms of wall angle (**Figures 5A,C,E,G**), although alveolar walls align with the direction of strain somewhat more rapidly in the analytical model because interactions between the nodes of the network model resist alignment to some degree. In particular, the analytical model assumes that the alveolar wall ends rotate according to the macroscopic strain; however, in the network model each node pulls on another wall which delays the alignment with strain. The strain distributions from the two models (**Figures 5B,D,F,H**) are less consistent than the angle distributions, although both models exhibit similar ranges of strain values. An important difference between the two models that may account for the discrepancies seen in the strain panels of **Figure 5** is that while alveolar walls can only increase in length with macroscopic strain in the analytical model, in the network model it is possible for two adjacent nodes in the network model to approach each with increasing strain if the nodes are aligned perpendicular to the direction of strain (as illustrated in **Figure 10B, Appendix B**). The network model considers such shortened walls to be flaccid, thus making no contribution to the strain energy.

Figure 6 shows fits from the analytical model to stress-strain measurements in rat lung tissue strips made under different tonicity conditions (**Figure 6A**) and between WT and MRTF-A KO mice (**Figure 6B**). The fitted model parameters are shown in **Table 1**. Alterations in tonicity had no statistically significant effect on Y_{ae}, but Y_{be} increased by 211% between normal and hypotonic conditions (p = 0.03) and showed a nearly significant (p = 0.09) decrease between normal and hypertonic conditions. On the other hand, Y_{ae} decreased significantly (p = 0.014) between WT and MRTF-A KO mice, while there was no significant change in Y_{be}. These differential effects of changes in tonicity vs. MRTF-A KO are as expected on the basis of altered proteoglycan charge density vs. reduced collagen I deposition in the tissue.

Figure 7 shows that age increases parenchymal tissue stiffness, and that the analytical model recapitulates this effect. The elastic moduli obtained by fitting the model to the young and old stress-strain relationships are given in **Table 2**. Values for Y_a and Y_b as well as the fiber tensile elastic modulus (Y_f) were estimated using literature values for the density of wall tissue in a parenchymal strip ($\delta_{V,w}$) and the density of fibers in an alveolar wall ($\delta_{V,f}$) obtained by Huang et al. (2007) in 2 and 20 month old C57BL/6 mice. They found that the tissue fraction was 35% independent of age, while the total fiber content (collagen plus elastin) decreased with age from 4 to 2.75%. The values of Y_{be} estimated by the analytical model did not change with age, but Y_{ae} increased by 34.4% from 4.4 to 5.9 kPa (p = 0.043). Y_f increased with age by 99.4% from 311 to 620 kPa (p = 0.001).

DISCUSSION

In this study, we developed an analytical model of lung parenchymal tissue mechanics that links uniaxial stress-strain behavior at the level of the tissue strip to the alignment and elongation of alveolar walls. By modeling this behavior, we were able to separate and estimate the tensile and bond-bending moduli of alveolar walls under different experimental conditions and biological processes such as aging.

The model replicated experimental stress-strain data from a variety of sources and provided average estimates of the tensile modulus of an average alveolar wall and the bond-bending modulus of the junction between walls (**Tables 1, 2**). Investigations of model behavior (**Figures 2, 3**) suggest that the

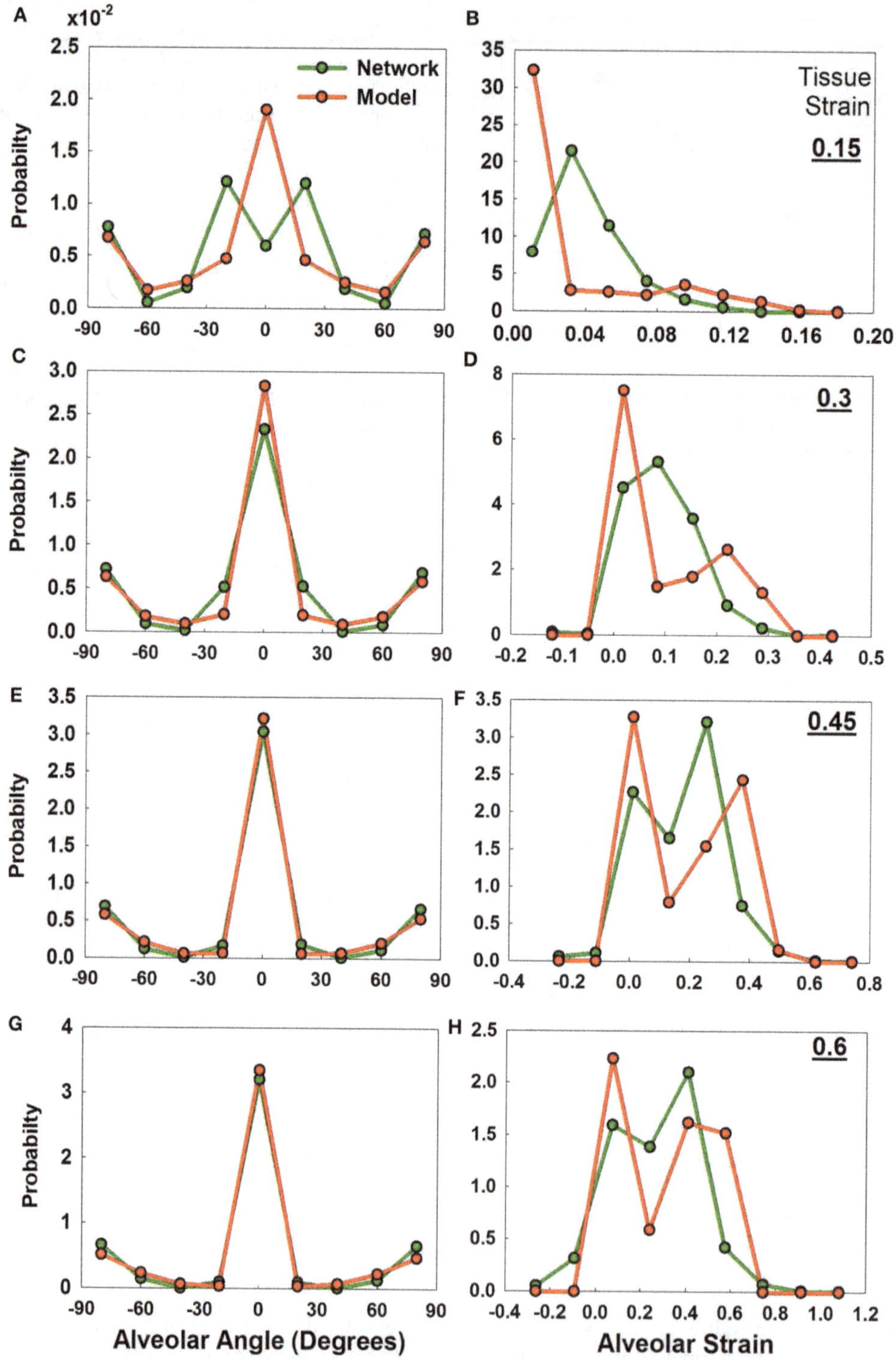

FIGURE 5 | Uniaxial analytical and the network model-based alveolar angle and strain distributions. The graphs show alveolar angle probability distribution functions **(A,C,E,G)** and alveolar strain probability distribution functions **(B,D,F,H)** from the analytical model and the network at four levels of tissue strains (0.15, 0.3, 0.45, and 0.6). Initial alveolar strains are zero. Initial angle distribution is shown in **Appendix B, Figure 9B** .

ratio of the tensile to the bond-bending elastic moduli must exceed 1 in order to account for the experimentally observed strain-stiffening properties of lung tissue (Fung, 1984; Karlinsky, 1992; Pinart et al., 2011; Suki and Bates, 2011; Yi et al., 2016; Polio et al., 2018). The stress-strain relationships predicted by the model become increasingly non-linear as the modulus ratio

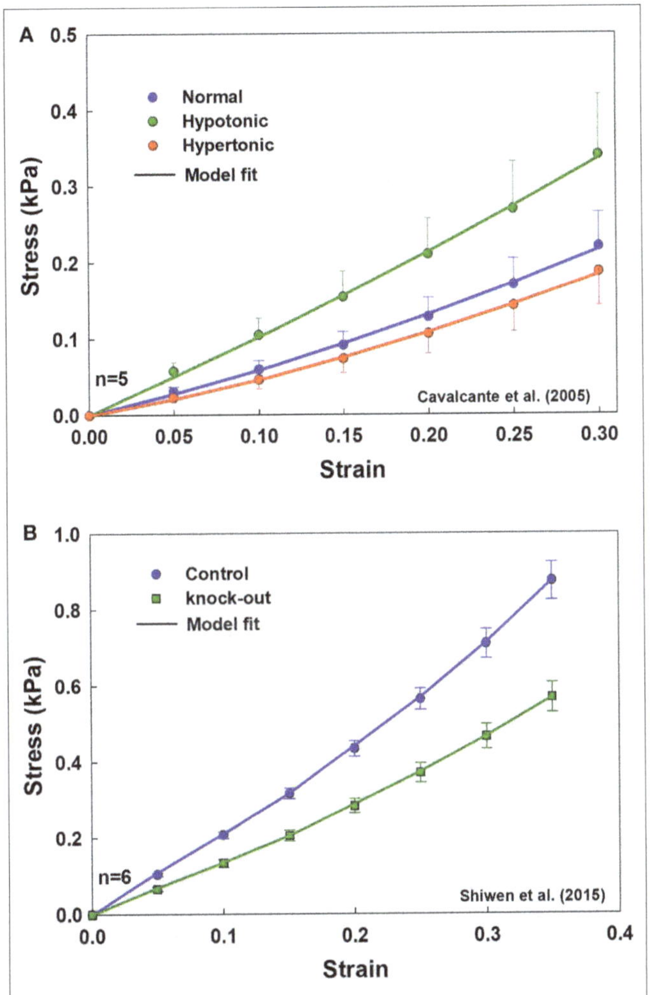

FIGURE 6 | Population mean and standard error, with model fits (solid lines) for the tissue strips for **(A)** three different tonicities (normal, hypertonic, and hypotonic) from rat lungs, and **(B)** from WT and MRTF-A KO mice.

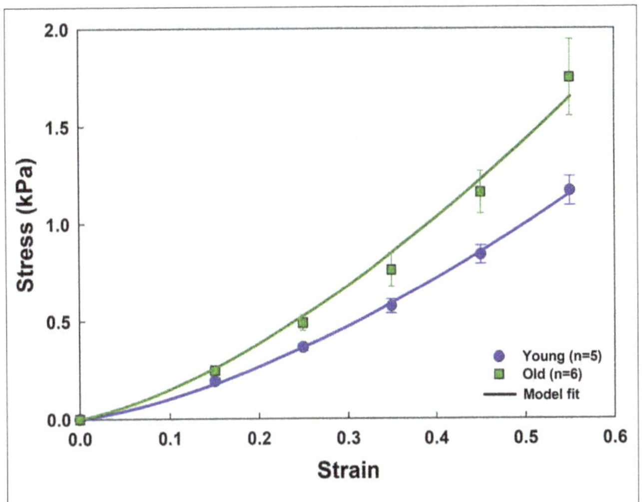

FIGURE 7 | Stress-strain curves and parameter estimation results for the aging data. Experimental data (mean and standard errors) for young and old mice are shown with symbols. Model fits are plotted as solid lines.

TABLE 1 | Model validation experimental results.

	Y_{ae} (kPa)	%Δ	*p*-value	Y_{be} (kPa)	%Δ	*p*-value
Tonicity—Rat Tissue Strips						
Normal	1.94 ± 1.07			0.27 ± 0.14		
Hypotonic	3.28 ± 1.75	69	0.11	0.84 ± 0.41	211	0.03
Hypertonic	1.78 ± 1.03	−8	0.11	0.11 ± 0.11	−60	0.09
Collagen Knockout—Mouse Tissue Strips						
Control	5.96 ± 1.39			1.28 ± 0.42		
Knock-out	3.94 ± 0.93	−34	0.014	0.84 ± 0.58	−34	0.165

Y_{ae} and Y_{be} values are mean ± standard deviation. %Δ is the percent difference with respect to the normal control.

increases. This is consistent with the notion that the alveolar walls and the embedded fibers are the main load bearing elements in the lung parenchyma (Romero et al., 1998; Yuan et al., 2000; Maina and West, 2005; Yi et al., 2016), and is supported by our finding that reducing collagen in the wall reduces tissue stiffness (**Figure 6B**). Furthermore, since the elastic modulus of an alveolar wall in the model is constant with stretch, the non-linearity of the predicted stress-strain relationships arises purely from alignment that allows the walls to align with the direction of macroscopic strain, which is essentially a recruitment process. Alignment also implies a certain capacity of the wall to oppose being stretched, something that is modulated by the ratio of Y_{ae} to Y_{be}. The higher the ratio, the stiffer the alveolar wall and the faster the alignment (**Figure 2B**). Ratios larger than 1 were obtained from the fitting (**Tables 1, 2**) which is expected on physiological grounds since the function of the wall, and particularly the fibers within it, is to provide a mechanically resilient structure within a very thin layer to support structural integrity and gas exchange (Weibel, 2009; Maina and West, 2005).

The estimated values of Y_{ae} (~5 kPa) and Y_f (~300 kPa for the young mice) obtained by fitting the analytical model to experimental stress-strain relationships match those reported in literature (**Table 2**). For example, Polio et al. (2018), measured Y_{ae} in porcine lung using cavitation rheology (6.1 ± 1.6 kPa), small amplitude oscillatory shear rheometry (3.3 ± 0.5), micro-indentation (1.4 ± 0.4), and uniaxial tension (3.4 ± 0.4) and showed that all these techniques provided values in the same range. Using AFM, Liu and Tschumperlin (2011) estimated a value around 5 kPa for mice, while Jorba et al. (2019) obtained values around 10 kPa at low strain in rats. Cavalcante et al. (2005) used their network model to estimate the effective alveolar wall stiffness to be ~5 kPa. Assuming that collagen fibers are the primary load bearing constituents of the wall, they also estimated fiber tensile elastic modulus to be ~300 kPa, which is similar to the average modulus in mice provided by our analytical model (**Table 2**) even though our estimate is an ensemble value including both elastin and collagen fibers. Furthermore, the elastic modulus of single elastin fibers is around 410 kPa (Aaron

TABLE 2 | Aging results showing mean and standard errors with respective *p*-values for young and old mice.

Modulus (kPa)	Young ($n = 5$)	Old ($n = 6$)	*p*-value
Y_{ae}	4.36 ± 0.45	5.86 ± 1.35	0.043
Y_{be}	0.114 ± 0.001	0.161 ± 0.066	0.77
Y_a	12.44 ± 1.14	15.49 ± 3.53	0.094
Y_b	0.42 ± 0.25	0.46 ± 0.17	0.77
Y_f	311 ± 29	620 ± 131	0.001

Model fitted values for Y_{ae} and Y_{be} were used to derive Y_a, Y_b, and Y_f. Y_a = average alveolar tensile elastic modulus; Y_b = average alveolar wall bond-bending elastic modulus; Y_f = average fiber tensile elastic modulus.

and Gosline, 1981). This is similar to the values of Y_f we obtained in mice in the present study (**Table 2**), perhaps because the delayed recruitment of flaccid collagen fibers causes elastin to be the primary determinant of stress at low strain (Mead, 1961).

The elastic moduli of the alveolar wall and the load-bearing fiber estimated by the analytical model both increased with age (**Table 2**), as did the stiffness of the tissue itself (**Figure 7**). Thus, even though the fiber content of the alveolar wall was reduced in the older mice, the fibers themselves were actually stiffer, something that can be attributed to the increased protein fiber cross-linking that is known to occur with age (Reiser et al., 1987; Snedeker and Gautieri, 2014). This implies that the increased lung compliance that occurs with age (Knudson et al., 1977; Suki and Bartolák-Suki, 2015) must be a reflection of age-related increase in airspace dimensions (Thurlbeck, 1967). More importantly, however, this finding also suggests that cells in the aging lung will experience an increased stiffening of the ECM substrate upon which they live, which has implications for cellular signaling and senescence (Suki and Bartolák-Suki, 2015).

Our analytical model thus recapitulates key experimental observations made in lung tissue strips and provides estimates of constitutive tissue properties that are consistent with experimental measurement and prediction by other models. These findings must nevertheless be viewed in light of the model limitations, which relate principally to the assumptions inherent in it. For example, a fundamental assumption of the model, made in the interests of mathematical tractability, is that alveolar walls can be represented as components that do not interact except insofar as to collaborate in the generation of bond-bending forces through their relative orientations. In other words, the orientation of a given wall is assumed not to influence the orientations of any of the neighboring walls to which it is connected. While this might seem open to question, the estimates of elastic modulus obtained by fitting the model to data generated by a numerical model compare well both to the parameters (**Figure 4**) and to wall angles and strains (**Figure 5**) in the numerical model even though the analytical model is not capable of recapitulating network effects that can take place in the numerical model.

Concerning validation by comparing the model to another model, we note the following. If an analytical model is developed with simplifying assumptions, it is often the case that such a model is compared to a more sophisticated numerical model that accounts for mechanisms that are necessarily omitted from the analytic approach. Since Cavalcante et al. (2005) did verify their model experimentally, we chose this model to investigate how network effects influenced the current model.

Another important simplifying assumption in the analytical model is that the stress-strain behavior of the alveolar wall is linear with a constant elastic modulus. A recent study used atomic force microscopy (AFM) to measure alveolar septal wall stiffness in decellularized rat lung tissue and found that indentation stiffness increased from about 10 kPa at 0 strain to about 80 kPa at 0.3 strain (Jorba et al., 2019). While the mechanism underlying this non-linear behavior remains unclear, one possibility is that it reflects the progressive straightening of flaccid fibers (Sobin et al., 1988; Mercer and Crapo, 1990; Toshima et al., 2004). Elastin fibers are generally presumed not to be flaccid under any conditions, so the flaccid fibers are probably collagen (Mercer and Crapo, 1990; Chen et al., 2013; Chow et al., 2014). Another possible explanation for the AFM results is geometric; the opposing force on a probe pushing perpendicular to a fiber under tension is due to the vector component of the tension in the fiber that is generated against the probe as the fiber bends. It is also possible that the stress-strain behavior of the fiber itself is actually non-linear. This behavior could be incorporated into the model at the expense of increased model complexity. As an example, the elastic moduli could be modeled using a polynomial equation to capture waviness or fiber stiffening. Even though this additional complexity might not have an analytical solution and thus would need to be solved numerically, the same geometrical considerations and energy minimization principles still hold and are applicable. Thus, in relation to the present study, it must be noted that the modulus parameters estimated by the analytical model represent averages of the tensile and bond-bending moduli of a large population of alveolar walls.

The analytical model also assumes affine kinematics, meaning that microstrains occurring in small parcels of tissue mirror the macrostrains of the tissue as a whole. This does not, however, apply to individual alveolar walls, which move according to their respective initial orientations. These orientations vary widely throughout the tissue, as they do in the numerical network model (Cavalcante et al., 2005), and also as found experimentally; alveolar wall segments violate the affine deformation assumption during uniaxial stretching (Brewer et al., 2003).

In summary, we have developed an analytical model that establishes a link between the mechanical behavior of lung tissue at the macroscopic tissue level and alveolar wall scale. Matching the model predictions to experimental data provides realistic values for the tensile and bond-bending moduli of individual alveolar walls, as well as their changes with age, collagen content, and matrix charge density. The model thus provides a potential platform upon which to understand how disease processes and aging affect lung function, and how interventions such as mechanical ventilation might be optimized to avoid damaging the tissue or avoid aberrant mechanotransduction of the cells contained within it.

AUTHOR CONTRIBUTIONS

SB, BS, and JB contributed to model development. AT collected data for the young and old mouse study. SB contributed to forward simulations and experimental data fitting. SB and BS contributed to data analysis. SB, BS, and JB contributed to writing the manuscript. All authors approved the submitted manuscript.

ACKNOWLEDGMENTS

The authors are also grateful to Dr. Xingbin Ai for providing isolated lungs from aged mice.

REFERENCES

Aaron, B. B., and Gosline, J. M. (1981). Elastin as a random-network elastomer: a mechanical and optical analysis of single elastin fibers. *Biopolymers* 20, 1247–1260. doi: 10.1002/bip.1981.360200611

Bachofen, H., and Schürch, S. (2001). Alveolar surface forces and lung architecture. *Comp. Biochem. Physiol. Part A Mol. Integr. Physiol.* 129, 183–193. doi: 10.1016/S1095-6433(01)00315-4

Brewer, K. K., Sakai, H., Alencar, A. M., Majumdar, A., Arold, S. P., Lutchen, K. R., et al. (2003). Lung and alveolar wall elastic and hysteretic behavior in rats: effects of *in vivo* elastase treatment. *J. Appl. Physiol.* 95, 1926–1936. doi: 10.1152/japplphysiol.00102.2003

Cavalcante, F. S. A., Ito, S., Brewer, K., Sakai, H., Alencar, A. M., Almeida, M. P., et al. (2005). Mechanical interactions between collagen and proteoglycans: implications for the stability of lung tissue. *J. Appl. Physiol.* 98, 672–679. doi: 10.1152/japplphysiol.00619.2004

Chalmers, G. W., Gosline, J. M., and Lillie, M. A. (1999). The hydrophobicity of vertebrate elastins. *J. Exp. Biol.* 202, 301–314.

Chen, H., Slipchenko, M. N., Liu, Y., Zhao, X., Cheng, J.-X., Lanir, Y., et al. (2013). Biaxial deformation of collagen and elastin fibers in coronary adventitia. *J. Appl. Physiol.* 115, 1683–1693. doi: 10.1152/japplphysiol.00601.2013

Chow, M.-J., Turcotte, R., Lin, C. P., and Zhang, Y. (2014). Arterial extracellular matrix: a mechanobiological study of the contributions and interactions of elastin and collagen. *Biophys. J.* 106, 2684–2692. doi: 10.1016/j.bpj.2014.05.014

Decraemer, W. F., Maes, M. A., and Vanhuyse, V. J. (1980). An elastic stress-strain relation for soft biological tissues based on a structural model. *J. Biomech.* 13, 463–468. doi: 10.1016/0021-9290(80)90338-3

Denny, E., and Schroter, R. C. (2006). A model of non-uniform lung parenchyma distortion. *J. Biomech.* 39, 652–663. doi: 10.1016/j.jbiomech.2005.01.010

Fung, Y. C. (1984). Structure and stress-strain relationship of soft tissues. *Am. Zool.* 24, 13–22. doi: 10.1093/icb/24.1.13

Huang, K., Mitzner, W., Rabold, R., Schofield, B., Lee, H., Biswal, S., et al. (2007). Variation in senescent-dependent lung changes in inbred mouse strains. *J. Appl. Physiol.* 102, 1632–1639. doi: 10.1152/japplphysiol.00833.2006

Jorba, I., Beltrán, G., Falcones, B., Suki, B., Farré, R., García-Aznar, J. M., et al. (2019). Nonlinear elasticity of the lung extracellular microenvironment is regulated by macroscale tissue strain. *Acta Biomater.* 92, 265–276. doi: 10.1016/j.actbio.2019.05.023

Karlinsky, J. B. (1992). Stress-strain characteristics of normal and emphysematous hamster lung strips. *Respir. Physiol.* 90, 251–260. doi: 10.1016/0034-5687(92)90106-7

Knudson, R. J., Clark, D. F., Kennedy, T. C., and Knudson, D. E. (1977). Effect of aging alone on mechanical properties of the normal adult human lung. *J. Appl. Physiol.* 43, 1054–1062. doi: 10.1152/jappl.1977.43.6.1054

Kohn, J. C., Lampi, M. C., and Reinhart-King, C. A. (2015). Age-related vascular stiffening: causes and consequences. *Front. Genet.* 6:112. doi: 10.3389/fgene.2015.00112

Lanir, Y. (1979). A structural theory for the homogeneous biaxial stress-strain relationships in flat collagenous tissues. *J. Biomech.* 12, 423–436. doi: 10.1016/0021-9290(79)90027-7

Liao, H., and Belkoff, S. M. (1999). A failure model for ligaments. *J. Biomech.* 32, 183–188. doi: 10.1016/S0021-9290(98)00169-9

Liu, F., and Tschumperlin, D. J. (2011). Micro-mechanical characterization of lung tissue using atomic force microscopy. *J. Vis. Exp.* e2911. doi: 10.3791/2911

Maina, J. N., and West, J. B. (2005). Thin and strong! The bioengineering dilemma in the structural and functional design of the blood-gas barrier. *Physiol. Rev.* 85, 811–844. doi: 10.1152/physrev.00022.2004

Maksym, G. N., and Bates, J. H. T. (1997). A distributed nonlinear model of lung tissue elasticity. *J. Appl. Physiol.* 82, 32–41. doi: 10.1152/jappl.1997.82.1.32

Maksym, G. N., Fredberg, J. J., and Bates, J. H. T. (1998). Force heterogeneity in a two-dimensional network model of lung tissue elasticity. *J. Appl. Physiol.* 85, 1223–1229. doi: 10.1152/jappl.1998.85.4.1223

Maroudas, A., and Bannon, C. (1981). Measurement of swelling pressure in cartilage and comparison with the osmotic pressure of constituent proteoglycans. *Biorheology* 18, 619–632. doi: 10.3233/BIR-1981-183-624

Mead, J. (1961). Mechanical properties of lungs. *Physiol. Rev.* 41, 281–330. doi: 10.1152/physrev.1961.41.2.281

Mercer, R. R., and Crapo, J. D. (1990). Spatial distribution of collagen and elastin fibers in the lungs. *J. Appl. Physiol.* 69, 756–765. doi: 10.1152/jappl.1990.69.2.756

Panwar, P., Lamour, G., Mackenzie, N. C. W., Yang, H., Ko, F., Li, H., et al. (2015). Changes in structural-mechanical properties and degradability of collagen during aging-associated modifications. *J. Biol. Chem.* 290, 23291–23306. doi: 10.1074/jbc.M115.644310

Parameswaran, H., Majumdar, A., and Suki, B. (2011). Linking microscopic spatial patterns of tissue destruction in emphysema to macroscopic decline in stiffness using a 3D computational model. *PLoS Comput. Biol.* 7:e1001125. doi: 10.1371/journal.pcbi.1001125

Pidaparti, R. M., Burnette, M., Heise, R. L., and Reynolds, A. (2013). Analysis for stress environment in the alveolar sac model. *J. Biomed. Sci. Eng.* 6, 901–907. doi: 10.4236/jbise.2013.69110

Pinart, M., Faffe, D. S., Sapiña, M. G., and Romero, P. V. C. (2011). Dynamic nonlinearity of lung tissue: effects of strain amplitude and stress level. *J. Appl. Physiol.* 110, 653–660. doi: 10.1152/japplphysiol.01115.2010

Polio, S. R., Kundu, A. N., Dougan, C. E., Birch, N. P., Aurian-Blajeni, D. E., Schiffman, J. D., et al. (2018). Cross-platform mechanical characterization of lung tissue. *PLoS ONE* 13:e0204765. doi: 10.1371/journal.pone.0204765

Reiser, K. M., Hennessy, S. M., and Last, J. A. (1987). Analysis of age-associated changes in collagen crosslinking in the skin and lung in monkeys and rats. *Biochim. Biophys. Acta.* 926, 339–348. doi: 10.1016/0304-4165(87)90220-0

Ritter, M. C., Jesudason, R., Majumdar, A., Stamenovic, D., Buczek-Thomas, J. A., Stone, P. J., et al. (2009). A zipper network model of the failure mechanics of extracellular matrices. *Proc. Natl. Acad. Sci. U.S.A.* 106, 1081–1086. doi: 10.1073/pnas.0808414106

Romero, F. J., Pastor, A., Lopez, J., and Romero, P. V. (1998). A recruitment-based rheological model for mechanical behavior of soft tissues. *Biorheology* 35, 17–35. doi: 10.1016/S0006-355X(98)00015-8

Sacks, M. S. (2003). Incorporation of experimentally-derived fiber orientation into a structural constitutive model for planar collagenous tissues. *J. Biomech. Eng.* 125, 280–287. doi: 10.1115/1.1544508

Shiwen, X., Stratton, R., Nikitorowicz-Buniak, J., Ahmed-Abdi, B., Ponticos, M., Denton, C., et al. (2015). A role of Myocardin Related Transcription Factor-A (MRTF-A) in scleroderma related fibrosis. *PLoS ONE* 10:e0126015. doi: 10.1371/journal.pone.0126015

Snedeker, J. G., and Gautieri, A. (2014). The role of collagen crosslinks in ageing and diabetes - the good, the bad, and the ugly. *Muscles Ligaments Tendons J.* 4, 303–308. doi: 10.32098/mltj.03.2014.07

Sobin, S. S., Fung, Y. C., and Tremer, H. M. (1988). Collagen and elastin fibers in human pulmonary alveolar walls. *J. Appl. Physiol.* 64, 1659–1675. doi: 10.1152/jappl.1988.64.4.1659

Suki, B., and Bartolák-Suki, E. (2015). "Biomechanics of the aging lung parenchyma," in *Mechanical Properties of Aging Soft Tissues*, eds B. Derby and R. Akhtar (Cham: Springer International Publishing), 95–133.

Suki, B., and Bates, J. H. T. (2011). Lung tissue mechanics as an emergent phenomenon. *J. Appl. Physiol.* (1985) 110, 1111–1118. doi: 10.1152/japplphysiol.01244.2010

Suki, B., Ito, S., Stamenović, D., Lutchen, K. R., and Ingenito, E. P. (2005). Biomechanics of the lung parenchyma: critical roles of collagen and mechanical forces. *J. Appl. Physiol.* 98, 1892–1899. doi: 10.1152/japplphysiol.01087.2004

Takahashi, A., Majumdar, A., Parameswaran, H., Bartolák-Suki, E., and Suki, B. (2014). Proteoglycans maintain lung stability in an elastase-treated mouse model of emphysema. *Am. J. Respir. Cell Mol. Biol.* 51, 26–33. doi: 10.1165/rcmb.2013-0179OC

Thurlbeck, W. M. (1967). The internal surface area of nonemphysematous lungs. *Am. Rev. Respir. Dis.* 95, 765–773.

Toshima, M., Ohtani, Y., and Ohtani, O. (2004). Three-dimensional architecture of elastin and collagen fiber networks in the human and rat lung. *Arch. Histol. Cytol.* 67, 31–40. doi: 10.1679/aohc.67.31

Weibel, E. R. (2009). What makes a good lung? *Swiss Med Wkly*, 139, 375–86.

Wilson, T. A., and Bachofen, H. (1982). A model for mechanical structure of the alveolar duct. *J. Appl. Physiol.* 52, 1064–1070. doi: 10.1152/jappl.1982.52.4.1064

Wuyts, F. L., Vanhuyse, V. J., Langewouters, G. J., Decraemer, W. F., Raman, E. R., and Buyle, S. (1995). Elastic properties of human aortas in relation to age and atherosclerosis: a structural model. *Phys. Med. Biol.* 40, 1577–1597. doi: 10.1088/0031-9155/40/10/002

Yi, E., Sato, S., Takahashi, A., Parameswaran, H., Blute, T. A., Bartolák-Suki, E., et al. (2016). Mechanical forces accelerate collagen digestion by bacterial collagenase in lung tissue strips. *Front Physiol* 7:287. doi: 10.3389/fphys.2016.00287

Yuan, H., Kononov, S., Cavalcante, F. S. A., Lutchen, K. R., Ingenito, E. P., and Suki, B. (2000). Effects of collagenase and elastase on the mechanical properties of lung tissue strips. *J. Appl. Physiol.* 89, 3–14. doi: 10.1152/jappl.2000.89.1.3

3

Three Alveolar Phenotypes Govern Lung Function in Murine Ventilator-Induced Lung Injury

Bradford J. Smith[1,2]*, Gregory S. Roy[3], Alyx Cleveland[3], Courtney Mattson[1], Kayo Okamura[1], Chantel M. Charlebois[3], Katharine L. Hamlington[2], Michael V. Novotny[4], Lars Knudsen[5,6], Matthias Ochs[7], R. Duncan Hite[4,8] and Jason H. T. Bates[3]

[1] Department of Bioengineering, College of Engineering, Design & Computing, University of Colorado Denver | Anschutz Medical Campus, Aurora, CO, United States, [2] Department of Pediatric Pulmonary and Sleep Medicine, School of Medicine, University of Colorado Anschutz Medical Campus, Aurora, CO, United States, [3] Vermont Lung Center, Larner College of Medicine, The University of Vermont, Burlington, VT, United States, [4] Lerner Research Institute, Cleveland Clinic, Cleveland, OH, United States, [5] Institute of Functional and Applied Anatomy, Hannover Medical School, Hanover, Germany, [6] Biomedical Research in Endstage and Obstructive Lung Disease Hannover (BREATH), Member of the German Center for Lung Research, Hanover, Germany, [7] Institute of Functional Anatomy, Charité Medical University of Berlin, Berlin, Germany, [8] Division of Pulmonary, Critical Care and Sleep Medicine, Department of Internal Medicine, College of Medicine, University of Cincinnati, Cincinnati, OH, United States

***Correspondence:**
Bradford J. Smith
Bradford.Smith@cuanschutz.edu

Mechanical ventilation is an essential lifesaving therapy in acute respiratory distress syndrome (ARDS) that may cause ventilator-induced lung injury (VILI) through a positive feedback between altered alveolar mechanics, edema, surfactant inactivation, and injury. Although the biophysical forces that cause VILI are well documented, a knowledge gap remains in the quantitative link between altered parenchymal structure (namely alveolar derecruitment and flooding), pulmonary function, and VILI. This information is essential to developing diagnostic criteria and ventilation strategies to reduce VILI and improve ARDS survival. To address this unmet need, we mechanically ventilated mice to cause VILI. Lung structure was measured at three air inflation pressures using design-based stereology, and the mechanical function of the pulmonary system was measured with the forced oscillation technique. Assessment of the pulmonary surfactant included total surfactant, distribution of phospholipid aggregates, and surface tension lowering activity. VILI-induced changes in the surfactant included reduced surface tension lowering activity in the typically functional fraction of large phospholipid aggregates and a significant increase in the pool of surface-inactive small phospholipid aggregates. The dominant alterations in lung structure at low airway pressures were alveolar collapse and flooding. At higher airway pressures, alveolar collapse was mitigated and the flooded alveoli remained filled with proteinaceous edema. The loss of ventilated alveoli resulted in decreased alveolar gas volume and gas-exchange surface area. These data characterize three alveolar phenotypes in murine VILI: flooded and non-recruitable alveoli, unstable alveoli that derecruit at airway pressures below 5 cmH_2O, and alveoli with relatively normal structure and function. The fraction of alveoli with each phenotype is reflected in the proportional changes in pulmonary system elastance at positive end expiratory pressures of 0, 3, and 6 cmH_2O.

Keywords: ventilator-induced lung injury, stereology, pulmonary surfactant, lung function, alveolar mechanics

INTRODUCTION

Mechanical ventilation is required for major surgery and resuscitation and in critical emergencies such as acute respiratory distress syndrome (ARDS) (Force et al., 2012), but this lifesaving therapy carries the risk of ventilator-induced lung injury (VILI). The mechanisms of VILI are well documented and include direct tissue injury from overdistension (volutrauma) (Webb and Tierney, 1974; Hernandez et al., 1989) and the cyclic collapse and reopening of small airways and alveoli (atelectrauma) (Muscedere et al., 1994). These injurious forces act at the microscale to damage the epithelial and endothelial cells that comprise the blood-gas barrier (Dreyfuss and Saumon, 1998; Hamlington et al., 2018b), allowing the ingress of proteinaceous edema into the distal airspace that is associated with changes in lung mechanics (Hamlington et al., 2016a).

Changes in the lung structure–function relationship during VILI are currently understood through the lens of organ-scale imaging techniques such as CT (Yen et al., 2019). However, the positive feedback mechanism between leak, surfactant function, altered mechanics, and injury occurs at the alveolar and acinar scales (Knudsen et al., 2018). As such, measurements of morphometry are necessary to bridge studies of cellular injury and alveolocapillary barrier disruption (Hamlington et al., 2018a) to organ-scale measurements of structure and function. Understanding how these mechanisms are associated across length scales is critical for developing approaches to mitigating them. Structure-function correlations may also improve clinical practice by defining the mechanistic basis for diagnostic parameters such as the driving pressure (Aoyama et al., 2018; Pereira Romano et al., 2020) and subject-specific computational models (Hamlington et al., 2016b; Mellenthin et al., 2019; Morton et al., 2019) that seek to optimize ventilation based on patient-specific alveolar mechanics.

To address this knowledge gap, we used design-based stereology to measure parenchymal structure over a range of air inflation pressures in a mouse model of VILI. The state of the pulmonary surfactant system was assessed by measuring minimum surface tension and surfactant composition. Organ-scale mechanical function was determined with the forced oscillation technique (FOT) to quantify stiffness, airway resistance, and tissue damping at different levels of lung inflation. Together, these data define the structure–function relationship in murine VILI.

MATERIALS AND METHODS

Animal Procedures

Eight to ten week old female BALB/c mice (Jackson Laboratories, Bar Harbor, ME, United States) weighing 17.1–22.3 g were studied under Institutional Animal Care and Use Committee (IACUC)-approved protocols. Mice were anesthetized with an intraperitoneal (IP) injection of 100 mg/kg ketamine and 16 mg/kg xylazine, tracheostomized with a 18 ga metal cannula, and ventilated using a flexiVent small animal ventilator (SCIREQ, Montreal, QC, Canada). Respiratory drive was suppressed *via* 0.8 mg/kg pancuronium bromide administered at the onset of mechanical ventilation. Alternating doses of 50 mg/kg ketamine and 50 mg/kg ketamine with 8 mg/kg xylazine were administered at 30-min intervals with 150 μL IP 5% dextrose lactated Ringer's solution. Fluid volume from the anesthetic was 10 μL/g. The electrocardiogram was monitored to assure that the rodents maintained a deep plane of anesthesia during paralysis.

Mechanical ventilation experiments to generate tissue for structural analysis were conducted at the University of Vermont and approved by the University of Vermont Institutional Animal Care and Use Committee (IACUC #14-056). Bronchoalveolar lavage fluid for surfactant analysis was collected under identical ventilation conditions by the same investigator at the University of Colorado Denver in experiments approved by the University of Colorado Denver Anschutz Medical Campus, IACUC (#00230).

Ventilation Protocol

All animals were ventilated for a 10-min stabilization period with a delivered tidal volume (Vt) = 10 ml/kg at a respiratory rate (RR) = 200 breaths/min and a positive end expiratory pressure (PEEP) = 3 cmH_2O (baseline ventilation). Recruitment maneuvers (RM) consisting of a 3 sec ramp to 30 cmH_2O followed by a 3 sec breath hold were applied to reopen regions that may have collapsed during the surgical procedure. Following the stabilization period, lung function was assessed. Testing consisted of an RM and a dynamic pressure-volume (PV) loop that ramped airway pressure (Paw) from 0 to 37.5 cmH_2O, held pressure for 3 sec, and ramped pressure back to zero over 3 sec. Derecruitability tests were then performed at PEEP = 6, 3, and 0 cmH_2O, denoted by D_{rec}^{PEEP6}, D_{rec}^{PEEP3}, and D_{rec}^{PEEP0}. Each test consisted of an RM and then Vt = 10 ml/kg and RR = 200 breaths/min at the specified PEEP. Nine multi-frequency FOT impedance measurements were recorded at 18 s intervals and fit to the constant phase model (Hantos et al., 1992) to determine respiratory system elastance (H), tissue damping (G), and Newtonian resistance (Rn). The total duration of the lung function assessment was 13 min. Lungs from the control group were then harvested for morphometric analysis. In a separate sub-group of animals, bronchoalveolar lavage fluid (BALF) was collected for surfactant analysis.

The VILI group was then subjected to repeated blocks of ventilation consisting of 4 min 45 s of injurious ventilation with a plateau pressure (Pplat) = 37.5 cmH_2O, RR = 50 breaths/min, inspiratory:expiratory ratio of 1:2, and PEEP = 0 cmH_2O. This Pplat was selected to generate severe VILI in an experimentally tractable timeframe without causing any pneumothoraces. At the end of each block a PV loop was recorded followed by two FOT measurements separated by 10 s of baseline ventilation. These 5-min ventilation blocks were applied until H doubled, at which point the lung function assessment was repeated prior to harvest for either morphometry or surfactant analysis. The mean duration of injurious mechanical ventilation was 87.3 min with a standard deviation of 17.5 min. Including with the 10 min stabilization period and two 13 min lung function assessments, the mean duration of ventilation for the VILI group was 123.3 min.

Surfactant Analysis

Bronchoalveolar lavage fluid was collected by instilling and suctioning back 1 ml warm normal saline three times and then centrifuging at 700 *g* at 4°C for 5 min. A total of 100 μl of the cell-free supernatant for each animal was separated, and the remainder of the BALF from three mice in the same treatment group was combined and centrifuged at 40,000 *g*. The ultracentrifuged supernatant containing the surfactant small aggregate (SA) was stored at −80°C for later analysis. The surfactant pellet, containing the large aggregate (LA) fraction, was washed twice by resuspending the pellet in 1 ml saline and centrifuging at 40,000 *g*. Finally, the LA pellet was resuspended in 100 μl saline and stored at −80°C for later analysis.

Quantitation of the surfactant recovered from the BAL was completed by measuring lipid phosphorous content in the LA and SA fractions as previously described (Rouser et al., 1970). Total surfactant recovery represents the combined amount of both fractions. Total BAL protein was quantified with a BCA assay (ThermoShandon-Pierce). Surfactant surface lowering activity was assessed by measuring minimal surface tension of the LA fraction *ex vivo* using a pulsating bubble surfactometer (General Transco) as described (Enhorning and Holm, 1993; Hite et al., 2005). Surfactant was preheated to 37°C at 2 mg (PL from LA)/ml in 150 mM NaCl, 5 mM $CaCl_2$, 5 mM Tris solution, and the samples were pulsated at 20 pulses/min for 20 min.

Lung Tissue Preparation

Lung structure was analyzed in a separate subgroup of mice that were not subjected to a bronchoalveolar lavage. The lungs were fixed through the vasculature while the air inflation pressure was held at a prescribed level (described below) to maintain surface tension effects and allow comparison to the lung function data (Gil et al., 1979; Bachofen et al., 1982). The fixation process was initiated during baseline ventilation by performing a bilateral thoracotomy and flushing the pulmonary circulation with 5 ml 100 U/ml heparinized saline with 3% 100 kDa dextran at a pressure of 25 cmH_2O. Three RMs were applied and then Paw increased to 30 cmH_2O over 3 s, held for 3 s, decreased to either 2, 5, or 10 cmH_2O, and the trachea was ligated. These pressures were selected based on our previous morphometric analysis of bleomycin-injured rats (Knudsen et al., 2018) where nearly all recruitable alveoli were open at Paw = 10 cmH_2O and approximately half the recruitable alveoli were closed at Paw = 5 cmH_2O. The lower limit of Paw = 2 cmH_2O was selected since PEEPs < 2 cmH_2O are not typically applied in lung-protective ventilation. Five animals were prepared at each airway pressure for the control and VILI groups. The lungs were then perfused with 1.5% glutaraldehyde, 1.5% paraformaldehyde in 0.15 M HEPES buffer for approximately 5 min before immersion fixation for at least 24 h.

Tissue processing and sampling was conducted using standardized protocols (Mühlfeld et al., 2013; Knudsen et al., 2018). Briefly, non-pulmonary tissue was removed, and the total lung volume determined using Archimedes principle. The first step of systematic uniform random sampling was conducted by cutting the lungs into 1.5 mm transverse sections and retaining either even or odd numbered slabs. The slabs were post-fixed with 1% OsO_4 in 0.1 M cacodylate buffer for 2 h and then overnight in half saturated aqueous uranyl acetate, dehydrated in a graded acetone series, and embedded in glycol methacrylate (Technovit 7100, Heraeus Kulzer, Wehrheim, Germany) to avoid tissue shrinkage (Schneider and Ochs, 2014). The first and fourth 1.5 μm sections from a consecutive series were mounted and stained with orcein and then used with the physical disector stereology probe to estimate alveolar number. Another 1.5 μm section was stained with toluidine blue to estimate volumes and surface areas.

Design-Based Stereology

The stereological analysis was conducted according to standards for lung structure quantification (Hsia et al., 2010). A majority of the systematic uniform random sampling and image acquisition was conducted using a Zeiss Axioscope II with a Ziess Axiocam AR camera (Zeiss, Thornwood, NY, United States) controlled with the Stereo Investigator software package (MBF Bioscience, Williston, VT, United States). Approximately 10% of the images (distributed randomly across groups and subjects) were recorded using an Olympus BX53 with a DP73 camera (Olympus, Waltham, MA, United States) controlled with the NewCast stereology software (Visiopharm, Hørsholm, Denmark). Stereological quantification of all images was performed using a custom MATLAB (Mathworks, Natick, MA, United States) graphical user interface.

A cascade sampling design was used starting with the volume fraction of parenchyma in the whole lung [Vv(par/lung)] that we define as areas contributing to gas exchange and excluding airways, vessels outside the septal walls, and peribronchiolar tissue. This, and all volume fractions, were measured using point counting. The percentage of the tissue section analyzed (the sampling fraction, S_F) for Vv(par/lung) was 100% at 5× magnification. The parenchyma was then subdivided into volume fractions of alveolar airspace [Vv(alvair/par)], alveolar duct airspace [Vv(ductair/par)], and non-air material [Vv(non-air/par)] that include tissue and airspace edema fluid. This assessment was performed at 20× magnification and S_F = 11%. Fields of view were selected for analysis using systematic uniform random sampling whereby the morphometry software selected a random starting location and images were then automatically sampled on a 1,200 × 1,200 μm grid over the entire tissue section. This approach blinds the investigator to the selection of the images used for analysis, thus removing the potential for bias. The non-air material in the parenchyma [Vv(non-air/par)] was then analyzed at 40× magnification (S_F = 2.8%, 1,200 μm grid spacing) to determine the volume fractions of septal tissue of patent alveoli [Vv(sep,air/par], total septal tissue [Vv(sep,total/par)], and airspace edema [Vv(edema/par)]. The volume of each compartment (demarcated with V in place of Vv) was determined by multiplying the volume fractions by the volume of the reference space. The surface area per volume available for gas exchange [Sv(alvair/par)] was estimated at 40× magnification (S_F = 2.8%, 1,200 μm grid spacing) by counting line intersections with aerated septal tissue that was not covered with alveolar edema. The gas exchange surface area

[S(alvair)] was determined by multiplying Sv(alvair/par) by the parenchymal volume [V(par)] and the mean septal thickness defined as $\tau(sep) = 2\ V(sep,air)/S(alvair)$. The physical disector method (Ochs et al., 2004) was used to determine the number of patent [N(alv)] and flooded [N(flood)] alveoli that we define as alveoli with visible architecture and alveolar edema fully blocking the alveolar mouth using 40× magnification (S_F = 6.25%, 800 μm grid spacing). The total number of alveoli is then N(alv,total) = N(alv) + N(flood), the number-weighted average alveolar volume V_n(alv) = V(alvair)/N(alv), and the alveolar surface area to volume ratio S/V(alv) = S(alvair)/V(alvair).

Statistical Analysis

Data were curated in MATLAB and statistical analysis was performed in R (The R Foundation). A Shapiro-Wilk test was used to assess normality. If the data were not significantly different from the normal distribution ($p > 0.05$) then an ANOVA was performed followed by pairwise comparisons using the lsmeans package (Lenth, 2016) and Tukey's adjustment for multiple comparisons. Data that failed the normality test was analyzed with a Kruskal-Wallis test followed by a rank-sum Conover–Iman test (PMCMR package) with the Holm correction for multiple comparisons.

The time series of lung function parameters H, G, and Rn measured during the derecruitability tests were analyzed using a linear mixed effects model (LME) (NLME package in R) on the natural logarithm of the time and parameter values. This is equivalent to fitting the equation $y = \alpha\ t^{\beta}$ to the time series of measurements as we have previously described (Smith et al., 2017). Fixed effects were derecruitability test PEEP (D_{rec}^{PEEP}), the time within the derecruitability test (*t*), and whether the measurement was recorded before or after VILI (*Injury*). The intercept for each animal was included as a random effect and the Akaike information criterion (AIC) was used to determine the most appropriate model. Temporal autocorrelation was accounted for with a first-order autocorrelation structure for the continuous time covariate grouped by animal, derecruitability test PEEP, and injury status (Pinheiro and Bates, 2000).

RESULTS

Pulmonary system elastance following an RM in the uninjured lungs (**Figure 1**, first row) was significantly different between the derecruitability tests at different PEEP levels, while the rate of change of H over time (the slope) remained consistent between PEEPs (**Table 1**). VILI (**Figure 1**, second row) increased the H intercept at all PEEPs with a proportionally greater increase occurring in D_{rec}^{PEEP0} where the elastance at the start of the derecruitability test was approximately doubled. The rate of elastance increase over time was also elevated in D_{rec}^{PEEP0} and, to a lesser extent, in D_{rec}^{PEEP3}. Tissue damping (G) increased monotonically with PEEP prior to injury (**Figure 2**, first row) and was independent of *t* (**Table 2**). Following VILI, G demonstrated a marked increase in D_{rec}^{PEEP0} that was similar in magnitude to the change in H. Central airway resistance (Rn) tended to decrease with PEEP (**Figure 3**) in both healthy and injured lung. Following VILI, Rn was slightly increased in D_{rec}^{PEEP0} and decreased in D_{rec}^{PEEP6}. The temporal dependence of Rn was not affected by VILI (**Table 2**).

The changes in lung function are associated with structural alterations in the perfusion-fixed lung tissue. Alveoli in the Control lungs (**Figure 4**, first row) remained patent from Paw = 10 cmH_2O (right column) down to airway pressures of 2 cmH_2O (left column). Note that these airway pressures are applied in open-chested mice, and the contributions of the chest wall are discussed below. By contrast, the VILI lungs exhibited diffuse alveolar edema (second row, asterisks) and retraction of the alveolar septa (second row, arrows) at Paw = 5 and 10 cmH_2O. At Paw = 2 cmH_2O, the injured parenchyma tended to consolidate into patches of flooded and collapsed alveoli with air remaining in the ductal space. These injured regions were interspersed between areas of parenchyma that appeared normal.

Quantitative structural changes with VILI included a significant decrease in V(alvair) (**Figure 5A**) in conjunction with reduced N(alv) (**Figure 6B**). The average alveolar volume [V_n(alv)] is defined as the ratio of these two quantities and indicates a modest stiffening of patent alveoli with injury (**Figure 6E**). By contrast, V(ductair) did not demonstrate significant alterations in VILI (**Figure 5B**), leading to a fractional shift of ventilation volume from the alveoli to the alveolar ducts with VILI (**Figure 5C**) that was significant at all airway pressures. The surface area available for gas exchange (**Figure 5D**) was significantly reduced across all airway pressures in VILI. This reduction is primarily due to a loss of ventilated alveoli and not to reduced surface area to volume ratio in the remaining patent units as indicated by increased S/V(alv) when comparing control and VILI at Paw = 2 cmH_2O (**Figure 6F**, lines). For comparison, **Figure 6F** shows the hypothetical surface area to volume ratios for perfectly spherical alveoli (symbols), and these values are less than those measured *in vivo* despite the reduction in area caused by the alveolar mouth. The increase in S/V(alv) at low Paw in VILI suggests that the alveolar geometry becomes more distorted in the injured lung. Injurious ventilation did not change V(sep, total) (**Figure 5E**) or τ(sep), and although septal thickness tended to increase with decreasing Paw there were no significant alterations (**Figure 6A**). Little to no airspace edema was observed in the control animals (**Figure 5F**), and V(edema) was constant across inflation pressures in VILI.

The number of ventilated alveoli [N(alv), **Figure 6B**] remained constant across inflation pressures in the Control animals, indicating an absence of derecruitment even at Paw = 2 cmH_2O. The VILI mice demonstrated a constant N(alv) at Paw = 5 and 10 cmH_2O that was significantly less than in the Controls. Reducing the inflation pressure to 2 cmH_2O in the VILI animals led to a significant reduction in aerated alveoli. Flooded alveoli [N(flood), **Figure 6C**] were defined as having a liquid meniscus fully spanning the alveolar mouth. N(flood) remained constant across inflation pressures in the VILI group, and no flooded alveoli were observed across the 15 control lungs analyzed (**Table 3**). **Figure 6D** shows that the total number of flooded and aerated alveoli [N(alv,total)] is consistent across all

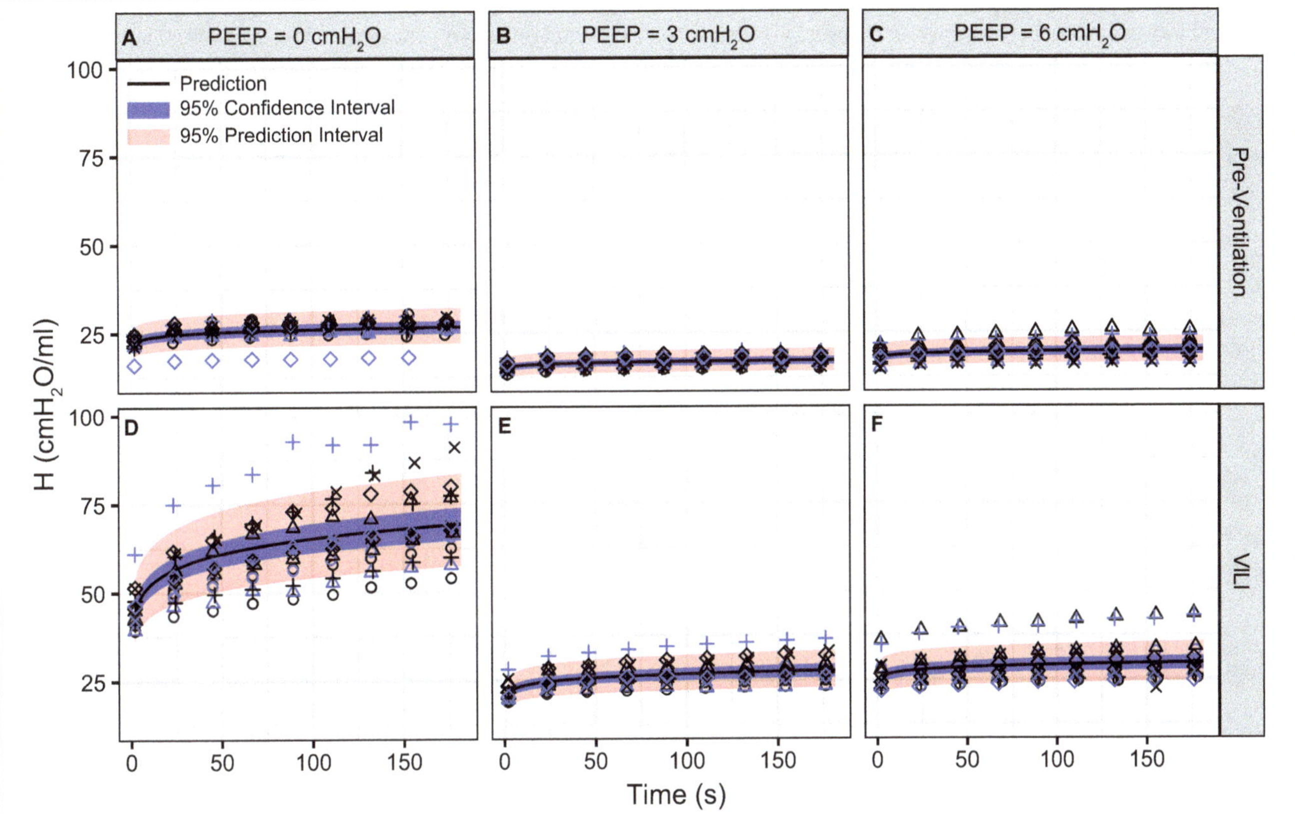

FIGURE 1 | Pulmonary system elastance (H) measured during derecruitability tests at PEEP = 0 **(A,D)**, 3 **(B,E)**, and 6 cmH$_2$O **(C,F)** before **(A–C)** and after injurious mechanical ventilation **(D–F)**. The LME model fit is shown with a black line, the 95% confidence interval is shown with a blue band, and the 95% prediction interval is shown with a red band. Symbols depict raw data for each animal and are consistent between **Figures 1–3**. Fifteen mice are in each group.

TABLE 1 | Pairwise comparison of the LME model using log-transformed lung function parameters, which is equivalent to fitting the equation $y = \alpha\, t^{\beta}$ to the raw data.

Pairwise comparison	Slope			Intercept		
	H	G	Rn	H	G	Rn
D_{rec}^{PEEP0} (Pre) – D_{rec}^{PEEP3} (Pre)	−0.012	0.002	−0.016	0.68	1.25	0.61
D_{rec}^{PEEP0} (Pre) – D_{rec}^{PEEP6} (Pre)	−0.013	0.001	−0.032	0.79	1.78	0.52
D_{rec}^{PEEP3} (Pre) – D_{rec}^{PEEP6} (Pre)	−0.001	−0.001	−0.016	1.17	1.42	0.85
D_{rec}^{PEEP0} (Pre) – D_{rec}^{PEEP0} (Post)	0.060	0.115	0.008	1.90	2.17	1.15
D_{rec}^{PEEP3} (Pre) – D_{rec}^{PEEP3} (Post)	0.029	0.022	0.009	1.40	1.06	0.97
D_{rec}^{PEEP6} (Pre) – D_{rec}^{PEEP6} (Post)	0.008	−0.018	−0.002	1.44	1.16	0.86
D_{rec}^{PEEP0} (Post) – D_{rec}^{PEEP3} (Post)	−0.042	−0.090	−0.013	0.50	0.61	0.51
D_{rec}^{PEEP0} (Post) – D_{rec}^{PEEP6} (Post)	−0.065	−0.090	−0.041	0.60	0.95	0.38
D_{rec}^{PEEP3} (Post) – D_{rec}^{PEEP6} (Post)	−0.022	−0.005	−0.028	1.21	1.55	0.75

The numeric values for slope indicate the change in β from the left-hand to the right-hand derecruitability test listed under "Pairwise Comparison." The numeric values provided for the intercepts indicate the fold change in the raw (not log transformed) intercept α. Gray cells indicate $p < 0.05$. Fifteen mice are in each group.

groups except at Paw = 2 cmH$_2$O where there is a striking decrease with VILI.

Figure 7 shows the pairwise relationships between the last elastance measurement in D_{rec}^{PEEP0}, D_{rec}^{PEEP3}, and D_{rec}^{PEEP6} and N(alv) at Paw = 2, 5, and 10 cmH$_2$O. Note that the mean pressure of the derecruitability tests is approximately 2–3 cmH$_2$O greater than the onset pressures so that the mechanics and structure are measured at roughly the same pressure. Elastance is strongly correlated with the number of patent alveoli (R^2 = 0.78), and the form of the regression was selected based on our prior computational simulations where elastance increases with the inverse of the lung open fraction (Smith et al., 2013, 2015; Hamlington et al., 2016b; Mellenthin et al., 2019).

The changes in lung structure and function are accompanied by alterations in the pulmonary surfactant system. BALF total phospholipid (PL) content (**Figure 8A**) significantly increased

TABLE 2 | Results from regression analysis predicting log-transformed H, G, or Rn from derecruitability test PEEP (D_{rec}^{PEEP}) with factors D_{rec}^{PEEP0}, D_{rec}^{PEEP3}, and D_{rec}^{PEEP6}; the log-transformed continuous time within the derecruitability test (*t*); and an *Injury* factor describing if the measurements were recorded at the start of the experiment (pre-ventilation) or after ventilation to a doubling of pulmonary system elastance (VILI).

	H		G		Rn	
Predictor	**Estimate (SE)**	***p*-value**	**Estimate (SE)**	***p*-value**	**Estimate (SE)**	***p*-value**
Intercept	3.083 (0.034)	<0.0001	0.500 (0.062)	<0.0001	−1.103 (0.057)	<0.0001
t	0.038 (0.006)	<0.0001	−0.002 (0.015)	0.8857	0.035 (0.009)	0.0002
D_{rec}^{PEEP3}	−0.386 (0.036)	<0.0001	0.228 (0.075)	0.0024	−0.499 (0.009)	<0.0001
D_{rec}^{PEEP6}	−0.229 (0.036)	<0.0001	0.580 (0.075)	<0.0001	−0.657 (0.047)	<0.0001
VILI	0.642 (0.036)	<0.0001	0.778 (0.075)	<0.0001	0.146 (0.047)	0.0021
$t \times D_{rec}^{PEEP3}$	−0.012 (0.008)	0.1529	0.002 (0.021)	0.8910	−0.016 (0.013)	0.2292
$t \times D_{rec}^{PEEP6}$	−0.014 (0.008)	0.1088	0.001 (0.021)	0.9627	−0.032 (0.013)	0.0138
$t \times$ VILI	0.060 (0.008)	<0.0001	0.115 (0.021)	<0.0001	0.008 (0.013)	0.5550
$D_{rec}^{PEEP3} \times$ VILI	−0.309 (0.051)	<0.0001	−0.710 (0.106)	<0.0001	−0.176 (0.067)	0.0089
$D_{rec}^{PEEP6} \times$ VILI	−0.279(0.051)	<0.0001	−0.623 (0.106)	<0.0001	−0.298 (0.067)	<0.0001
$t \times D_{rec}^{PEEP3} \times$ VILI	−0.031 (0.012)	0.0100	−0.093 (0.030)	0.0015	0.002 (0.019)	0.9034
$t \times D_{rec}^{PEEP6} \times$ VILI	−0.051 (0.012)	<0.0001	−0.097 (0.030)	0.0009	−0.009 (0.019)	0.6143

Fifteen mice are in each group.

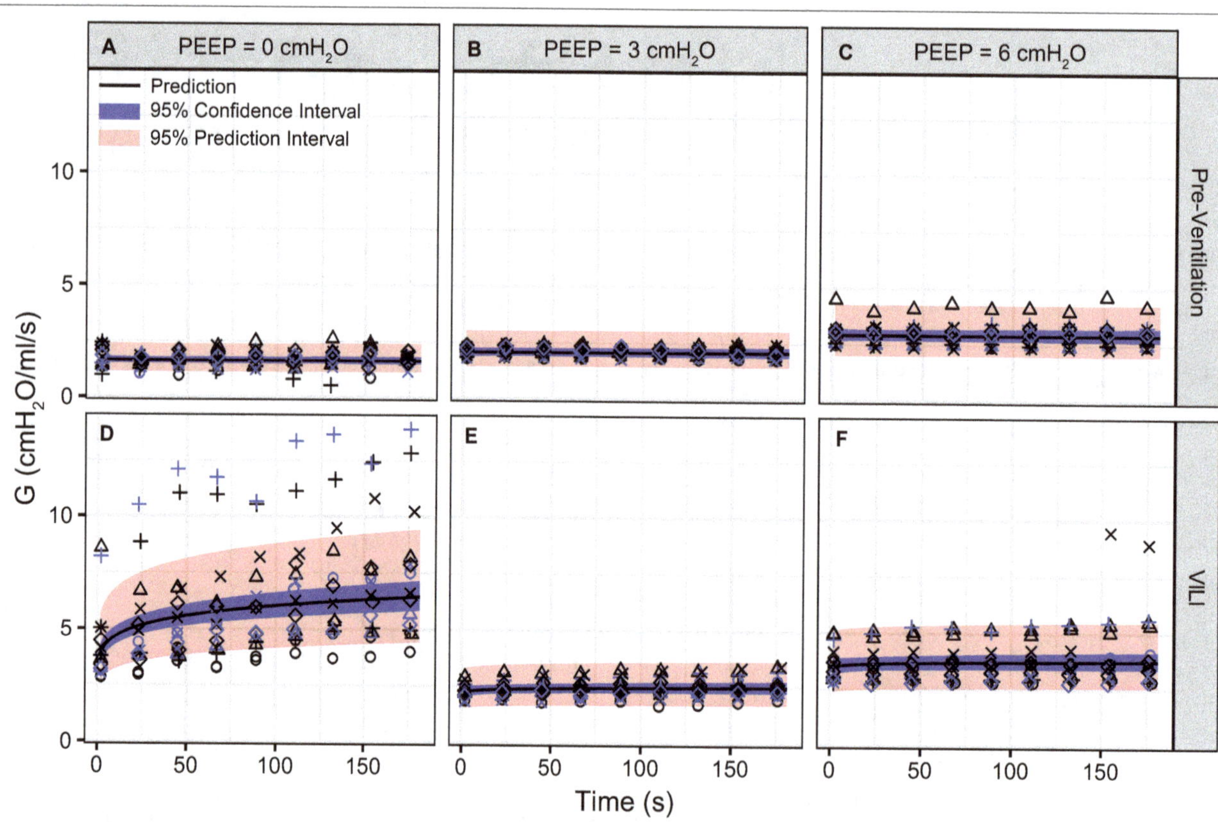

FIGURE 2 | Tissue damping (G) measured during derecruitability tests at PEEP = 0 **(A,D)**, 3 **(B,E)**, and 6 cmH$_2$O **(C,F)** (columns) before **(A–C)** and after injurious mechanical ventilation **(D–F)**. The LME model fit is shown with a black line, the 95% confidence interval is shown with a blue band, and the 95% prediction interval is shown with a red band. Symbols depict raw data for each animal and are consistent between **Figures 1–3**. Fifteen mice are in each group.

following high tidal volume ventilation due primarily to an increase in SA, which are less surface active. The increase in SA fraction also resulted in a striking and significant decrease in the LA/SA ratio (**Figure 8B**), a frequent marker of surfactant degradation, turnover, and/or injury. The fraction of the most surface-active LA was unchanged after VILI, but the functional quality of the LA pellet was significantly disrupted as demonstrated by a marked increase in minimum surface tension

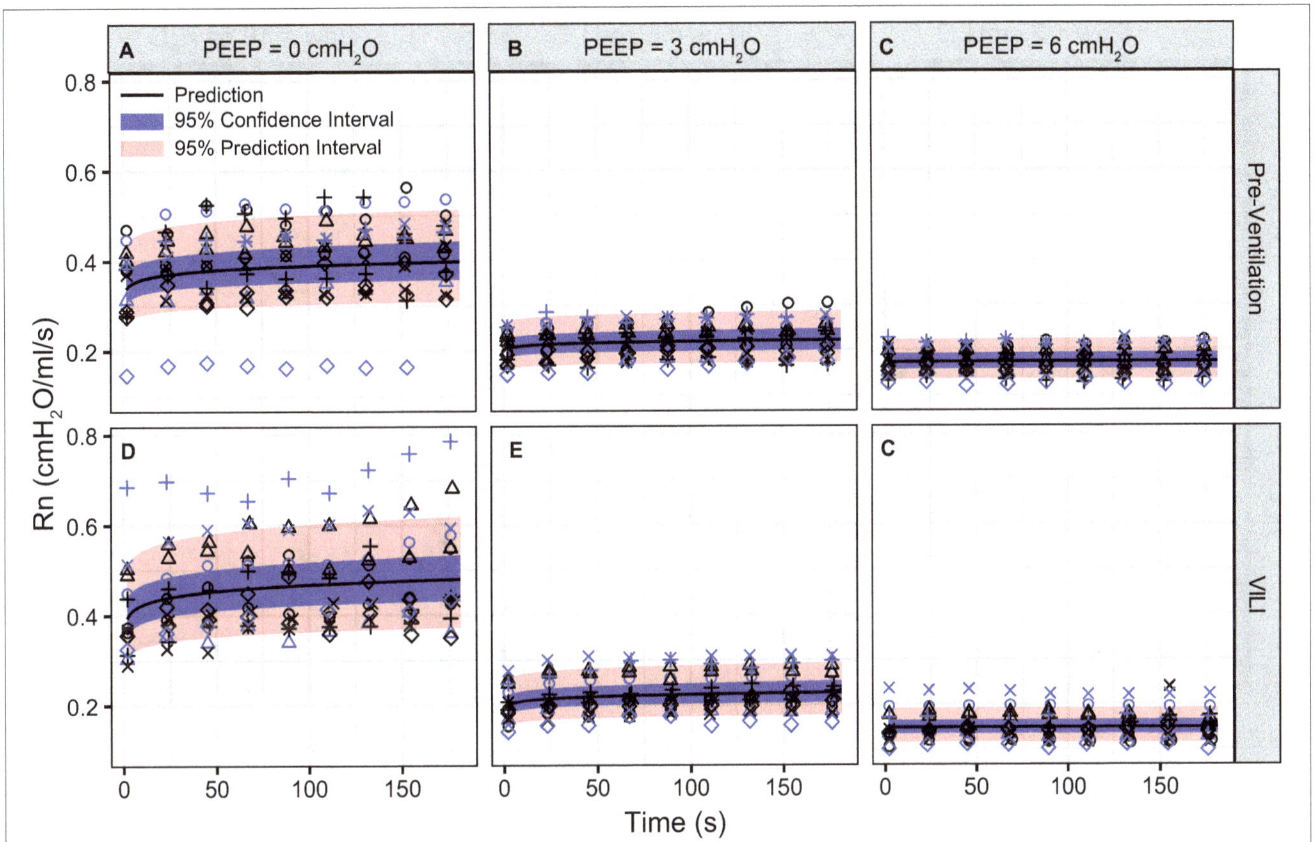

FIGURE 3 | Newtonian resistance (Rn) measured during derecruitability tests at PEEP = 0 **(A,D)**, 3 **(B,E)**, and 6 cmH$_2$O **(C,F)** before **(A–C)** and after injurious mechanical ventilation **(D–F)**. The LME model fit is shown with a black line, the 95% confidence interval is shown with a blue band, and the 95% prediction interval is shown with a red band. Symbols depict raw data for each animal and are consistent between **Figures 1–3**. Fifteen mice are in each group.

(**Figure 8D**), which translates *in vivo* to reduced surface tension lowering activity and reduced overall surfactant function. The airspace of the injured lung contained eightfold more protein (**Figure 8C**), which likely represents a combination of proteins released by the lung parenchyma and serum protein extravasation across a disrupted alveolocapillary barrier.

DISCUSSION

The macroscale pressures and flows applied at the trachea during mechanical ventilation result in microscale parenchymal injury (Dreyfuss and Saumon, 1998). The resulting ingress of protein-rich edema into the parenchymal airspace causes changes in alveolar dynamics at the microscale that are then reflected in macroscale alterations in lung function (Hamlington et al., 2018b). Macro- to micro-scale interactions in VILI thus take place in both directions, which we investigated by correlating VILI-induced changes in mouse lung microstructure to changes in lung function. Understanding the link between structure and function at both micro and macro levels of scale is crucial for developing optimized mechanical ventilation strategies that interrupt the vicious cycle of surfactant degradation and inactivation (Agassandian and Mallampalli, 2013), mechanical injury, inflammation, and altered lung function that drives VILI pathogenesis.

The most striking alterations in VILI-related organ-scale function are seen at low lung volumes (**Figure 1**, column 1), where we observe an approximately twofold increase in the first value of elastance measured at PEEP = 0 cmH$_2$O immediately following an RM in VILI compared to controls (**Table 1**, intercept). This is attributable to the loss of roughly half the ventilated alveoli [N(alv), **Figure 6B**], due both to derecruitment that is reversible with an RM and the flooding of alveoli [N(flood), **Figure 6C**] that are not recruitable. H then continues to increase over the subsequent three minutes of D_{rec}^{PEEP0} at a rate that is greater in the injured lungs (**Table 1**, slope). Although we cannot assess time-dependent alveolar collapse in fixed tissue, our previous studies indicate that this increased rate of lung stiffening is a consequence of accelerated alveolar derecruitment (Smith et al., 2015) that we would ascribe, in the current study, to elevated minimum surface tension (**Figure 8D**).

The PEEP = 3 and 6 cmH$_2$O derecruitability tests also show progressive increases in H, although of substantially smaller magnitudes than at PEEP = 0 cmH$_2$O (**Table 1**), no doubt because airway pressures remained above the derecruitment pressures of most of the unstable alveoli at the higher PEEP levels. This is borne out by our stereological analysis, which shows a decrease

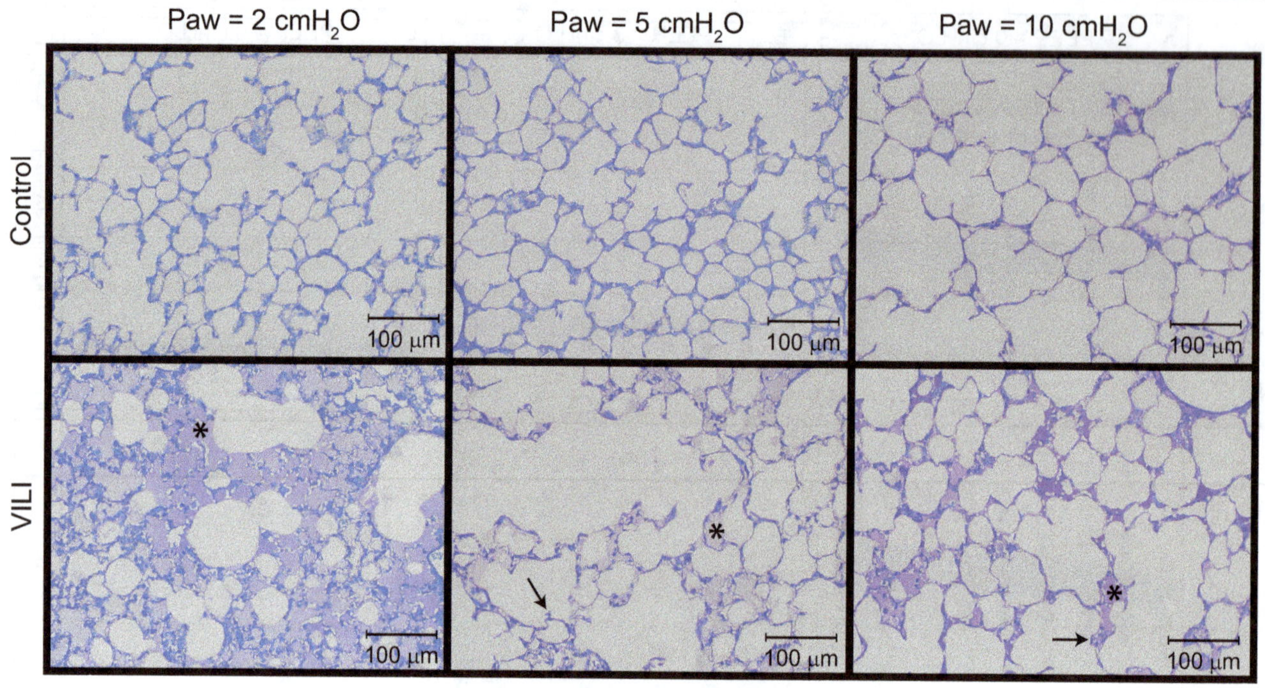

FIGURE 4 | Representative micrographs for control (first row) and VILI (second row) mice that were perfusion fixed at an airway pressure Paw = 2 cmH_2O (first column), Paw = 5 cmH_2O (second column), and Paw = 10 cmH_2O (third column). Asterisk indicates alveolar edema and arrows denote retracted alveolar septa.

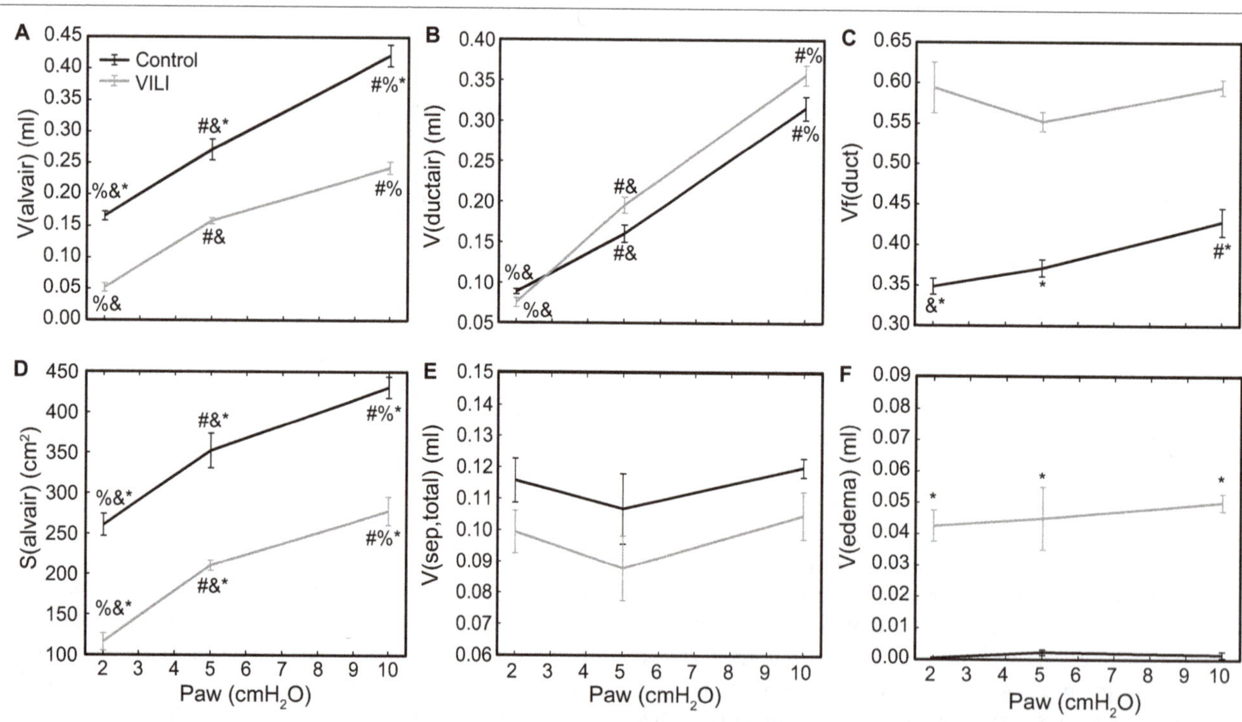

FIGURE 5 | Volume of air in the alveoli V(alvair) **(A)**, volume of air in the alveolar ducts V(ductair) **(B)**, volume fraction of parenchymal air in the alveolar ducts Vf(duct) **(C)**, gas-exchanging surface area S(alvair) **(D)**, total septal tissue volume V(sep,tot) **(E)**, and alveolar edema volume V(edema) **(F)** for the control (black lines) and VILI (gray lines) mice fixed at airway pressures Paw = 2, 5, and 10 cmH_2O. Significant differences from Paw = 2 cmH_2O (#), Paw = 5 cmH_2O (%), Paw = 10 cmH_2O (&) in the same treatment group. Significant difference at the same airway pressure between treatment groups is shown with asterisks. $n = 5$ for each point and the error bars show standard error.

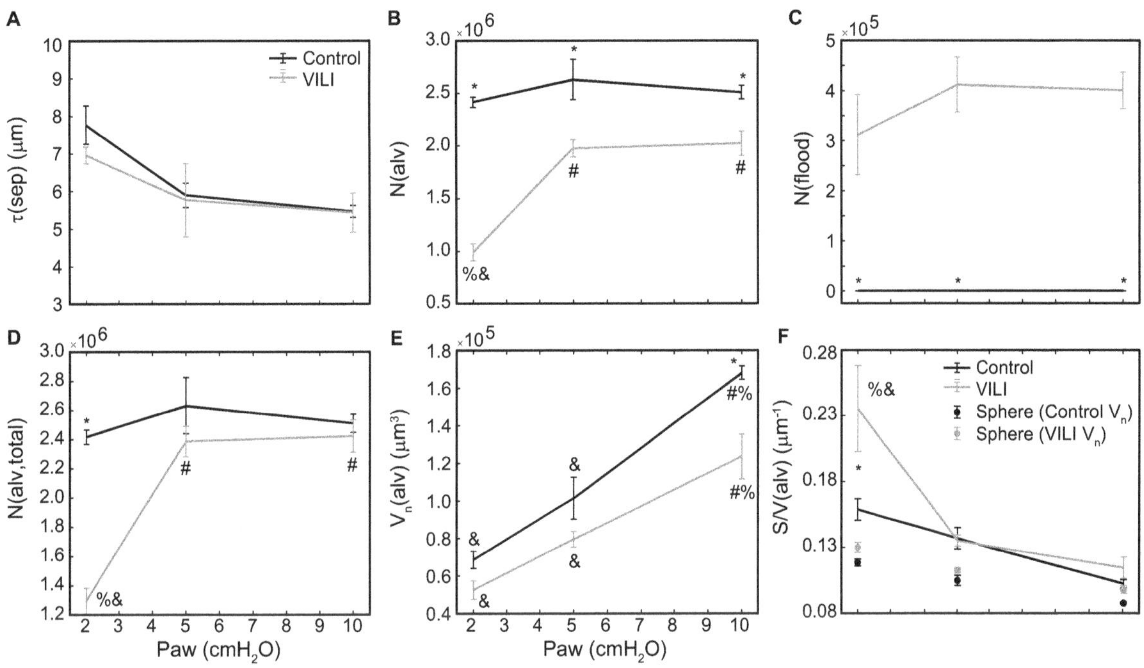

FIGURE 6 | Average alveolar septal wall thickness **(A)**, number of patent alveoli N(alv) **(B)**, number of flooded alveoli N(flood) **(C)**, total number of alveoli with discernable structure N(alv,total) = N(alv) + N(flood) **(D)**, and the number-weighted mean alveolar volume V_n(alv) **(E)** for the control (black lines) and VILI (gray lines) mice fixed at airway pressures Paw = 2, 5, and 10 cmH_2O. Points plotted with the alveolar surface area to volume ratio [S/V(alv), **(F)**] depict the S/V for a sphere with volume V_n(alv). Significant differences from Paw = 2 cmH_2O (#), Paw = 5 cmH_2O (%), Paw = 10 cmH_2O (&) in the same treatment group. Significant difference at the same airway pressure between treatment groups is shown with asterisks. n = 5 for each point and the error bars show standard error.

in N(alv) at the higher PEEP levels that is commensurate with the corresponding rates of increase in H. However, the total number of alveoli, N(alv,total), which includes both patent and flooded units, was unchanged in the VILI animals compared to controls at Paw = 5 and 10 cmH_2O. This indicates that the increase in elastance in D_{rec}^{PEEP3} and D_{rec}^{PEEP6} is primarily due to the accumulation of flooded, non-recruitable alveoli rather than recruitment-resistant atelectasis or small airway closure. **Figure 7** shows that the H values measured at the end of the derecruitability tests in all animals are inversely related to the fraction of patent alveoli (the "open fraction"), as we have previously postulated in our modeling studies of ventilator and acute lung injury in rodents (Smith et al., 2013, 2015; Hamlington et al., 2016b). This type of relationship was also observed during the acute phase of bleomycin injury in rats (Lutz et al., 2015; Knudsen et al., 2018) and lends strong support to the notion that the increases in lung stiffness seen in the acutely injured lung are largely reflective of loss of lung units through various derecruitment mechanisms. This has the important corollary that the dynamics of recruitment and derecruitment in the injured lung may be inferred directly from observed changes in H.

As expected, the loss of ventilated alveoli with VILI was accompanied by corresponding losses in V(alvair) at all pressures (**Figure 5A**). Less expected was the reduction in V_n(alv) (**Figure 6E**), because we previously observed mean alveolar volume to increase during the first 3 days of bleomycin injury in rats (Knudsen et al., 2018). Bleomycin-treated rats experience similar changes in minimum surface tension (Lutz et al., 2015) to those we found in the present study, so the differences in alveolar volume behavior cannot be attributed to differences in surfactant function. On the other hand, there may have been differences in the way that alveoli became derecruited in the two models. Finite element simulations indicate that the degree of alveolar enlargement caused by tethering forces from adjacent derecruited regions of the lung is greater when the adjacent alveoli are collapsed as opposed to being merely flooded (Albert et al., 2019). The later stages of bleomycin injury are characterized by widespread alveolar collapse that is resistant to reopening even at high airway pressures (Knudsen et al., 2018), which may explain why the mean volume of open alveoli was increased in this model. In contrast, in the VILI model of the present study the collapsed alveoli could be reopened by an RM, and the alveoli remained patent down to Paw = 5 cmH_2O, which would have reduced the tethering forces. Furthermore, at Paw = 2 cmH_2O the VILI lungs were characterized by extensive areas of both flooded and collapsed alveoli interspersed with regions of normal-appearing alveoli, so that tethering-induced alveolar volume increases would be confined to the boundaries between the collapsed and open regions.

The surface area available for gas exchange (**Figure 5D**) followed the same trend as V(alvair), increasing with Paw and decreasing with VILI. However, the mean surface area-to-volume ratio of an individual alveolus (**Figure 6F**) showed a striking increase with VILI at Paw = 2 cmH_2O, indicating that the

TABLE 3 | Summarized stereological data from control and VILI lungs.

Paw cmH_2O	V(alvair) ml	V(ductair) ml	V(edema) ml	V(sep,air) ml	V(sep,total) ml	S(alvair) cm^2	τ (sep) μm	N(alv)	N(flood)	N(alv,total)	V_n(alv) μm^3
Control											
2	$0.166^{\%,\&,*}$	$0.089^{\%,\&}$	0.000^*	0.101^*	0.116	$260.6^{\%,\&,*}$	7.8	$2,416,000^*$	0^* (0)	$2,416,000^*$	$68,660^\&$
	(0.016)	(0.007)	(0.000)	(0.019)	(0.016)	(30.4)	(1.1)	(110,815)		(110,815)	(10,074)
5	$0.272^{\#,\&,*}$	$0.161^{\#,\&}$	0.002^*	0.105^*	0.107	$352.3^{\#,\&,*}$	5.9	$2,632,000^*$	0^* (0)	2,632,000	$101,420^\&$
	(0.037)	(0.024)	(0.002)	(0.025)	(0.025)	(47.4)	(0.7)	(431,010)		(431,010)	(25,039)
10	$0.421^{\#,\%,*}$	$0.316^{\#,\%}$	0.002^*	0.118^*	0.120	$431.1^{\#,\%,*}$	5.5	$2,510,000^*$	0^* (0)	2,510,000	$168,200^{\#,\%,*}$
	(0.038)	(0.032)	(0.002)	(0.008)	(0.007)	(29.1)	(0.3)	(140,712)		(140,712)	(8,106)
VILI											
2	$0.052^{\%,\&,*}$	$0.075^{\%,\&}$	0.043^*	0.040^*	0.099	$116.1^{\%,\&,*}$	6.9	$991,800^{\%,\&,*}$	$312,020^*$	$1,294,000^{\%,\&,*}$	$52,540^\&$
	(0.016)	(0.013)	(0.011)	(0.009)	(0.015)	(24.0)	(0.5)	(182,486)	(178,976)	(202,745)	(11,141)
5	$0.158^{\#,\&,*}$	$0.196^{\#,\&}$	0.045^*	0.062^*	0.088	$210.5^{\#,\&,*}$	5.8	$1,976,000^{\#,*}$	$412,200^*$	$2,386,800^\#$	$79,540^\&$
	(0.011)	(0.022)	(0.022)	(0.027)	(0.023)	(14.1)	(2.2)	(184,201)	(122,873)	(235,812)	(9,362)
10	$0.243^{\#,\%,*}$	$0.357^{\#,\%}$	0.050^*	0.075^*	0.105	$278.4^{\#,\%,*}$	5.4	$2,024,000^{\#,*}$	$400,400^*$	$2,423,400^\#$	$123,520^{\#,\%,*}$
	(0.022)	(0.027)	(0.006)	(0.015)	(0.017)	(39.0)	(1.2)	(259,962)	(81,048)	(247,958)	(26,696)

Lungs were perfusion fixed at airway pressures Paw = 2, 5, and 10 cmH_2O. Values are given as mean (standard deviation). Significant differences from Paw = 2 cmH_2O (#), Paw = 5 cmH_2O (%), Paw = 10 cmH_2O (&) in the same treatment group. Significant difference at the same airway pressure between treatment groups is shown with asterisks. Each pressure in control and VILI includes n = 5 mice.

alveoli themselves had become less spherical and the alveolar septa possibly more convoluted. This is generally what one might expect in a deflating alveolus (Knudsen and Ochs, 2018), particularly if the alveolar walls become stiffer in VILI. Alveolar wall thickness was essentially unchanged by VILI (**Figure 6A**), however, so the stiffening was more likely due to increased surface tension.

The effect of alveolar stiffness on macro-scale mechanics was secondary to the loss of ventilated alveoli due to collapse and flooding (**Figure 7**). Our data indicate that the degradation of mechanical function with VILI follows the same path as in ARDS where different alveolar phenotypes have been postulated to define three distinct lung zones (Gattinoni et al., 1987): Zone D is comprised of damaged alveoli that cannot be recruited, corresponding to N(flood) in the current study. Zone R is comprised of unstable alveoli that are injured but recruitable, represented by the decrease in N(alv) between Paw = 5 and 2 cmH_2O in VILI (**Figure 6D**). This represents an VILI-induced upward shift of the distribution of alveolar derecruitment pressures (i.e., alveolar instability) since there is no change in N(alv) between Paw = 5 and 2 cmH_2O in the controls. Zone H comprises the remaining open alveoli (i.e., the "baby lung") that remain aerated at low Paw. Our microscale analysis shows that the mechanics of these open alveoli are not entirely normal since V_n(alv) and S/V(alv) are altered in VILI, but these alterations are secondary contributors to organ-scale mechanics when compared to the loss of ventilated alveoli. These three alveolar phenotypes have different dynamic behaviors that are reflected in the time- and pressure-dependence of H. It is important to note that while these three alveolar phenotypes are generally stable there may be variability between respiratory cycles. *In vivo* confocal microscopy shows that flooded alveoli are typically stable but may occasionally expel their edematous contents and become re-aerated (Wu et al., 2017). Likewise, nearby alveoli may alternately collapse on subsequent respiratory cycles (Broche et al., 2017) so that on subsequent breaths a single alveolus my either be collapsed or open.

The correlation between alveolar recruitment and elastance (**Figure 7**) may provide a mechanistic basis for identifying optimally lung-protective ventilation strategies. **Figure 6** shows alveolar recruitment occurring between pressures of 2 and 5 cmH_2O and, as such, H decreases as PEEP is increased from 0 to 3 cmH_2O (**Figure 1**). By contrast, further increasing PEEP to 6 cmH_2O causes a modest increase in elastance (and thus driving pressure) that is indicative of parenchymal overdistension. Taken together, these data suggest that the optimal PEEP based on lung elastance (or driving pressure) for these VILI mice lies between 3 and 6 cmH_2O to recruit the recruitable alveoli (Zone R) without causing tissue overdistension by applying excessive PEEP in a futile attempt to recruit the Zone D alveoli that, in our VILI model, are flooded with edema.

Tissue damping is challenging to interpret through the lens of fixed tissue because it describes the viscous losses in the parenchyma that are, by definition, dynamic processes. The fractional changes in G during the derecruitability tests were, for the most part, rather similar to the corresponding fractional changes in H (**Table 1**), which is most readily interpreted as being

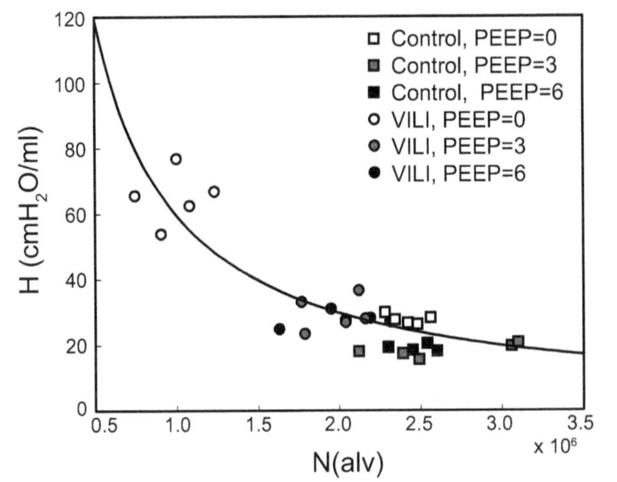

FIGURE 7 | Pulmonary system elastance *H* at the end of D_{rec}^{PEEP0} plotted against the number of alveoli N(alv) at Paw = 2 cmH_2O (white symbols, *n* = 10) for control (squares) and VILI (circles). Gray symbols (*n* = 10) show the final elastance measurement in D_{rec}^{PEEP3} against N(alv) at Paw = 5 cmH_2O (*n* = 10); black symbols show the final elastance measurement in D_{rec}^{PEEP6} against N(alv) at Paw = 10 cmH_2O. The best-fit line (R^2 = 0.78, $p < 10^{-13}$) has the equation $H = 24.40/(N(alv)/2.44 \times 10^6)$.

due simply to derecruitment of lung units, although it could also reflect an intrinsic coupling of the elastic and dissipative properties of lung parenchyma (Kaczka and Smallwood, 2012). Nevertheless, the largest alteration in G caused by VILI was an approximately twofold increase during D_{rec}^{PEEP0} (**Figure 2D**) that was slightly larger than the corresponding relative increase in H (**Figure 1D**). This may have been due to an increase in some form of dissipative process in the lung, such as intra-tidal recruitment (Kaczka et al., 2005, 2011), movement of fluid within and between partially flooded alveoli, or the folding and unfolding of septal pleats as suggested by an increased S/V(alv). In contrast, at PEEP = 3 and 6 cmH_2O the VILI-induced changes in G were relatively less than those in H. This contrasts with findings in open-chest but otherwise healthy mice in which tissue hysteresivity = G/H remained constant with lung volume (Sly et al., 2003). Theoretical analysis, however, shows that reductions in hysteresivity can arise if ongoing recruitment and derecruitment of lung units occurs while lung impedance is being measured by the FOT (Bates and Allen, 2006), as might easily be the case in severely injured lungs.

The decrease in airway resistance with PEEP (**Figure 3**) is readily attributable to the increase in airway caliber caused by airway-parenchymal tethering forces. This mechanism may also explain the modest VILI-induced decrease in Rn during D_{rec}^{PEEP6}, since flooded alveoli near the airways would be unable to expand normally during lung inflation and thus would cause tethering-forces on the airway to be correspondingly increased. Similarly, reduced or compressive tethering forces in atelectatic regions might explain why Rn was increased after VILI during D_{rec}^{PEEP0}. However, these changes in Rn were relatively minor, and were even non-existent during D_{rec}^{PEEP3}, indicating that central airway structure was not substantially affected by injurious ventilation. Indeed, stereological analysis revealed only occasional edema in the airways, and we did not find any airways that were either partially buckled or fully collapsed.

The structural and functional changes detailed above are associated with changes to the alveolar fluid-mechanical microenvironment that oppose alveolar inflation and promote collapse. The increased volume of fluid (**Figure 5F**) in partially flooded alveoli decreases the interfacial radius of curvature, which increases the pressure differential across the air–liquid interface and causes the lining fluid to exert a greater inward force that facilitates collapse. Furthermore, the functionality of the surfactant system is compromised (**Figure 8C**) from an apparent increase in surfactant degradation (increased SA fraction and decreased LA/SA ratio) and inactivation of PLs in the LA aggregates. The degradation of surface-active LA (Yamada et al., 1990) into surface-inactive SA (**Figure 8A**) may be attributed to

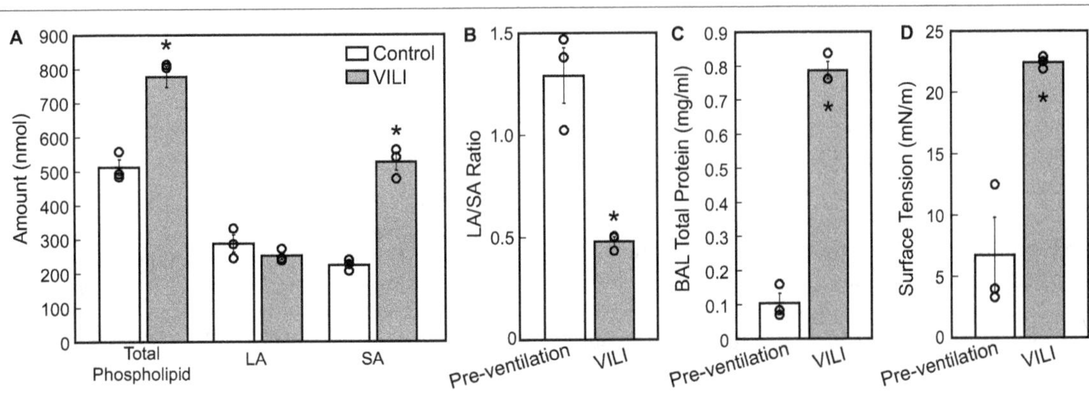

FIGURE 8 | Total phospholipid content (**A**, white bars) is increased following ventilation and was accompanied by an increase in small aggregate (SA) and slight decrease in large aggregate (LA) causing a decrease in the LA/SA ratio **(B)**. The total protein content in the BAL **(C)** is significantly increased in the VILI animals and the minimum surface tension measured using the pulsating bubble surfactometer (PBS) was significantly higher post-injury. Significant differences are indicated with asterisks and individual datapoints representing the pooled analysis of three animals are indicated with circles. BALF from three mice was pooled for each of the three datapoints. Error bars show standard error.

large cyclic strains imposed by high-volume, PEEP = 0 cmH_2O ventilation (Greenfield et al., 1964) that severely compresses the interfacial film so that it ruptures on re-expansion (Wyszogrodski et al., 1975). These mechanical effects can occur in the first 5 min of high tidal-volume ventilation (McClenahan and Urtnowski, 1967; Forrest, 1972). Therefore, in the present study, ventilation-induced surfactant degradation may have been the first step in the vicious cycle of altered alveolar dynamics, collapse, atelectrauma, and volutrauma that lead to eventually fatal VILI.

The mechanism for inactivation of the LA fraction is less clear and may very well be multifactorial. Airspace protein content is elevated (**Figure 8C**) due to alveolar surface damage (Dreyfuss et al., 1988; Hamlington et al., 2018b) and the resulting alveolocapillary leak (Hamlington et al., 2018a). Alveolar surface damage increases the BALF concentration of epithelial proteins such as E-cadherin while alveolocapillary leak accounts for the presence of serum proteins including albumin and immunoglobulin (IgG) in the BALF of mice ventilated under similar conditions (Smith et al., 2017). Our surface tension analysis includes the effects of BAL proteins that migrate with the PLs of the LA fraction during ultracentrifugation and inhibit surface lowering activity through disruption of phospholipid packing in the molecular films at the air–liquid interface. Furthermore, changes to the LA composition including phospholipids, surfactant-associate proteins or both may be present, and were not explored in these studies. Preliminary studies examining the presence of secretory phospholipases capable of targeting surfactant PLs revealed no significant changes in the BAL during this VILI model (data not shown) (Hite et al., 1998).

Our study has a number of limitations. First, the lungs were prepared for morphometric analysis with the chest wall retracted, which means that at high inflation pressures the lung volumes would have been greater than in closed-chest animals due to absence of constraint by the thorax. Conversely, at low inflation pressures the absence of the chest wall would have resulted in lower lung volumes due to the absence of the negative pleural pressure that opposes collapse. Based on lung volumes, airway pressures, and esophageal pressures measured in mice of equivalent age and weight to those used in the current study (Lai and Chou, 2000) we estimate that our morphometry data recorded at Paw = 2 cmH_2O corresponds to Paw = 1.5 cmH_2O in the intact mouse, an open-chested Paw = 10 cmH_2O is equivalent to 12 cmH_2O with the chest wall present, and at Paw = 5 cmH_2O the contribution of the chest wall is approximately zero. In addition, our morphometry was conducted on fixed tissue sections and this limits the analysis to static conditions following a prolonged breath hold. As such, we are unable to offer any insights into the intra-breath alveolar and acinar dynamics, which could provide important insights into, for example, how the elastance of an individual alveolus is altered by VILI. Phase contrast synchrotron computed tomography offers a pathway to analyze alveolar dynamics in future studies (Chang et al., 2015; Morgan et al., 2020). Another limitation is that the high inspiratory pressures and zero PEEP used to generate VILI in the current study are far outside clinical guidelines for safe ventilation. Indeed, they were specifically chosen to provide the volutrauma and atelectrauma necessary for VILI pathogenesis, while reducing the potential for deleterious metabolic effects occurring over long periods of ventilation (Wilson and Takata, 2019). Accordingly, our analysis is limited to the direct effects of VILI without the contribution of downstream inflammatory effects that take longer to manifest. Finally, the fact that our analysis was conducted in mice must be considered when applying our findings to ARDS and VILI in human subjects. Since the mouse lung is quite small, the effect of the gravitational gradient on lung structure and function is reduced in comparison to human subjects. Intrinsic structural differences are also present, including the pattern of branching which is monopodial (asymmetric) in mice and dichotomous (symmetric) in humans.

CONCLUSION

Three alveolar phenotypes typically develop with VILI: (1) flooded alveoli that cannot be recruited at any pressure, (2) unstable alveoli that are open at high pressures but readily collapse as pressure is reduced, and (3) relatively normal alveoli that remain open at low pressures. The relative proportions of each phenotype can be estimated using derecruitability tests that quantify time-dependent alveolar derecruitment as a function of PEEP. These correlations between lung structure and function could provide insights into optimally lung-protective ventilation strategies.

AUTHOR CONTRIBUTIONS

BS, GR, KH, LK, MO, RH, and JB contributed to the conception and design of the study. BS, GR, AC, CM, KO, CC, and MN acquired the experimental data. BS, KH, RH, and JB analyzed and interpreted the data. BS drafted the manuscript. CM, KO, RH, and JB wrote sections of the manuscript. All authors contributed to the article and approved the submitted version.

REFERENCES

Agassandian, M., and Mallampalli, R. K. (2013). Surfactant phospholipid metabolism. *Biochim. Biophys. Acta* 1831, 612–625. doi: 10.1016/j.bbalip.2012.09.010

Albert, R. K., Smith, B., Perlman, C. E., and Schwartz, D. A. (2019). Is progression of pulmonary fibrosis due to ventilation-induced lung injury?. *Am. J. Respir. Crit. Care Med.* 200, 140–151. doi: 10.1164/rccm.201903-0497PP

Aoyama, H., Pettenuzzo, T., Aoyama, K., Pinto, R., Englesakis, M., and Fan, E. (2018). Association of driving pressure with mortality among ventilated patients with acute respiratory distress syndrome: a systematic review and meta-analysis. *Crit. Care Med.* 46, 300–306. doi: 10.1097/ccm.0000000000002838

Bachofen, H., Ammann, A., Wangensteen, D., and Weibel, E. R. (1982). Perfusion fixation of lungs for structure-function analysis: credits and limitations. *J. Appl. Physiol. Respir. Environ. Exerc. Physiol.* 53, 528–533. doi: 10.1152/jappl.1982.53.2.528

Bates, J. H., and Allen, G. B. (2006). The estimation of lung mechanics parameters in the presence of pathology: a theoretical analysis. *Ann. Biomed. Eng.* 34, 384–392. doi: 10.1007/s10439-005-9056-6

Broche, L., Perchiazzi, G., Porra, L., Tannoia, A., Pellegrini, M., Derosa, S., et al. (2017). Dynamic mechanical interactions between neighboring airspaces determine cyclic opening and closure in injured lung. *Crit. Care Med.* 45, 687–694. doi: 10.1097/Ccm.0000000000002234

Chang, S., Kwon, N., Kim, J., Kohmura, Y., Ishikawa, T., Rhee, C. K., et al. (2015). Synchrotron X-ray imaging of pulmonary alveoli in respiration in live intact mice. *Sci. Rep.* 5:8760. doi: 10.1038/srep08760

Dreyfuss, D., and Saumon, G. (1998). Ventilator-induced lung injury: lessons from experimental studies. *Am. J. Respir. Crit. Care Med.* 157, 294–323. doi: 10.1164/ajrccm.157.1.9604014

Dreyfuss, D., Soler, P., Basset, G., and Saumon, G. (1988). High inflation pressure pulmonary edema. Respective effects of high airway pressure, high tidal volume, and positive end-expiratory pressure. *Am. Rev. Respir. Dis.* 137, 1159–1164. doi: 10.1164/ajrccm/137.5.1159

Enhorning, G., and Holm, B. A. (1993). Disruption of pulmonary surfactant's ability to maintain openness of a narrow tube. *J. Appl. Physiol.* 74, 2922–2927. doi: 10.1152/jappl.1993.74.6.2922

Force, A. D. T., Ranieri, V. M., Rubenfeld, G. D., Thompson, B. T., Ferguson, N. D., Caldwell, E., et al. (2012). Acute respiratory distress syndrome: the Berlin Definition. *JAMA* 307, 2526–2533. doi: 10.1001/jama.2012.5669

Forrest, J. B. (1972). The effect of hyperventilation on pulmonary surface activity. *Br. J. Anaesth.* 44, 313–320. doi: 10.1093/bja/44.4.313

Gattinoni, L., Pesenti, A., Avalli, L., Rossi, F., and Bombino, M. (1987). Pressure-volume curve of total respiratory system in acute respiratory failure. Computed tomographic scan study. *Am. Rev. Respir. Dis.* 136, 730–736. doi: 10.1164/ajrccm/136.3.730

Gil, J., Bachofen, H., Gehr, P., and Weibel, E. R. (1979). Alveolar volume-surface area relation in air- and saline-filled lungs fixed by vascular perfusion. *J. Appl. Physiol. Respir. Environ. Exerc. Physiol.* 47, 990–1001. doi: 10.1152/jappl.1979.47.5.990

Greenfield, L. J., Ebert, P. A., and Benson, D. W. (1964). Effect of positive pressure ventilation on surface tension properties of lung extracts. *Anesthesiology* 25, 312–316. doi: 10.1097/00000542-196405000-00009

Hamlington, K. L., Bates, J. H. T., Roy, G. S., Julianelle, A. J., Charlebois, C., Suki, B., et al. (2018a). Alveolar leak develops by a rich-get-richer process in ventilator-induced lung injury. *PLoS One* 13:e0193934. doi: 10.1371/journal.pone.0193934

Hamlington, K. L., Smith, B. J., Dunn, C. M., Charlebois, C. M., Roy, G. S., and Bates, J. H. T. (2018b). Linking lung function to structural damage of alveolar epithelium in ventilator-induced lung injury. *Respir. Physiol. Neurobiol.* 255, 22–29. doi: 10.1016/j.resp.2018.05.004

Hamlington, K. L., Dunn, C. M., Roy, G. S., Smith, B. J., and Bates, J. H. T. (2016a). Linking alveolar epithelial barrier disruption to function in ventilator-induced lung injury. *Am. J. Respir. Crit. Care Med.* 193:A4826.

Hamlington, K. L., Smith, B. J., Allen, G. B., and Bates, J. H. (2016b). Predicting ventilator-induced lung injury using a lung injury cost function. *J. Appl. Physiol.* 121, 106–114. doi: 10.1152/japplphysiol.00096.2016

Hantos, Z., Daroczy, B., Suki, B., Nagy, S., and Fredberg, J. J. (1992). Input impedance and peripheral inhomogeneity of dog lungs. *J. Appl. Physiol.* 72, 168–178. doi: 10.1152/jappl.1992.72.1.168

Hernandez, L. A., Peevy, K. J., Moise, A. A., and Parker, J. C. (1989). Chest wall restriction limits high airway pressure-induced lung injury in young-rabbits. *J. Appl. Physiol.* 66, 2364–2368. doi: 10.1152/jappl.1989.66.5.2364

Hite, R. D., Seeds, M. C., Bowton, D. L., Grier, B. L., Safta, A. M., Balkrishnan, R., et al. (2005). Surfactant phospholipid changes after antigen challenge: a role for phosphatidylglycerol in dysfunction. *Am. J. Physiol. Lung Cell Mol. Physiol.* 288, L610–L617. doi: 10.1152/ajplung.00273.2004

Hite, R. D., Seeds, M. C., Jacinto, R. B., Balasubramanian, R., Waite, M., and Bass, D. (1998). Hydrolysis of surfactant-associated phosphatidylcholine by mammalian secretory phospholipases A2. *Am. J. Physiol.* 275, L740–L747. doi: 10.1152/ajplung.1998.275.4.L740

Hsia, C. C., Hyde, D. M., Ochs, M., and Weibel, E. R. (2010). Ats Ers Joint Task Force on Quantitative Assessment of Lung Structure. An official research policy statement of the American Thoracic Society/European Respiratory Society: standards for quantitative assessment of lung structure. *Am. J. Respir. Crit. Care Med.* 181, 394–418. doi: 10.1164/rccm.200809-1522ST

Kaczka, D. W., Cao, K. L., Christensen, G. E., Bates, J. H. T., and Simon, B. A. (2011). Analysis of regional mechanics in canine lung injury using forced oscillations and 3d image registration. *Ann. Biomed. Eng.* 39, 1112–1124. doi: 10.1007/s10439-010-0214-0

Kaczka, D. W., Hager, D. N., Hawley, M. L., and Simon, B. A. (2005). Quantifying mechanical heterogeneity in canine acute lung injury: impact of mean airway pressure. *Anesthesiology* 103, 306–317.

Kaczka, D. W., and Smallwood, J. L. (2012). Constant-phase descriptions of canine lung, chest wall, and total respiratory system viscoelasticity: effects of distending pressure. *Respir. Physiol. Neurobiol.* 183, 75–84. doi: 10.1016/j.resp.2012.06.008

Knudsen, L., Lopez-Rodriguez, E., Berndt, L., Steffen, L., Ruppert, C., Bates, J. H. T., et al. (2018). Alveolar Micromechanics in Bleomycin-induced Lung Injury. *Am. J. Respir. Cell Mol. Biol.* 59, 757–769. doi: 10.1165/rcmb.2018-0044OC

Knudsen, L., and Ochs, M. (2018). The micromechanics of lung alveoli: structure and function of surfactant and tissue components. *Histochem. Cell Biol.* 150, 661–676. doi: 10.1007/s00418-018-1747-9

Lai, Y. L., and Chou, H. (2000). Respiratory mechanics and maximal expiratory flow in the anesthetized mouse. *J. Appl. Physiol.* 88, 939–943. doi: 10.1152/jappl.2000.88.3.939

Lenth, R. V. (2016). Least-Squares Means: the R Package lsmeans. *J. Stat. Softw.* 69, 1–33. doi: 10.18637/jss.v069.i01

Lutz, D., Gazdhar, A., Lopez-Rodriguez, E., Ruppert, C., Mahavadi, P., Günther, A., et al. (2015). Alveolar derecruitment and collapse induration as crucial mechanisms in lung injury and fibrosis. *Am. J. Respir. Cell Mol. Biol.* 52, 232–243. doi: 10.1165/rcmb.2014-0078oc

McClenahan, J. B., and Urtnowski, A. (1967). Effect of ventilation on surfactant, and its turnover rate. *J. Appl. Physiol.* 23, 215–220. doi: 10.1152/jappl.1967.23.2.215

Mellenthin, M. M., Seong, S. A., Roy, G. S., Bartolak-Suki, E., Hamlington, K. L., Bates, J. H. T., et al. (2019). Using injury cost functions from a predictive single-compartment model to assess the severity of mechanical ventilator-induced lung injuries. *J. Appl. Physiol.* 127, 58–70. doi: 10.1152/japplphysiol.00770.2018

Morgan, K. S., Parsons, D., Cmielewski, P., McCarron, A., Gradl, R., Farrow, N., et al. (2020). Methods for dynamic synchrotron X-ray respiratory imaging in live animals. *J. Synchrotr. Radiat.* 27(Pt 1), 164–175. doi: 10.1107/S1600577519014863

Morton, S. E., Knopp, J. L., Chase, J. G., Moller, K., Docherty, P., Shaw, G. M., et al. (2019). Predictive virtual patient modelling of mechanical ventilation: impact of recruitment function. *Ann. Biomed. Eng.* 47, 1626–1641. doi: 10.1007/s10439-019-02253-w

Mühlfeld, C., Knudsen, L., and Ochs, M. (2013). "Stereology and morphometry of lung tissue," in *Methods in Molecular Biology*, eds D. J. Taatjes, and B. T. Mossman, (Totowa, NJ: Humana Press).

Muscedere, J. G., Mullen, J. B. M., Gan, K., and Slutsky, A. S. (1994). Tidal Ventilation at Low Airway Pressures Can Augment Lung Injury. *Am. J. Respir. Crit. Care Med.* 149, 1327–1334. doi: 10.1164/ajrccm.149.5.8173774

Ochs, M., Nyengaard, L., Jung, A., Knudsen, L., Voigt, M., Wahlers, T., et al. (2004). The number of alveoli in the human lung. *Am. J. Respir. Crit. Care Med.* 169, 120–124. doi: 10.1164/rccm.200308-1107OC

Pereira Romano, M. L., Maia, I. S., Laranjeira, L. N., Damiani, L. P., Paisani, D. M., Borges, M. C., et al. (2020). Driving pressure-limited strategy for patients with acute respiratory distress syndrome. A pilot randomized clinical trial. *Ann. Am. Thorac. Soc.* 17, 596–604. doi: 10.1513/AnnalsATS.201907-506OC

Pinheiro, J. C., and Bates, D. M. (2000). *Mixed-Effects Models in S and S-PLUS.* New York, NY: Springer.

Rouser, G., Fleischer, S., and Yamamoto, A. (1970). Two dimensional thin layer chromatographic separation of polar lipids and determination of phospholipids by phosphorus analysis of spots. *Lipids* 5, 494–496. doi: 10.1007/bf02531316

Schneider, J. P., and Ochs, M. (2014). Alterations of mouse lung tissue dimensions during processing for morphometry: a comparison of methods. *Am. J. Physiol. Lung Cell Mol. Physiol.* 306, L341–L350. doi: 10.1152/ajplung.00329.2013

Sly, P. D., Collins, R. A., Thamrin, C., Turner, D. J., and Hantos, Z. (2003). Volume dependence of airway and tissue impedances in mice. *J. Appl. Physiol.* 94, 1460–1466. doi: 10.1152/japplphysiol.00596.2002

Smith, B. J., Bartolak-Suki, E., Suki, B., Roy, G. S., Hamlington, K. L., Charlebois, C. M., et al. (2017). Linking ventilator injury-induced leak across the blood-gas barrier to derangements in murine lung function. *Front. Physiol.* 8:466. doi: 10.3389/fphys.2017.00466

Smith, B. J., Grant, K. A., and Bates, J. H. (2013). Linking the development of ventilator-induced lung injury to mechanical function in the lung. *Ann. Biomed. Eng.* 41, 527–536. doi: 10.1007/s10439-012-0693-2

Smith, B. J., Lundblad, L. K., Kollisch-Singule, M., Satalin, J., Nieman, G., Habashi,

N., et al. (2015). Predicting the response of the injured lung to the mechanical breath profile. *J. Appl. Physiol.* 118, 932–940. doi: 10.1152/japplphysiol.00902.2014

Webb, H. H., and Tierney, D. F. (1974). Experimental pulmonary-edema due to intermittent positive pressure ventilation with high inflation pressures. Protection by positive end-expiratory pressure. *Am. Rev. Respir. Dis.* 110, 556–565.

Wilson, M., and Takata, M. (2019). Mechanical ventilation in mice: does longer equal better? *Am. J. Respir. Cell Mol. Biol.* 60, 137–138. doi: 10.1165/rcmb.2018-0308ED

Wu, Y., Nguyen, T. L., and Perlman, C. E. (2017). Accelerated deflation promotes homogeneous airspace liquid distribution in the edematous lung. *J. Appl. Physiol.* 122, 739–751. doi: 10.1152/japplphysiol.00526.2016

Wyszogrodski, I., Kyei-Aboagye, K., Taeusch, H. W. Jr., and Avery, M. E. (1975). Surfactant inactivation by hyperventilation: conservation by end-expiratory pressure. *J. Appl. Physiol.* 38, 461–466. doi: 10.1152/jappl.1975.38.3.461

Yamada, T., Ikegami, M., and Jobe, A. H. (1990). Effects of surfactant subfractions on preterm rabbit lung function. *Pediatr. Res.* 27, 592–598. doi: 10.1203/00006450-199006000-00011

Yen, S., Preissner, M., Bennett, E., Dubsky, S., Carnibella, R., O'Toole, R., et al. (2019). The link between regional tidal stretch and lung injury during mechanical ventilation. *Am. J. Respir. Cell Mol. Biol.* 60, 569–577. doi: 10.1165/rcmb.2018-0143OC

4

Modeling Lung Derecruitment in VILI Due to Fluid-Occlusion: The Role of Emergent Behavior

Vitor Mori[1,2], Bradford J. Smith[3], Bela Suki[4] and Jason H. T. Bates[1]*

[1] Department of Medicine, Vermont Lung Center, Larner College of Medicine, The University of Vermont, Burlington, VT, United States, [2] Department of Telecommunications and Control Engineering, University of São Paulo, São Paulo, Brazil, [3] Department of Bioengineering, College of Engineering, Design & Computing, University of Colorado Denver, Aurora, CO, United States, [4] Department of Biomedical Engineering, Boston University, Boston, MA, United States

***Correspondence:**
Vitor Mori
vitor.mori@uvm.edu

Ventilator-induced lung injury (VILI) is driven by the processes of volutrauma and atelectrauma, which can act synergistically to compromise the blood-gas barrier. We have postulated that this synergy arises through a rich-get-richer mechanism whereby atelectrauma causes holes to form in the blood-gas barrier while concomitant volutrauma causes susceptible holes to progressively enlarge as VILI worsens. We previously developed an analytical model based on this idea that accurately predicts the progressive increases in lung elastance seen immediately following a recruitment maneuver as VILI progresses over the course of hours. In the present study we extend this model to account for the rate of change of elastance, due to closure of lung units, in the minutes following a recruitment maneuver. We found that the distribution of unit closing velocities throughout the lung can be described by a power law with an exponent of −2 that matches previously published power laws associated with the dynamics of lung recruitment. Our model thus reveals lung collapse as an example of emergent complex behavior and links the dynamics of altered function in the injured lung to structural damage in a way that explains the mechanisms of injury progression arising from the ongoing stresses and strains applied by mechanical ventilation.

Keywords: acute lung injury, analytical model, alveolar flooding, surface tension, lung elastance

INTRODUCTION

Mechanical ventilation plays a major role in critical care, providing life support to patients in respiratory failure. However, because of the stresses and strains it imposes on the tissues of the lung, mechanical ventilation can also cause ventilator-induced lung injury (VILI) (Dos Santos and Slutsky, 2000; Gattinoni et al., 2003; Slutsky and Ranieri, 2013). The two principle injury mechanisms of VILI are over-distension of the tissues that gives rise to volutrauma, and cyclic recruitment and derecruitment of lung units that gives rise to atelectrauma (Parker et al., 1993; Dreyfuss and Saumon, 1998). Volutrauma and atelectrauma are both involved in compromising the blood-bas barrier of the lung, which allows plasma-derived fluid and proteins to leak into the airspaces. This disrupts surfactant function, which then decreases lung compliance and thus increases the tissue stresses associated with mechanical ventilation, making the leak worse. At the same time, the lung becomes progressively more derecruited, which places the remaining open lung regions at greater risk of over-distension

(Gattinoni and Pesenti, 2006; Gattinoni et al., 2016). Patients with pre-existing lung injury, particularly acute respiratory system distress syndrome (ARDS), are highly susceptible to VILI (Slutsky and Ranieri, 2000; Dreyfuss and Hubmayr, 2016). Various ventilation strategies have been proposed to manage ARDS and prevent VILI, but once underway it is difficult to break out of the vicious cycle of progressing injury (Slutsky and Ranieri, 2013).

We have shown in a number of studies in mice (Seah et al., 2011; Smith et al., 2013, 2017) that the nature and degree of lung injury is reflected in what we term the *derecruitability* of the lung. Derecruitability is measured by applying a recruitment maneuver (deep inflation) to maximally open closed airspaces followed immediately by a period (typically 3 min) of mechanical ventilation at a designated tidal volume (V_t) and level of positive end-expiratory pressure (PEEP). Lung stiffness (H) rises progressively during the ventilation period to a degree that is modest (perhaps 20%) in a normal lung, but is dramatically enhanced in the injured lung to an extent that reflects the degree of injury (Smith et al., 2013). Some of the post-recruitment increase in H in the normal lung likely reflects changes in surface tension arising from the dynamics of surfactant at the air-liquid interface and viscoelastic adaptation of tissue stress, but the highly exaggerated increases in H seen in the injured lung are largely the result of progressive derecruitment of airspaces (Massa et al., 2008; Smith et al., 2017; Hamlington et al., 2018b).

We denote as D_{rate} the mean rate of increase in H over the 3 min following recruitment, while H_1 is the first measurement of H made immediately after recruitment (Smith and Bates, 2013; Smith et al., 2013). Both D_{rate} and H_1 increase with the severity of lung injury, but they do not mirror each other exactly. D_{rate} quantifies derecruitment dynamics that manifest over a timescale of minutes, probably reflecting instabilities in the fluid layer lining the small airways and alveoli (Smith et al., 2013). H_1, on the other hand, quantifies either much more rapid derecruitment phenomena or an inability to recruit at all, more likely explicable on the basis of rapid alveolar flooding by accumulated edema fluid and/or unstable collapse of lung units caused by high surface tension in the air-liquid interface (Smith et al., 2013). D_{rate} and H_1 together thus comprise a pair of sensitive biomarkers of lung injury (Smith et al., 2013).

We have previously shown in mice that, as VILI develops, the time-course of H_1 can be accurately accounted for in terms of the accumulated leak of plasma-derived material through holes in the blood-gas barrier (Mori et al., 2018). These holes appear to be generated by both atelectrauma and volutrauma acting synergistically in a rich-get-richer fashion (Hamlington et al., 2018a). The rate of accumulation of edema in the airspaces, and thus the displacement of air that results, is a function of the number and sizes of these holes, both of which increase with time during injurious mechanical ventilation. In the present study, we extend this analysis to D_{rate} in order to establish a consistent theory of derecruitability of the injured lung that links both H_1 and D_{rate} to the biophysical processes taking place during the development of VILI.

MATERIALS AND METHODS

Model Development

In the following model development we take a similar analytical approach to our previous study of the dependence of H_1 on degree of lung injury, this time focusing on the complementary parameter D_{rate}. To account for the progressive increase in D_{rate} that accompanies the development of VILI, it is necessary to model events taking place over two different scales of time. The longer time scale, on the order to minutes to hours, concerns the progression of VILI itself. The shorter time scale, on the order of seconds to minutes, involves the dynamic recruitment and derecruitment of alveoli and small airways that are reflected in our periodic assessments of VILI. In order to avoid ambiguity between these two time scales in the following mathematical development, events taking place over the shorter time scale (seconds to a few minutes) will be referenced to time denoted by τ while events taking place over the longer time scale (many minutes to hours) will be referenced to time denoted by t.

We first consider the short time-scale assessment of VILI, which is based on the computational model of recruitment/derecruitment dynamics proposed by Bates and Irvin (2002) consisting of a parallel distribution of lung units. Each unit has its own airway to which is applied the same pressure. The units open and close according to their randomly assigned critical opening and closing airway pressures (P_o and P_c, respectively). These pressures are drawn from probability distribution $f_{P_o}(P_o)$ and $f_{P_c}(P_c)$, respectively. However, a unit does not necessarily open or close as soon as it traverses its particular value of either P_o or P_c. Rather, a latency is built into the process by associating with each unit a *virtual trajectory* variable x that can assume any value between 0 (corresponding to the unit being definitively closed) and 1 (definitively open). An open unit remains open until $x = 0$, while a closed unit remains closed until $x = 1$. Movement of x along the virtual trajectory occurs to the right (i.e., toward increasing values of x) when $P > P_o$, and to the left when $P < P_c$, with the rate of change x being proportional to the amount by which P either exceeds P_o or is less than P_c. The constants of proportionality that determine the velocity of x rightward and leftward are s_0 and s_c, respectively. That is,

$$\begin{aligned} \frac{dx}{d\tau} &= (P - P_o)\, s_o; \quad \text{for } P \geq P_o \\ &= (P - P_c)\, s_c; \quad \text{for } P \leq P_c \\ &= 0; \quad \text{for } P_c < P < P_o \end{aligned} \tag{1}$$

where $0 \leq x < 1$. The velocity constants s_0 and s_c for each unit are drawn from probability distributions $f_{s_o}(s_0)$ and $f_{s_c}(s_c)$, respectively.

Following the original model (Bates and Irvin, 2002), we assume that P_o and P_c are distributed according to Gaussians with variances σ_0 and σ_c, and means μ_0 and μ_c, respectively. In accord with the findings of Massa et al. (2008) in acid-injured mice, we set the two variances to be equal (i.e., $\sigma_0 = \sigma_c = \sigma$) and the two means separated by δP such that the opening pressures are greater than the closing pressures (i.e., $\mu_0 = \mu_c + \delta P$)

$$f_{P_c}(P_c) = \frac{1}{\sigma\sqrt{2\pi}} e^{-\frac{1}{2}\left(\frac{P_c-\mu_c}{\sigma}\right)^2} \tag{2}$$

and

$$f_{P_o}(P_o) = \frac{1}{\sigma\sqrt{2\pi}} e^{-\frac{1}{2}\left(\frac{P_o-\mu_c-\delta P}{\sigma}\right)^2} \tag{3}$$

We assume that σ and δP do not change with increasing injury, so the progression of VILI is reflected entirely in the way that μ_c increases with time.

The velocity distributions $f_{s_o}(s_0)$ and $f_{s_c}(s_c)$ were originally specified on purely empirical grounds as conforming to hyperbolic functions (Bates and Irvin, 2002), motivated by the ubiquitous appearance of such functions in naturally occurring complex systems (West, 1990; Robertson et al., 2000; West et al., 2000). Solving the model analytically using such functions is not possible, however, because hyperbolas are not finite-integrable over $s \in (0, \infty)$, but finite integrals can be obtained by having the exponent of the power law be different from unity and by specifying a small positive lower limit, s_m, for integration. Accordingly, we set

$$f_{s_c}(s_c) = \frac{\alpha - 1}{s_m}\left(\frac{s_c}{s_m}\right)^{-\alpha} \tag{4}$$

where $0 < s_m < s_c < \infty$ and $\alpha > 1$.

When modeling how the fraction of closed lung, F_{closed}, changes during a derecruitability test, we avoid having to consider $f_{s_o}(s_0)$ specifically by assuming, as did Albert et al. (2009), that it is only derecruitment that takes place to any significant extent during the 3 min following a recruitment maneuver. That is, we assume that the fully recruited lung derecruits progressively during these 3 min as if exposed to an effective pressure, $P_{\text{derecruit}}$, that is fixed throughout the breath and that reflects the mean airway pressure applied by the mechanical ventilator. $P_{\text{derecruit}}$ is determined by the applied level of PEEP plus some positive ΔP that depends on the ventilation regimen that is applied on top of the PEEP. As the lung becomes progressively more injured, and thus stiffer, mean airway pressure increases. This pressure increase is offset to some extent, however, by the compliance of the gas in the piston and connecting tubing of the flexiVent ventilator (Scireq, Montreal, Canada) that was used to collect the experimental data. While the effect of this compliance on calculation of H was compensated for digitally (Schuessler and Bates, 1995), it still absorbed an increasing fraction of the pressure increases as the lung stiffened (Smith et al., 2013). Mean airway pressure also increases somewhat over the course of a single derecruitability test. However, in order to obtain an analytical solution to our model we assumed that $P_{\text{derecruit}}$ remains unchanged over each of the 3 min derecruitment maneuvers. This is clearly not precisely the case, but we take it to be a reasonable first-order approximation since tidal volume is quite low during the tests.

For a unit to have the possibility of closing during a derecruitability test it must therefore satisfy the condition $P_c > P_{\text{derecruit}}$. Whether or not a particular unit actually closes during the test, however, depends on whether it moves along its virtual trajectory rapidly enough for x to reach a value of 0 before the 3 min test is complete and that there is no significant retrograde motion of x during the inspiratory portions of the test. If the duration of the test were to continue indefinitely, the asymptotic value to which F_{closed} would tend is that which satisfies the above condition, which is

$$F_{\text{closed}}(\infty) = \int_{P_{\text{derecruit}}}^{\infty} \left[\frac{1}{\sigma\sqrt{2\pi}} e^{-\frac{1}{2}\left(\frac{P_c-\mu_c}{\sigma}\right)^2}\right] dP_c \tag{5}$$

This situation is never actually achieved, of course, because the derecruitability test is terminated after 3 min.

We assume that the recruitment maneuver establishes an initial condition for which all units open and are positioned at $x = 1$ along their respective virtual trajectories. As derecruitment proceeds during the test, the various units in the model close sequentially. The time, τ, at which a given unit closes is determined by how quickly it traverses the length of its virtual trajectory from $x = 1$ to $x = 0$, which is given by

$$\tau = \frac{1}{s_c\,|P_{\text{derecruit}} - P_c|} \tag{6}$$

which means that the units that have closed by time τ are those that have closing pressures satisfying $\frac{1}{\tau(P_c-P)} < s_c$. Assuming, as did Albert et al. (2009), that $f_{P_c}(P_c)$ and $f_{s_c}(s_c)$ are statistically independent, $F_{\text{closed}}(P, \tau)$ is given by

$$F_{\text{closed}}(P, \tau) = \int_P^{\infty} \int_{[(P_c-P)\tau]^{-1}}^{\infty} \frac{1}{\sigma\sqrt{2\pi}} e^{-\frac{1}{2}\left(\frac{P_c-\mu_c}{\sigma}\right)^2} \cdot \frac{\alpha-1}{s_m}\left(\frac{s_c}{s_m}\right)^{-\alpha} dP_c ds_c \tag{7}$$

A detailed step-by-step solution of Eq.7 is presented in the **Supplementary Material.**

Solving Eq. 7 we find that $\alpha = 2$ and Eq. 4 of thus becomes

$$f_{s_c}(s_c) = \frac{1}{s_m}\left(\frac{s_c}{s_m}\right)^{-2} \tag{8}$$

Massa et al. (2008) found $\sigma = 3$ in mice with acute lung injury caused by hydrochloric acid instillation. Smith et al. (2013) found $\mu_c(t) = kt$, where k is a constant, in injuriously ventilated mice. Since PEEP is zero and H is measured using small-amplitude perturbations in lung volume, we assume that $P = 0$ to a first approximation (Mori et al., 2018). D_{rate} can thus be written as:

$$D_{\text{rate}}(t) = \frac{H_1(t)\, s_m}{\sqrt{2\pi}}\left[\sqrt{\frac{\pi}{2}}3kt\left(erf\left(\frac{kt}{3\sqrt{2}}\right)+1\right) + 9e^{-\frac{1}{2}\left(\frac{kt}{3}\right)^2}\right] \tag{9}$$

From our previous proposed model (Mori et al., 2018) we can relate Eq. 9 to H_1 when t is sufficiently large:

$$\lim_{t\to\infty} D_{\text{rate}}(t) = 3ks_m\frac{1}{\sqrt{a}}\left(H_1(t) - \frac{H_0}{2}\right) \tag{10}$$

Experimental Data

We tested the predictions of the above model against a set of data collected in mice and published previously (Smith et al., 2013). A detailed description of the experimental method used, as well as animals ethics approval, are given in this previous publication. Briefly, healthy 8- to 10-week-old female BALB/c mice (18.3–24.4 g) were anesthetized with 90 mg/kg intraperitoneal sodium pentobarbital and then connected to a computer-controlled mechanical ventilator (flexiVent, Scireq, Montreal, Canada). Following paralysis (0.5 ml/kg IP injection of pancuronium bromide) animals received a 21 min protocol starting with 16.5 min of injurious ventilation delivered at zero PEEP with a very large V_t (1.0, 1.1, 1.2, and 1.3 ml in 4 different groups of animals) followed by a derecruitability test (4.5 min protocol consisting of a deep inflation followed by ventilation at zero PEEP with V_t = 0.25 ml during which elastance was measured every 20 s). This 21 min protocol was repeated continuously for 4 h or until the animal died. The way that the lungs derecruit over time during the derecruitment test is reflected in the way that H increases with time (Allen and Bates, 2004). Finally, the resulting estimations of D_{rate} from the derecruitability tests were fitted to Eq. 15, and the 95% joint confidence regions for s_m and k were determined as described by Mori et al. (2018).

It should be pointed out that we also measured parameters related to the resistance of both the conducting airways and the respiratory system tissues in these mice. We focus here exclusively on the elastance parameter H in our model because it scales inversely with the fraction of lung that remains open, provided intrinsic tissue stiffness does not change, thus serving as a convenient biomarker of derecruitment. Lung tissue resistance scales similarly to elastance (Smith et al., 2020) and therefore adds no new information, so we did not include it in our model. Airway resistance tends to correlate less well with lung derecruitment because the proximal branches of the airway tree, which contribute much to airway resistance, mostly remain patent even when significant portions of the lung periphery derecruit (Smith et al., 2020).

Model Fitting

The model described by Eq. 9 was fit to the elastance data versus time collected within each derecruitment maneuver with MATLAB (The Mathworks, Natick, MA, United States) using a non-linear least squares method (trust-region algorithm) for each animal individually in all 4 groups, resulting in a pair of values of s_m and k for each animal. The maximum number of evaluations and iterations were set to 600 and 400, respectively, and the termination tolerance value of the cost function (mean squared residual) was 10^{-6}. Finally, the 95% joint confidence regions for s_m and k were determined as described by Mori et al. (2018).

RESULTS

Figure 1 shows the fits of Eq. 9 to experimental data from four groups of over-ventilated mice (V_t = 1.0, 1.1, 1.2, and 1.3 ml, with zero PEEP), together with the experimental data. The model fits pass within one standard error either side of the data points in most cases, and are very close to these ranges in the other cases. The R^2 values for all fits were greater than 0.85. This demonstrates that the model accurately accounts for the way that injury, as reflected by H, accelerates over time and how this acceleration increases with increasing V_t.

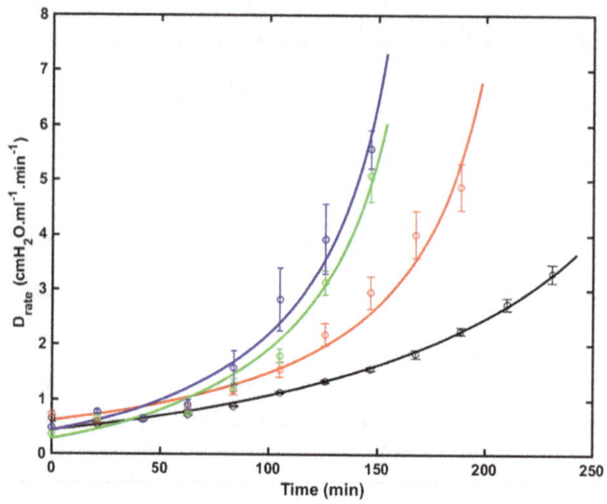

FIGURE 1 | D_{rate} (average ± SE) versus time as VILI developed in the 4 groups of mice (symbols) together with the model fits to Eq. 9 (lines). Black: V_t = 1.0 ml (RMSE = 0.35); Red: V_t = 1.1 ml (RMSE = 0.64); Green: V_t = 1.2 ml (RMSE = 0.36); Blue: V_t = 1.3 ml (RMSE = 0.65). The data were collected in a previous study (Smith et al., 2013) (RMSE – root mean squared residual.).

Figure 2 shows the two model parameters in Eq. 9, s_m and k, versus V_t. There was no dependence of s_m on V_t by ANOVA (p = 0.11, **Figure 2A**), whereas k was significantly greater for the lungs exposed to the two higher V_t compared to the two lower V_t ($p < 0.001$, **Figure 2B**). Normality of the distributions of all parameter groups was supported by the Shapiro-Wilk test ($p > 0.05$). The Bonferroni *post hoc* test was performed to assess inter-groups differences for k. All statistical tests were performed in MATLAB 2019b (The Mathworks, Natick, MA, United States).

The joint 95% confidence intervals show clean separation between the parameter pairs for the four groups of mice (**Figure 3**).

Figure 4 shows plots of $D_{rate}(t)$ versus H_1 for all animals studied. Also shown are the model predictions of $D_{rate}(t)$ from Eq. 9 versus H_1 calculated according to Mori et al. (2018). Lastly, **Figure 5** shows, in a Bland-Altman plot, the difference between modeled and measured D_{rate} values as a function of H_1.

DISCUSSION

We have developed an analytical model of the time-course of derecruitment in the injured lung that mimics observations of how lung derecruitability evolves during the development of VILI. This analytical model is based on our previous numerical approach of ascribing recruitment and derecruitment dynamics

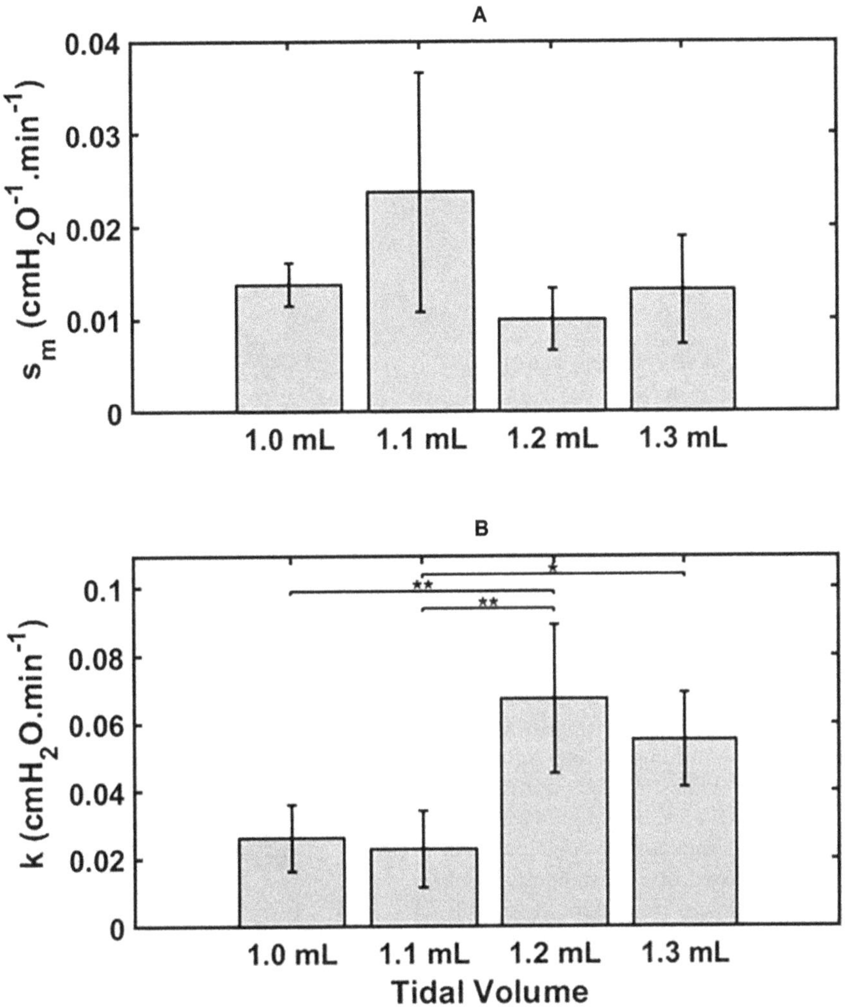

FIGURE 2 | Mean ± 2 SEM for the two key model parameters s_m **(A)** and k **(B)** and for the 4 groups, 1.0 ml (n = 6), 1.1 ml (n = 6), 1.2 ml (n = 5) and 1.3 ml (n = 4). Statistically significant differences between groups are indicated by: $^*P < 0.05$), $^{**}P < 0.01$.

to the behavior of a virtual trajectory associated with various lung units (Bates and Irvin, 2002; Massa et al., 2008). This model uses a similar analytic approach to our recent study that examined how H measured immediately after a recruitment maneuver (H_1) increases as a function of worsening lung injury (Mori et al., 2018). In this sense, the present study complements our previous model analysis since together they provide a complete analytic description of how a deep inflation of the injured lung recruits closed lung units and then how these units derecruit again over time as governed by the values of the three fixed parameters α, s_m, and k, where α and k depend on V_t. The model of the present study accurately predicts the manner in which the temporal evolution of D_{rate} varies with both time and injurious V_t (**Figure 1**), dependencies that are embodied in a single parameter, k, thought to largely reflect how surface tension increases with time (**Figure 2**). Surface tension elevation is a consequence of surfactant dysfunction, itself caused either by direct damage to the surfactant or by the presence of material that has leaked from the vasculature into the airspaces of the lung. H can also increase as a result of accumulated fluid that floods alveoli. This model thus links developments in physical injury of the parenchyma tissue to the dynamics of lung function derangement via the physiologic mechanism of airspace derecruitment.

Analytical models generally do not have the same flexibility as numerical models to describe the complex details of experimental data. On the other hand, when the model equations are based on putative underlying mechanisms, as in the present case, analytical models may offer insight of a general nature that more empirical nature of numerical models cannot. In this regard, the model in the present study supports the suitability of a power-law function as describing the velocity distribution along virtual trajectories (Eq. 4). The parameter s_m sets the minimum closing velocity, which corresponds to those units that close so slowly they remain open throughout the entire derecruitability test. It is possible that these units would eventually close if the derecruitability tested lasted long

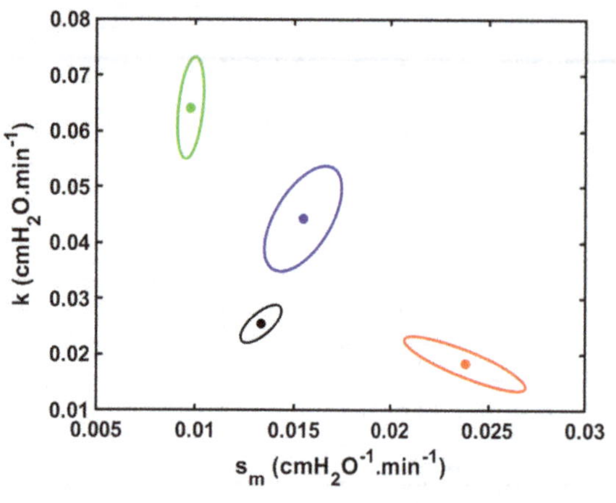

FIGURE 3 | Joint paired 95% confidence regions for the model parameters. The optimum parameter values (those that minimize the root mean squared difference between measured and modeled D_{rate}) are located at the centers of the ellipses. Black: V_t = 1.0 ml; Red: V_t = 1.1 ml; Green: V_t = 1.2 ml; Blue: V_t = 1.3 ml.

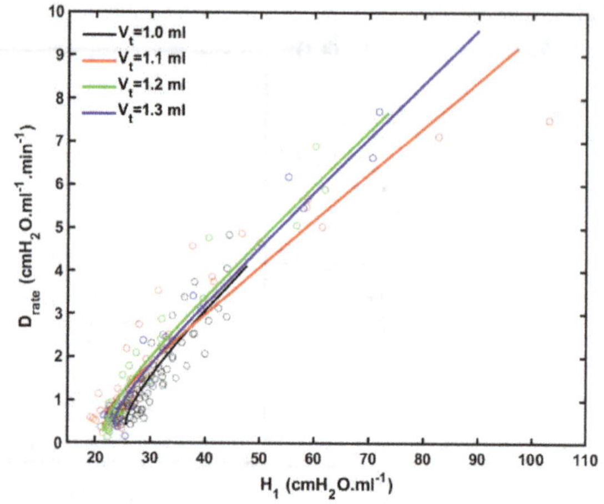

FIGURE 4 | Rate of change of lung stiffness (D_{rate}) versus initial measurement of post-recruitment stiffness (H_1) measured in the 4 groups of mice (symbols) together with the model fits (lines). Black: V_t = 1.0 ml; Red: V_t = 1.1 ml; Green: V_t = 1.2 ml; Blue: V_t = 1.3 ml.

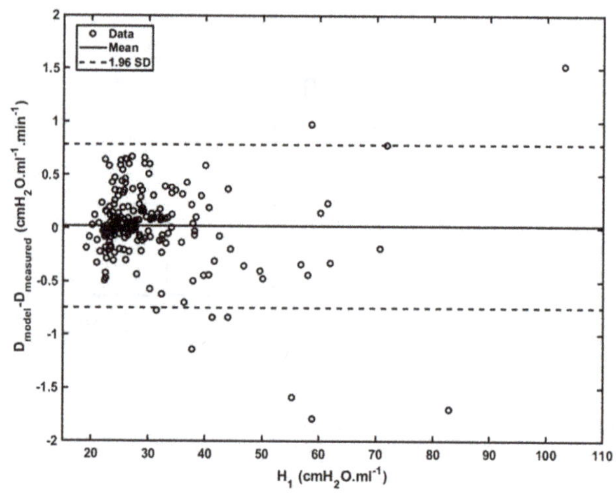

FIGURE 5 | Difference between modeled and measured D_{rate} as a function of H_1 (open dots). Mean is represented by the full line whereas 95% interval (± 1.96 SD) is represented by dashed lines.

enough, but they make no contribution to the data when the tests last only 3 min. Interestingly, the exponent of the power law was found to be −2 purely on the basis of the empirically observed linear increase in lung stiffness following a recruitment maneuver at zero PEEP. In other words, this exponent value comes from the qualitative behavior of the data rather than the fit of a particular model. This is significant because power laws have been invoked in a previous model of lung recruitment during lung inflation to account for avalanches of sequential opening events along the airway tree that are triggered when critical opening pressures are surpassed (Suki et al., 1994, 2000). Moreover, both inter-crackle intervals and terminal air space sizes that are linked by avalanches throughout the airway tree are characterized by power-law distributions having an exponent of −2 (Suki et al., 2000; Alencar et al., 2001). The similarity between the probability distribution for s_c and these other avalanche-based mechanisms in the lung might not be a coincidence, but rather might follow in some way from the fractal branching structure of the airway tree. Thus, although our model consists of a parallel collection of respiratory units that cannot open in the kinds of cascades observed in the airway tree (Suki, 2002), the fractal structure of the lung is embedded in our model through the power-law form of the distribution of s_c (Eq. 4) and thus conforms to previous work by Suki et al. (1994, 2000), Alencar et al. (2001), and Suki (2002).

Having the geometry of the airway tree be implicit in our model in the functional form for s_c could also explain the findings of Massa et al. (2008) that $f_{s_o}(s_O)$ and $f_{s_c}(s_C)$ are unchanged following lung injury. That is, although lung injury would be expected to damage the alveolar parenchyma and the airway epithelium, there is no reason to suppose it would alter the branching structure of the airway tree, which would leave the functional form for s_c preserved. On the other hand, we do expect that injury would increase the mean values of the distributions for P_c and P_o (Eqs 2 and 3, respectively) on the basis of increases in surface tension at the air-liquid interface within the lungs as a result of blood-gas barrier perforation and the subsequent airspace accumulation of fluid and protein (Massa et al., 2008; Smith et al., 2013). This conveniently allows us to account for the progression of lung injury largely in terms of the evolution of the value of a single parameter, k in Eq. 9 (**Figures 2, 3**).

We previously reported an apparent master relationship between and D_{rate} and H_1 (Smith et al., 2013). The model developed in the present study, however, suggests this is not quite the case because rate of change of D_{rate} with injury (Eq. 10) is predicted to depend on k, which depends on V_t (**Figure 2B**), even though the initial value of D_{rate} (Eq. 10

of the **Supplementary Material**) does not (**Figure 2A**). On the other hand, the dependence of dD_{rate}/dH_0 on V_t is rather subtle (**Figure 4**), and is easily masked by noise in the data, so the notion of a single master relationship may still be a useful approximation. Also, both H_1 (Mori et al., 2018) and D_{rate} (**Figure 4**) exhibit exponential growth over the time-scale of our experiment (up to 4 h), but they are unlikely to continue to increase indefinitely beyond this point because this would correspond to derecruitment of the entire lung. Even if this was a possibility, however, forcing a sizeable V_t into an ever shrinking lung would eventually lead to pressures that would cause rupture of the tissues. In any case, it appears that neither eventually would ever be realized because the mice died when about 75% of the lung became derecruited, at which point H_1 and D_{rate} were still increasing exponentially.

Another feature of the relationship between D_{rate} and H_1 is the early transient seen in **Figure 4**, which shows that D_{rate} to begin to increase early in the development of lung injury before H_1 changes noticeably. We have previously postulated (Smith et al., 2013) that increases in D_{rate} are due to increases in surface tension that give rise to derecruitment dynamics manifesting over a timescale of minutes, while increases in H_1 reflect flooded alveoli that have become permanently derecruited. This being the case, the relationship between D_{rate} and H_1 in **Figure 4** suggests that surfactant deactivation by plasma-derived fluid and proteins starts to occur as soon as this material arrives in the airspaces whereas a certain volume of fluid as to accumulate in the airspaces before it can cause noticeable alveolar flooding. It also suggests that D_{rate} is more directly related to the "rich-get-richer" hypothesis of VILI that we have previously advanced (Hamlington et al., 2018a; Mori et al., 2018) and thus may be the more sensitive marker of the onset of lung injury. On the other hand, even though the model errors for D_{rate} do not appear to depend on H_1 (**Figure 5**), at large t, D_{rate}, and H_1 become linearly dependent on each other (Eq. 10) suggesting that both variables ultimately embody the same pathophysiological information, although the fits of the present study are not as good at this end of the data range compared to those of our previous study (Smith et al., 2013) which curve over and follow the data better. Regardless, both D_{rate} and H_1 are increased by fluid accumulation in the airspaces, so some kind of monotonic relationship between the two parameters is to be expected.

Our model has a number of limitations. For example, although we have characterized derecruitability of the lung in terms of only two parameters, H_1 and D_{rate}, the increase in H with time during a derecruitability test is only approximately linear in its early stages; eventually, H begins to plateau (Allen et al., 2002; Allen and Bates, 2004; Massa et al., 2008). Such a plateau is inevitable as only those lung units for which $P < P_c$ will eventually close as $\tau \to \infty$. D_{rate} is thus an empirical characterization of only part of a more complex relationship. We also neglected intra-breath variations in the pressures applied to the lungs by mechanical ventilation, as well as the way they depend on the degree of lung injury. We assumed a constant pressure for derecruitment in order to be able to solve the model equations analytically (Eq. 7) and so gain the benefits of insight that a closed-form solution provides. In reality of course, these pressures are not constant because mean airway pressure rises for a given V_t as the lung becomes progressively more consolidated, so more quantitatively accurate predictions would require the numerical solution of a computational model in which airway pressures are allowed to vary in a realistic manner. This may partly explain why the ellipse areas of the joint parameter confidence regions in **Figure 3** tend to be greater for larger V_t (i.e., greater VILI); we would generally expect a simple analytical model to fit better to data from normal or mildly injured lungs compared to those that are severely injured. We also waived details concerning alveolar micromechanics such as interactions between neighboring respiratory units, although we recognize the potentially important role of such interactions in lung injury (Knudsen and Ochs, 2018). Finally, we have assumed that the dynamics of derecruitability in the lung are accurate indicators of the degree of lung injury, but they are not direct measures of such. Nevertheless, numerous prior studies from our laboratory have established a tight link between derecruitability and direct measures of damage to the blood-gas barrier (Allen and Bates, 2004; Allen et al., 2005; Smith et al., 2017; Hamlington et al., 2018a,b).

In summary, we have developed an analytical version of our previously developed computational model of the dynamics of lung derecruitment following a recruitment maneuver. We found that the distribution of velocity constants defining rates of movement along the virtual trajectories associated with the pulmonary airways follows a power-law with the same exponent of −2 as found in other investigations into the dynamics of lung recruitment and derecruitment. We speculate that this may reflect the fractal-like structure of the airway tree throughout which recruitment and derecruitment may take place as cascades of open and closing events. Our study also suggests that the rate of change in lung stiffness represented by the parameter D_{rate}, to the extent that this remains constant during a 3 min derecruitability test, is a particularly sensitive marker of the degree of lung injury.

AUTHOR CONTRIBUTIONS

VM developed the model analysis, coded the simulations, and drafted the manuscript. BJS, BS, and JB contributed to the development of the model concept, checked the mathematics, and edited and approved the manuscript. All authors contributed to the article and approved the submitted version.

REFERENCES

Albert, S. P., Dirocco, J., Allen, G. B., Bates, J. H., Lafollette, R., Kubiak, B. D., et al. (2009). The role of time and pressure on alveolar recruitment. *J. Appl. Physiol.* 106, 757–765. doi: 10.1152/japplphysiol.90735.2008

Alencar, A. M., Buldyrev, S. V., Majumdar, A., Stanley, H. E., and Suki, B. (2001). Avalanche dynamics of crackle sound in the lung. *Phys. Rev. Lett.* 87: 088101.

Allen, G., and Bates, J. H. (2004). Dynamic mechanical consequences of deep inflation in mice depend on type and degree of lung injury. *J. Appl. Physiol.* 96, 293–300. doi: 10.1152/japplphysiol.00270.2003

Allen, G., Lundblad, L. K., Parsons, P., and Bates, J. H. (2002). Transient mechanical benefits of a deep inflation in the injured mouse lung. *J. Appl. Physiol.* 93, 1709–1715. doi: 10.1152/japplphysiol.00473.2002

Allen, G. B., Pavone, L. A., Dirocco, J. D., Bates, J. H., and Nieman, G. F. (2005). Pulmonary impedance and alveolar instability during injurious ventilation in rats. *J. Appl. Physiol.* 99, 723–730. doi: 10.1152/japplphysiol.01339.2004

Bates, J. H., and Irvin, C. G. (2002). Time dependence of recruitment and derecruitment in the lung: a theoretical model. *J. Appl. Physiol.* 93, 705–713. doi: 10.1152/japplphysiol.01274.2001

Dos Santos, C., and Slutsky, A. (2000). Invited review: mechanisms of ventilator-induced lung injury: a perspective. *J. Appl. Physiol.* 89, 1645–1655. doi: 10.1152/jappl.2000.89.4.1645

Dreyfuss, D., and Hubmayr, R. (2016). What the concept of VILI has taught us about ARDS management. *Intens. Care Med.* 42, 811–813. doi: 10.1007/s00134-016-4287-6

Dreyfuss, D., and Saumon, G. (1998). Ventilator-induced lung injury: lessons from experimental studies. *Am. J. Respir. Crit. Care Med.* 157, 294–323. doi: 10.1164/ajrccm.157.1.9604014

Gattinoni, L., Carlesso, E., Cadringher, P., Valenza, F., Vagginelli, F., and Chiumello, D. (2003). Physical and biological triggers of ventilator-induced lung injury and its prevention. *Eur. Respir. J.* 22, 15s–25s.

Gattinoni, L., Marini, J. J., Pesenti, A., Quintel, M., Mancebo, J., and Brochard, L. (2016). The "baby lung" became an adult. *Intens. Care Med.* 42, 663–673. doi: 10.1007/s00134-015-4200-8

Gattinoni, L., and Pesenti, A. (2006). "The concept of baby lung," in *Applied Physiology in Intensive Care Medicine*, (Berlin: Springer), 303–311. doi: 10.1007/3-540-37363-2_44

Hamlington, K. L., Bates, J. H., Roy, G. S., Julianelle, A. J., Charlebois, C., Suki, B., et al. (2018a). Alveolar leak develops by a rich-get-richer process in ventilator-induced lung injury. *PLoS One* 13:e0193934. doi: 10.1371/journal.pone.0193934

Hamlington, K. L., Smith, B. J., Dunn, C. M., Charlebois, C. M., Roy, G. S., and Bates, J. H. T. (2018b). Linking lung function to structural damage of alveolar epithelium in ventilator-induced lung injury. *Respir. Physiol. Neurobiol.* 255, 22–29. doi: 10.1016/j.resp.2018.05.004

Knudsen, L., and Ochs, M. (2018). The micromechanics of lung alveoli: structure and function of surfactant and tissue components. *J. Histochem. Cell Biol.* 150, 661–676. doi: 10.1007/s00418-018-1747-9

Massa, C. B., Allen, G. B., and Bates, J. H. (2008). Modeling the dynamics of recruitment and derecruitment in mice with acute lung injury. *J. Appl. Physiol.* 105, 1813–1821. doi: 10.1152/japplphysiol.90806.2008

Mori, V., Smith, B. J., Suki, B., and Bates, J. H. (2018). Linking physiological biomarkers of ventilator-induced lung injury to a rich-get-richer mechanism of injury progression. *Ann. Biomed. Eng.* 47, 638–645. doi: 10.1007/s10439-018-02165-1

Parker, J. C., Hernandez, L. A., and Peevy, K. J. (1993). Mechanisms of ventilator-induced lung injury. *Crit. Care Med.* 21, 131–143. doi: 10.3109/9781420019261-9

Robertson, H. T., Altemeier, W. A., and Glenny, R. W. (2000). Physiological implications of the fractal distribution of ventilation and perfusion in the lung. *Ann. Biomed. Eng.* 28, 1028–1031. doi: 10.1114/1.1310215

Schuessler, T. F., and Bates, J. H. (1995). A computer-controlled research ventilator for small animals: design and evaluation. *IEEE Trans. Biomed. Eng.* 42, 860–866. doi: 10.1109/10.412653

Seah, A. S., Grant, K. A., Aliyeva, M., Allen, G. B., and Bates, J. H. (2011). Quantifying the roles of tidal volume and PEEP in the pathogenesis of ventilator-induced lung injury. *Ann. Biomed. Eng.* 39, 1505–1516. doi: 10.1007/s10439-010-0237-6

Slutsky, A. S., and Ranieri, V. M. (2000). Mechanical ventilation: lessons from the ARDSNet trial. *Respirat. Res.* 1:2.

Slutsky, A. S., and Ranieri, V. M. (2013). Ventilator-induced lung injury. *New Engl. J. Med.* 369, 2126–2136.

Smith, B. J., Bartolak-Suki, E., Suki, B., Roy, G. S., Hamlington, K. L., Charlebois, C. M., et al. (2017). Linking ventilator injury-induced leak across the blood-gas barrier to derangements in murine lung function. *Front. Physiol.* 8:466. doi: 10.3389/fphys.2017.00466

Smith, B. J., and Bates, J. H. (2013). Assessing the progression of ventilator-induced lung injury in Mice. *IEEE Trans. Biomed. Eng.* 60, 3449–3457. doi: 10.1109/tbme.2013.2267151

Smith, B. J., Grant, K. A., and Bates, J. H. (2013). Linking the development of ventilator-induced injury to mechanical function in the lung. *Ann. Biomed. Eng.* 41, 527–536. doi: 10.1007/s10439-012-0693-2

Smith, B. J., Roy, G. S., Cleveland, A., Mattson, C., Okamura, K., Charlebois, C. M., et al. (2020). Three alveolar phenotypes govern lung function in murine ventilator-induced lung injury. *Front. Physiol.* 11:660. doi: 10.3389/fphys.2020.00660

Suki, B. (2002). Fluctuations and power laws in pulmonary physiology. *Am. J. Respirat. Crit. Care Med.* 166, 133–137. doi: 10.1164/rccm.200202-152pp

Suki, B., Alencar, A. M., Tolnai, J., Asztalos, T., Peták, F., Sujeer, M. K., et al. (2000). Size distribution of recruited alveolar volumes in airway reopening. *J. Appl. Physiol.* 89, 2030–2040. doi: 10.1152/jappl.2000.89.5.2030

Suki, B., Barabási, A.-L., Hantos, Z., Peták, F., and Stanley, H. E. (1994). Avalanches and power-law behaviour in lung inflation. *Nature* 368:615. doi: 10.1038/368615a0

West, B. J. (1990). Physiology in fractal dimensions: error tolerance. *Ann. Biomed. Eng.* 18, 135–149. doi: 10.1007/bf02368426

West, G. B., Brown, J. H., and Enquist, B. J. (2000). "The origin of universal scaling laws in biology," in *Scaling in Biology*, eds J. H. Brown and G. B. West (Oxford: Oxford University Press), 87–112.

5

Age-Related Structural and Functional Changes in the Mouse Lung

*Henri Schulte[1], Christian Mühlfeld[1,2,3] and Christina Brandenberger[1,2,3]**

[1] *Institute of Functional and Applied Anatomy, Hannover Medical School, Hanover, Germany,* [2] *Cluster of Excellence REBIRTH (From Regenerative Biology to Reconstructive Therapy), Hanover, Germany,* [3] *Biomedical Research in Endstage and Obstructive Lung Disease Hannover (BREATH), Member of the German Center for Lung Research (DZL), Hanover, Germany*

***Correspondence:**
Christina Brandenberger
brandenberger.christina@mh-hannover.de

Lung function declines with advancing age. To improve our understanding of the structure-function relationships leading to this decline, we investigated structural alterations in the lung and their impact on micromechanics and lung function in the aging mouse. Lung function analysis was performed in 3, 6, 12, 18, and 24 months old C57BL/6 mice (n = 7–8/age), followed by lung fixation and stereological sample preparation. Lung parenchymal volume, total, ductal and alveolar airspace volume, alveolar volume and number, septal volume, septal surface area and thickness were quantified by stereology as well as surfactant producing alveolar epithelial type II (ATII) cell volume and number. Parenchymal volume, total and ductal airspace volume increased in old (18 and 24 months) compared with middle-aged (6 and 12 months) and young (3 months) mice. While the alveolar number decreased from young (7.5×10^6) to middle-aged (6×10^6) and increased again in old (9×10^6) mice, the mean alveolar volume and mean septal surface area per alveolus conversely first increased in middle-aged and then declined in old mice. The ATII cell number increased from middle-aged (8.8×10^6) to old (11.8×10^6) mice, along with the alveolar number, resulting in a constant ratio of ATII cells per alveolus in all age groups (1.4 ATII cells per alveolus). Lung compliance and inspiratory capacity increased, whereas tissue elastance and tissue resistance decreased with age, showing greatest changes between young and middle-aged mice. In conclusion, alveolar size declined significantly in old mice concomitant with a widening of alveolar ducts and late alveolarization. These changes may partly explain the functional alterations during aging. Interestingly, despite age-related lung remodeling, the number of ATII cells per alveolus showed a tightly controlled relation in all age groups.

Keywords: pulmonary aging, micromechanics, stereology, late alveolarization, alveolar epithelial type II cells

INTRODUCTION

Lung aging is accompanied by functional, micromechanical and structural alterations (Chan and Welsh, 1998; Sharma and Goodwin, 2006; Pinkerton et al., 2014). In the elderly (>65 years of age), lung diseases like chronic obstructive pulmonary disease (COPD; Ito and Barnes, 2009; Provinciali et al., 2011), fibrosis/IPF (Raghu et al., 2006; Collard, 2010; Fell et al., 2010; Thannickal, 2013), cancer (Howlader et al., 2019) or acute respiratory distress syndrome (ARDS; Ely et al., 2002; Rubenfeld et al., 2005) occur more frequently and with greater severity than in younger individuals.

These pathologies are also associated with alterations in pulmonary structure and function. For better comprehension of pathological changes with age, it is therefore important to understand the changes of lung function, micromechanics, and structure during normal aging.

Lung function is described by parameters of physiological breathing (Becklake and Crapo, 1991; Pellegrino et al., 2005) that were observed to decline in the elderly (Janssens et al., 1999). For example, studies have shown an increased residual volume (RV) and functional reserve volume (FRV), as well as decreased values of forced expiratory volume in one second (FEV1) in elderly individuals (Kerstjens et al., 1997; Janssens et al., 1999; Turner et al., 2017). Moreover, static lung compliance was found to increase with age (Wahba, 1983; Levitzky, 1984). These changes lead to increased respiratory impairment in the elderly (Vaz Fragoso and Gill, 2012). The mechanical properties of the lung tissue that influence lung function are described by different parameters, such as lung stiffness and elastance (Suki et al., 2011; Suki, 2014; Suki and Bartolák-Suki, 2014). Investigations on age-related changes in lung micromechanics have shown that the elastic recoil pressure decreases in the elderly (Janssens et al., 1999; Turner et al., 2017), possibly due to changes in tissue composition and remodeling (Mercer and Crapo, 1990; Toshima et al., 2004; Subramaniam et al., 2017). Changes in micromechanics are furthermore closely related to structural alterations in the human lung. Structural remodeling and airspace enlargement in aging human lungs was shown qualitatively (D'Errico et al., 1989) as well as quantitatively, by estimation of mean linear intercept [L_m] (Verbeken et al., 1992a). In an MRI-based study with hyperpolarized ^3He gas, Quirk et al. (2016) further confirmed an increase of L_m as well as decreasing alveolar depth and larger alveolar ductal radius in aging human lungs. These findings show that lung function, micromechanics and structure are closely linked and age-dependent. However, most studies on lung function and micromechanics in humans are cross-sectional and non-invasive and cannot provide the informational quality as research conducted under controlled laboratory conditions. Furthermore, histological samples of healthy human lung tissue are difficult to obtain and often not suited for quantitative structural analysis by means of stereology (Hsia et al., 2010) due to inadequate sample preparation. Thus, studies investigating lung aging are frequently performed under controlled laboratory conditions in animal models to correlate functional and structural parameters in the lung (Zosky, 2015).

In mice, the assessment of lung function and micromechanics is often done by forced ventilation techniques and measurements of pressure-volume changes (Vanoirbeek et al., 2010; De Vleeschauwer et al., 2011; Robichaud et al., 2017). Previous studies on lung function over different time courses of maturation and aging provided evidence of an increased inspiratory capacity (IC) (including tidal volume and inspiratory reserve volume) or static lung compliance with age (Huang et al., 2007; Veldhuizen et al., 2019). Major changes in lung function were further found in early adulthood and to a lesser extent later in life (Zosky, 2015; Elliott et al., 2016). Micromechanically, elastic recoil pressure and airway resistance were shown to decrease with age in mice, whereas lung tissue stiffness tended to increase (Huang et al., 2007; Elliott et al., 2016; Veldhuizen et al., 2019).

Structural changes of the mouse lung with maturation and age included stereological quantification of parameters that are relevant for lung function such as lung volume, alveolar volume and number as well as septal surface area and thickness. However, results on structural changes with age are controversial. For example, Pozarska et al. (2017) found the highest alveolar numbers in 9 months old (mo) mice and biggest alveoli in 22 mo mice in an experimental study covering an age range of 2, 9, and 22 mo mice, whereas another study found no difference in alveolar number in 6 and 24 mo mice (Glassberg et al., 2014). Moreover, little is known about changes in parenchymal airspaces, alveolar septal surface area and volume in the course of aging. These parameters contribute to intact lung function and mechanics and changes may affect the integrity of the lung (Subramaniam et al., 2017; Knudsen and Ochs, 2018). At cellular level, alveolar epithelial type II (ATII) cells play an important role for intact lung function as they produce alveolar surface tension reducing surfactant to prevent alveolar collapsing during breathing (Bachofen and Schürch, 2001). However, no data is available on ATII cell number and size in pulmonary aging. Additionally, although structural investigation by design-based stereology is considered as the gold-standard for morphometric lung research (Hsia et al., 2010), little information is available linking lung functional and micromechanical measurements with profound stereological analyses of the aging mouse lung.

Thus, the aim of this study was to contribute to a comprehensive understanding of age-related structural changes in the mouse lung and linking the findings to functional and micromechanical parameters. As most investigations on lung aging are based on only two age groups (Glassberg et al., 2014; Kling et al., 2017; Veldhuizen et al., 2019), the understanding of gradual changes in lung aging is still limited. The present study investigated age-related changes in lung function, micromechanics and structure in male C57/BL6JRj mice aged 3, 6, 12, 18, or 24 months to provide a more comprehensive picture of the developmental process from young adulthood to later stages of life.

MATERIALS AND METHODS

Animal Model

Male C57BL/6JRj mice were ordered from Janvier Labs (France) at an age of 3, 6, 12, 18, or 24 months, including 7–8 animals per age group. Before experimental start the animals were allowed to acclimate for 1 week at the local housing facility (Zentrales Tierlaboratorium, Hannover Medical School) with food and water *ad libitum*. The experiments included lung function measurements and quantitative light microscopic analysis (stereology) of the lung. Animal procedures were authorized by the responsible authorities at LAVES (Niedersächsisches Landesamt für Verbraucherschutz und Lebensmittelsicherheit) and are in accordance with the German law for animal protection

(TierSchG; BGBl. I, p. 1206 with corr. on p. 1313) and with the European directive, 2010/63/EU.

Lung Function and Micromechanics Measurements

Before lung function testing, mice were injected with 80 mg/kg body weight ketamine (Anesketin 100 mg/ml, Eurovet Animal Health B.V.) and 5 mg/kg body weight xylazine (Rompun 2%, Bayer Vital GmbH) intraperitoneally. Under deep anesthesia, tracheotomy was performed and the animals were ventilated by a mechanical ventilation system (flexiVent® FX Module 1 for mice, SCIREQ® Scientific Respiratory Equipment Inc.) at 100 breaths/min and a tidal volume of 10 ml/kg body weight. To suppress spontaneous breathing during lung function measurements, the mice received 0.8 mg/kg body weight pancuronium bromide (Pancuronium-Actavis 2 mg/ml, Actavis GmbH) intraperitoneally. Lung function measurements were taken at a constant positive end-expiratory pressure (PEEP) of 3 cmH_2O after two recruitment maneuvers. In a different set of animals aged 3, 6, or 18 months ($n = 7$/age), derecruitability maneuvers were performed with increasing PEEPs of 1, 3, 6, and 10 cmH_2O. The aim of this experiment was to test for age differences in micromechanical behavior under non-physiological conditions. Static compliance (Cst) was computed by the Salazar-Knowles equation (Salazar and Knowles, 1964). Micromechanical parameters such as tissue resistance (G) and tissue elastance (H) were assessed by forced oscillations following an established protocol (Lutz et al., 2015; Lopez-Rodriguez et al., 2016). Tissue hysteresivity (η) was computed as the ratio of G/H and hysteresis was calculated as the area between the inflation and deflation limbs of the pressure-volume curve.

Lung Fixation and Sample Preparation

After lung function measurements mice were killed and the lungs were fixed by tracheal instillation at a pressure of 20 cmH_2O with aldehyde fixative, containing 1.5% paraformaldehyde (Sigma-Aldrich) and 1.5% glutaraldehyde (Sigma-Aldrich) in 0.15 M HEPES buffer (Merck Millipore). Afterward the heart–lungs-package was excised from the body and stored in the fixative for at least 24 h. Lung volume [V(lung)] was estimated using the Archimedes principle (Scherle, 1970; Schneider and Ochs, 2013). After lung volume measurements, lungs were consecutively sectioned into slices. Every other slice was embedded in glycol methacrylate (Technovit® 7100, Kulzer GmbH), while the remaining samples were subsampled and embedded in epoxy resin (Glycid ether 100 for electron microscopy, SERVA Electrophoresis GmbH). Both embedding protocols were conducted as previously described in detail (Schneider and Ochs, 2014).

From the glycol methacrylate embedded samples 1.5 μm thick sections were cut and stained with toluidine blue (Toluidinblau O, C.I. 52040, Carl Roth GmbH) and eosin-orcein (Eosin G, C.I. 45380, Sigma-Aldrich and Orcein, C.I. Natural Red 28, Sigma-Aldrich), respectively. From the epoxy resin embedded samples sections with a thickness of 1 μm were cut and stained with toluidine blue.

Design-Based Stereology

Design-based stereology is the gold standard for quantitative morphometric analyses of the lung due to its accuracy, efficiency, and precision (Hsia et al., 2010) and was applied throughout the entire study. The investigator was blinded to the group identity of the samples during the analysis. The tissue slides were digitalized with a light-microscopic slide scanner (AxioScan.Z1, Carl Zeiss Microscopy GmbH). Systematic uniform random sampling (SURS) (Gundersen and Jensen, 1987; Gundersen et al., 1999; Nyengaard and Gundersen, 2006; Hsia et al., 2010) for stereological analysis was performed with the newCAST™ software (version 5.3.1.1640, Visiopharm®). The following parameters were estimated by stereology: volumes of lung parenchyma, non-parenchyma, septum, parenchymal airspace, alveolar airspace, and ductal airspace. Moreover, septal surface area, number of alveoli, and number and volume of ATII cells were quantified as previously described in detail (Brandenberger et al., 2015).

The estimation of the parenchymal lung volume [V(par,lung)] and non-parenchymal lung volume [V(non-par,lung)] was done by point counting on toluidine blue stained, glycol methacrylate embedded sections. SURS was performed with the Visiopharm® software at a magnification of 5× and a sampling fraction of 15–25%. Sampling fractions were dependent on the size of the embedded lung sections and kept constant within one animal. A stereological test grid with 36 sampling points was used (**Supplementary Figure 1A**). Calculation was done by multiplication of the volume density [V_V(par/lung)] with the total lung volume [V(lung)] as shown in Eq. 1:

$$V(\text{par,lung}) = \sum P(\text{par}) / \sum P(\text{tot}) \cdot V(\text{lung}) \qquad (1)$$

While $\Sigma P(\text{tot})$ represents all points falling on lung tissue, $\Sigma P(\text{par})$ represents the points on parenchymal tissue. Corresponding calculations were performed for non-parenchymal volume estimation.

Total parenchymal airspace volume [V(airtot,par)], septal volume [V(sept,par)], total septal surface area [S(sept,par)] and mean septal thickness [$\bar{\tau}$(sept)] were quantified on toluidine blue stained, glycol methacrylate embedded sections, scanned with an objective lens magnification of 20×. SURS was performed at sampling fractions of 1.25 to 3.5% per animal using a 20× magnification. The stereological test system contained 12 test lines with 24 test points and a length per point [l/p] of 9.4 μm (**Supplementary Figure 1B**). Point counting was applied to estimate septal volume density [V_V(sept/par)] and total parenchymal airspace volume density [V_V(airtot/par)]. Septal volume [V(sept,par)] and total airspace volume [V(airtot,par)] were achieved by multiplying the respective volume densities with V(par,lung).

The septal surface density [S_V(sept/par)] was estimated by counting intersections (I) of test lines with the septal surface. S(sept,par) was calculated by multiplying S_V(sept/par) with the reference volume as described previously (Weibel, 1979; Cruz-Orive and Weibel, 1990; Mayhew, 1991; Howard and Reed, 1998; Schneider and Ochs, 2013) and shown in Eq. 2:

$$\mathrm{S(sept,par)} = 2 \cdot \sum \mathrm{I(sept)}/(\mathrm{l/p} \cdot \sum \mathrm{P(tot)}) \cdot \mathrm{V(par,lung)} \quad (2)$$

Last, the septal thickness [$\bar{\tau}$(sept)] was calculated as shown in Eq. 3:

$$\bar{\tau}\mathrm{(sept)} = 2 \cdot \mathrm{V_V(sept/par)}/\mathrm{S_V(sept/par)} \quad (3)$$

To distinguish alveolar airspace [V(airalv,par)] and ductal airspace [V(airduct,par)], a further investigation was done on toluidine blue stained, glycol methacrylate embedded sections scanned with an objective lens magnification of 20×. SURS was performed at a sampling fraction of 2.5–6% per animal and a magnification of 10×. The stereological test grid contained 36 points (**Supplementary Figure 1C**). Calculations of ductal volume density [V_V(airduct,par)] and volume V(airduct,par) were done analogously to parenchymal volume estimations, as shown in Eq. 1. The alveolar airspace volume [V(airalv,par)] was calculated by subtraction of V(airduct,par) from V(airtot,par).

For the unbiased estimation of alveolar number [N(alv,par)] and ATII cell number [N(ATII,par)], the physical disector was used (Sterio, 1983; Ochs, 2006). This method allows the estimation of numbers in a test volume by creating a 3D test system from two planar and parallel cut sections. An unbiased counting frame was used for number estimations (Gundersen, 1977).

Alveoli are assumed to have one entrance to alveolar ducts which is enclosed by a ring of elastin fibers (Mercer and Crapo, 1990; Toshima et al., 2004; Meyerholz et al., 2017). The number of alveoli can be estimated by the Euler number, which describes the connectivity of the alveolar network (Hyde et al., 2004; Ochs et al., 2004). In principle, three topological events are possible to describe a network: bridges, islands, and holes. In the case of alveoli, the Euler number can be reduced to bridges as the other topological items occur very rarely (islands) or never (holes) (Gundersen et al., 1993). Thus, a counting event was the appearance of a closed alveolar elastin "bridge" [B(alv)] on one section and two elastin tips (=open alveolar entrance ring) on the other section. For this analysis, glycol methacrylate embedded and eosin-orcein stained sections of two serial tissue sections with a disector height [h] of 3 μm were used (Ochs, 2006). This staining dyes elastin fibers in red-brown and thereby improves the visualization of bridges (Ochs, 2006). The slices were scanned with an objective lens magnification of 20× and further processed via SURS at a magnification of 20×. Sampling fractions of 2–4.75% per animal were used. The area of the counting frame [A] was 35,570 μm^2 (**Supplementary Figures 2A,B**). Parenchymal reference space was measured using point counting [P(par)] on the lower left and upper right corners of the reference section. To increase efficiency, counting was applied in both directions of the image pair. Alveolar number was calculated by multiplying alveolar number density [N_V(alv/par)] by the reference volume as shown in Eq. 4:

$$\mathrm{N(alv,par)} = \sum \mathrm{B(alv)}/(\sum \mathrm{P(par)} \cdot \mathrm{A} \cdot \mathrm{h}) \cdot \mathrm{V(par,lung)} \quad (4)$$

The number-weighted mean alveolar volume [$\bar{v}_N$(alv)] was calculated as in Eq. 5:

$$\bar{v}_\mathrm{N}\mathrm{(alv)} = \mathrm{V(airalv,par)}/\mathrm{N(alv,par)} \quad (5)$$

just like the number-weighted mean alveolar septal surface area [$\overline{\mathrm{S(sept)/N(alv)}}$].

For the quantification of ATII cell numbers, nuclei of ATII cells [N(ATII)] were counted for the disector analysis as unique counting events per cell. Cells were counted, if their nucleus only appeared on one section of the disector image pair. Toluidine blue stained tissue sections of epoxy resin embedded samples were cut with a disector height [h] of 3 μm. Slices were scanned with an objective lens magnification of 40× and further processed via SURS at a magnification of 40×. Approximately 180 image pairs per animal (60 per slice) were generated and evaluated. The area of the counting frame [A] was 12,000 μm^2 (**Supplementary Figures 2C,D**). The number of ATII cells [N(ATII,par)] was calculated by multiplication of the ATII cell number density [N_V(ATII/par)] by the reference volume, as shown in Eq. 6:

$$\mathrm{N(ATII,par)} = \sum \mathrm{N(ATII)}/(\sum \mathrm{P(par)} \cdot \mathrm{A} \cdot \mathrm{h}) \cdot \mathrm{V(par,lung)} \quad (6)$$

Simultaneously, the number-weighted mean volume of ATII cells [$\bar{v}_N$(ATII)] was estimated using the planar rotator (Vedel-Jensen and Gundersen, 1993). Only cells sampled within the disector pairs were subjected to the rotator, using the nucleus as reference point. From the individual estimations, the arithmetic mean was calculated to obtain the number-weighted mean volume of the cells.

Statistical Analysis

All statistical analyses were performed using SigmaPlot® software, version 13.0.0.83 (SYSTAT® Software Inc.). Data were tested for normality by Shapiro–Wilk test and for equal variance by Brown-Forsythe test. If the data passed both tests, a one-way ANOVA was performed with a pairwise comparison by Bonferroni's *t*-test. If the equal variance or normality test failed, data were ln transformed and a one-way ANOVA was performed afterward. For lung function measurements with increasing PEEPs, a repeated measures ANOVA with Bonferroni *t*-test was applied. No outlier tests were performed and no data were excluded from the study. Differences were regarded as significant if $p < 0.05$.

RESULTS

Lung Function and Micromechanics Change Greatest in Early Mouse Adulthood

The greatest changes in lung function such as inspiratory capacity (IC) and static compliance (Cst) were observed in the early period of adulthood, between young (3 mo) and middle-aged (6 and 12 mo) mice. Both, IC and Cst increased by 25% from 3 to 6 mo mice and reached their maximum values at 18 months (**Figures 1A,B**). However, body weight also increased with age, showing biggest changes between young and middle-aged mice (**Table 1**) and therefore, Cst and IC per body weight remained quite stable in the course of aging (**Figures 1C,D**). Only a small but significant increase in IC per body weight was found between 3 and 12 mo mice. Tissue resistance (G) and tissue elastance (H) decreased significantly from 3 to 6 months by 21 and 27%, respectively (**Figures 1E,F**), but no significant changes were found between middle-aged and old (18 and 24 mo) mice. Hysteresivity (η) showed no significant changes during aging (**Figure 1G**), whereas hysteresis increased significantly from 3 and 6 to 18 mo mice by approximately 50% (**Figure 1H**). All lung function measurement data are further displayed in **Supplementary Table 1**. Results of lung function measurements with increasing PEEPs of 1, 3, 6, and 10 cmH_2O did not provide any further insights in age-related changes in micromechanics (**Supplementary Figure 3**).

Lung Parenchyma: Widening of Alveolar Ducts in Old Mice

Pulmonary histology of lung tissue revealed a normal lung parenchyma with absence of any pathological findings such as inflammation or fibrosis. Lung parenchyma from young and middle-aged mice appeared compact with many collateral alveoli surrounding narrow alveolar ducts (**Figures 2A–C**), whereas parenchyma of old mice appeared less densely packed due to wider alveolar ducts (**Figures 2D,E**). Stereological quantification revealed that lung volume, parenchymal volume as well as the volume of the parenchymal airspace increased approximately one third from middle-aged to old mice (**Figures 2F–H**), while the volume densities of these parameters remained almost constant (**Table 1**). The increase in the volume of the parenchymal airspace during aging was mainly driven by an increase in ductal airspace volume that occurred between 12 (249 mm^3) and 18 mo (460 mm^3) mice (**Figure 2I**), whereas the volume of the alveolar airspace just increased by 16% (**Figure 2J**). While the volume density of septal tissue remained constant in all age groups, the total septal volume increased from young to old mice (**Table 1**). Notably, no significant changes in total parenchymal, ductal and alveolar airspace volumes were measured between 18 and 24 mo mice.

Increasing Number and Decreasing Size of Alveoli in Old Mice

Histology of alveolar structures showed small and densely packed alveoli in young mice (**Figure 3A**), while the alveoli in middle-aged and old mice were more distended (**Figures 3B–E**). In eosin-orcein stained sections alveolar openings can be well detected due to brown staining of elastin tips at the end of septal borders. The septa oriented toward the alveolar duct thereby appeared shorter in old mice in comparison with middle-aged and young mice (**Figures 3A–E**). Stereologically, the number density of alveoli showed greatest and significant changes between young and middle-aged mice, decreasing with age (**Figure 3F**). The absolute number of alveoli on the other hand first decreased from young to middle-aged mice and then increased from middle-aged to old mice by approximately 50% (**Figure 3G**). The total septal surface area increased significantly from young to middle-aged and to old (18 mo) mice (**Figure 3H**). However, the septal surface density declined significantly between middle-aged and old (24 mo) mice (**Table 1**). Accordingly, the mean septal surface area per alveolus was approximately one third bigger in middle-aged compared to young or old (24 mo) mice (**Figure 3I**). Similarly, the number-weighted mean alveolar volumes were biggest in middle-aged mice ($\sim$ 88,000 μm^3) and significantly smaller in young ($\sim$ 64,000 μm^3) or old ($\sim$ 69,000 μm^3) mice (**Figure 3J**). The mean septal thickness remained relatively constant over the time course of aging at around 3 μm (**Table 1**).

ATII Cell Number Density Remains Constant in Middle-Aged and Old Mice

Representative light micrographs of toluidine blue stained, epoxy resin embedded tissue sections with ATII cells are shown in **Figures 4A–E**. The ATII cells here are clearly distinguishable due to the metachromatic staining behavior of surfactant storing lamellar bodies. ATII cells were mostly localized in the "corners" of alveoli, near to branching septa and were part of the alveolar septum. Individual cell morphology at light microscopic level remained qualitatively uniform with age. In young mice (**Figure 4A**), the density of ATII cells was slightly higher compared to older mice (**Figures 4B–E**). This observation was also supported by stereological findings, as the number density of ATII cells was highest in 3 mo mice and significantly decreased with age, showing an approximately 20% lower density in old mice (**Figure 4F**). However, the absolute number of ATII cells increased from middle-aged (8.8×10^6) to old mice (11.7×10^6) (**Figure 4G**). Interestingly, the number of ATII cells per alveolus remained almost constant at a count of approximately 1.4 over the time course of aging (**Figure 4H**). The number of ATII cells per septal surface area declined from 3 to 12 months of age and increased again from 12 to 24 mo mice (**Figure 4I**). The mean volume of ATII cells, estimated by the planar rotator, stayed constant over lifetime at approximately 280 μm^3 (**Figure 4J**).

DISCUSSION

The aim of this study was to investigate lung aging with respect to structure and function. The results show detailed structural and functional alterations in the mouse lungs over a broad time course from young adult to old mice. In summary, changes in lung function [inspiratory capacity (IC) and static compliance Cst], micromechanics (tissue resistance G and tissue elastance H) and alveolar number and size were greatest in early adulthood

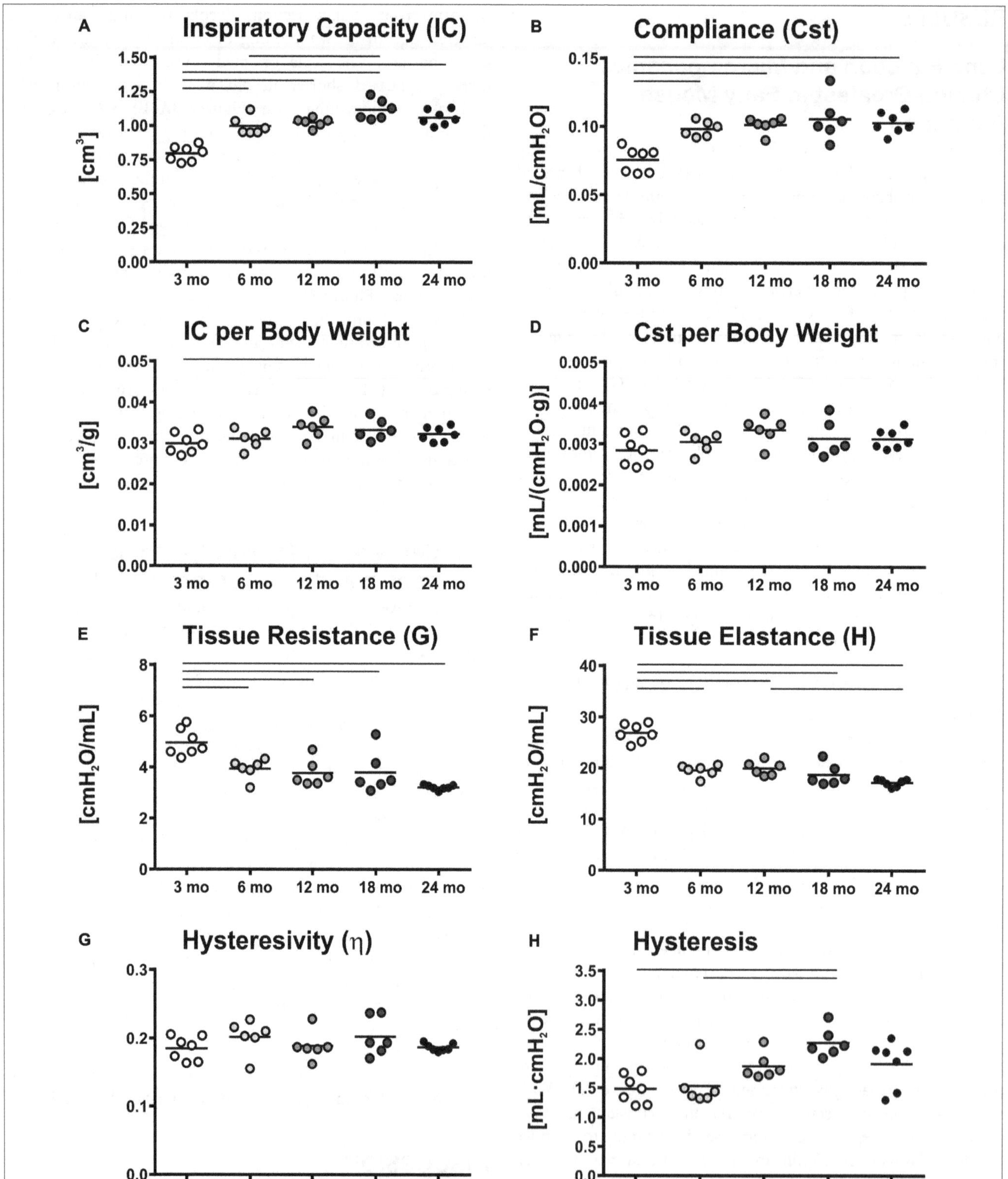

FIGURE 1 | Lung function and micromechanics. Inspiratory capacity (IC) **(A)** and static compliance (Cst) **(B)** showed significant increases from young to middle-aged and old mice, respectively. However, IC and Cst corrected for body weight remained rather constant over lifetime **(C,D)**. Tissue resistance (G) **(E)** and tissue elastance (H) **(F)** changed most in early mouse adulthood. Hysteresivity (η) remained constant during aging **(G)**, whereas hysteresis increased from 3 and 6 mo mice to 18 mo mice **(H)**. Each point represents one animal; bars show means and lines indicate statistically significant differences between age groups (one-way ANOVA with Bonferroni t-test, $p < 0.05$).

TABLE 1 | Data of body weight, lung volume, and stereological parameters regarding parenchymal volumes and alveolar septum.

Parameter	3 mo	6 mo	12 mo	18 mo	24 mo
m(body) [g]	26.7 (1.1)	32.4* (1.5)	29.9* (1.6)	33.8*‡ (3.0)	32.7* (2.0)
V(lung) [cm^3]	0.97 (0.12)	1.01 (0.07)	1.02 (0.05)	1.35*†‡ (0.14)	1.31*†‡ (0.07)
V(lung)/m(body) [10^{-2} cm^3/g]	3.65 (0.53)	3.13 (0.29)	3.42 (0.16)	4.04† (0.54)	4.01† (0.38)
V_V(par/lung)	0.873 (0.025)	0.856 (0.023)	0.839 (0.034)	0.878 (0.027)	0.855 (0.025)
V_V(non-par/lung)	0.120 (0.025)	0.139 (0.023)	0.156 (0.034)	0.116 (0.025)	0.140 (0.025)
V_V(other/lung)	0.0074 (0.0037)	0.0062 (0.0016)	0.0067 (0.0036)	0.0063 (0.0029)	0.0063 (0.0030)
V_V(airtot/par)	0.906 (0.013)	0.902 (0.012)	0.902 (0.011)	0.914 (0.008)	0.911 (0.012)
V_V(airduct/par)	0.344 (0.029)	0.296* (0.039)	0.291* (0.016)	0.386†‡ (0.034)	0.368†‡ (0.018)
V_V(sept/par)	0.094 (0.013)	0.098 (0.012)	0.098 (0.011)	0.086 (0.008)	0.089 (0.012)
V(par,lung) [mm^3]	847 (101)	865 (71)	858 (69)	1190*†‡ (130)	1119*†‡ (77)
V(non-par,lung) [mm^3]	117 (30)	140 (24)	158 (31)	157 (35)	182* (31)
V(airtot,par) [mm^3]	767 (88)	781 (71)	774 (67)	1087*†‡ (121)	1019*†‡ (73)
V(airduct,par) [mm^3]	292 (44)	257 (38)	249 (17)	460*†‡ (74)	413*†‡ (44)
V(airalv,par) [mm^3]	475 (55)	525 (59)	525 (55)	627*†‡ (66)	606* (34)
V(sept,par) [mm^3]	79.9 (16.7)	84.1 (6.5)	83.7 (8.1)	102.5* (13.7)	99.7* (13.7)
S_V(sept/par) [mm^{-1}]	63.8 (5.5)	65.0 (5.7)	66.6 (5.6)	59.7 (3.4)	56.1†‡ (6.4)
S(sept,par) [10^3 mm^2]	54.1 (8.7)	56.1 (5.6)	57.0 (5.4)	71.1*†‡ (10.1)	62.7 (7.8)
$\bar{\tau}$(sept) [μm]	2.94 (0.22)	3.01 (0.29)	2.95 (0.33)	2.89 (0.19)	3.19 (0.31)

*Data are expressed as mean (SD). *$p < 0.05$ for 3 mo vs. 6, 12, 18, 24 mo; †$p < 0.05$ for 6 mo vs. 12, 18, 24 mo; ‡$p < 0.05$ for 12 mo vs. 18, 24 mo.*

from 3 to 6 mo mice, whereas most other morphological parameters exhibited greatest alterations with progressing age in old mice. Particularly, the ductal airspace volume increased in old mice. Additionally, late alveolarization was observed as well as alveoli with shorter septa and a reduced alveolar depth. The number of ATII cells increased along with alveolar number in old mice.

Lung Function and Micromechanics in Aging Mice

Greatest changes of lung function and micromechanics were observed in the early adulthood, between 3 and 6 months of age. This has also been shown by others for BALB/c (Ranga et al., 1979) and C57BL/6 mice (Elliott et al., 2016). While Huang et al. suggested a linear decline (Huang et al., 2007), our data supported a non-linear change in lung function and micromechanics in aging C57BL/6 mice, similarly as also shown by Elliott et al. (2016). They observed greatest alterations in early adulthood between 2 and 6 months of age, including increases in IC and Cst by 36% and decreases of G and H by 38% and 34%, respectively, but little changes were observed later in life (Elliott et al., 2016). These findings are consistent with our data showing similar increases for IC (+25%), Cst (+30%), G (−21%), and H (−27%) between 3 and 6 mo mice. Additionally, an increase in hysteresis was found from young and middle-aged (6 mo) to old (18 mo) mice (**Figure 1H**). Similarly, increases in hysteresis were found in elastase-induced emphysematous mouse lungs (Brewer et al., 2003; Vanoirbeek et al., 2010; Robichaud et al., 2017). Hysteresis is mainly affected by surfactant and the properties of extracellular matrix (ECM) (Suki et al., 2011). Little is known regarding surfactant function in later life, but in a previous study a decrease in septal elastin fibers and an increase in septal collagen fibers were measured between young (3 months) and old (18 months) mice (Kling et al., 2017), most likely contributing to the changes in pulmonary micromechanics with age.

In humans, Sicard et al. (2018) estimated the elastic modulus in different anatomical regions of the lungs via atomic force microscopy and found age-related increases in the stiffness of lung parenchyma and vessels. Furthermore, in humans many lung function parameters such as FEV1, forced vital capacity (FVC) and vital capacity (VC) show a decline with age (Ware et al., 1990; Verbeken et al., 1992b; Janssens et al., 1999; Sharma and Goodwin, 2006), while static lung compliance increases in the elderly (Wahba, 1983; Levitzky, 1984). The inter-species translation of lung function and micromechanics measurements from mice to humans or vice versa is difficult because of the different analytical procedures (Miller et al., 2005; Lopez-Rodriguez et al., 2016). Nevertheless, it seems as lung micromechanics are similarly altered in humans and mice with age.

Structural Changes in the Lung Parenchyma With Progressing Age

Lung volumes increased with age, particularly in older mice (**Figure 2F**). This is in line with other studies in mice (Elliott et al., 2016; Pozarska et al., 2017). In humans, lung growth was reported to be mainly restricted to initial lung development and not occurring later in life (de Jong et al., 2006; Copley et al., 2009; Zach et al., 2012; Herring et al., 2014), except after hemi-pneumonectomy (Butler et al., 2012). This finding, however, suggests that lung growth can occur throughout lifetime.

Accompanied by an increase in lung volume in old mice, an enlargement of alveolar ducts was observed (**Figure 2I**). This has been described before in aging mammalian lungs. Beside qualitative observations (D'Errico et al., 1989; Kerr et al., 1990; Yamamoto et al., 2003; Glassberg et al., 2014), mean linear

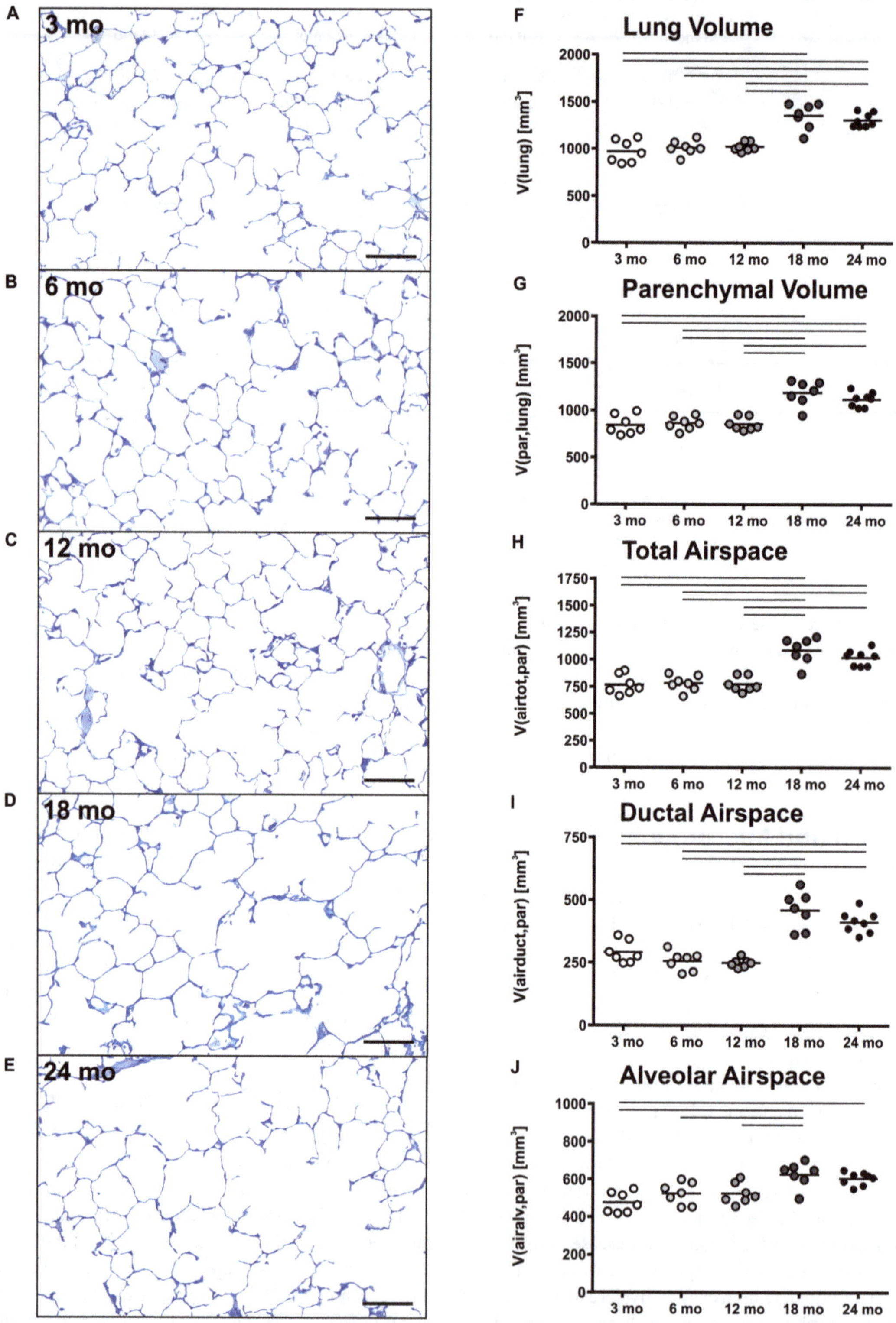

FIGURE 2 | Lung parenchymal airspace volumes. **(A–E)** Representative light micrographs of each age group stained with toluidine blue show pulmonary histology. No inflammation or fibrosis was observed qualitatively at any time point. The light micrographs of 3 **(A)**, 6 **(B)**, and 12 **(C)** mo mice show a compact, regular lung parenchyma, whereas the light micrographs of 18 **(D)** and 24 **(E)** mo mice reveal visible widening of alveolar ducts causing a less compact appearance of the parenchyma. Scale bar = 100 μm. **(F–J)** Graphs show lung volume **(F)** and stereological results of parenchymal volume **(G)**, total parenchymal airspace volume **(H)**, ductal airspace volume **(I)**, and alveolar airspace volume **(J)**. Each point represents one animal; bars show means and lines indicate statistically significant differences between age groups (one-way ANOVA with Bonferroni *t*-test, $p < 0.05$).

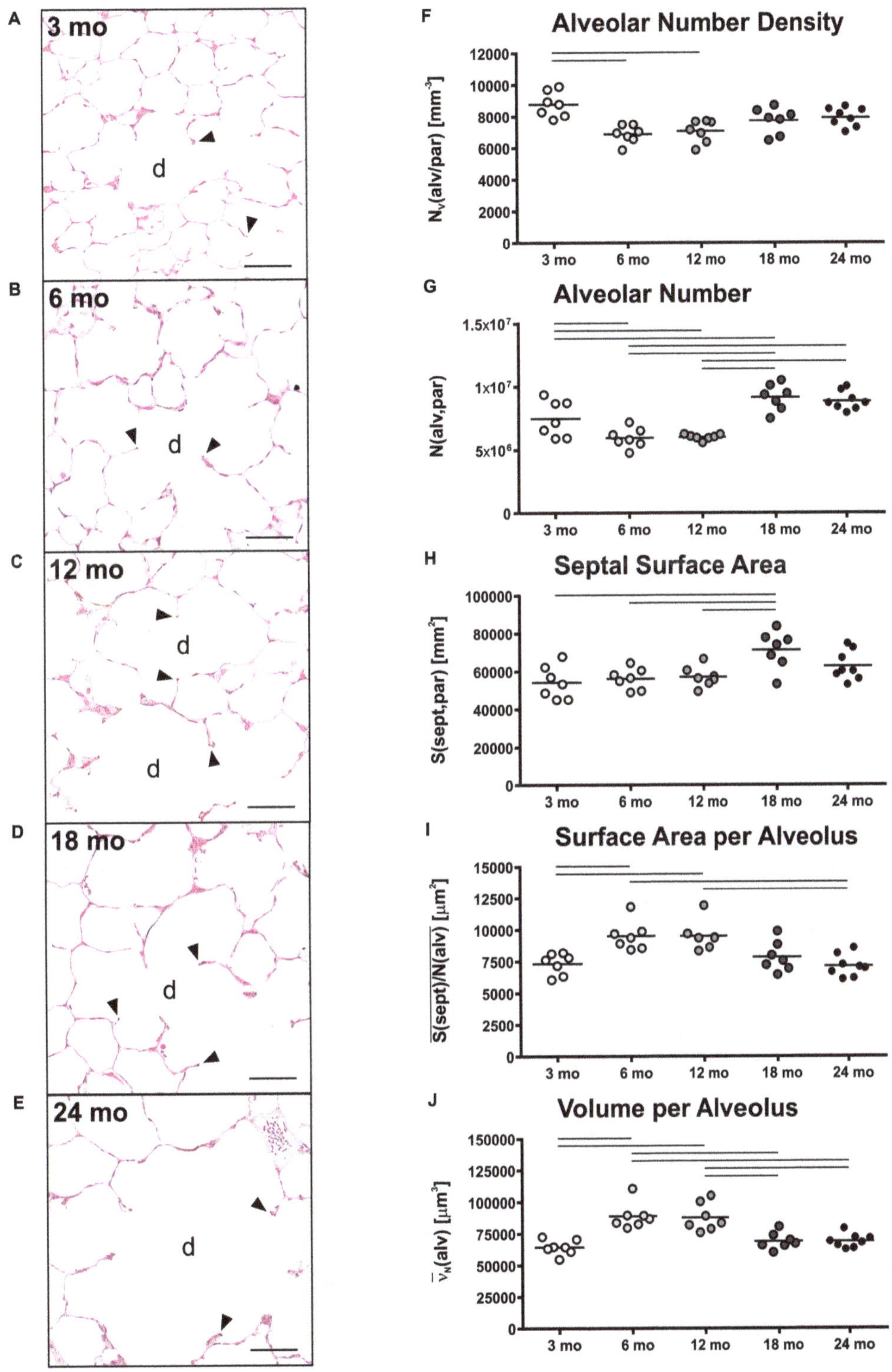

FIGURE 3 | Alveolar changes with age. **(A–E)** Representative light micrographs of each age group show pulmonary histology of eosin-orcein stained lungs. Arrowheads indicate alveolar septal border tips as part of the alveolar entrance ring. Septal border tips are dyed brown by orcein, demonstrating elastin accumulation around the alveolar entrances. Alveolar ducts are indicated by "d." At 3 months **(A)**, a high density of small alveoli and narrow alveolar ducts can be observed. The light micrographs of 6 **(B)** and 12 **(C)** mo mice show similar narrow alveolar ducts, but alveoli appear less dense. In 18 **(D)** and 24 **(E)** mo mice, the alveolar density seems to remain constant compared to middle-aged mice. The alveolar ducts, however, appear wider and alveolar septal borders seem to be shorter. Scale bar = 50 μm. **(F–J)** Graphs show stereological results of alveolar number density **(F)**, alveolar number **(G)**, total alveolar septal surface area **(H)**, mean septal surface area per alveolus **(I)**, and mean alveolar volume **(J)**. Each point represents one animal; bars show means and lines indicate statistically significant differences between age groups (one-way ANOVA with Bonferroni *t*-test, $p < 0.05$).

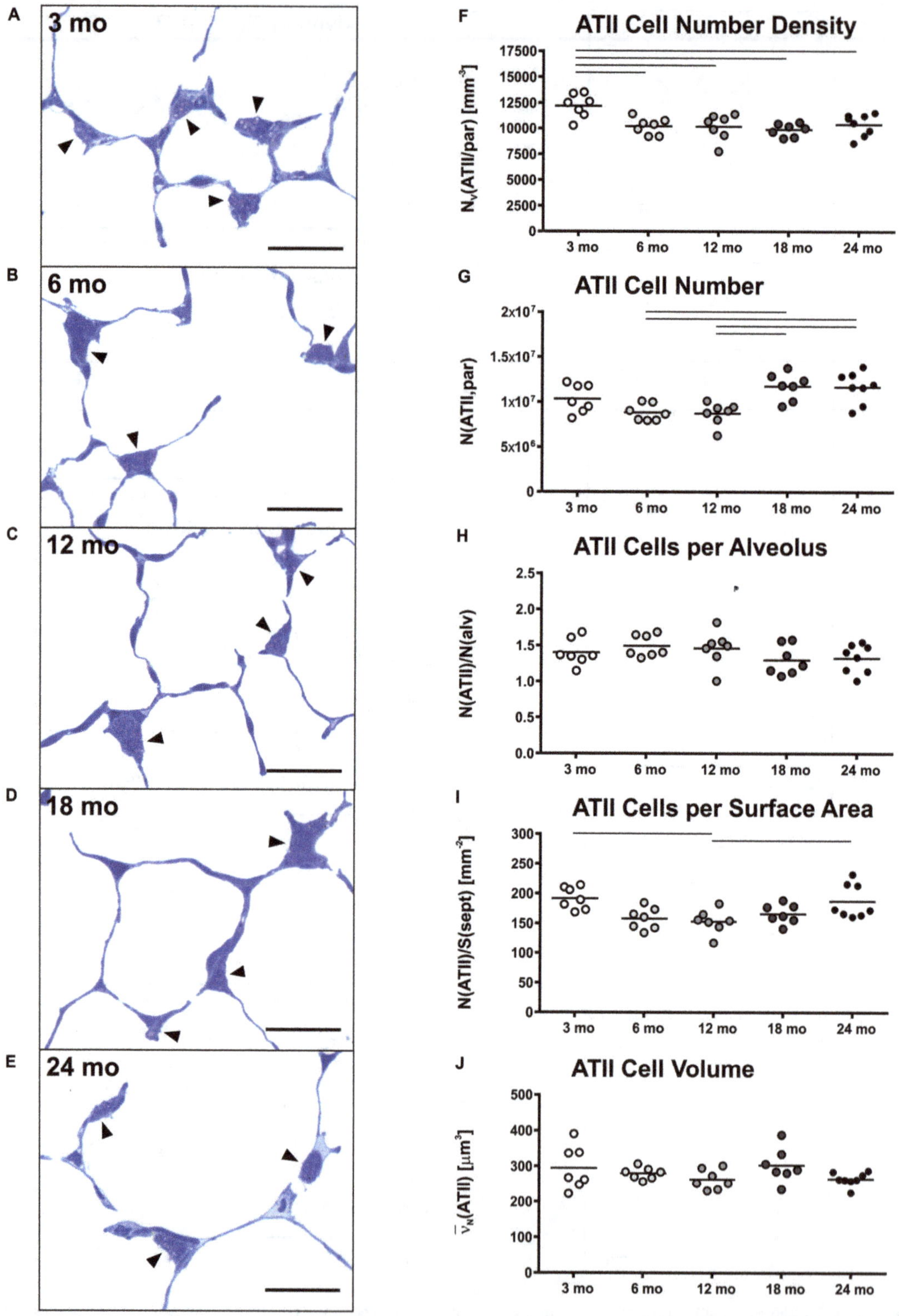

FIGURE 4 | Alveolar epithelial type II (ATII) cell characteristics. **(A–E)** Representative light micrographs of each age group show pulmonary histology. Tissue sections were stained with toluidine blue. Arrowheads indicate ATII cells, typically located in alveolar "corners". Intracellular lamellar bodies appear violet due to a metachromatic staining behavior. The ATII cells look quite homogeneous at any age in light microscopic images. However, the cell number density seems to be highest in 3 mo mice **(A)**. Scale bar = 20 µm. **(F–J)** Graphs show stereological results of ATII cell number density **(F)** and ATII cell number **(G)** as well as mean ATII cell number per alveolus **(H)**, mean ATII cell number per alveolar septal surface area **(I)**, and mean ATII cell volume **(J)**. Each point represents one animal; bars show means and lines indicate statistically significant differences between age groups (one-way ANOVA with Bonferroni *t*-test, $p < 0.05$).

intercept [L_m] is a frequently used parameter to estimate the mean chord length of the complete acinar airspace complex (Verbeken et al., 1992a; Huang et al., 2007; Elliott et al., 2016; Quirk et al., 2016). L_m is inversely related to S/V as $4/L_m$ and expresses the mean free length between two intersections of alveolar septal surface with an unbiased test line system of straight lines (Knudsen et al., 2010). Although this parameter is easy to assess, it cannot reflect different compartments of air-filled spaces. Furthermore, L_m is susceptible to bias as it does not consider shape and critically depends on the execution of lung inflation, lung volume measurement, and (unbiased) sampling procedures in histological studies, as reviewed in Weibel et al. (2007). Therefore, L_m cannot be stated as a sufficient parameter for parenchymal airspace alterations (Weibel et al., 2007; Mühlfeld and Ochs, 2013). Only with estimation of alveolar number and by differentiating between alveolar and ductal airspace, the correct and unbiased conclusions can be drawn on changes in alveolar size and ductal airspace (Mühlfeld and Ochs, 2013). Nevertheless, comparing our results of septal surface density S_V(sept/par) or, practically, S/V in older mice with studies in aging C57BL/6 mice estimating L_m (Huang et al., 2007; Elliott et al., 2016), their findings of increasing L_m with age is in line with our data of decreasing S_V(sept/par). Considering a concomitant increase in alveolar number density N_V(alv/par) with age, this provides evidence of declining alveolar size, which is coherent with enlargement of the alveolar ducts.

Age-Related Changes in Alveolarization

Alveolarization is mainly a postnatal process and occurs as early "bulk" and a late "continued" alveolarization (Schittny, 2017). Late alveolarization is discussed as the formation of new alveoli after the maturation of the alveolar septum which outlasts later periods of lung development (Burri, 2006; Schittny et al., 2008; Tschanz et al., 2014). Alveolarization has been shown to continue until young adulthood in humans (Narayanan et al., 2012; Herring et al., 2014), rats (Tschanz et al., 2014) and mice (Mund et al., 2008; Pozarska et al., 2017), however, little is known about late alveolarization in the elderly or in aged rodents.

The investigations showed that the number of alveoli increased from middle-aged to old mice, suggesting a late alveolarization in the old animals. Similarly, a study comparing 3 and 20 mo mice via microCT showed an increased number of alveoli per acinus in old mice (Vasilescu et al., 2012), supporting the idea of late alveolarization as well. In this study, the mean septal surface area per alveolus increased by approximately 15% from 3 to 20 mo mice, which is coherent with our data displaying a slight, non-significant increase of 7% from 3 to 18 mo mice. However, the point in time with the most prominent late alveolarization in our study, occurring from middle-aged to old mice, was not covered in their study. Others also reported different findings. For example, Glassberg et al. (2014) found no age-related changes in alveolar number in 6 and 24 mo female C57BL/6 mice. Furthermore, a study from Pozarska et al. (2017), investigating postnatal lung alveolarization in juvenile and adult mice of both sexes with an age of 2, 9, or 22 months as adult groups, showed highest numbers of alveoli in 9 mo mice. Moreover, the study found alveoli to have greatest volumes in 22 mo mice, whereas our results showed a decrease in alveolar size in old mice. The opposing observations may occur due to strain and sex differences. Furthermore, the study presumably included the total parenchymal airspace volume V(airtot,par) comprising alveolar and ductal airspace volumes to estimate the number-weighted mean alveolar volume $\bar{\upsilon}_N$(alv) (Pozarska et al., 2017). In comparison, we only used the total alveolar airspace volume V(airalv,par) without ductal airspace to estimate $\bar{\upsilon}_N$(alv). This has a direct impact on the estimation of the mean alveolar volume. By excluding ductal airspace from the estimation of alveolar volume, changes in ductal airspace will have no impact on alveolar volume calculations (**Table 2**). Here, in our study we therefore found a decrease in number-weighted mean alveolar volume in old mice, while the total number of alveoli was still increasing with age.

The findings of alveolar duct widening and smaller alveoli in old mice compared to middle-aged mice suggest a shortening of alveolar septal borders leading to a reduced alveolar depth, as described previously for aging human lungs (Quirk et al., 2016). The qualitative findings in pulmonary histology support this assumption (**Figures 3D,E**). As discussed by Quirk et al. (2016), the decreasing alveolar depth is concomitant with an increasing radius of alveolar ducts during aging in

TABLE 2 | Data of stereological parameters regarding alveoli and ATII cells.

Parameter	3 mo	6 mo	12 mo	18 mo	24 mo
N_V(alv/par) [10^3 mm^{-3}]	8.77 (0.81)	6.87* (0.57)	7.04* (0.71)	7.72 (0.84)	7.91 (0.59)
N(alv,par) [10^6]	7.48 (1.44)	5.95* (0.78)	6.00* (0.23)	$9.14^{*†‡}$ (1.05)	$8.84^{†‡}$ (0.72)
N_V(ATII/par) [10^3 mm^{-3}]	12.21 (1.17)	10.21* (0.81)	10.18* (1.28)	9.88* (0.62)	10.41* (1.07)
N(ATII,par) [10^6]	10.34 (1.57)	8.82 (0.93)	8.73 (1.26)	$11.76^{†‡}$ (1.50)	$11.68^{†‡}$ (1.73)
$\bar{\upsilon}_N$(ATII) [μm^3]	295 (61)	280 (17)	263 (28)	303 (48)	265 (19)
V(airalv,par)/N(alv,par) = $\bar{\upsilon}_N$(alv) [10^3 μm^3]	64.5 (5.9)	88.8* (10.2)	87.7* (11.1)	$69.0^{†‡}$ (6.5)	$68.9^{†‡}$ (5.3)
V(airtot,par)/N(alv,par) [10^3 μm^3]	104.1 (10.2)	132.2* (12.1)	129.3* (14.7)	119.7 (13.8)	115.7 (8.9)
S(sept,par)/N(alv,par) = $\overline{S(sept)/N(alv)}$ [10^3 μm^2]	7.32 (0.8)	9.51* (1.2)	9.52* (1.2)	7.83 (1.2)	$7.12^{†‡}$ (0.9)
N(ATII,par)/S(sept,par) [mm^{-2}]	192 (19)	158 (18)	153* (20)	166 (16)	$187^{‡}$ (28)
N(ATII,par)/N(alv,par)	1.40 (0.18)	1.49 (0.15)	1.46 (0.24)	1.30 (0.21)	1.33 (0.20)

*Data are expressed as mean (SD). *$p < 0.05$ for 3 mo vs. 6, 12, 18, 24 mo; $^{†}p < 0.05$ for 6 mo vs. 12, 18, 24 mo; $^{‡}p < 0.05$ for 12 mo vs. 18, 24 mo.*

human lungs at 19–71 years of age. It is assumed that these observations correspond with decreasing elastic recoil pressure and increasing shear modulus of the lung tissue (Verbeken et al., 1992a; Subramaniam et al., 2017; Knudsen and Ochs, 2018). Furthermore, alterations in septal elastin and collagen fiber distribution are considered to contribute to these observations in old mice (Toshima et al., 2004; Subramaniam et al., 2017).

It has to be mentioned that age-related changes in mechanical behavior of the lungs, as observed in Cst, could also affect structural parameters such as alveolar size. This holds particularly true, if lungs are instillation fixed under a constant pressure. In our study, Cst increased from 3 mo mice to older mice (**Figure 1C**), therefore, it is possible that changes in Cst affected alveolar size differences between 3 mo and older mice. However, in middle-aged and old mice Cst remained quite constant (**Figure 1C**). Hence in these groups, we consider the results in alveolar size measurements comparable, showing an age-related decline in alveolar size in old mice.

Alterations of ATII Cell Numbers With Progressing Age

ATII cells play an important role for the functionality of the lung, as they serve as progenitor cells for alveolar epithelial type I (ATI) cells, stabilize intra-alveolar surface tension by producing surfactant and have an immunological function (reviewed in Fehrenbach, 2001). While transcriptomics and proteomics were done in ATII cells of young and old mice (Angelidis et al., 2019) and age-related changes were assessed in ATII cells as reviewed in Brandenberger and Mühlfeld (2017), there is no research on the absolute ATII cell number at multiple time points of adulthood yet. Stereological ATII cell quantification is very time consuming due to the necessity of the disector, but is superior to other quantification methods like flow cytometry (Jansing et al., 2017; Dzhuraev et al., 2019) or planimetry (Jansing et al., 2017). Nevertheless, there is a lot of research quantifying ATII cells stereologically in human (Crapo et al., 1982; Stone et al., 1992), rat (Crapo et al., 1980; Stone et al., 1992) and mouse (Stone et al., 1992; Dzhuraev et al., 2019) lungs for one age group.

Our results showed slightly higher total and alveolar surface-related ATII cell numbers for young compared to middle-aged mice (**Figures 4F,I**). This is in line with investigations in early postnatal rat lung development, showing a decline in ATII cells in the first days of life (Kauffman et al., 1974) and appears biologically consistent, as ATII cells serve as progenitor cells for alveolar epithelial type I (ATI) cells (Evans et al., 1975). From middle-aged to old mice, the ATII cell number density remained quite constant (**Figure 4G**), whereas, unexpectedly, the total number of ATII cells increased significantly (**Figures 4G,I**). We hypothesized that ATII cell number would further decrease with age or remain at least constant due to progenitor cell senescence with aging (Alder et al., 2015; Chen et al., 2015). However, our results indicate that ATII cell number concomitantly increased with lung volume in old mice. The constant ratio of ATII cells per alveolus during aging supports this finding (**Figure 4H**). It appears possible that a constant ATII cell number per alveolus contributes to a maintaining surfactant secretion, preserving lung function in old mice (Hills, 1999; Fehrenbach, 2001). However, further research is needed to address this hypothesis.

Developing and Aging of the Mouse Lung

C57BL/6 mice are commonly used for geriatric research (Miller and Nadon, 2000; Huang et al., 2007; Elliott et al., 2016; Kling et al., 2017; Angelidis et al., 2019). The median lifespan of male C57BL/6 mice is approximately 900 days or 29 months (Yuan et al., 2009). Flurkey et al. (2007) recommend using animals aged onto 85–90% of survivorship as oldest group for geriatric research, which would count for approximately 24 mo C57BL/6 mice. We summarized the 5 age groups of this study into 3 groups, because this classification reflected changes of almost all parameters and supported comprehension of the results: one young adult (3 mo), two middle-aged (6 and 12 mo), and two old (18 and 24 mo) mice groups. However, Flurkey et al. (2007) categorized 3–6 mo mice as mature adults and 10–14 mo mice as middle-aged. In recent aging studies with C57BL/6 (Kling et al., 2017; Brandenberger et al., 2018) and BALB/c (Gomez et al., 2007; Chen et al., 2014) mice, 3 and 18 mo groups are frequently used to represent young and old, respectively. Lung development occurs until young adulthood (Schittny, 2017). We found great changes in lung function, micromechanics, and structure between 3 and 6 months of age, suggesting lung development to continue beyond pubertal maturation. Supportively, Miller and Nadon (2000) discussed using mice of 4–6 months of age for young groups to avoid influences of post-pubertal maturation processes. Nevertheless, we considered it important to include also young adult mice of 3 months into our study to have the full range of adult life covered.

CONCLUSION

In summary, this study provides comprehensive insights on structural alterations in the aging C57BL/6JRj mouse lung, linking it with changes in lung function and micromechanics. Age-related structural alterations mainly appeared between middle-aged and old mice and were characterized by lung growth accompanied by a widening of alveolar ducts. Moreover, late alveolarization occurred, concomitant with decreasing alveolar size, most likely due to reduced alveolar depth. Quite constant relations of ATII cells to alveolar number and alveolar surface area were observed. However, lung function and micromechanics altered most between young and middle-aged mice.

AUTHOR CONTRIBUTIONS

HS, CB, and CM designed the research, interpreted the results of experiments, edited and revised the manuscript, and approved final version of the manuscript. HS and CB performed the experiments, analyzed the data, and prepared the figures. HS drafted the manuscript.

ACKNOWLEDGMENTS

We would like to thank Lars Knudsen for the constructive discussions, and Susanne Kuhlmann, Rita Lichatz, and Christa Lichtenberg for their excellent technical assistance.

REFERENCES

Alder, J. K., Barkauskas, C. E., Limjunyawong, N., Stanley, S. E., Kembou, F., Tuder, R. M., et al. (2015). Telomere dysfunction causes alveolar stem cell failure. *Proc. Natl. Acad. Sci. U.S.A.* 112, 5099–5104. doi: 10.1073/pnas.1504780112

Angelidis, I., Simon, L. M., Fernandez, I. E., Strunz, M., Mayr, C. H., Greiffo, F. R., et al. (2019). An atlas of the aging lung mapped by single cell transcriptomics and deep tissue proteomics. *Nat. Commun.* 10:963. doi: 10.1038/s41467-019-08831-9

Bachofen, H., and Schürch, S. (2001). Alveolar surface forces and lung architecture. *Comp. Biochem. Physiol. A Mol. Integr. Physiol.* 129, 183–193. doi: 10.1016/S1095-6433(01)00315-4

Becklake, M., and Crapo, R. O. (1991). Lung function testing: selection of reference values and interpretative strategies. *Am. Rev. Respir. Dis.* 144, 1202–1218. doi: 10.1164/ajrccm/144.5.1202

Brandenberger, C., Kling, K. M., Vital, M., and Christian, M. (2018). The role of pulmonary and systemic immunosenescence in acute lung injury. *Aging Dis.* 9, 553–565. doi: 10.14336/ad.2017.0902

Brandenberger, C., and Mühlfeld, C. (2017). Mechanisms of lung aging. *Cell Tissue Res.* 367, 469–480. doi: 10.1007/s00441-016-2511-x

Brandenberger, C., Ochs, M., and Mühlfeld, C. (2015). Assessing particle and fiber toxicology in the respiratory system : the stereology toolbox. *Part. Fibre Toxicol.* 12, 1–15. doi: 10.1186/s12989-015-0110-8

Brewer, K. K., Sakai, H., Alencar, A. M., Majumdar, A., Arold, S. P., Lutchen, K. R., et al. (2003). Lung and alveolar wall elastic and hysteretic behavior in rats: effects of in vivo elastase treatment. *J. Appl. Physiol.* 95, 1926–1936. doi: 10.1152/japplphysiol.00102.2003

Burri, P. H. (2006). Structural aspects of postnatal lung development - alveolar formation and growth. *Biol. Neonate* 89, 313–322. doi: 10.1159/000092868

Butler, J. P., Loring, S. H., Patz, S., Tsuda, A., Yablonskiy, D. A., and Mentzer, S. J. (2012). Evidence for adult lung growth in humans. *N. Engl. J. Med.* 367, 244–247. doi: 10.1056/nejmoa1203983

Chan, E. D., and Welsh, C. H. (1998). Geriatric respiratory medicine. *Chest* 114, 1704–1733. doi: 10.1378/chest.114.6.1704

Chen, M. M., Palmer, J. L., Plackett, T. P., Deburghgraeve, C. R., and Kovacs, E. J. (2014). Age-related differences in the neutrophil response to pulmonary *Pseudomonas* infection. *Exp. Gerontol.* 54, 42–46. doi: 10.1016/j.exger.2013.12.010

Chen, R., Zhang, K., Chen, H., Zhao, X., Wang, J., Li, L., et al. (2015). Telomerase deficiency causes alveolar stem cell senescence-associated low-grade inflammation in lungs. *J. Biol. Chem.* 290, 30813–30829. doi: 10.1074/jbc.M115.681619

Collard, H. R. (2010). The age of idiopathic pulmonary fibrosis. *Am. J. Respir. Crit. Care Med.* 181, 771–772. doi: 10.1164/rccm.201001-0049ED

Copley, S. J., Wells, A. U., Hawtin, K. E., Gibson, D. J., Hodson, J. M., Jacques, A. E. T., et al. (2009). Lung morphology in the elderly: comparative CT study of subjects over 75 years old versus those under 55 years old. *Radiology* 251, 566–573. doi: 10.1148/radiol.2512081242

Crapo, J. D., Barry, B. E., Foscue, H. A., and Shelburne, J. (1980). Structural and biochemical Changes in rat lungs occurring during exposures to lethal and adaptive doses of oxygen. *Am. Rev. Respir. Dis.* 122, 123–143. doi: 10.1164/arrd.1980.122.1.123

Crapo, J. D., Barry, B. E., Gehr, P., Bachofen, M., and Weibel, E. R. (1982). Cell number and Cell characteristics of the normal human lung. *Am. Rev. Respir. Dis.* 126, 332–337. doi: 10.1164/arrd.1982.126.2.332

Cruz-Orive, L. M., and Weibel, E. R. (1990). Recent stereological methods for cell biology: a brief survey. *Am. J. Physiol. Cell. Mol. Physiol.* 258, L148–L156. doi: 10.1152/ajplung.1990.258.4.l148

de Jong, P. A., Long, F. R., Wong, J. C., Merkus, P. J., Tiddens, H. A., Hogg, J. C., et al. (2006). Computed tomographic estimation of lung dimensions throughout the growth period. *Eur. Respir. J.* 27, 261–267. doi: 10.1183/09031936.06.00070805

De Vleeschauwer, S. I., Rinaldi, M., De Vooght, V., Vanoirbeek, J. A., Vanaudenaerde, B. M., Verbeken, E. K., et al. (2011). Repeated invasive lung function measurements in intubated mice: an approach for longitudinal lung research. *Lab. Anim.* 45, 81–89. doi: 10.1258/la.2010.010111

D'Errico, A., Scarani, P., Colosimo, E., Spina, M., Grigioni, W. F., and Mancini, A. M. (1989). Changes in the alveolar connective tissue of the ageing lung. *Virchows Arch. A Pathol. Anat. Histopathol.* 415, 137–144. doi: 10.1007/bf00784351

Dzhuraev, G., Rodríguez-Castillo, J. A., Ruiz-Camp, J., Salwig, I., Szibor, M., Vadász, I., et al. (2019). Estimation of absolute number of alveolar epithelial type 2 cells in mouse lungs: a comparison between stereology and flow cytometry. *J. Microsc.* 275, 36–50. doi: 10.1111/jmi.12800

Elliott, J. E., Mantilla, C. B., Pabelick, C. M., Roden, A. C., and Sieck, G. C. (2016). Aging-related changes in respiratory system mechanics and morphometry in mice. *Am. J. Physiol. Cell. Mol. Physiol.* 311, L167–L176. doi: 10.1152/ajplung.00232.2016

Ely, E. W., Wheeler, A. P., Thompson, B. T., Ancukiewicz, M., Steinberg, K. P., and Bernard, G. R. (2002). Recovery Rate and Prognosis in Older Persons Who Develop Acute Lung Injury and the Acute Respiratory Distress Syndrome. *Ann. Intern. Med.* 136, 25–36. doi: 10.7326/0003-4819-136-1-200201010-00007

Evans, M. J., Cabral, L. J., Stephens, R. J., and Freeman, G. (1975). Transformation of alveolar type 2 cells to type 1 cells following exposure to NO2. *Exp. Mol. Pathol.* 22, 142–150. doi: 10.1016/0014-4800(75)90059-3

Fehrenbach, H. (2001). Alveolar epithelial type II cell: defender of the alveolus revisited. *Respir Res.* 2, 33–46. doi: 10.1186/rr36

Fell, C. D., Martinez, F. J., Liu, L. X., Murray, S., Han, M. L. K., Kazerooni, E. A., et al. (2010). Clinical predictors of a diagnosis of idiopathic pulmonary fibrosis. *Am. J. Respir. Crit. Care Med.* 181, 832–837. doi: 10.1164/rccm.200906-0959OC

Flurkey, K., Currer, J. M., and Harrison, D. E. (2007). "Mouse models in aging research," in *The Mouse in Biomedical Research*, eds J. G. Fox, M. T. Davisson, F. W. Quimby, S. W. Barthold, C. E. Newcomer, and A. L. Smith, (Amsterdam: Elsevier Inc), 637–672. doi: 10.1016/b978-012369454-6/50074-1

Glassberg, M. K., Choi, R., Manzoli, V., Shahzeidi, S., Rauschkolb, P., Voswinckel, R., et al. (2014). 17β-estradiol replacement reverses age-related lung disease in estrogen-deficient C57BL/6J mice. *Endocrinology* 155, 441–448. doi: 10.1210/en.2013-1345

Gomez, C. R., Hirano, S., Cutro, B. T., Birjandi, S., Baila, H., Nomellini, V., et al. (2007). Advanced age exacerbates the pulmonary inflammatory response after lipopolysaccharide exposure. *Crit. Care Med.* 35, 246–251. doi: 10.1097/01.CCM.0000251639.05135.E0

Gundersen, H. J. G. (1977). Notes on the estimation of the numerical density of arbitrary profiles: the edge effect. *J. Microsc.* 111, 219–223. doi: 10.1111/j.1365-2818.1977.tb00062.x

Gundersen, H. J. G., Boyce, R. W., Nyengaard, J. R., and Odgaard, A. (1993). The connEulor: unbiased estimation of connectivity using physical disectors under projection. *Bone* 14, 217–222. doi: 10.1016/8756-3282(93)90144-Y

Gundersen, H. J. G., and Jensen, E. B. (1987). The efficiency of systematic sampling in stereology and its prediction. *J. Microsc.* 147, 229–263. doi: 10.1111/j.1365-2818.1987.tb02837.x

Gundersen, H. J. G., Jensen, E. B., Kieu, K., and Nielsen, J. (1999). The efficiency of systematic sampling in stereology - reconsidered. *J. Microsc.* 193, 199–211. doi: 10.1046/j.1365-2818.1999.00457.x

Herring, M. J., Putney, L. F., Wyatt, G., Finkbeiner, W. E., and Hyde, D. M. (2014). Growth of alveoli during postnatal development in humans based on stereological estimation. *Am. J. Physiol. Cell. Mol. Physiol.* 307, L338–L344. doi: 10.1152/ajplung.00094.2014

Hills, B. A. (1999). An alternative view of the role(s) of surfactant and the alveolar model. *J. Appl. Physiol.* 87, 1567–1583. doi: 10.1152/jappl.1999.87.5.1567

Howard, C. V., and Reed, M. G. (1998). *Unbiased Stereology.* Oxford: BIOS Scientific Publishers Limited.

Howlader, N., Noone, A. M., Krapcho, M., Miller, D., Brest, A., Yu, M., et al. (2019). *SEER Cancer Statistics Review, 1975–2016*, Bethesda, MD: National Cancer Institute, Available at: https://seer.cancer.gov/csr/1975_2016/, based on November 2018 SEER data submission, posted to the SEER web site, April 2019 (accessed August 7, 2019).

Hsia, C. C. W., Hyde, D. M., Ochs, M., and Weibel, E. R. (2010). An official research policy statement of the american thoracic society/european respiratory society: standards for quantitative assessment of lung structure. *Am. J. Respir. Crit. Care Med.* 181, 394–418. doi: 10.1164/rccm.200809-1522ST

Huang, K., Rabold, R., Schofield, B., Mitzner, W., and Tankersley, C. G. (2007). Age-dependent changes of airway and lung parenchyma in C57BL/6J mice. *J. Appl. Physiol.* 102, 200–206. doi: 10.1152/japplphysiol.00400.2006

Hyde, D. M., Tyler, N. K., Putney, L. F., Singh, P., and Gundersen, H. J. G. (2004). Total number and mean size of alveoli in mammalian lung estimated using fractionator sampling and unbiased estimates of the Euler characteristic of alveolar openings. *Anat. Rec. A Discov. Mol. Cell. Evol. Biol.* 277, 216–226. doi: 10.1002/ar.a.20012

Ito, K., and Barnes, P. J. (2009). COPD as a disease of accelerated lung aging. *Chest* 135, 173–180. doi: 10.1378/chest.08-1419

Jansing, N. L., McClendon, J., Henson, P. M., Tuder, R. M., Hyde, D. M., and Zemans, R. L. (2017). Unbiased quantitation of alveolar type II to alveolar type I cell transdifferentiation during repair after lung injury in mice. *Am. J. Respir. Cell Mol. Biol.* 57, 519–526. doi: 10.1165/rcmb.2017-0037MA

Janssens, J., Pache, J. C., and Nicod, L. P. (1999). Physiological changes in respiratory function associated with ageing. *Eur. Respir. J.* 13, 197–205. doi: 10.1034/j.1399-3003.1999.13a36.x

Kauffman, S. L., Burri, P. H., and Weibel, E. R. (1974). The postnatal growth of the rat lung II. *Autoradiogr. Anat. Rec.* 180, 63–76. doi: 10.1002/ar.1091800108

Kerr, J. S., Yu, S. Y., and Riley, D. J. (1990). Strain specific respiratory air space enlargement in aged rats. *Exp. Gerontol.* 25, 563–574. doi: 10.1016/0531-5565(90)90022-T

Kerstjens, H. A. M., Rijcken, B., Schouten, J. P., and Postma, D. S. (1997). Decline of FEV1 by age and smoking status: facts, figures, and fallacies. *Thorax* 52, 820–827. doi: 10.1136/thx.52.9.820

Kling, K. M., Lopez-Rodriguez, E., Pfarrer, C., Mühlfeld, C., and Brandenberger, C. (2017). Aging exacerbates acute lung injury-induced changes of the air-blood barrier, lung function, and inflammation in the mouse. *Am. J. Physiol. Cell. Mol. Physiol.* 312, L1–L12. doi: 10.1152/ajplung.00347.2016

Knudsen, L., and Ochs, M. (2018). The micromechanics of lung alveoli : structure and function of surfactant and tissue components. *Histochem. Cell Biol.* 150, 661–676. doi: 10.1007/s00418-018-1747-9

Knudsen, L., Weibel, E. R., Gundersen, H. J. G., Weinstein, F. V., and Ochs, M. (2010). Assessment of air space size characteristics by intercept (chord) measurement: an accurate and efficient stereological approach. *J. Appl. Physiol.* 108, 412–421. doi: 10.1152/japplphysiol.01100.2009

Levitzky, M. G. (1984). Effects of aging on the respiratory system. *Physiologist* 27, 102–107.

Lopez-Rodriguez, E., Boden, C., Echaide, M., Perez-Gil, J., Kolb, M., Gauldie, J., et al. (2016). Surfactant dysfunction during overexpression of TGF-β1 precedes profibrotic lung remodeling in vivo. *Am. J. Physiol. Cell. Mol. Physiol.* 310, L1260–L1271. doi: 10.1152/ajplung.00065.2016

Lutz, D., Gazdhar, A., Lopez-Rodriguez, E., Ruppert, C., Mahavadi, P., Günther, A., et al. (2015). Alveolar derecruitment and collapse induration as crucial mechanisms in lung injury and fibrosis. *Am. J. Respir. Cell Mol. Biol.* 52, 232–243. doi: 10.1165/rcmb.2014-0078OC

Mayhew, T. M. (1991). The new stereological methods for interpreting functional morphology from slices of cells and organs. *Exp. Physiol.* 76, 639–665. doi: 10.1113/expphysiol.1991.sp003533

Mercer, R. R., and Crapo, J. D. (1990). Spatial distribution of collagen and elastin fibers in the lungs. *J. Appl. Physiol.* 69, 756–765. doi: 10.1152/jappl.1990.69.2.756

Meyerholz, D. K., Suarez, C. J., Dintzis, S. M., and Frevert, C. W. (2017). "Respiratory system," in *Comparative Anatomy and Histology*, eds P. M. Treuting, S. M. Dintzis, and K. S. Montine, (Amsterdam: Elsevier Inc), 147–162. doi: 10.1016/B978-0-12-802900-8.00009-9

Miller, M. R., Hankinson, J., Brusasco, V., Burgos, F., Casaburi, R., Coates, A., et al. (2005). Standardisation of spirometry. *Eur. Respir. J.* 26, 319–338. doi: 10.1183/09031936.05.00034805

Miller, R. A., and Nadon, N. L. (2000). Principles of animal use for gerontological research. *J. Gerontol. Biol. Sci.* 55A, B117–B123. doi: 10.1093/gerona/55.3.B117

Mühlfeld, C., and Ochs, M. (2013). Quantitative microscopy of the lung: a problem-based approach. *Part* 2: stereological parameters and study designs in various diseases of the respiratory tract. *Am. J. Physiol. Cell. Mol. Physiol.* 305, L205–L221. doi: 10.1152/ajplung.00427.2012

Mund, S. I., Stampanoni, M., and Schittny, J. C. (2008). Developmental alveolarization of the mouse lung. *Dev. Dyn.* 237, 2108–2116. doi: 10.1002/dvdy.21633

Narayanan, M., Owers-Bradley, J., Beardsmore, C. S., Mada, M., Ball, I., Garipov, R., et al. (2012). Alveolarization continues during childhood and adolescence. *Am. J. Respir. Crit. Care Med.* 185, 186–191. doi: 10.1164/rccm.201107-1348oc

Nyengaard, J. R., and Gundersen, H. J. G. (2006). Sampling for stereology in lungs. *Eur. Respir. Rev.* 15, 107–114. doi: 10.1183/09059180.00010101

Ochs, M. (2006). A brief update on lung stereology. *J. Microsc.* 222, 188–200. doi: 10.1111/j.1365-2818.2006.01587.x

Ochs, M., Nyengaard, J. R., Jung, A., Knudsen, L., Voigt, M., Wahlers, T., et al. (2004). The number of alveoli in the human lung. *Am. J. Respir. Crit. Care Med.* 169, 120–124. doi: 10.1164/rccm.200308-1107OC

Pellegrino, R., Viegi, G., Brusasco, V., Crapo, R. O., Burgos, F., Casaburi, R., et al. (2005). Interpretative strategies for lung function tests. *Eur. Respir. J.* 26, 948–968. doi: 10.1183/09031936.05.00035205

Pinkerton, K. E., Herring, M. J., Hyde, D. M., and Green, F. H. Y. (2014). "Normal aging of the lung," in *The Lung*, eds K. E. Pinkerton, and R. Harding, (Amsterdam: Elsevier Inc), 265–285. doi: 10.1016/B978-0-12-799941-8.00014-6

Pozarska, A., Rodríguez-Castillo, J. A., Surate Solaligue, D. E., Ntokou, A., Rath, P., Mižíková, I., et al. (2017). Stereological monitoring of mouse lung alveolarization from the early postnatal period to adulthood. *Am. J. Physiol. Cell. Mol. Physiol.* 312, L882–L895. doi: 10.1152/ajplung.00492.2016

Provinciali, M., Cardelli, M., and Marchegiani, F. (2011). Inflammation, chronic obstructive pulmonary disease and aging. *Curr. Opin. Pulm. Med.* 17, S3–S10. doi: 10.1097/01.mcp.0000410742.90463.1f

Quirk, J. D., Sukstanskii, A. L., Woods, J. C., Lutey, B. A., Conradi, M. S., Gierada, D. S., et al. (2016). Experimental evidence of age-related adaptive changes in human acinar airways. *J. Appl. Physiol.* 120, 159–165. doi: 10.1152/japplphysiol.00541.2015

Raghu, G., Weycker, D., Edelsberg, J., Bradford, W. Z., and Oster, G. (2006). Incidence and prevalence of idiopathic pulmonary fibrosis. *Am. J. Respir. Crit. Care Med.* 174, 810–816. doi: 10.1164/rccm.200602-163OC

Ranga, V., Kleinerman, J., Ip, M. P., and Sorensen, J. (1979). Age-related changes in elastic fibers and elastin of lung. *Am. Rev. Respir. Dis.* 119, 369–376. doi: 10.1164/arrd.1979.119.3.369

Robichaud, A., Fereydoonzad, L., Limjunyawong, N., Rabold, R., Allard, B., Benedetti, A., et al. (2017). Automated full-range pressure-volume curves in mice and rats. *J. Appl. Physiol.* 123, 746–756. doi: 10.1152/japplphysiol.00856.2016

Rubenfeld, G. D., Caldwell, E., Peabody, E., Weaver, J., Martin, D. P., Neff, M., et al. (2005). Incidence and outcomes of acute lung injury. *N. Engl. J. Med.* 353, 1685–1693. doi: 10.1056/NEJMoa050333

Salazar, E., and Knowles, J. H. (1964). An analysis of pressure-volume characteristics of the lungs. *J. Appl. Physiol.* 19, 97–104. doi: 10.1152/jappl.1964.19.1.97

Scherle, W. (1970). A simple method for volumetry of organs in quantitative stereology. *Mikroskopie* 26, 57–60.

Schittny, J. C. (2017). Development of the lung. *Cell Tissue Res.* 367, 427–444. doi: 10.1007/s00441-016-2545-0

Schittny, J. C., Mund, S. I., and Stampanoni, M. (2008). Evidence and structural mechanism for late lung alveolarization. *Am. J. Physiol. Cell. Mol. Physiol.* 294, L246–L254. doi: 10.1152/ajplung.00296.2007

Schneider, J. P., and Ochs, M. (2013). "Stereology of the lung," in *Methods in Cell Biology*, ed. P. M. Conn, (Cambridge, MA: Academic Press Inc), 257–294. doi: 10.1016/B978-0-12-407239-8.00012-4

Schneider, J. P., and Ochs, M. (2014). Alterations of mouse lung tissue dimensions during processing for morphometry: a comparison of methods. *Am. J. Physiol. Cell. Mol. Physiol.* 306, L341–L350. doi: 10.1152/ajplung.00329.2013

Sharma, G., and Goodwin, J. (2006). Effect of aging on respiratory system physiology and immunology. *Clin. Interv. Aging* 1, 253–260. doi: 10.2147/ciia.2006.1.3.253

Sicard, D., Haak, A. J., Choi, K. M., Craig, A. R., Fredenburgh, L. E., and Tschumperlin, D. J. (2018). Aging and anatomical variations in lung tissue stiffness. *Am. J. Physiol. Cell. Mol. Physiol.* 314, L946–L955. doi: 10.1152/ajplung.00415.2017

Sterio, D. C. (1983). The unbiased estimation of number and sizes of arbitrary particles using the disector. *J. Microsc.* 134, 127–136. doi: 10.1111/j.1365-2818.1984.tb02501.x

Stone, K. C., Mercer, R. R., Gehr, P., Stockstill, B., and Crapo, J. D. (1992). Allometric Relationships of Cell Numbers and Size in the Mammalian Lung. *Am. J. Respir. Cell Mol. Biol.* 6, 235–243. doi: 10.1165/ajrcmb/6.2.235

Subramaniam, K., Kumar, H., and Tawhai, M. H. (2017). Evidence for age-dependent air-space enlargement contributing to loss of lung tissue elastic recoil pressure and increased shear modulus in older age. *J. Appl. Physiol.* 123, 79–87. doi: 10.1152/japplphysiol.00208.2016

Suki, B. (2014). Assessing the functional mechanical properties of bioengineered organs with emphasis on the lung. *J. Cell. Physiol.* 229, 1134–1140. doi: 10.1002/jcp.24600

Suki, B., and Bartolák-Suki, E. (2014). "Biomechanics of the aging lung parenchyma," in *Mechanical Properties of Aging Soft Tissues*, eds B. Derby, and R. Akhtar, (New York, NY: Springer International Publishing), 95–133. doi: 10.1007/978-3-319-03970-1_5

Suki, B., Stamenović, D., and Hubmayr, R. (2011). Lung parenchymal mechanics. *Compr. Physiol.* 1, 1317–1351. doi: 10.1002/cphy.c100033

Thannickal, V. J. (2013). Mechanistic links between aging and lung fibrosis. *Biogerontology* 14, 609–615. doi: 10.1007/s10522-013-9451-6

Toshima, M., Ohtani, Y., and Ohtani, O. (2004). Three-dimensional architecture of elastin and collagen fiber networks in the human and rat lung. *Arch. Histol. Cytol.* 67, 31–40. doi: 10.1679/aohc.67.31

Tschanz, S. A., Salm, L. A., Roth-Kleiner, M., Barré, S. F., Burri, P. H., and Schittny, J. C. (2014). Rat lungs show a biphasic formation of new alveoli during postnatal development. *J. Appl. Physiol.* 117, 89–95. doi: 10.1152/japplphysiol.01355.2013

Turner, J. M., Mead, J., and Wohl, M. E. (2017). Elasticity of human lungs in relation to age. *J. Appl. Physiol.* 25, 664–671. doi: 10.1152/jappl.1968.25.6.664

Vanoirbeek, J. A. J., Rinaldi, M., De Vooght, V., Haenen, S., Bobic, S., Gayan-Ramirez, G., et al. (2010). Noninvasive and invasive pulmonary function in mouse models of obstructive and restrictive respiratory diseases. *Am. J. Respir. Cell Mol. Biol.* 42, 96–104. doi: 10.1165/rcmb.2008-0487OC

Vasilescu, D. M., Gao, Z., Saha, P. K., Yin, L., Wang, G., Haefeli-Bleuer, B., et al. (2012). Assessment of morphometry of pulmonary acini in mouse lungs by nondestructive imaging using multiscale microcomputed tomography. *Proc. Natl. Acad. Sci. U.S.A.* 109, 17105–17110. doi: 10.1073/pnas.1215112109

Vaz Fragoso, C. A., and Gill, T. M. (2012). Respiratory impairment and the aging lung: a novel paradigm for assessing pulmonary function. *J. Gerontol. Ser. A Biol. Sci. Med. Sci.* 67, 264–275. doi: 10.1093/gerona/glr198

Vedel-Jensen, E. B., and Gundersen, H. J. (1993). The rotator. *J. Microsc.* 170, 35–44. doi: 10.1111/j.1365-2818.1993.tb03321.x

Veldhuizen, R. A. W., McCaig, L. A., Pape, C., and Gill, S. E. (2019). The effects of aging and exercise on lung mechanics, surfactant and alveolar macrophages. *Exp. Lung Res.* 45, 113–122. doi: 10.1080/01902148.2019.1605633

Verbeken, E. K., Cauberghs, M., Mertens, I., Clement, J., Lauweryns, J. M., and Van de Woestijne, K. P. (1992a). The senile lung - 1. *Structural Aspects. Chest* 101, 793–799. doi: 10.1378/chest.101.3.793

Verbeken, E. K., Cauberghs, M., Mertens, I., Clement, J., Lauweryns, J. M., and Van de Woestijne, K. P. (1992b). The senile lung - 2. *Funct. Aspects. Chest* 101, 800–809. doi: 10.1378/chest.101.3.800

Wahba, W. M. (1983). Influence of aging on lung function - clinical significance of changes from age twenty. *Anesth. Analg.* 62, 764–776. doi: 10.1213/00000539-198308000-00011

Ware, J. H., Dockery, D. W., Louis, T. A., Xu, X., Ferris, B. G., and Speizer, F. E. (1990). Longitudinal and cross-sectional estimates of pulmonary function decline in never-smoking adults. *Am. J. Epidemiol.* 132, 685–700. doi: 10.1093/oxfordjournals.aje.a115710

Weibel, E. R. (1979). *Stereological Methods*, Vol. 1. Cambridge, MA: Academic Press Inc.

Weibel, E. R., Hsia, C. C. W., and Ochs, M. (2007). How much is there really? Why stereology is essential in lung morphometry. *J. Appl. Physiol.* 102, 459–467. doi: 10.1152/japplphysiol.00808.2006

Yamamoto, Y., Tanaka, A., Kanamaru, A., Tanaka, S., Tsubone, H., Atoji, Y., et al. (2003). Morphology of aging lung in F344/N rat: alveolar size, connective tissue, and smooth muscle cell markers. *Anat. Rec. A Discov. Mol. Cell. Evol. Biol.* 272, 538–547. doi: 10.1002/ar.a.10172

Yuan, R., Tsaih, S.-W., Petkova, S. B., De Evsikova, C. M., Xing, S., Marion, M. A., et al. (2009). Aging in inbred strains of mice: study design and interim report on median lifespans and circulating IGF1 levels. *Aging Cell* 8, 277–287. doi: 10.1111/j.1474-9726.2009.00478.x

Zach, J. A., Newell, J. D., Schroeder, J., Murphy, J. R., Curran-Everett, D., Hoffman, E. A., et al. (2012). Quantitative computed tomography of the lungs and airways in healthy nonsmoking adults. *Invest. Radiol.* 47, 596–602. doi: 10.1097/RLI.0b013e318262292e

Zosky, G. R. (2015). "Aging of the normal lung," in *Comparative Biology of the Normal Lung*, ed. R. A. Parent, (Amsterdam: Elsevier Inc), 185–204. doi: 10.1016/B978-0-12-404577-4.00013-8

6

Alveolar Dynamics and Beyond – The Importance of Surfactant Protein C and Cholesterol in Lung Homeostasis and Fibrosis

Kirsten Sehlmeyer[1,2†], Jannik Ruwisch[1,2†], Nuria Roldan[3] and Elena Lopez-Rodriguez[1,2,4]*

[1] *Institute of Functional and Applied Anatomy, Hannover Medical School, Hanover, Germany,* [2] *Biomedical Research in Endstage and Obstructive Lung Disease Hannover, Member of the German Centre for Lung Research, Hanover, Germany,* [3] *Alveolix AG and ARTORG Center, University of Bern, Bern, Switzerland,* [4] *Institute of Functional Anatomy, Charité – Universitätsmedizin Berlin, Berlin, Germany*

***Correspondence:**
Elena Lopez-Rodriguez
elena.lopez-rodriguez@charite.de

† These authors have contributed equally to this work

Surfactant protein C (SP-C) is an important player in enhancing the interfacial adsorption of lung surfactant lipid films to the alveolar air-liquid interface. Doing so, surface tension drops down enough to stabilize alveoli and the lung, reducing the work of breathing. In addition, it has been shown that SP-C counteracts the deleterious effect of high amounts of cholesterol in the surfactant lipid films. On its side, cholesterol is a well-known modulator of the biophysical properties of biological membranes and it has been proven that it activates the inflammasome pathways in the lung. Even though the molecular mechanism is not known, there are evidences suggesting that these two molecules may interplay with each other in order to keep the proper function of the lung. This review focuses in the role of SP-C and cholesterol in the development of lung fibrosis and the potential pathways in which impairment of both molecules leads to aberrant lung repair, and therefore impaired alveolar dynamics. From molecular to cellular mechanisms to evidences in animal models and human diseases. The evidences revised here highlight a potential SP-C/cholesterol axis as target for the treatment of lung fibrosis.

Keywords: surfactant protein C, pulmonary fibrosis, alveolar dynamics, lipid metabolism, alveolar macrophages, cholesterol, metaflammation

WHY IS CHOLESTEROL PRESENT IN THE LUNG?

As recently reviewed by Zuniga-Hertz and Patel (2019), 2.32 billion years ago, the atmospheric oxygen raised (Bekker et al., 2004) leading to many changes in life. One of these changes may have been the appearance of sterols, around 2.7 billion years ago (Brocks et al., 1999; French et al., 2015) after the GOE (Great Oxygen Event) as suggested by fossil evidences. However, which is the connection between oxygen and sterols? It has been proposed that sterols emerged as an evolutionary strategy to reduce oxygen diffusion through cellular membranes, probably in a world where organisms were not ready to respond to oxidative stress yet. Interestingly, sterol biosynthesis is highly dependent on oxygen (DeBose-Boyd, 2008).

How can sterols, such as cholesterol, regulate oxygen diffusion through biological membranes? The molecular mechanism by which cholesterol can influence small solute permeation and diffusion through lipid membranes is not well understood. However, it has been proposed that the interactions between cholesterol and the acyl carbon chains in phospholipids (stabilized by Van der Waals' forces) (Wennberg et al., 2012) create tightly packed arrangements that limits small molecule diffusion (Zocher et al., 2013). By decreasing trans-gauche rotation of the phospholipid acyl chains, membrane rigidity increases (Cassera et al., 2002; Molugu and Brown, 2019) leading to less free volume and free pockets which may accommodate oxygen, therefore reducing its flux (its partition and diffusion) through membranes (Zuniga-Hertz and Patel, 2019).

Mammals developed sophisticated organs to optimize the uptake of oxygen during the life essential breathing cycle. From conducting airways to the second biggest surface exposed to the environment, the alveolar human surface (Ochs et al., 2004). In addition, the first membrane that oxygen encounters in the mammalian lungs is a complex mixture of lipids (mainly phosphatidylcholines (PC), such as dipalmitoylphosphatidylcholine (DPPC), up to a 90%) and proteins (10%) with a 5–10% of cholesterol (14–20% mol) (Zuo et al., 2008; Bernhard, 2016), called lung surfactant (surface active agent). Interestingly two surfaces in the human body present with abnormally higher cholesterol molar ratio, and both of them are in contact with the environment tightly regulating the uptake of oxygen. On the one hand, as previously explained, lung surfactant presents around a 14–20% mol cholesterol in its composition. On the other hand the eye lens surface contains up to 35% mol of cholesterol (Raguz et al., 2008; Mainali et al., 2013), compared to a normal cell plasma membrane with a 0.5 phospholipid to cholesterol molar ratio (van Meer et al., 2008; Widomska et al., 2017). Although the main function of lung surfactant has not been related to oxygen flux control, it has been described to accelerate oxygen diffusion through a water layer (Olmeda et al., 2010), reflecting the importance of lung surfactant as potential oxygen flux regulator. The main function of lung surfactant is to reduce surface tension in order to prevent alveolar collapse during expiration and therefore stabilizing open alveoli allowing oxygen to diffuse through the lung tissue to the blood (Knudsen et al., 2017; Bates and Smith, 2018; Knudsen and Ochs, 2018). Alveolar parenchyma is thin enough to allow oxygen diffusion and is composed of a minimum of three components: (1) alveolar epithelium, where alveolar epithelial type I cells (AE1C) cover 60% of the surface with a small cytoplasm but in a long and thin disposition, whereas alveolar type II cells (AE2C) are in charge of synthesizing, secreting and regulating surfactant composition; (2) both cells sit on a very thin basal membrane; (3) to which a thin endothelium is attached on the opposite side, creating a thin but extensive air-blood barrier. The last step oxygen encounters in its way to the rest of the organs is the erythrocyte membrane. Red blood cells present a rather high cholesterol content, which comprises a 1:1 phospholipid to cholesterol ratio (Zuniga-Hertz and Patel, 2019). In addition, it has been described that oxygen diffusion through red blood cell membranes is decreased in the presence of increased cholesterol content (Buchwald et al., 2000). And therefore, reduction of cholesterol content in those membranes (such as after the use of Simvastatin for 12 weeks) improves oxygen diffusion rate (Menchaca et al., 1998).

In the long way of oxygen through the human body this review focuses on the first barrier, lung surfactant and how its components may impact the normal function of the lung. There is a particular interest in the relevance of the role of cholesterol, and more specifically, in the long described potential relation between surfactant protein C (SP-C) and cholesterol content in lung surfactant. Here, we described the state of the art at the molecular level, contrasting with data from animal models and human patients, where lung mechanics and alveolar dynamics is affected during SP-C deficiency related disease.

IS THERE A RELATIONSHIP BETWEEN SP-C AND CHOLESTEROL?

Known Functions of SP-C

SP-C is the smallest (4.2 kDa) and most hydrophobic protein in lung surfactant. It accounts for ~1% of lung surfactant mass, becoming the most abundant protein in molar terms. SP-C appeared relatively late in evolution and its sequence has remained highly conserved among species (Potter et al., 2007). The lack of any known homologous protein and its confined expression (Korfhagen et al., 1990), makes it a specific marker associated with the differentiation of lung tissue, and particularly of AE2C. SP-C exists as a 35 amino acid transmembrane protein expressed as a larger precursor (21 kDa) in AE2C cells. Structurally, it adopts a metastable α-helical structure, although its high proportion of branched residues makes it prone to adopt β-sheet structures and fibrillogenic amyloid-like aggregates (Johansson, 2001; Johansson et al., 2004;

Abbreviations: α-SMA, alpha smooth muscle actin; aaAMs, alternatively activated alveolar macrophages; ABCA1, ATP binding cassette transporter A1; ABCG1, ATP binding cassette transporter G1; ADA, adenosine-deaminase; ADP, adenosine diphosphate; AEC, alveolar epithelial cell; AE1C, alveolar epithelial type 1 cell; AE2C, alveolar epithelial type 2 cell; ALI, acute lung injury; AM, alveolar macrophages; AMP, adenosine monophosphate; ApoA1, apolipoprotein A1; ApoE, apolipoprotein E; ARDS, acute respiratory distress syndrome; Arg-1, arginase 1; ASC, apoptosis speck-like protein; ATP, adenosine triphosphate; BALF, bronchoalveolar lavage fluid; Ca^{2+}, calcium; caAMs, classically activated alveolar macrophages; CARD, caspase recruitment domain; chILD, Children Interstitial Lung Disease; DAMPs, damage associated molecular patterns; D_{LCO}, diffusion capacity for carbon monoxide; DPPC, dipalmitoylphosphatidylcholine; EC, extracellular; ECM, extracellular matrix; EMT, epithelial to mesenchymal transition; ER, endoplasmic reticulum; FEV1, forced expiratory pressure in 1 second; FRC, forced residual capacity; GOE, great oxygen event; HCl, chloride acid; HPS, Hermansky–Pudlak syndrome; HRCT, high resolution computed tomography; ILD, interstitial lung disease; IPF, idiopathic pulmonary fibrosis; LA, large aggregate; LAP-1, latency associated peptide 1; LDL, low-density lipoprotein; LPS, lipopolysaccharide; LTP-1, latency TGF-β1 binding protein-1; mRNA, messenger ribonucleic acid; MMP-9, matrix-metalloprotease 9; MMP-13, matrix-metalloprotease 13; MyD88, myeloid differentiation primary response 88; NFκβ, necrosis factor-kappa-beta; NLRP3 NOD-, LRR- and pyrin domain-containing protein 3; NOS-2, inducible nitric oxide synthase; NRDS, neonatal respiratory distress syndrome; PAP, pulmonary alveolar proteinosis; PC, phosphatydilcholine; PEEP, positive end-expiratory pressure; P2XR7, P2X purinoreceptor 7; P2 × 4R, P2X purinoreceptor 4; P2Y2R, P2Y purinoreceptor 2; Relm-α, resistin-like alpha; ROS, reactive oxygen species; RSV, respiratory syncytial virus; SA, small aggregate; SHH, sonic hedgehog; SP-B, surfactant protein B; SP-C, surfactant protein C; SFTPC, surfactant protein C gene; TGF-b1, transforming growth factor beta 1; TIMP1, tissue-metalloprotease inhibitor 1; TLC, total lung capacity; TLR-4, Toll-like receptor 4; TNF-α, tumor necrosis factor alpha; UIP, unusual interstitial pneumonia; VILI, ventilation induced lung injury; YM1, chitinase-like protein 1.

Chou and Fasman, 2006), a common feature in several interstitial lung diseases such as pulmonary fibrosis. SP-C greatly alters lipid packing in membranes influencing lipid motion and lateral distribution (Morrow et al., 1993; Dico et al., 1997). As described before, this may also influence the availability of free volume and free pockets, which may accommodate oxygen. However, a direct study of SP-C content and oxygen diffusion through surfactant membranes has not been assessed so far. SP-C also increases membrane permeability (Plasencia et al., 2004; Parra et al., 2011, 2013) and promotes interfacial lipid adsorption and lipid transfer among different lipid structures (Creuwels et al., 1993; Possmayer et al., 2001; Wang et al., 2005). SP-C is responsible for the reversible formation of multilayered stacks connected to the interfacial monolayer (Amrein et al., 1997; Wang et al., 2005). Doing so, it allows the capture of surfactant material presumably squeezed out during exhalation (area compression) and surfactant re-spreading upon inhalation (area expansion). In this process, protein palmitoylation seems to be relevant to sustain protein association to the highly compressed interfacial films reached during exhalation (Plasencia et al., 2001; Lukovic et al., 2012).

SP-C-associated functions overlap in many cases with surfactant protein B (SP-B) activity, at least when assayed in different *in vitro* models. This includes facilitating lipid adsorption (Creuwels et al., 1993; Possmayer et al., 2001; Wang et al., 2005) into the air-liquid interface or generating 3D structures that serve as a surfactant reservoir (Amrein et al., 1997; Wang et al., 2005), which store newly secreted surfactant complexes and surfactant molecules squeezed out from the interface upon compression. In this context, SP-C could be figured as a supporting molecule for SP-B function rather than an element competent by itself to assist specific features of the complex and dynamic surfactant functionality. Nevertheless, considering the extensive processing of SP-C to its mature form, its extremely conserved sequence and tissue-specific localization, and the difficulties that a cell must overcome to produce and store such a hydrophobic molecule, it is unlikely that this peptide appeared evolutionarily just as an alternative strategy to assist SP-B activities.

SP-C and Cholesterol Relationships in the Lung Surfactant Context

Surfactant cholesterol represents a paradox regarding its origin (Orgeig and Daniels, 2001; Lopez-Rodriguez et al., 2017). Some works have suggested that it is supplied by the low and high-density lipoproteins present in blood circulation (Olmeda et al., 2017). However, other studies have failed to prove that circulating cholesterol ends up forming part of surfactant complexes (Orgeig and Daniels, 2001; Milos et al., 2016), suggesting that other possible sources must be taken into account. It is remarkable that cholesterol levels in surfactant are tightly regulated to ensure a proper breathing function, and they are able to increase and decrease extremely fast in response to changes in temperature or breathing rate (Doyle et al., 1994; Orgeig et al., 2011). This seems to imply that a cholesterol reservoir might exist in order to provide cholesterol at fast rates when an increase is required. A specific cell type, the lipofibroblast, has been suggested as a reservoir of cholesterol (Besnard et al., 2009; Torday and Rehan, 2011), although further validation is required to confirm its presence through different organisms and whether it constitutes a surfactant cholesterol storage. AE2C cells are able of producing cholesterol in peroxisomes (Batenburg and Haagsman, 1998), but alveolar macrophages (AMs) also exhibit enzymes involved in cholesterol synthesis (Baker et al., 2010b). Elucidating how cholesterol levels are regulated in the context of surfactant physiology is key to understand responses associated with several respiratory pathologies, especially those characterized by the incorporation in surfactant of abnormal cholesterol amounts such as the acute respiratory distress syndrome (ARDS) (Vockeroth et al., 2009) or pulmonary alveolar proteinosis (PAP).

The presence of cholesterol induces a marked segregation of fluid phases in surfactant (Bernardino de la Serna et al., 2004; Keating et al., 2007), and variations in cholesterol levels are known to adapt surfactant structures extremely fast to defined physiological situations (Doyle et al., 1994; Orgeig and Daniels, 2001). This evidence highlights cholesterol as a structural modulator of surfactant membranes and films. Besides, mechanisms involved in cholesterol sensing and mobilization may be evolutionary conserved to regulate cholesterol levels in surfactant. On the other hand, some studies suggest that SP-C might be involved in cholesterol regulation (Gómez-Gil et al., 2009a,b; Baumgart et al., 2010; Roldan et al., 2016, 2017), which could also be linked to the role of SP-C in lung homeostasis. Therefore, the role of SP-C in cholesterol mobilization and dynamics could be tracked back to a combined effect of protein- and cholesterol-induced alterations on membrane structure. In fact, an increase in cholesterol motion was described upon incorporation of SP-C into lung surfactant-derived vesicles (Roldan et al., 2016), an effect potentially associated to SP-C-promoted membrane-fragmenting effect (Parra et al., 2011, 2013; Roldan et al., 2016). Besides, SP-C and cholesterol have been also related to modulating membrane architecture responding in a coordinate manner to temperature changes (Roldan et al., 2017), suggesting that SP-C is involved in cholesterol mobilization by altering membrane structure (Roldan et al., 2016). In addition, taking into account that SP-C supplementation restores the functionality of cholesterol-containing films in a dynamic context (Gómez-Gil et al., 2009b; Baumgart et al., 2010), we could hypothesize that SP-C could be related to the compositional refinement of lung surfactant films from less surface-active molecules, involving cholesterol and other unsaturated phospholipids. Interestingly, observations made by Leonenko et al. (2007) could support this hypothesis. The incorporation of increasing amounts of cholesterol in a surfactant clinical preparation resulted in structurally and functionally different interfacial films (Gunasekara et al., 2005; Leonenko et al., 2007). Compression-expansion isotherms allowed the determination of lipid loss from the interfacial film upon compression, which were considerably low for physiological cholesterol amounts, permitting the re-establishment of a functional interfacial film (Gunasekara et al., 2005; Leonenko et al., 2007). Shifting that to SP-C function, lipid loss occurring for physiological cholesterol levels could be associated with a

SP-C-dependent cholesterol refinement, in which SP-C-induced lipid reorganizations could be involved. However, lipid loss increased substantially for cholesterol concentrations beyond physiological levels, showing a markedly different film structure and impaired functionality (Gunasekara et al., 2005; Leonenko et al., 2007). For these supra-physiological cholesterol levels, the SP-C amount present in a clinical surfactant preparation like the one tested in this study (~1 wt%), could be likely insufficient to overcome cholesterol impairing effects and the irreversible film collapse. Supplementation of these films with different SP-C amounts would provide valuable information to confirm SP-C effects on cholesterol mobilization.

SP-C/cholesterol relationships might be involved in surfactant refinement with a homeostatic purpose in the lung. Both, cholesterol-loaded vesicles, as well as their combination with SP-C, led to a higher lipid engulfment by AMs (Ruwisch et al., 2020). Increased cholesterol content, however, seemed to increase lipid uptake by AMs regardless of the presence of SP-C. Vesicle size and membrane fluidity can affect lipid uptake by AMs (Justice et al., 2014), and thus, the combined effect of cholesterol and SP-C on membrane structure and fluidity (Roldan et al., 2016, 2017) is a factor that must be taken into account. The study of the transcriptional response of MH-S cells to lipid administration revealed that genes associated to lipid metabolism and cholesterol transport were altered upon lipid uptake. Changes in gene expression appear to depend on lipid composition, including the presence or absence of SP-C and/or cholesterol. However, specific effects of cholesterol and SP-C require a thorough and extensive analysis, which also warrant a deeper exploration of the poorly studied pathways for cholesterol synthesis, degradation and mobilization in AMs.

SP-C could then be considered as a pivotal molecule linking cholesterol and lipid homeostasis, lung immunity, lung surfactant biophysical activity and potentially oxygen diffusion regulation, which would explain its particular features, lung tissue specific localization and sequence conservation along evolution. Several questions remain to be answered, including how SP-C effects are coordinated with SP-B function to modulate surfactant activity; which are the molecular mechanisms and SP-C structural determinants involved in membrane reorganizations and how cholesterol levels in surfactant are sensed and regulated regarding SP-C function by both AE2C and AMs. Future research assessing these questions would constitute an essential piece to understand the molecular mechanisms ruling lung surfactant behavior and its implication in respiratory pathologies, generating valuable information useful to improve the current clinical preparations applied for surfactant replacement therapy.

SP-C, CHOLESTEROL AND ALVEOLAR MICROMECHANICS

SP-C Deficiency Predisposes to Alveolar Instability

According to LaPlace law, the intra-alveolar pressure of and idealized isotropic alveolus is inversely proportional to its radius. Therefore, at end-expiration, the breathing stage in which the intra-alveolar volume reaches its minimum (ignoring rare occurring phenomena like Pendelluft; Tabuchi et al., 2016), the intra-alveolar pressure reaches its maximum. Under physiologic conditions, end-expiratory pressure is homogenously distributed among the alveoli and surface tension is low enough preventing alveolar collapse. To maintain alveolar pressure throughout the lung constant, surface tension also changes accordingly to alveolar radius (**Figure 1**).

However, during expiration the surfactant film collapses and thus, end-expiratory surface tension may drastically increase and lead to higher intra-alveolar pressures as well as a rather heterogeneous inter-alveolar pressure distribution. As the intra-alveolar pressure is *per se* higher in small-radius alveoli (relative to its larger neighbors) by its anatomy, this may increase the likelihood of alveolar collapse. Hence, it has been described that the result of surfactant dysfunction in a murine model of AE2C apoptosis is ductal airspace over distension together with alveolar collapse (Mouded et al., 2009). On the one hand, this may explain the increased vulnerability of small subpleural alveoli to surfactant dysfunction. On the other hand, points toward an essential role of alveolar collapse in fibrotic remodeling, as collapsing alveoli was proposed to be the initiating hotspot in pulmonary fibrogenesis (Mai et al., 2016; Knudsen et al., 2017; Petroulia et al., 2018).

Alveolar Collapse – The Springboard for Lung Mechanic Impairment

The central role of alveolar collapse in the development of diseases such as lung fibrosis is not a novel finding and was already stated by Myers and Katzenstein (1988). Moreover, alveolar collapse induced by surfactant dysfunction has also been well described in the field of ARDS and acute lung injury (ALI) (Bates and Smith, 2018; Nieman G.F. et al., 2018). Although the increase in surface tension and alveolar instability is much more pronounced in ARDS (Smith et al., 2017; Autilio and Pérez-Gil, 2018) than under SP-C deficiency, leading to a rather acute than chronic respiratory pathology, ARDS as well as rather chronic lung fibrosis may be associated with a similar underlying disease mechanism. This is highlighted by the fact that alveolar collapse, respiratory distress and concomitant ventilation in-homogeneities haven been demonstrated to be present in patients from both diseases (Todd et al., 2015; Al-Saiedy et al., 2018; Autilio and Pérez-Gil, 2018; Petroulia et al., 2018). Moreover, pulmonary fibrosis is also seen in later disease stage of ARDS patients, resembling an aberrant pulmonary repair mechanism in response to lung injury (Hasan et al., 2017), which has also been stated to be the major mechanism of disease in idiopathic pulmonary fibrosis (IPF) patients (Snijder et al., 2019).

Atelectrauma and volutrauma are two mechanism contributing to tissue injury in ARDS (**Figure 2**). In the injured lung, repetitive alveolar collapse (atelectrauma) is caused by increased surface tension (induced by various agents). During the inspiration phase, the transpulmonary pressure gradient increases until the alveolar pressure of the closed (de-recruited) alveolus is exceeded and is re-opened (recruited). If the maximal

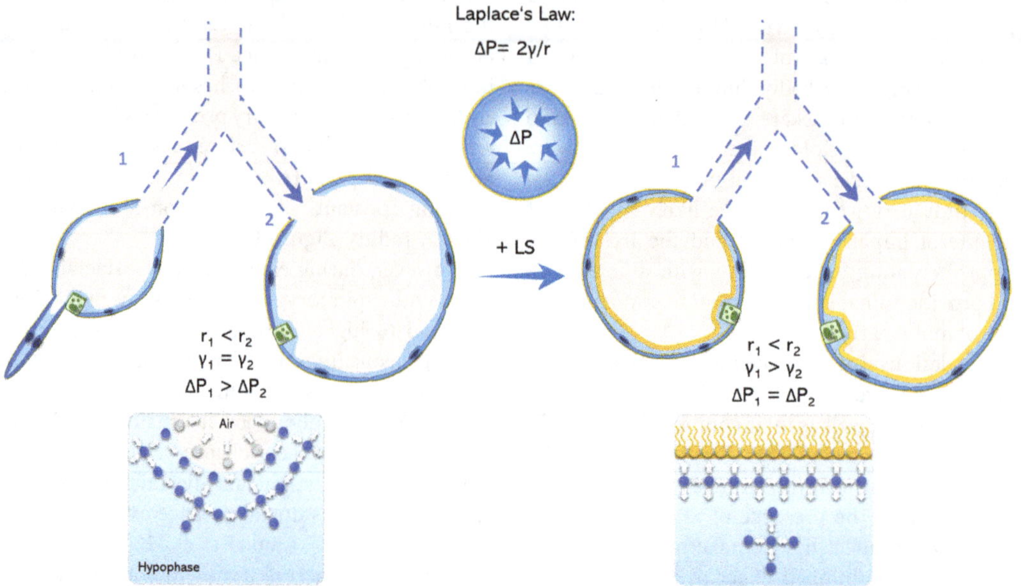

FIGURE 1 | Schematic model of Young-La Place law in the acinar airways. The inner pressure of an idealized spherical alveolus is defined by the Young-La Place law as $\Delta P = 2\gamma/r$. Therefore, alveoli with small radius (alveolus 1) comprise higher internal pressures in relation to alveoli with larger radius (alveolus 2). Accordingly, alveolus 1 would tend to collapse toward alveolus 2 under the absence of a functional surfactant film, what permits alveolar size heterogeneity **(left panel)**. However, in the presence of surfactant, surface tension is reduced as intermolecular forces are homogenously generated between water-water- and water-air phase, avoiding bending of the air-liquid interface and avoiding alveolar collapse **(right panel)**. LS, lung surfactant.

generated transpulmonary pressure fails to exceed the intra-alveolar pressure, the alveolus remains collapsed and its alveolar walls stay adjacent to each other. This model is supported by findings of Bachofen and Schürch, who described alveolar wall stretching and ductal airspace over distension on electron microscopic images resulting from surfactant inactivation-induced alveolar collapse (Bachofen and Schürch, 2001). Considering the mechanism of atelectrauma, the alveolar lining fluid should not be neglected. Weibel and Gil first described the alveolar lining lavage as an interfacial film and sub-interfacial liquid reservoir defined as the hypophase (Weibel and Gil, 1968). As the alveolus deflates during expiration, its defining septa start to fold. The folding septal branches are continuously filled with this alveolar lining fluid during expiration (Rühl et al., 2019). Under increased surface tensions the alveolus is further de-recruited leading to more pronounced septal folding and enhanced inter-septal liquid accumulation. During inspiration, an increasing transpulmonary pressure is generated by the respiratory muscles (Mead et al., 1970; Gattinoni et al., 2017). As soon as this pressure exceeds the end-expiratory intra-alveolar pressure, a bubble of air is forced through the lining fluid between the septal folds in order increase alveolar volume by forcing septal de-folding. During this process mechanical axial shear stresses are generated with the air-bubble moving toward the lining fluid, leading to injurious deformation of AEC2 (Bilek et al., 2003). Of note, the cell damaging force vectors strongly increase with rising surface tension at the interface of the lining fluid, as the speed of the bubble is highly reduced (Cassidy et al., 1999; Ghadiali and Gaver, 2008). Meanwhile, AEC2 injury impairs the epithelial functional integrity resulting in accumulation of alveolar edema and reduced rates of surfactant production. Thus, starting a vicious cycle leading to continuously increasing surface tension and epithelial injury, resulting in AEC2 hyperplasia and fibrosis (Fehrenbach, 2001; Mouded et al., 2009; Sisson et al., 2010) (**Figure 2**).

In the healthy parenchymal lung architecture, tissue stress and stretch occurring during breathing are homogenously distributed. However, if certain alveolar regions become atelectatic, homogenous ventilation is significantly impaired. Alveolar collapse leads to microscale air redistribution, resulting in an inhomogeneous alveolar size distribution before inspiration (Mead et al., 1970). According to alveolar anatomy, single septal walls usually build the parenchymal border of two neighboring alveoli, also known as alveolar interdependence (Knudsen and Ochs, 2018). If one of these alveoli collapses, septal distortion of the adjacent alveoli leads to rising mechanical stresses (Mead et al., 1970). Hence, atelectatic alveoli act as stress concentrators and amplify the applied stresses and strains of their neighbors (Bates and Smith, 2018). During inspiration and increasing lung volumes, this phenomenon becomes even more relevant: transpulmonary pressures generated during inspiration will initially rather lead to over inflation of the already enlarged, distorted alveoli than reopening the atelectatic ones. This causes further alveolar over distension during inspiration. During over distension, an alveolus is first fully de-folded before its wall is stretched. Therefore, the effective septal deformation (= strain) strongly depends on the inspired/applied tidal volume and the alveolar "baseline" shape during resting expiratory position. Usually mechanical stretch primarily occurs under rather high pressures reaching over the upper inflection

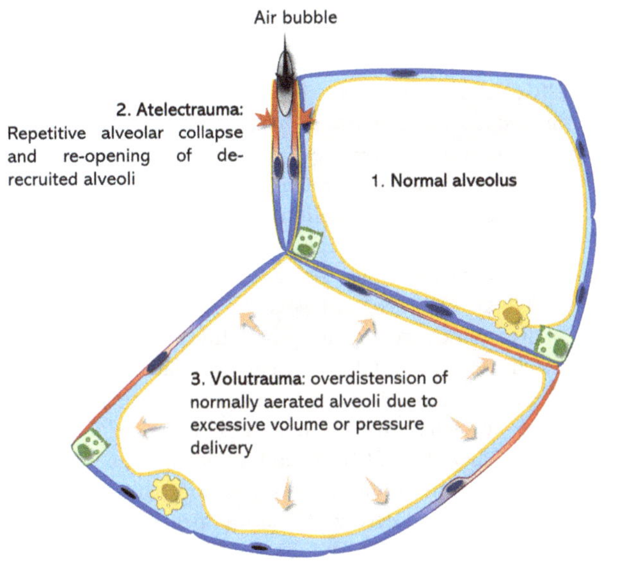

FIGURE 2 | Surfactant dysfunction related atelectrauma and volutrauma. According to the La Place law (**Figure 1**) surfactant dysfunction predisposes alveoli for collapse. Alveolar micro-atelectasis causes septal distortion of neighboring alveoli due septal, interalveolar architectural dependence. Thereby the collapsed alveolus acts as a stress concentrator leading to injurious mechanical deformation of neighboring epithelial cells (blue-red color transition) during the breathing cycle (volutrauma). Meanwhile, every time a bubble of air is forced into the atelectatic, lining-fluid filled alveolus during inspiration, as a result of increasing transpulmonary pressures, extremely damaging shear stresses are generated on the epithelium (atelectrauma), further potentiating damage of the alveolar epithelium (Bates and Smith, 2018; Rühl et al., 2019).

point of the pulmonary pressure-volume curve (Knudsen and Ochs, 2018). However, when inflating a healthy lung beyond total lung capacity (TLC) of 80% the extracellular matrix components of the alveolar septa, collagen and elastin, become the major stress bearing components, thus mechanical forces start acting on the septal interstitium (Bachofen et al., 1987; Knudsen and Ochs, 2018). Moreover, single vulnerable alveoli in proximity to stress concentrators, may already get stretched at physiologic low tidal volumes (Mead et al., 1970). In line with this, Kollisch-Singule et al. (2015) found pulmonary injury in surfactant depleted pig lungs already at physiologic tidal volumes (6 ml/kg bodyweight), while pigs with maintained surfactant function, required a drastically higher degree of volutrauma to induce relevant lung injury (30 ml/kg bodyweight). In the ARDS lung atelectrauma and volutrauma act synergistically to induce vascular leakage. Smith et al. (2013, 2017) elegantly demonstrated that initial epithelial injury by atelectrauma predisposes septal walls for volutrauma, leading to significant leakage of the gas-blood barrier. Ventilated mice lungs only developed high concentrations of BALF protein levels, an indicator for gas-blood barrier integrity, when ventilated at PEEP (positive end-expiratory pressure) of 0cmH2O (atelectrauma) in combination with mid or high tidal volumes (volutrauma) (see **Figure 2**). Meanwhile, neither atelectrauma nor volutrauma alone were sufficient to induce pulmonary edema (Smith et al., 2017). As alveolar epithelial cell (AEC) damage has been demonstrated to precede edema formation (Rühl et al., 2019), the absence of alveolar edema in the SP-C deficient lung (Ruwisch et al., 2020), does not rule out the relevance of this protein in preventing alveolar collapse and alveolar over distension, which commonly lead to microscale tissue injuries. Interestingly, hyperplastic AEC2 are present in a global SP-C knock out (KO) mouse model, which may resemble a reaction to chronic mechanical stress (Glasser et al., 2003; Ruwisch et al., 2020). Moreover, surfactant dysfunction in a chronic murine model of AEC injury impressively demonstrated the long-term effects of chronic airway instability to cause microarchitectural air re-distribution resulting in an emphysema-like phenotype, which is characterized by collapsed alveoli and enlarged alveolar ducts (Mouded et al., 2009). Furthermore, repetitive insults during dynamic strain have been related to more harmful properties on AEC integrity than constant high static strains (Nieman G. et al., 2018). This may further emphasize the relevance of airway instabilities, in the absence of volutrauma, in a rather chronic setting, as occurs in IPF patients, where recruitment/de-recruitment cycles take place over a long period of time. In line with this, "velcro-crackles" have been often described to precede computer tomographic changes in IPF lungs. Indeed, they are considered the auditory correlate of damaging energy-rich alveolar re-openings during inspiration, supporting the clinical relevance of impaired alveolar micromechanics in fibrosing lung diseases (Vyshedskiy et al., 2009).

At the lung mechanical macroscale level, alveolar collapse and surfactant dysfunction exhibit notable influence on the lung's viscoelastic properties. Collapsed airways require high amounts of energy to be reopened, while dysfunctional surfactant increases the hysteresis effect in inflating lungs by rising surface tension. This effect results in parenchymal stiffening, increasing levels of pulmonary tissue elastance (Smith et al., 2013; Birkelbach et al., 2015). During inspiration, the energy applied is rather dissipated creating injurious axial force vectors on the airway epithelium than being stored in the septal elastic fiber network. Therefore, pulmonary tissue damping rises accordingly. In line with this, data from our group demonstrated a significant increase in tissue damping and tissue elastance in 10 weeks old SP-C deficient mice in contrast to age-matched control mice, supporting the concept of alveolar collapse as an initial trigger (Ruwisch et al., 2020). During aging, redistribution of air as well as ECM (Extracellular Matrix) remodeling may alter lung mechanics consistent with findings of Glasser et al. (2001, 2003). Indeed, this work emphasized aberrant tissue hysteresivity (the quotient of energy dissipative forces and lung elastance) at low PEEP, a condition where alveoli are prone to collapse. At those low lung volumes, surfactant becomes the major defining factor of pulmonary breathing mechanics (Bachofen et al., 1987). Moreover, pressure-volume loops demonstrated an increased pulmonary hysteresis, which also reflects increased energy dissipation during inflation of the lung. Gattinoni et al. (2017) already suggested this energy to be potentially harmful for the pulmonary tissue, as it is not reused for elastic recoil properties. Persistent septal micro injury may be, in turn, a relevant factor for altered AEC2 biology, aberrant wound repair, pulmonary inflammation and interstitial fibrotic remodeling. Phenomena described in a number of children suffering interstitial lung disease (chILD), who showed reduced or absent levels of mature SP-C (Cong et al., 2017), as described in the next sections.

Establishing Injurious Mechanical Stress as a Driving Factor for Fibrogenesis

Under healthy conditions and homogenously distributed lung stress, plasma membrane injury of AEC is normally seen. Indeed, AEC are highly capable of Ca^{2+} and lysosome dependent repair mechanisms as well as membrane folds for preventing cellular damage (Cong et al., 2017). However, lysosomal stress as seen in Hermansky-Pudlack Syndrome (HPS) patients may impair cellular repair, favoring profibrotic wound repair and the development of unusual interstitial pneumonia (UIP) (Ozyilmaz et al., 2013; Kook et al., 2016). Moreover, if high parenchymal stress leads to plasma membrane defects of more than 1 μm, aberrant AEC wound repair cascades are induced (Cong et al., 2017). Very high strains induced by pressure above $40cmH_2O$ have been shown to be sufficient to cause membrane blebbing and cellular apoptosis (Dreyfuss et al., 1999).

Typically, AEC injury response includes signaling of several mechano-transduction pathways including the transforming growth factor β1 (TGF-β1), Wnt β-catenin, sonic hedgehog (Shh), and the Notch-midkine signaling pathways as well as induction of endoplasmic reticulum (ER) stress. Interestingly, all these pathways have been interlinked with the induction of profibrotic genes, epithelial-to-mesenchymal transition (EMT) or increased ECM deposition. Moreover, ER stress is known to compromise the secretory capacity of AEC2, impairing surfactant metabolism, which initiates a vicious cycle of alveolar instability and stress-mediated AEC injury (Cong et al., 2017). In a murine model of chloride acid (HCl) induced surfactant depletion, impaired lung mechanics was characterized by increased tissue elastance. This was followed by an increased expression of various mesenchymal markers, such as α-smooth muscle actin (α-SMA) and vimentin in AEC2, whereas the expression of epithelial cell markers, including pro-SP-B, were reduced (Cabrera-Benítez et al., 2012; Mao et al., 2017). Consequently, EMT may be a potent second hit even further compromising: (1) surfactant function and; (2) the regenerative capacitiy of the pulmonary epithelium further directing the damage response toward fibrosis. TGF-β1 is expressed by both AECs as well as resident inflammatory cells like AM (Saito et al., 2018). In addition, a large pool of latent-inactive TGF-β1 is located as a complex with latency associated peptide 1 (LAP-1) and latency TGF-β1 binding protein-1 (LTP-1) in the ECM (Hinz and Suki, 2016; Saito et al., 2018). In the healthy lung, during inspiration, ECM fiber stretching is not sufficient to release active TGF-β1 from its inhibitory binding complex. However, as soon as pulmonary tissue stiffening occurs, interstitial fibroblasts are primed toward myofibroblast differentiation by expressing contractile actin-myosin elements (Zhou et al., 2013). This drastically increases the likelihood of TGF-β1 release upon parenchymal strain, as myofibroblast are able to bind LAP-1 via αV-integrins (Hinz, 2012; Hinz and Suki, 2016). Interestingly, increased epithelial injury resulted in increased expression of epithelial αVß6-integrins, further potentiating the release of TGF-β1 by mechano-transduction (Sheppard, 2015). In line with this, Froese et al. (2016) showed increased expression and release of TGF-β1 in fibrotic IPF lungs, which are characterized by parenchymal stiffening. Importantly the pressures generated by Froese and his team rather reflected gradients comparable to pressure induced by spontaneous breathing than high unphysiological gradients, emphasizing the role of spontaneous breathing as a relevant source of mechanical stress-released active TGF-β1 (Hinz and Suki, 2016). Nevertheless, the role of non-fibrotic but rather collapse-induced parenchymal stiffening in the context of extracellular (EC) TGF-β1 release to date has not been clarified. Finally, TGF-β1 overexpressing mice have been shown to develop surfactant dysfunction and high surface tension (Lopez-Rodriguez et al., 2016) including down-regulation of SP-C expression, by interfering with its transcription factor activity. In this context, considering the afore mentioned section, it becomes clear that an EC TGF-β1 pool bears the potential of an additional devastating loop by further compromising lung mechanics, potentiating epithelial injury.

Inflammatory Response Under Impaired Lung Mechanics – Where Sterols Come Into Play

The role of inflammation and inflammatory cells in fibrogenesis has been controversial over the last decades. Although anti-inflammatory medications have produced devastating clinical results in a IPF clinical trials (Raghu et al., 2006; Idiopathic Pulmonary Fibrosis Clinical Research Network et al., 2012), the role of immune cells, like AMs, in lung fibrogenesis and pulmonary tissue repair has been repetitively underscored (Wynn and Barron, 2010; Wynn et al., 2013; Romero et al., 2014; Jin et al., 2018; Smigiel and Parks, 2018; Puttur et al., 2019). A promising link between mechanical stretch and inflammatory response may be the release of adenosine triphosphate (ATP) (Cong et al., 2017; Hasan et al., 2017). Physiologically, mechanical stretch of AEC1 transmits the release of ATP via P2XR7, functioning as a stretch sensor (Patel et al., 2005; Mishra et al., 2011). However, under prolonged alveolar injury concentrations of ATP and its related nucleotides sharply rise, finally overwhelming the degradative enzymatic machinery. Hence, levels of ATP continuously stay high in the early exudative stage of ARDS until the expression of its degrading ecto-enzyme catches up (Hasan et al., 2017). Under these circumstances, ATP and its metabolites act as damage associated molecular patterns (DAMPs). This results in pro-inflammatory signaling on the one hand, but interestingly also in the induction of various profibrotic pathways on the other hand. In fact, high levels of EC ATP enhanced TGF-β1 expression and deposition of collagen 1 and fibronectin in fibroblasts via P2XR7 signaling *in vitro* (Wang et al., 2003; Qu et al., 2009). Meanwhile, ATP signaling via the same receptor enhanced the release of profibrotic tissue-metalloprotease inhibitor 1 (TIMP1), which attenuates the function of ECM-degrading enzymes, resulting in increased interstitial amounts of ECM, a hallmark of lung fibrosis (Gu and Wiley, 2006). Interestingly, elevated levels of TIMP1 have also been observed in bronchoalveolar lavage fluid (BALF) of IPF patients, whereas expression of Timp1 was induced in 10 weeks old SP-C deficient mice (Beeh et al., 2003). In addition, both Ca^{2+} and ATP are well-known stimulating agents of surfactant secretion (Voyno-Yasenetskaya et al., 1991; Dico et al., 1997; Patel et al., 2005; Dietl et al., 2012). This may reflect a counteracting response, where surfactant secretion may be enhanced during high release of ATP and Ca^{2+}, during injury.

Alternatively activated alveolar macrophages (aaAMs) are mainly characterized by expression of resistin-like alpha (Relm-α), chitinase-like proteins (YM1), inducible nitric oxide synthase (NOS-2) or arginase 1 (Arg-1) (Wynn and Barron, 2010). Their profibrotic potential derives primarily through expression of TGF-β1 and the activation of latent TGF-β1 via matrix-metalloproteases (e.g., MMP-9) (Xing et al., 1997; Schmid-Kotsas et al., 1999; Cameron et al., 2001; Karlmark et al., 2009; Lin et al., 2009). Moreover, aaAMs haven been shown in topographic proximity to myofibroblasts, being highly capable of collagen secretion (Ramm et al., 1998; Leicester et al., 2004; Thompson et al., 2008). Finally, aaAMs prime the alveolar micromilieu toward fibrosis by secreting various pro-fibrotic cytokines including IL-4, IL-10, IL-13 and the rather pro-inflammatory cytokine IL-1β. Of note, induced expression of YM1, a chitinase-like protein 1 (Bargagli et al., 2007; Terèelj et al., 2009; Wynn and Barron, 2010), but also in SP-C deficient mice (Glasser et al., 2003). Increased accumulation of macrophages with induced TGF-β1 expression was seen in bleomycin-challenged SP-C deficient mice in areas with significant parenchymal distortion. This further emphasizes the link between mechanical stress and macrophage regulation (Lawson et al., 2005). Interestingly, this misbalance between classical and alternative differentiation was not solely dependent on SP-C deficiency, but also specific to the genetic 129/Sv6 background. The 129/Sv6 strain is characterized by an increased dietary cholesterol accumulation and has been described to develop foamy, lipid-laden macrophages with highly induced YM1 expression with age (Jolley et al., 1999; Hoenerhoff et al., 2006). Curiously, SP-C deficient mice as well as patients suffering mutant SP-C derived interstitial lung diseases (ILDs) related to mutations of SP-C, showed similar foamy macrophages in BALF and tissue as well as abundant cholesterol clefts (Glasser et al., 2003; Hamvas et al., 2004; Abou Taam et al., 2009; Ruwisch et al., 2020). Taken together, this suggests a SP-C deficiency and cholesterol induced axis resulting in dysregulated macrophage metabolism and in misbalanced alternative differentiation (**Figure 3**). Cholesterol clefts are present in aging 129/Sv4 mice (Hoenerhoff et al., 2006), SP-C deficient mice (Glasser et al., 2003; Ruwisch et al., 2020) or aaAMs in human herpes virus (HHV)-induced lung fibrosis (Mora et al., 2006). Hence, this may be a potential morphological biomarker of dysregulated alternative activation and an indicator for lung fibrosis. However, the exact interplay between cholesterol and SP-C and macrophage regulation has not been yet elucidated. Nevertheless, studies from our group, suggested SP-C to be necessary for maintaining cholesterol homeostasis in an AM cell line (MHS cells) (Ruwisch et al., 2020). In line with this, Romero and colleagues recently proposed the profibrotic potential of a lipid related paracrine axis between macrophages and epithelial cells (Romero et al., 2014). Interestingly, their team demonstrated the presence of foamy, lipid-laden macrophages overexpressing YM1 and TGF-β1 in bleomycin induced lung injury, which has been already associated with reduced expression of the *Sftpc* and *Sftpb* gene (Schmidt et al., 2004; Lutz et al., 2015). Romero's team further showed oxidized phospholipids to be another crucial inductor of foam cell formation and alternative differentiation. The role of oxidized lipid species to induce foam cell formation in macrophages has been extensively studied in the field of atherosclerosis (Ertunc and Hotamisligil, 2016). Circulatory macrophages located in atherosclerotic plaques are frequently challenged with oxidized low-density lipoprotein (LDL), oxysterols or cholesterol. These lipids are endocytosed via various receptors, including CD36 and scavenger receptors. Accumulation of toxic lipid species decompensates the metabolic capacity of those macrophages, leading to cholesterol cleft formation and induction of necrotic factor kappa beta (NFκB) related cellular stress pathways. One central element in the so called "metaflammatory" process. This is the formation of the NOD-, LRR- and pyrin domain-containing protein 3 (NLRP3) inflammasome, resulting in the production of pro-inflammatory cytokines including IL-1β and IL-18 (Duewell et al., 2010; Ramji and Davies, 2015). Importantly, macrophage derived IL-1β and inflammasome activation have been referred to as key features in various forms of lung fibrosis including IPF (Zhang et al., 1993; Kolb et al., 2001; Gasse et al., 2007; Wynn and Barron, 2010; Eldridge et al., 2017).

In addition, cholesterol-induced "metaflammation" in macrophages may also be not only important in development of atherosclerosis but seems to be also highly relevant in the lung. For example, AMs are central elements in surfactant catabolism (comprehensively reviewed in Lopez-Rodriguez et al., 2017), and are continuously challenged with various phospho- and neutral lipids. Therefore, knocking down cholesterol transporters, such as ATP binding cassette transporter A1 (ABCA1) and G1 (ABCG1) leads to impaired cellular cholesterol efflux and cholesterol accumulation. In addition, those animal models showed respiratory distress, impaired surfactant metabolism and cholesterol cleft containing, lipid-laden AMs (Thomassen et al., 2007; Baker et al., 2010a; Chai et al., 2017; Fessler, 2017). Moreover, impaired reverse cholesterol transport in apolipoprotein E (ApoE) and apolipoprotein A1 (ApoA1) deficient mice was also linked to increased pulmonary oxidative stress and inflammation (in ApoE KO mice) as well as to foam cell formation and lung fibrogenesis (in ApoA1 KO mice) (Yao et al., 2016). Interestingly, surfactant function as well as metabolic integrity of AM was restored after application of cyclodextrin, a cholesterol sequestering-drug, underlining the injurious potential of cholesterol for surfactant function and pulmonary lipid homeostasis (Gunasekara et al., 2010). The finding of cholesterol clefts and lipid laden macrophages in patients with SP-C mutations suggests impaired cholesterol homeostasis to be of relevance for development of lung disease in these patients (Hamvas et al., 2004; Abou Taam et al., 2009; Mechri et al., 2010; Cottin and Cordier, 2011; Litao et al., 2017).

Cholesterol overloaded macrophages exhibited an increased Toll-like receptor 4 (TLR-4) signaling mediated immune

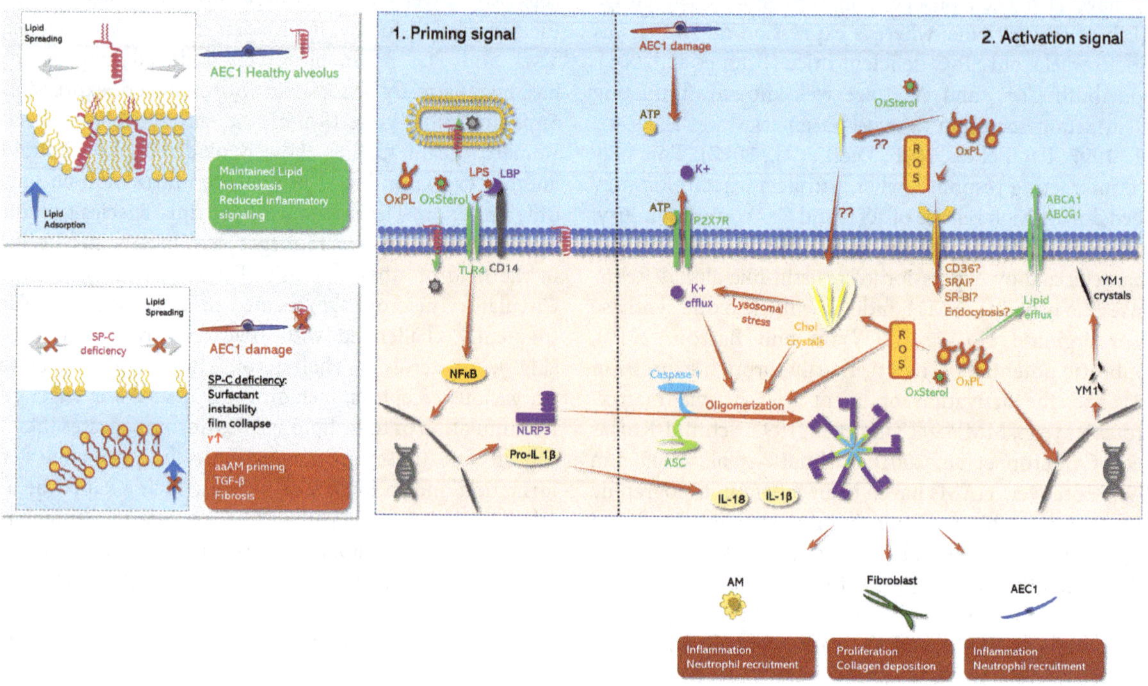

FIGURE 3 | Schematic role of SP-C in pulmonary metaflammation. **(Left panel)** comparison between the status of AE1C in the presence (healthy alveolus, top panel) or absence (damaged alveolus, bottom panel) of SP-C. **(Right panel: 1) Priming signal:** TLR4 signaling is abrogated under the presence of mature SP-C. On the one hand, SP-C interferes with the complex formation of LBP and CD14 potentially attenuating TLR4 mediated NLPR3 priming in response DAMP/PAMP stimuli. This ant-inflammatory effect may be further potentiated by the N-terminal segment of SP-C transferring TLR4 activators either into neighboring phospholipid microsomes or directly to the cytoplasmic compartment of the macrophage (Chaby et al., 2005; Garcia-Verdugo et al., 2009). Moreover, maintained surfactant homoeostasis/surfactant catabolism counteracts the accumulation/formation of oxidized lipid species and cholesterol clefts on the one hand, and minimizes atelec- and volutrauma on the other hand (Ruwisch et al., 2020), likely diminishing the release of DAMPS like ATP on the other hand. Together this prevents the buildup of inflammasome oligomerizing stimuli, what may at least partly explain the aberrant inflammatory response of SP-C KO mice to various inflammatory stimuli in contrast to WT mice (Glasser et al., 2008, 2013a). **(Right panel: 2) Activating signal:** NLRP3 inflammasome comprises an initial NFκβ related priming phase, preceding a secondary activation signal (Swanson et al., 2019): In the first step various proinflammatory DAMPS (oxysterols, oxidized PL species) or PAMPS (LPS) activate macrophages via TLR-4 signaling via an either LPS binding protein (LBP)/CD14 dependent or independent way (Chaby et al., 2005; Garcia-Verdugo et al., 2009). Thereby, LBP facilitates the binding of e.g., LPS to CD14, what accelerates LPS related TLR4 signaling. TLR4 signaling in turn drives NFκB-mediated expression of NLRP3, pro-IL-β1 and proIL-18 (Priming phase) (Gasse et al., 2007; Swanson et al., 2019). In the second step, multiple potential hits including PAMPS like extracellular ATP (Mariathasan et al., 2006; Swanson et al., 2019), intracellular cholesterol clefts (Ertunc and Hotamisligil, 2016), oxysterols and oxidized phospholipid derived mitochondrial oxidative stress (Fessler, 2017; Manon et al., 2018) induce previously synthetized NLRP3 to form oligomers with caspase 1 and ASC leading to mature inflammasome formation. Thereby, increased level of extracellular ATP may be derived from mechanically stressed AEC1 (Hasan et al., 2017), leading to an inflammasome activating K^+ efflux via P2X7R. Meanwhile, SP-C deficiency related dysfunctional surfactant catabolism and surfactant dysfunction may favor the generation of oxidized PL species and the formation of cholesterol clefts (Fessler and Summer, 2016; Ruwisch et al., 2020). Likewise, these cholesterol crystals cause lysosomal stress, which in turn resembles another potent driving factor of inflammasome formation via induction of a K^+ efflux. Finally, the active NLRP3 inflammasome converts inactive proIL-1β and proIL-18 into their active form IL-1β and IL-18. IL-1β promotes fibrotic remodeling (Gasse et al., 2007; Cassel et al., 2008; Wree et al., 2014; Lv et al., 2018). Meanwhile, another effect of accumulation of injurious lipid species inside the macrophages may also prime their hosts toward a profibrotic aaAM-phenotype (Romero et al., 2014) via induction of several aaAM related genes including, chitinase-like-3 (YM1), which has also been described to form electron dense crystals in various alternative activation of macrophages-disease models (Hoenerhoff et al., 2006; Mora et al., 2006), what may result in a profibrotic feed-forward loop (Smigiel and Parks, 2018).

response as well as elevated expression levels of IL-1β, emphasizing a potential role of NLRP3 inflammasome activation in pulmonary macrophages (Fessler, 2017). The NLRP3-inflammasome consists of three elements including the NLRP3, procaspase 1 and the apoptosis speck-like protein (ASC) containing a caspase recruitment domain (CARD), which links NLRP3 with procaspase 1 (Robert et al., 2016). In order to generate full activation of the inflammasome complex usually two independent signals are needed (**Figure 3**): (1) a NFκβ priming signal TLR-4 signaling [enhanced by lipopolysaccharide (LPS) or oxidized phospholipid species] or the presence of cholesterol crystals (Bauernfeind et al., 2009; Ertunc and Hotamisligil, 2016; Fessler and Summer, 2016; Nakayama, 2018; Saito et al., 2019) and; (2) purinergic signaling as may result from mechanical stress induced AEC1 injury (Hasan et al., 2017). Elevated levels of ATP have been found in BALF of patients with lung fibrosis, further supporting the idea of EC ATP as a potential inflammasome co-activator (Riteau et al., 2010). Hence, the NLRP3 inflammasome may resemble a crucial link between impaired lung mechanics and aberrant lipid metabolism in fibrosing lung diseases. Interestingly, IPF patients have been described to have elevated levels of unsaturated PC, a PC variant which highly susceptible for oxidative stress (Fessler and Summer, 2016). In combination with the fact, that IPF occurs predominantly in the elderly and has been interlinked with cigarette smoking, mitochondrial stress and cellular senescence, factors driving the generation of reactive oxygen species (ROS). Thus, the IPF lung appears as a hotspot for lipid oxidation (Lederer and Martinez, 2018). Elevated levels of ROS and increased levels of cholesterol in surfactant are also present in bleomycin-induced lung fibrosis (Allawzi et al., 2019), highlighting the relevance of ROS, surfactant oxidation and foam cell formation in fibrogenesis. This is further supported by the presence foamy, Oil-Red-O positive cells in BALF of patients not only with *Sftpc* mutations, but also in patients with sporadic interstitial fibrosis (Basset-Léobon et al., 2010).

Nevertheless, SP-C deficiency may play a distinct role in foam cell formation. Not only is SP-C crucial for stabilizing cholesterol-containing surfactant films (Gómez-Gil et al., 2009a,b) and maintaining physiologic mechanical lung properties but also it seems to interfere with TLR-4 signaling. *In vitro* studies demonstrated that SP-C attenuates LPS induced cytokine production via TLR-4 signaling in a macrophage cell line, suggesting SP-C to play a role in innate immunity (Augusto et al., 2003). Thereby, SP-C seems to compromise the affinity of TLR-4 to LPS via a complex interplay with CD14 (Chaby et al., 2005). However, Garcia-Verdugo et al. (2009) also proposed a CD14 independent mechanism, by which the transfer of LPS into liposomes mediated by the N-terminal SP-C segment would prevent LPS binding to TLR4. This results in a reduced cytokine production upon LPS stimulation (Garcia-Verdugo et al., 2009). In line with these findings, SP-C KO mice exhibited an increased inflammatory response upon LPS challenge characterized by increased macrophage accumulation and higher expression levels of IL-1β, IL-6 and tumor necrosis factor alpha (TNF-α) (Glasser et al., 2013a). Interestingly, SP-C containing phospholipid vesicles reduced TLR-4 signaling in these mice. Noteworthy, this immunomodulatory role of SP-C seems to not to be restricted to LPS and bacteria-induced inflammation, as SP-C also demonstrated an anti-inflammatory role under pathogen-free conditions (Jin et al., 2018). Taken all together, this suggest that SP-C may not only orchestrate the activation of TLR-4 in an infectious setting, but it also has an impact on TLR-4 signaling in macrophages induced by oxidized surfactant lipids, a question that, to date, remains unclear.

Assuming this hypothesis (**Figure 3**), SP-C deficiency could predispose to TLR-4 activation by various oxidized cholesterol and PL species as well as their uptake. This results in proinflammatory signaling and NLRP3 inflammasome activation in macrophages (Ertunc and Hotamisligil, 2016). Impaired lung mechanics induced by SP-C deficiency may further promote inflammasome activation by ATP release and at the same time, lead to accelerated surfactant aggregate conversion (Veldhuizen et al., 1996, 1997; Vazquez De Anda et al., 2000; Maitra et al., 2002). Reduced amounts of surface-tension lowering large aggregates (LA) of surfactant, resulting from pronounced aggregate conversion to inactive small aggregates (SA), were accompanied by larger amounts of ROS susceptible phospholipid species (Fessler and Summer, 2016). Increased uptake of SA by AMs in combination with SP-C disrupted cholesterol metabolism, which may partly explain the presence of foamy macrophages in the SP-C deficient lung and lung diseases related to SP-C mutated forms (Glasser et al., 2003; Hamvas et al., 2004; Lawson et al., 2004; Stevens et al., 2005; Henderson et al., 2013; Liptzin et al., 2015; Salerno et al., 2016).

The relevance of inflammasome activation and IL-1β signaling in fibrotic parenchyma remodeling has been shown for silica induced- ILDs (Cassel et al., 2008), bleomycin-induced lung fibrosis (Gasse et al., 2007) and various other organ systems (Vilaysane et al., 2010; Wree et al., 2014; Lv et al., 2018). NLRP3 associated IL-1β release mediates NFκβ activation via IL-1R1/myeloid differentiation primary response 88 (MyD88) related signal transduction in fibroblasts. This results in a misbalance between TIMP-1 and matrix-metalloprotease 9 (MMP-9) and 13 (MMP-13) promoting interstitial collagen deposition and fibrosis (So et al., 2007; Ertunc and Hotamisligil, 2016). Furthermore, genetic deletion of NLRP3-inflammasome associated genes in a ventilated-induced fibrosis model resulted in decreased rates of stretch-induced EMT, which was accompanied by ameliorated fibrotic lung remodeling (Lv et al., 2018).

SP-C, CHOLESTEROL AND LUNG MECHANICS. EVIDENCES FROM ANIMAL MODELS AND HUMAN PATIENTS

All the molecular and cellular mechanisms explained in the previous sections impact the health and mechanical properties of the lungs. We described in this section the results of deleting the expression or mutating SP-C in animal models (**Table 1**). In addition, we present here evidences from ILD patients, described to have different mutations in SP-C (**Table 2**).

SP-C Modifications in Animal Models

Glasser et al. (2001, 2003) reported the generation of SP-C null mutant mice deficient in the expression of *Sftpc* in a Swiss black background. SP-C deficient mice were viable at birth and did grow and reproduce normally with only mild alterations in lung mechanics. In addition, *in vitro* studies of the SP-C deficient derived surfactant proved reduced stability of small bubbles but normal activity at normal bubble size using a captive bubble surfactometer (Glasser et al., 2001, 2003). In contrast, in 129/Sv background, SP-C deficient mice presented with severe morphological changes including enlargement of alveoli, AE2C hyperplasia and interstitial thickening together with a peribronchiolar and perivascular monocyte infiltration in some animals. Although areas of thickened alveolar septa stained positive for alpha-smooth muscle actin and blue in trichrome staining, septa were thinner in regions of airspace enlargement and total lung hydroxyproline remained unaffected (Glasser et al., 2003; Ruwisch et al., 2020). Importantly, lung structure was normal at birth, but emphysema and remodeling developed upon aging suggesting a process of ongoing injury and repair. Investigation of pulmonary mechanics exhibited increased lung volumes at higher pressures as well as increased hysteresivity

TABLE 1 | SP-C related mouse models.

Mouse model		General results	Lung morphology	BALF	Lung mechanics
SP-C null mutants					
Glasser et al., 2001	Generation of SP-C null mutant mice, Swiss black background	Viable, normal growth and reproducibility Reduced stability of small bubbles but normal activity at standard bubble size	Indistinguishable from controls		Reduced hysteresitivity at each end-expiratory pressure
Glasser et al., 2003	SP-C null mutant mice, 129/Sv background	Reduced health and fecundity	From 2 months: enlargement of alveoli, irregular alveolar septation, multifocal cellular infiltrates. From 6 month: type 2 cell hyperplasia, interstitial thickening, peribronchiolar and perivascular monocytic infiltration Intracellular lipid inclusions in macrophages and AE2C, cystoplasmic crystals in macrophages	Increased macrophage number	Increased lung volumes at higher pressures, increased hysteresivity, increased airway resistance and tissue damping
2nd hit models					
Lawson et al., 2005	Intratracheal bleomycin application, Swiss black background	Higher mortality and weight loss, more pronounced fibrosis and delayed resolution	Increased number of inflammatory cells, fibrotic foci (collagen, fibroblasts, destroyed septa), enhanced collagen deposition; delayed resolution of fibrosis	Increased neutrophil counts	
Madala et al., 2011	Bleomycin and rapamycin, S129S6 background	Preventive and therapeutic treatment with rapamycin failed to reduce bleomycin induced tissue inflammation and collagen deposition			
Glasser et al., 2008	Instillation of *Pseudomonas aeruginosa*, 129S6 and FVB/N strain	Reduced survival of 2-week-old mice, increased bacterial colony counts in 2-week-old 129S6 but not in FVB/N mice	Increased inflammation, tissue and airway infiltrates (neutrophils and enlarged macrophages with cytoplasmic inclusions)	Increased total cell counts: neutrophils; large foamy macrophages	
Glasser et al., 2009	Respiratory syncytial virus infection, 129S6 and FVB/N	Higher susceptibility to RSV and delayed resolution of induced changes in lung morphology in both strains	More extensive interstitial thickening, air space consolidation, goblet cell hyperplasia.	Increased total cell counts: polymorphonuclear leucocytes, lymphocytes, enlarged foamy mononuclear cells	
Glasser et al., 2013b	RSV infection, expression of SP-C inducible by doxycycline (on 129S6; *55.3/Sftpc-/-*)	SP-C expression reduced RSV-induced tissue inflammation and inflammatory cell counts and increased viral clearance	Diffuse alveolar and interstitial infiltrates in doxycycline untreated mice, reduced inflammation in doxycycline treated mice	Reduced total cell counts and percentage of neutrophil counts in doxycycline -treated mice	
Glasser et al., 2013a	LPS challenge, 129S6 background	More intense airway and airspace inflammation, delayed resolution of tissue inflammation	More intense cellular infiltration, perivascular edema, fragmentation of alveolar septa; residual inflammation 30 days post LPS exposure	Increased total cell counts without LPS challenge (reduced by application of Survanta)	
Models with incomplete proSP-C processing					
Conkright et al., 2002	Expression of SP-C_{24-57} HA, FVB/N	Delayed/arrested lung development and lethal neonatal respiratory distress syndrome			

(Continued)

TABLE 1 | Continued

Mouse model		General results	Lung morphology	BALF	Lung mechanics
Bridges et al., 2003	Deletion of exon 4	Not viable	Fetal lung tissue: disrupted lung organogenesis, branching morphogenesis, dose-dependent cell cytotoxicity		
Lawson et al., 2011	Conditional expression of L188Q upon doxycycline; intratracheal bleomycin	No spontaneous pulmonary fibrosis; more extensive fibrosis in response to bleomycin	Increased apoptosis, total lung collagen, higher number of myofibroblasts after bleomycin	Cell numbers unaltered in bleomycin treated WT and mutant mice	More reduced static lung compliance in bleomycin treated L188Q mice than challenged controls
Nureki et al., 2018	Conditional mouse mutant, constitutive and inducible I73T expression (by Tamoxifen), C57BL/6J	Increased early mortality, spontaneous acute alveolitis, parenchymal injury, fibrotic remodeling	Constitutive I73T expression: diffuse parenchymal lung remodeling; disrupted embryonic lung architecture Induced expression: acute, diffuse lung injury after tamoxifen, partial recovery but development of fibrotic phenotype	Constitutive expression: age-dependent increases in BALF cellularity induced expression: increased total cell counts, early macrophage accumulation, followed by polymorphonuclear cells and eosinophilia, milder increase in total lymphocytes	Induced expression: restrictive pattern (PV loops), decreased static compliance
Venosa et al., 2019	Conditional mouse mutant, I73T expression induced by Tamoxifen; Local and i.v application of clodronate	Multiphasic and multicellular alveolitis; local clodronate application reduced survival, i.v. clodronate improved survival and reduced eosinophilia		Early reduction of macrophages, followed by accumulation of immature macrophages, neutrophils and eosinophils	
Katzen et al., 2019	Constitutive and conditional C121G mutant inducible by tamoxifen, C57BL/6J	Constitutive expression: lethal postnatal respiratory failure Conditional expression in adult mice: dose-dependent morbidity and mortality, multiphasic polycellular alveolitis with increased BALF cell counts	Constitutive: distorted architecture, enlarged airspaces, interstitial widening, inflammatory infiltrates, proteinaceous fluid conditional expression: acute diffuse lung injury, partial recovery but spontaneous fibrotic lung remodeling	Conditional expression: polycellular alveolitis, increased total cell counts, early macrophage increase, followed by neutrophils and eosinophils, milder increase in lymphocytes	Restrictive pattern: decline in static lung compliance
Jin et al., 2018	Sterile injury model (surfactant protein C-thymidine kinase) induced by ganciclovir in presence (SPC-TK) and absence (SPC-TK/SPC-KO) of SP-C expression	Increased injury and higher mortality in absence than in presence of SP-C expression	Diffuse alveolar damage qualitatively similar but more pronounced in SPC-TK/SPC-KO	Total cell counts unaltered in SPC-TK/SPC-KO and SPC-TK, higher neutrophils and lymphocyte cell counts in SPC-TK/SPC-KO	

in SP-C deficient mice. Abnormal intracellular lipid inclusions and crystals were observed in macrophages and AE2C (Glasser et al., 2001, 2003). While phospholipid content was normal in SP-C deficient lungs on the swiss black background, it was 2-fold elevated in 129/Sv background. In addition, lung mechanics showed increased lung volume at high pressure, tissue damping and hysteresivity in 129Sv background. Together, both studies show strain specific influences on the severity of the pulmonary phenotype (Glasser et al., 2001, 2003). Interestingly, as mentioned before, the 129Sv strain demonstrates an increased absorption of dietary cholesterol (Jolley et al., 1999) which might also contribute to the strain specific phenotype in *Sftpc* null mice.

Further investigations included additional hits aggravating the effects of SP-C deficiency (Lawson et al., 2005; Glasser et al., 2008, 2009, 2013a,b). Intratracheal application of bleomycin led to higher mortality, more pronounced weight loss, increased neutrophil counts and enhanced collagen deposition in SP-C deficient mice compared to controls. Increased fibrosis as additionally indicated by morphological parameters went along with a delayed resolution of bleomycin-induced fibrosis

TABLE 2 | Lung mechanics and BALF cells data from patients.

Variant	BALF cells	Lung mechanics	Reference
L188Q		TLC 52%, DLCo 51% (male patient, onset 20 years); FVC 21% (female patient, onset 17 years)	Thomas et al., 2002
I73T	85% M, 12% L, 3% N		Tredano et al., 2004
R167Q	84% M, 11% L, 5% N		
I73T	92% M, 7% N, 1% L, 0% E	FRC: 69% (8 months), 77% (13 years) DLCo: 25% (8 months), 51% (13 years)	Abou Taam et al., 2009
I73T	30% M, 60% N, 10% L, 0% E (Moraxella catarrhalis)	FRC: 138% (36 months), DLCo: 111% (33 months), 128% (36 months), 156% (42 months)	
I73T	82% M, 13% N, 3% L, 2% E	FRC: 120% (26 months), 128% (35 months), 73% (39 months) DLCo: 98% (26 months), 89% (35 months), 164% (39 months)	
I73T	84% M, 5% N, 11% L, 0% E		
I73T	93% M, 1% N, 6% L, 0% E	FRC 112% (26 months), DLCo: 87% (26 months)	
15x I73T, 1x V39A, c.325- 1G > A, c.424delC, c.435G > C (Q145H), L188P, C189Y, L194P	70 ± 5% M, 8 ± 2% L, 18 ± 4% N, total: 379 ± 56 × 10^3	82% patients with SpO_2 testing <95%	Thouvenin et al., 2010
I73T	40% M, 57% N, 3% L (mother 32 years)	FVC 62%, TLC 77%, FEV1 83%, RV 108%, DLCo 33%, PaO_2 room air 11.3 kPa, PaO_2 after 10 min exercise (35W): 7.3 kPa	Cottin et al., 2011
	74% M, 20% N, 4% L, 2% E (child, 3 months)		
G100S	BAL cell count (100.000 cells/ml): 2.4, 90% M, 7.5% L, 2.5% N, 0% E, CD4/CD8 ratio: 1,7	VC 72.2%, FEV1 84.1% DLCo: 69.3%	Ono et al., 2011
	BAL cell count (100.000 cells/ml): 2, 86% M, 12% L, 1% N, 1% E, CD4/CD8 ratio: 1.6	VC 85%, FEV1 90.3% DLCo: not available	
	BAL cell count (100.000 cells/ml): 1.4, 91% M, 5.8% L, 2.4% N, 0.8% E; CD4/CD8 ratio: 1.5	VC 96.6%, FEV1 85% DLCo: 65.2%	
	BAL cell count(100.000 cells/ml): 1.21,: 54.2% M, 10.1% L, 34.5% N, 1.2% E, CD4/CD8 ratio: 0.25	VC 42.5%, FEV1 92.9% DLCo: 38.5%	
	BAL cell count (100.000 cells/ml): 3.85, 80% M, 17.3% L, 1.1% N, 1.6% E, CD4/CD8 ratio: 0.6 (time diagnosis)	VC 65.3%, FEV1 83.3% DLCo: not available (at time diagnosis)	
Y104H	91% M, 8% L, 1% N	FVC 85%, DLCo 89%, oxygen saturation 97% to 95% (with exercise)	Kuse et al., 2013
I73T		16 years: 90% FVC, 86% TLC, 96% DLCo, 96% VO_2 max; 37 years: FVC 65%, TLC 91%, DLCo 42%, VO_2max: 5	Avital et al., 2014
I38F		14 years: FVC 77%, TLC 90%, DLCo 108%, VO_2 max 78%; 32 years: FVC 94%, TLC 96%, DLCo 82%, VO_2max 69%, high breathing reserve: 115 l/min, saturation 100% at peak exercise	
I73T		7 years: FVC 59%, TLC 95% DLCo not available, VO_2max 80%, 28 years: FVC 46%, TLC 48%, DLCo 58%, VO_2max 79%	
I73T		8 years: FVC 69%, TLC 100%, DLCo 107%, VO_2 max 83%, 29 years: FVC 102%, TLC 106%, DLCo 95%, VO_2max 83%	
V39L		16 years: FVC 88%, TLC 95%, DLCo 109%, VO_2max 93%; 37 years: 94% FVC, 96% TLC, 82% DLCo, 91% VO_2max	
C121F	Infiltration of granulocytes and alveolar macrophages		van Hoorn et al., 2014
I73T		4 months: 88% oxygen saturation, respiratory rate 85, V_T 6.0 ml/kg, V_E 507 ml/min/kg, Crs 2.96 ml/cmH_2O, Crs/kg 0.76/kg, VC 92 ml(52%), TLC 196 ml(74%), FRC 128 ml(110%), RV 104 ml(99%), V_{max}FRC 416 ml/s (263%), FEF_{75} 410 ml/s (207%), FEF_{85} 295 ml/s (258%)	Hevroni et al., 2015

(Continued)

TABLE 2 | Continued

Variant	BALF cells	Lung mechanics	Reference
I38F		3.3 months: 91% oxygen saturation, respiratory rate 77, V_T 6.3 ml/kg, V_E 484 ml/min/kg, Crs 2.26 ml/cmH_2O, Crs/kg 0.59/kg, VC 28 ml(69%), TLC 211 ml(94%), FRC 138 ml(125%), RV 108 ml(109%), V_{max}FRC 343 ml/s (245%), FEF_{75} 579 ml/s (334%), FEF_{85} 477 ml/s (476%)	
I73T	Normal cytology and lipid index lipid-laden alveolar macrophages		Salerno et al., 2016
L188E		Normal lung volumes, diffusion capacity 18% of predicted	Chibbar et al., 2004
E66K	Increased cellularity with foamy mononuclear cell		Stevens et al., 2005

Summary of data from patients suffering fibrosis related to a SP-C mutation. Changes in BALF cells and lung mechanics are summarized for the available data. Crs, respiratory system compliance; PaO_2, partial pressure of oxygen; RV, residual volume; VC, vital capacity; V_E, minute ventilation; V_T, tidal volume; VO_2 max, maximal oxygen uptake; FEF_{75}, Forced expiratory flow at 75% of forced vital capacity; FEF_{85}, Forced expiratory flow at 85% of forced vital capacity. M, macrophage; N, neutrophil; L, lymphocyte; E, eosinophil.

(Lawson et al., 2005). Preventive and therapeutic treatment with rapamycin failed to reduce bleomycin induced tissue inflammation and collagen deposition in SP-C deficiency (Madala et al., 2011). Instillation of *Pseudomonas aeruginosa* increased pulmonary injury and bacterial colony counts in SP-C deficient mice compared to control mice. As for unchallenged SP-C deficient mice, sensitivity to *Pseudomonas* challenge seemed to be strain specific since bacterial cell counts were enhanced in 129/Sv6 strain but unaltered in age-matched FVB/N mice. Further, neutrophils and enlarged macrophages with cytoplasmic inclusions were observed upon *Pseudomonas aeruginosa* challenge in absence of SP-C whereby the phagocytic index of macrophages in the SP-C deficient mouse model was reduced (Glasser et al., 2008). Similarly, SP-C deficient mice were more susceptible to respiratory syncytial virus (RSV) infection and resolution of RSV-induced alterations in lung morphology was delayed. Mice exhibited more extensive interstitial thickening, air space consolidation and goblet cell hyperplasia. Polymorphonuclear and macrophage cell counts were increased in BALF obtained from SP-C deficient mice as well as viral titers in lung homogenate (Glasser et al., 2008, 2009). In contrast to challenge with *Pseudomonas aeruginosa*, increased susceptibility of SP-C deficient mice to RSV was not restricted to 129/Sv6 strain but also observed in FVB/N background (Glasser et al., 2008, 2009). However, induction of SP-C expression in compound transgenic mice could reduce RSV-induced tissue inflammation and inflammatory cell counts (Glasser et al., 2013b). LPS-challenged mice develop more intense airway and airspace inflammation in the absence of SP-C. While control mice demonstrate a rapid resolution of LPS-induced cellular and tissue inflammation, inflammation persisted longer in SP-C deficient mice. Cell culture experiments further demonstrated increased LPS-induced cytokine expression of SP-C deficient AE2C compared to those from controls (Glasser et al., 2013b).

The model studied by Glasser et al. (2001, 2008) represents a null mutant mouse model without sufficient *Sftpc* expression leading to the absence of SP-C and proSP-C. Other models include mutations that cause aberrant accumulation of SP-C precursor proteins. Deletion of exon 4 (g.1728 G3A), a mutation detected in human SFTPC, resulted in a truncated form of SP-C (SP-CΔexon4) and incomplete pro-protein processing. Affected mice exhibited disrupted lung organogenesis, branching morphogenesis and expression-depended epithelial cell cytotoxicity (Bridges et al., 2003). Further, transgenic mice that express the mutant L188Q SP-C did not develop pulmonary fibrosis spontaneously, despite induction of ER stress, but developed a more extensive pulmonary fibrosis with reduced compliance and enhanced AEC apoptosis in response to bleomycin and authors suggested alveolar epithelial ER stress to play a crucial role in enhanced disease development (Lawson et al., 2011). Recently, Nureki et al. (2018) developed a conditional mouse mutant in which the expression of I73T, the most common SFTPC mutation found in human patients, is regulated by tamoxifen. In their study, expression of the human mutation induced a spontaneous acute alveolitis, followed by parenchymal injury and fibrotic remodeling in mice (Nureki et al., 2018). Tamoxifen controlled expression of isoleucin to threonine substitution at codon 73 in *Sftpc* (I73T) results in misprocessed proSP-C and leads to increased mortality at day 7 to 14 and acute diffuse parenchymal lung injury with polycellular alveolitis. An early influx of polymorphonuclear cells and macrophages was followed by eosinophilia. Partial recovery from acute injury was followed by aberrant remodeling, collagen deposition and AE2C cell hyperplasia and mechanical abnormalities. Pressure-volume curves displayed a restrictive pattern at 4 to 6 weeks post-tamoxifen and static compliance was reduced at week 4 but rose with resolution of inflammation. However, the fibrotic phenotype was preceded by TGF-β1 (Nureki et al., 2018). A detailed analysis of the same model showed an early reduction of macrophages, followed by an accumulation of immature macrophages and neutrophils before onset of eosinophilia at week 2 in combination with shift from proinflammatory to anti-inflammatory/profibrotic activation state in mRNA BALF cell analysis (Venosa et al., 2019). Total inspiratory capacity and static compliance were reduced in transgenic mice following the induction of the mutant protein whereas tissue damping was elevated, all together suggesting an enhanced tissue stiffness. While local clodronate application diminishing resident macrophages led to reduced survival, intravenous application of clodronate decreased accumulation of immature macrophages, improved survival and reduced eosinophilia (Venosa et al., 2019). Expression of another mutant protein, C121G, resulted in postnatal respiratory failure due to disrupted lung morphogenesis with enlargement of airspaces and interstitial widening in mice constitutively expressing C121G whereas a tamoxifen-mediated expression in adult mice induced acute parenchymal lung injury and a multiphasic polycellular alveolitis with increased BALF cell counts. Similar to the I73T model, an early increase of macrophages and neutrophils was followed by a later influx of eosinophils. Overall, lung mechanics showed a restrictive impairment indicated by a decline in static lung compliance (Katzen et al., 2019).

SP-C Mutations in Human Patients

Since Nogee et al. (2001) described the first case of a *Sftpc* mutation in an infant girl and her mother diagnosed with ILD (Nogee et al., 2001), several studies have been conducted to provide a link between variants in *SFTPC* and the manifestation of ILDs in adults or children. Since previous groups have already performed systematic reviews describing detected mutations, clinical parameters and radiographic as well as histological findings (Ono et al., 2011; Litao et al., 2017), we decided to focus on the work that reported either BALF cell counting or data on lung mechanics in their study (**Table 2**). In general, lung mechanics display a restrictive pattern (Thomas et al., 2002; Ono et al., 2011; Kuse et al., 2013; Avital et al., 2014; Hevroni et al., 2015). In particular, vital capacity, forced vital capacity were markedly reduced in some patients (Ono et al., 2011; Kuse et al., 2013; Avital et al., 2014; Hevroni et al., 2015) whereas mild reductions in forced expiratory pressure in 1 s (FEV1) (Cottin et al., 2011; Ono et al., 2011) were attributable to a generally reduced lung volume and not indicative of an obstruction. However, the reported residual volumes were high to normal (Cottin et al., 2011; Hevroni et al., 2015). Changes in functional residual capacity (FRC) were unspecific. While some patients demonstrated a reduced FRC, other studies reported elevated or normal values. Gas exchange as indicated by diffusing capacity for carbon monoxide exhibited distinct impairment in most (Thomas et al., 2002; Abou Taam et al., 2009; Cottin et al., 2011; Ono et al., 2011; Avital et al., 2014) resulting in a generally reduced oxygen (Thouvenin et al., 2010; Hevroni et al., 2015). However, Abou Taam and coworkers reported normal and increased diffusion capacity for carbon monoxide (D_{LCO}) in two patients (Abou Taam et al., 2009) and oxygenation was sufficient in another patient reported by Avital et al. (2014). Hence, heterogeneity of the disease is also reflected in lung function. While the majority of studies linked SFTPC mutations to the familial form of pulmonary fibrosis, genetic mutations in SFTPC were also detected in a subset of patients suffering from sporadic IPF (Lawson et al., 2004). Interestingly, sporadic patients also demonstrate with mixed pattern as reported by Cottin et al. (2011). Indeed, they reported a case of combined pulmonary fibrosis and emphysema in a patient with the most common I73T mutation.

As explained before, pulmonary fibrosis and especially IPF was linked to an AE2C dysfunction and increased ER stress response due to aberrant protein accumulation. Hyperplastic AE2C in histological examination are a common finding (Nogee et al., 2001; Chibbar et al., 2004; Hamvas et al., 2004; Cameron et al., 2005; Stevens et al., 2005; Soraisham et al., 2006; Mechri et al., 2010; Thouvenin et al., 2010; Citti et al., 2013; Litao et al., 2017; Park et al., 2018) and enhanced ER stress is a widely acknowledged pathomechanism in IPF (Korfei et al., 2008). However, reduced transcription of SFTPC due to promotor variant were associated with neonatal respiratory distress syndrome in late preterm infants (Wambach et al., 2010) and SP-C was absent in BALF samples of a family with chronic ILDs, together with reduced pro-SP-C staining, though no mutation was identified (Amin et al., 2001). While the majority of mutations leads to the onset of ILDs already in childhood (Chibbar et al., 2004; Hamvas et al., 2004; Tredano et al., 2004; Rosen and Waltz, 2005; Stevens et al., 2005; Bullard and Nogee, 2007; Guillot et al., 2009; Mechri et al., 2010; Cottin et al., 2011; Citti et al., 2013; Henderson et al., 2013; Hepping et al., 2013; Turcu et al., 2013; Akimoto et al., 2014; Avital et al., 2014; van Hoorn et al., 2014; Kroner et al., 2015; Liptzin et al., 2015; Peca et al., 2015; Griese et al., 2016; Liu et al., 2016; Hayasaka et al., 2018) a subset of variants results in a manifestation in later child- or adulthood (Lawson et al., 2004; Setoguchi et al., 2006; Markart et al., 2007; van Moorsel et al., 2010; Cottin et al., 2011; Ono et al., 2011; Kuse et al., 2013) suggesting a chronic process.

Besides to AE2C hyperplasia, cholesterol clefts are frequently detected on lung biopsy in context of an SFTPC mutations (Hamvas et al., 2004; Abou Taam et al., 2009; Mechri et al., 2010; Cottin et al., 2011; Litao et al., 2017) or on lung specimen from ILD patients lacking SP-C (Amin et al., 2001). Macrophages were often described as foamy (Lawson et al., 2004; Stevens et al., 2005; Henderson et al., 2013) or lipid-laden (Liptzin et al., 2015; Salerno et al., 2016). When analyzing BALF cells, the majority of cells usually consists of macrophages (Abou Taam et al., 2009; Thouvenin et al., 2010; Ono et al., 2011). However, some samples showed a marked increase in neutrophil (Thouvenin et al., 2010; Cottin et al., 2011) or lymphocyte (Ono et al., 2011) cell counting in the absence of an infection. Whether immune cell infiltration occurs in reaction to abnormal histological findings or rather causes alterations remains unclear in view of single time point studies in human patients. In addition, a detailed characterization of macrophages was not provided by the majority of studies, but different activation could have distinct effects on fibrogenesis.

LUNG FIBROSIS AND CHOLESTEROL

Recently, we have described the accumulation of cholesterol crystals in AMs of SP-C deficient animals (Ruwisch et al., 2020). We also showed similar crystals accumulated in the lung of an IPF patient. Looking through the literature this feature is commonly described (Glasser et al., 2003; Hoenerhoff et al., 2006; Mora et al., 2006) but no further investigated. Therefore, the role of cholesterol or accumulation of cholesterol in the form of crystals in cells is yet not well understood and often overlooked. As explained before, cholesterol is also involved in many processes apart from regulating membrane biophysical properties. Not many experimental data are available in the context of the influence of cholesterol in lung diseases. However, in the clinic settings, it is not surprising that certain patients are suffering from comorbidities that should be treated such as hypercholesterolemia. In fact, it is known that IPF increases the risk of heart diseases. Thus, it is common for IPF patients to receive medications aimed at reducing cardiovascular risk, including statins, which lower cholesterol levels (Kreuter et al., 2018). Data in this regard is still quite controversial. While, 3-hydroxy-3-methylglutaryl-coenzyme A reductase inhibitors (statins) aggravated pulmonary fibrosis in mice by increased production of mitochondrial ROS and NLRP3 inflammasome activation in macrophages. Statins, as potent inhibitors of the endogenous cholesterol synthesis have been associated with a lower decline in FVC in a cohort of untreated IPF patients (Kreuter et al., 2018). In line with this, diet induced systemic hyperlipidemia resulted in altered surfactant phospholipid composition leading to increased alveolar collapsibility, providing evidence that pulmonary lipid homeostasis is strongly related to the blood circulation (Baritussio et al., 1980). As approximately 83% of surfactant cholesterol has been stated to be derived from blood plasma (Turley et al., 1981), statins could contribute in preventing deleterious high levels of cholesterol in surfactant films, providing surfactant film stability and avoiding alveolar collapse. In addition, evaluation of lung function showed that patients receiving statin therapy and Ofev had less decline in pulmonary capacity, compared with a placebo (Kreuter et al., 2018). The yardstick that researchers used was patients' annual rate of decline in forced vital capacity (FVC). The results suggested that statins do not diminish Ofev's effectiveness (Kreuter et al., 2018).

Statins may also have an anti-inflammatory effect in the lung (Liao and Laufs, 2004; Jain and Ridker, 2005), thus a multifactorial mechanism may play an important role in their use. In conclusion, more experimental evidence is needed to support the use of cholesterol lowering drugs for the treatment of lung diseases such as fibrosis. In addition, the role of cholesterol and SP-C has to be further described and understood in order to develop new therapies. However, there is already promising data in this regard, opening a new pathway to target.

CONCLUSION

Summing up there are various potential either direct or indirect mechanisms how SP-C is able to interfere and modulate fibrogenesis in the lung. While SP-C deficiency mediated surfactant dysfunction and impaired lung mechanics are likely contributors in the generation of local mechanical stresses and strains, its biophysical interplay with cholesterol on the one hand, and its modulation of TLR-4 signaling on the other hand, highlights SP-C as a key element in a complex profibrotic network. Thereby SP-C deficiency comes into play not only in animal models, but also in patients with familial and non-familial forms of lung fibrosis such as IPF. Further research is needed in order to determine the potential of cholesterol lowering drugs as treatment or combined with anti-fibrotic drugs to find a better therapy for IPF patients.

AUTHOR CONTRIBUTIONS

KS, JR, NR, and EL-R contributed to the review, writing, and revising of the manuscript.

REFERENCES

Abou Taam, R., Jaubert, F., Emond, S., le Bourgeois, M., Epaud, R., Karila, C., et al. (2009). Familial interstitial disease with I73T mutation: a mid- and long-term study. *Pediatr. Pulmonol.* 44, 167–175. doi: 10.1002/ppul.20970

Akimoto, T., Cho, K., Hayasaka, I., Morioka, K., Kaneshi, Y., Furuta, I., et al. (2014). Hereditary interstitial lung diseases manifesting in early childhood in Japan. *Pediatr. Res.* 76, 453–458. doi: 10.1038/pr.2014.114

Allawzi, A., Elajaili, H., Redente, E. F., and Nozik-Grayck, E. (2019). Oxidative toxicology of bleomycin: role of the extracellular redox environment. *Curr. Opin. Toxicol.* 13, 68–73. doi: 10.1016/j.cotox.2018.08.001

Al-Saiedy, M., Gunasekara, L., Green, F., Pratt, R., Chiu, A., Yang, A., et al. (2018). Surfactant dysfunction in ARDS and bronchiolitis is repaired with cyclodextrins. *Mil. Med.* 183, 207–215. doi: 10.1093/milmed/usx204

Amin, R. S., Wert, S. E., Baughman, R. P., Tomashefski, J. F., Nogee, L. M., Brody, A. S., et al. (2001). Surfactant protein deficiency in familial interstitial lung disease. *J. Pediatr.* 139, 85–92. doi: 10.1067/mpd.2001.114545

Amrein, M., von Nahmen, A., and Sieber, M. (1997). A scanning force- and fluorescence light microscopy study of the structure and function of a model pulmonary surfactant. *Eur. Biophys. J.* 26, 349–357. doi: 10.1007/s002490050089

Augusto, L. A., Synguelakis, M., Espinassous, Q., Lepoivre, M., Johansson, J., and Chaby, R. (2003). Cellular antiendotoxin activities of lung surfactant protein C in lipid vesicles. *Am. J. Respir. Crit. Care Med.* 168, 335–341. doi: 10.1164/rccm.200212-1440OC

Autilio, C., and Pérez-Gil, J. (2018). Understanding the principle biophysics concepts of pulmonary surfactant in health and disease. *Arch. Dis. Child Fetal Neonat. Ed.* 104, F443–F451. doi: 10.1136/archdischild-2018-315413

Avital, A., Hevroni, A., Godfrey, S., Cohen, S., Maayan, C., Nusair, S., et al. (2014). Natural history of five children with surfactant protein C mutations and interstitial lung disease. *Pediatr. Pulmonol.* 49, 1097–1105. doi: 10.1002/ppul.22971

Bachofen, H., and Schürch, S. (2001). Alveolar surface forces and lung architecture. *Compar. Biochem. Physiol. Mol. Integr. Physiol.* 129, 183–193. doi: 10.1016/S1095-6433(01)00315-314

Bachofen, H., Schurch, S., Urbinelli, M., and Weibel, E. R. (1987). Relations among alveolar surface tension, surface area, volume, and recoil pressure. *J. Appl. Physiol.* 62, 1878–1887. doi: 10.1152/jappl.1987.62.5.1878

Baker, A. D., Malur, A., Barna, B. P., Ghosh, S., Kavuru, M. S., Malur, A. G., et al. (2010a). Targeted PPARγ deficiency in alveolar macrophages disrupts surfactant catabolism. *J. Lipid Res.* 51, 1325–1331. doi: 10.1194/jlr.m001651

Baker, A. D., Malur, A., Barna, B. P., Kavuru, M. S., Malur, A. G., and Thomassen, M. J. (2010b). PPARγ regulates the expression of cholesterol metabolism genes in alveolar macrophages. *Biochem. Biophys. Res. Commun.* 393, 682–687. doi: 10.1016/j.bbrc.2010.02.056

Bargagli, E., Margollicci, M., Luddi, A., Nikiforakis, N., Grazia Perari, M., Grosso, S., et al. (2007). Chitotriosidase activity in patients with interstitial lung diseases.

Respirat. Med. 101, 2176–2181. doi: 10.1016/j.rmed.2007.05.008

Baritussio, A., Enzi, G., Inelmen, E. M., Schiavon, M., de Biasi, F., Allegra, L., et al. (1980). Altered surfactant synthesis and function in rats with diet-induced hyperlipidemia. *Metabolism* 29, 503–510. doi: 10.1016/0026-0495(80)90075-X

Basset-Léobon, C., Lacoste-Collin, L., Aziza, J., Bes, J. C., Jozan, S., and Courtade-Saïdi, M. (2010). Cut-off values and significance of Oil Red O-positive cells in bronchoalveolar lavage fluid. *Cytopathology* 21, 245–250. doi: 10.1111/j.1365-2303.2009.00677.x

Batenburg, J. J., and Haagsman, H. P. (1998). The lipids of pulmonary surfactant: dynamics and interactions with proteins. *Progress Lipid Res.* 37, 235–276. doi: 10.1016/S0163-7827(98)00011-13

Bates, J. H. T., and Smith, B. J. (2018). Ventilator-induced lung injury and lung mechanics. *Ann. Transl. Med.* 6:378. doi: 10.21037/atm.2018.06.29

Bauernfeind, F. G., Horvath, G., Stutz, A., Alnemri, E. S., MacDonald, K., Speert, D., et al. (2009). Cutting edge: NF-κB activating pattern recognition and cytokine receptors license NLRP3 inflammasome activation by regulating NLRP3 expression. *J. Immunol.* 183, 787–791. doi: 10.4049/jimmunol.0901363

Baumgart, F., Ospina, O. L., Mingarro, I., Rodríguez-Crespo, I., and Pérez-Gil, J. (2010). Palmitoylation of pulmonary surfactant protein SP-C Is critical for its functional cooperation with SP-B to sustain compression/expansion dynamics in cholesterol-containing surfactant films. *Biophys. J.* 99, 3234–3243. doi: 10.1016/J.BPJ.2010.08.070

Beeh, K. M., Beier, J., Kornmann, O., and Buhl, R. (2003). Sputum matrix metalloproteinase-9, tissue inhibitor of metalloprotinease-1, and their molar ratio in patients with chronic obstructive pulmonary disease, idiopathic pulmonary fibrosis and healthy subjects. *Respirat. Med.* 97, 634–639. doi: 10.1053/rmed.2003.1493

Bekker, A., Holland, H. D., Wang, P.-L., Rumble, D., Stein, H. J., Hannah, J. L., et al. (2004). Dating the rise of atmospheric oxygen. *Nature* 427, 117–120. doi: 10.1038/nature02260

Bernardino de la Serna, J., Perez-Gil, J., Simonsen, A. C., and Bagatolli, L. A. (2004). Cholesterol rules: direct observation of the coexistence of two fluid phases in native pulmonary surfactant membranes at physiological temperatures. *J. Biol. Chem.* 279, 40715–40722. doi: 10.1074/jbc.M404648200

Bernhard, W. (2016). Lung surfactant: function and composition in the context of development and respiratory physiology. *Ann. Anat. Anatomischer Anzeiger* 208, 146–150. doi: 10.1016/J.AANAT.2016.08.003

Besnard, V., Wert, S. E., Stahlman, M. T., Postle, A. D., Xu, Y., Ikegami, M., et al. (2009). Deletion of Scap in alveolar type II cells influences lung lipid homeostasis and identifies a compensatory role for pulmonary lipofibroblasts. *J. Biol. Chem.* 284, 4018–4030. doi: 10.1074/jbc.m805388200

Bilek, A. M., Dee, K. C., and Gaver, D. P. (2003). Mechanisms of surface-tension-induced epithelial cell damage in a model of pulmonary airway reopening. *J. Appl. Physiol.* 94, 770–783. doi: 10.1152/japplphysiol.00764.2002

Birkelbach, B., Lutz, D., Ruppert, C., Henneke, I., Lopez-Rodriguez, E., Günther, A., et al. (2015). Linking progression of fibrotic lung remodeling and ultrastructural alterations of alveolar epithelial type II cells in the amiodarone mouse model. *Am. J. Physiol. Lung Cell. Mol. Physiol.* 309, L63–L75.

Bridges, J. P., Wert, S. E., Nogee, L. M., and Weaver, T. E. (2003). Expression of a human surfactant protein C mutation associated with interstitial lung disease disrupts lung development in transgenic mice. *J. Biol. Chem.* 278, 52739–52746. doi: 10.1074/jbc.m309599200

Brocks, J. J., Logan, G. A., Buick, R., and Summons, R. E. (1999). Archean molecular fossils and the early rise of eukaryotes. *Science* 285, 1033–1036. doi: 10.1126/science.285.5430.1033

Buchwald, H., O'Dea, T. J., Menchaca, H. J., Michalek, V. N., and Rohde, T. D. (2000). Effect of plasma cholesterol on red blood cell oxygen transport. *Clin. Exp. Pharmacol. Physiol.* 27, 951–955. doi: 10.1046/j.1440-1681.2000.03383.x

Bullard, J. E., and Nogee, L. M. (2007). Heterozygosity for ABCA3 mutations modifies the severity of lung disease associated with a surfactant protein C gene (SFTPC) mutation. *Pediatr. Res.* 62, 176–179. doi: 10.1203/PDR.0b013e3180a72588

Cabrera-Benítez, N. E., Parotto, M., Post, M., Han, B., Spieth, P. M., Cheng, W. E., et al. (2012). Mechanical stress induces lung fibrosis by epithelial-mesenchymal transition. *Crit. Care Med.* 40, 510–517. doi: 10.1097/CCM.0b013e31822f09d7

Cameron, H. S., Somaschini, M., Carrera, P., Hamvas, A., Whitsett, J. A., Wert, S. E., et al. (2005). A common mutation in the surfactant protein C gene associated with lung disease. *J. Pediatr.* 146, 370–375. doi: 10.1016/j.jpeds.2004.10.028

Cameron, R. G., Blendis, L. M., and Neuman, M. G. (2001). Accumulation of macrophages in primary sclerosing cholangitis. *Clin. Biochem.* 34, 195–201. doi: 10.1016/S0009-9120(01)00215-216

Cassel, S. L., Eisenbarth, S. C., Iyer, S. S., Sadler, J. J., Colegio, O. R., Tephly, L. A., et al. (2008). The Nalp3 inflammasome is essential for the development of silicosis. *Proc. Natl. Acad. Sci. U.S.A.* 105, 9035–9040. doi: 10.1073/pnas.0803933105

Cassera, M. B., Silber, A. M., and Gennaro, A. M. (2002). Differential effects of cholesterol on acyl chain order in erythrocyte membranes as a function of depth from the surface. An electron paramagnetic resonance (EPR) spin label study. *Biophys. Chem. Biophys. Chem.* 99, 117–127. doi: 10.1016/S0301-4622(02)00139-134

Cassidy, K. J., Halpern, D., Ressler, B. G., and Grotberg, J. B. (1999). Surfactant effects in model airway closure experiments. *J. Appl. Physiol.* 87, 415–427. doi: 10.1152/jappl.1999.87.1.415

Chaby, R., Garcia-Verdugo, I., Espinassous, Q., and Augusto, L. A. (2005). Interactions between LPS and lung surfactant proteins. *J. Endotoxin. Res.* 11, 181–185. doi: 10.1179/096805105X37358

Chai, A. B., Ammit, A. J., and Gelissen, I. C. (2017). Examining the role of ABC lipid transporters in pulmonary lipid homeostasis and inflammation. *Respirat. Res.* 18:41. doi: 10.1186/s12931-017-0526-529

Chibbar, R., Shih, F., Baga, M., Torlakovic, E., Ramlall, K., Skomro, R., et al. (2004). Nonspecific interstitial pneumonia and usual interstitial pneumonia with mutation in surfactant protein C in familial pulmonary fibrosis. *Mod. Pathol.* 17, 973–980. doi: 10.1038/modpathol.3800149

Chou, P. Y., and Fasman, G. D. (2006). Prediction of the secondary structure of proteins from their amino acid sequence. *Adv. Enzymol. Relat. Areas Mol. Biol.* 47, 45–48. doi: 10.1002/9780470122921.ch2

Citti, A., Peca, D., Petrini, S., Cutrera, R., Biban, P., Haass, C., et al. (2013). Ultrastructural characterization of genetic diffuse lung diseases in infants and children: a cohort study and review. *Ultrastruct. Pathol.* 37, 356–365. doi: 10.3109/01913123.2013.811454

Cong, X., Hubmayr, R. D., Li, C., and Zhao, X. (2017). Plasma membrane wounding and repair in pulmonary diseases. *Am. J. Physiol. Lung Cell. Mol. Physiol.* 312, L371–L391. doi: 10.1152/ajplung.00486.2016

Conkright, J. J., Na, C.-L., and Weaver, T. E. (2002). Overexpression of surfactant protein-c mature peptide causes neonatal lethality in transgenic mice. *Am. J. Respir. Cell Mol. Biol.* 26, 85–90. doi: 10.1165/ajrcmb.26.1.4686

Cottin, V., and Cordier, J.-F. (2011). SFTPC mutations in patients with familial pulmonary fibrosis: combined with emphysema? *Am. J. Respir. Crit. Med.* 183:1113. doi: 10.1164/ajrccm.183.8.1113

Cottin, V., Reix, P., Khouatra, C., Thivolet-Béjui, F., Feldmann, D., and Cordier, J.-F. (2011). Combined pulmonary fibrosis and emphysema syndrome associated with familial SFTPC mutation. *Thorax* 66, 918–919. doi: 10.1136/thx.2010.151407

Creuwels, L. A., Demel, R. A., van Golde, L. M., Benson, B. J., and Haagsman, H. P. (1993). Effect of acylation on structure and function of surfactant protein C at the air-liquid interface. *J. Biol. Chem.* 268, 26752–26758.

DeBose-Boyd, R. A. (2008). Feedback regulation of cholesterol synthesis: sterol-accelerated ubiquitination and degradation of HMG CoA reductase. *Cell Res.* 18, 609–621. doi: 10.1038/cr.2008.61

Dico, A. S., Taneva, S., Morrow, M. R., and Keough, K. M. (1997). Effect of calcium on phospholipid interaction with pulmonary surfactant protein C. *Biophys. J.* 73, 2595–2602. doi: 10.1016/S0006-3495(97)78289-78284

Dietl, P., Haller, T., and Frick, M. (2012). Spatio-temporal aspects, pathways and actions of Ca(2+) in surfactant secreting pulmonary alveolar type II pneumocytes. *Cell Calcium* 52, 296–302. doi: 10.1016/j.ceca.2012.04.010

Doyle, I. R., Jones, M. E., Barr, H. A., Orgeig, S., Crockett, A. J., McDonald, C. F., et al. (1994). Composition of human pulmonary surfactant varies with exercise and level of fitness. *Am. J. Respir. Crit. Med.* 149, 1619–1627. doi: 10.1164/ajrccm.149.6.8004321

Dreyfuss, D., Martin-Lefèvre, L., and Saumon, G. (1999). Hyperinflation-induced lung injury during alveolar flooding in rats: effect of perfluorocarbon instillation. *Am. J. Respir. Crit. Care Med.* 159, 1752–1757. doi: 10.1164/ajrccm.159.6.9805018

Duewell, P., Kono, H., Rayner, K. J., Sirois, C. M., Vladimer, G., Bauernfeind, F. G., et al. (2010). NLRP3 inflammasomes are required for atherogenesis and activated by cholesterol crystals. *Nature* 464, 1357–1361. doi: 10.1038/nature08938

Eldridge, W. B., Zhang, Q., Faro, A., Sweet, S. C., Eghtesady, P., Hamvas, A., et al. (2017). Outcomes of lung transplantation for infants and children with genetic disorders of surfactant metabolism. *J. Pediatr.* 184, 157–164. doi: 10.1016/J.JPEDS.2017.01.017

Ertunc, M. E., and Hotamisligil, G. S. (2016). Lipid signaling and lipotoxicity in metaflammation: indications for metabolic disease pathogenesis and treatment. *J. Lipid Res.* 57, 2099–2114. doi: 10.1194/jlr.R066514

Fehrenbach, H. (2001). Alveolar epithelial type II cell: defender of the alveolus revisited. *Respir. Res.* 2, 33–46. doi: 10.1186/rr36

Fessler, M. B. (2017). A new frontier in immunometabolism cholesterol in lung health and disease. *Ann. Am. Thorac. Soc.* 14, S399–S405. doi: 10.1513/AnnalsATS.201702-136AW

Fessler, M. B., and Summer, R. S. (2016). Surfactant lipids at the host-environment interface. metabolic sensors, suppressors, and effectors of inflammatory lung disease. *Am. J. Respir. Cell Mol. Biol.* 54, 624–635. doi: 10.1165/rcmb.2016-0011PS

French, K. L., Hallmann, C., Hope, J. M., Schoon, P. L., Zumberge, J. A., Hoshino, Y., et al. (2015). Reappraisal of hydrocarbon biomarkers in archean rocks. *Proc. Natl. Acad. Sci. U.S.A.* 112, 5915–5920. doi: 10.1073/pnas.1419563112

Froese, A. R., Shimbori, C., Bellaye, P.-S., Inman, M., Obex, S., Fatima, S., et al. (2016). Stretch-induced activation of transforming growth factor-β1 in pulmonary fibrosis. *Am. J. Respir. Crit. Care Med.* 194, 84–96. doi: 10.1164/rccm.201508-1638OC

Garcia-Verdugo, I., Garcia de Paco, E., Espinassous, Q., Gonzalez-Horta, A., Synguelakis, M., Kanellopoulos, J., et al. (2009). Synthetic peptides representing the N-terminal segment of surfactant protein C modulate LPS-stimulated TNF-α production by macrophages. *Innate Immun.* 15, 53–62. doi: 10.1177/1753425908100500

Gasse, P., Mary, C., Guenon, I., Noulin, N., Charron, S., Schnyder-Candrian, S., et al. (2007). IL-1R1/MyD88 signaling and the inflammasome are essential in pulmonary inflammation and fibrosis in mice. *J. Clin. Invest.* 117, 3786–3799. doi: 10.1172/JCI32285

Gattinoni, L., Marini, J. J., Collino, F., Maiolo, G., Rapetti, F., Tonetti, T., et al. (2017). The future of mechanical ventilation: Lessons from the present and the past. *Crit. Care* 21:183. doi: 10.1186/s13054-017-1750-x

Ghadiali, S. N., and Gaver, D. P. (2008). Biomechanics of liquid-epithelium interactions in pulmonary airways. *Respir. Physiol. Neurobiol.* 163, 232–243. doi: 10.1016/j.resp.2008.04.008

Glasser, S. W., Burhans, M. S., Korfhagen, T. R., Na, C.-L. L., Sly, P. D., Ross, G. F., et al. (2001). Altered stability of pulmonary surfactant in SP-C-deficient mice. *Proc. Natl. Acad. Sci. U.S.A.* 98, 6366–6371. doi: 10.1073/pnas.101500298

Glasser, S. W., Detmer, E. A., Ikegami, M., Na, C.-L., Stahlman, M. T., and Whitsett, J. A. (2003). Pneumonitis and emphysema in sp-C gene targeted mice. *J. Biol. Chem.* 278, 14291–14298. doi: 10.1074/jbc.m210909200

Glasser, S. W., Maxfield, M. D., Ruetschilling, T. L., Akinbi, H. T., Baatz, J. E., Kitzmiller, J. A., et al. (2013a). Persistence of LPS-induced lung inflammation in surfactant protein-C-deficient mice. *Am. J. Respir. Cell Mol. Biol.* 49, 845–854. doi: 10.1165/rcmb.2012-0374oc

Glasser, S. W., Senft, A. P., Maxfield, M. D., Ruetschilling, T. L., Baatz, J. E., Page, K., et al. (2013b). Genetic replacement of surfactant protein-C reduces respiratory syncytial virus induced lung injury. *Respir. Res.* 14:19. doi: 10.1186/1465-9921-14-19

Glasser, S. W., and Senft, A. (2009). "Pulmonary surfactant homeostasis and altered macrophage function," in *Lung Macrophages in Health And Disease*, ed. S. Hodge (Bentham: Science Publisher Ltd), 1–13. doi: 10.2174/978160805020810901010001

Glasser, S. W., Senft, A. P., Whitsett, J. A., Maxfield, M. D., Ross, G. F., Richardson, T. R., et al. (2008). Macrophage dysfunction and susceptibility to pulmonary *pseudomonas aeruginosa* infection in surfactant protein C-deficient mice. *J. Immunol.* 181, 621–628. doi: 10.4049/jimmunol.181.1.621

Glasser, S. W., Witt, T. L., Senft, A. P., Baatz, J. E., Folger, D., Maxfield, M. D., et al. (2009). Surfactant protein C-deficient mice are susceptible to respiratory syncytial virus infection. *Am. J. Physiol. Lung Cell. Mol. Physiol.* 297, L64–L72.

Gómez-Gil, L., Pérez-Gil, J., and Goormaghtigh, E. (2009a). Cholesterol modulates the exposure and orientation of pulmonary surfactant protein SP-C in model surfactant membranes. *Biochim. Biophys. Acta Biomemb.* 1788, 1907–1915. doi: 10.1016/J.BBAMEM.2009.05.011

Gómez-Gil, L., Schürch, D., Goormaghtigh, E., and Pérez-Gil, J. (2009b). Pulmonary surfactant protein SP-C counteracts the deleterious effects of cholesterol on the activity of surfactant films under physiologically relevant compression-expansion dynamics. *Biophys. J.* 97, 2736–2745. doi: 10.1016/J.BPJ.2009.08.045

Griese, M., Lorenz, E., Hengst, M., Schams, A., Wesselak, T., Rauch, D., et al. (2016). Surfactant proteins in pediatric interstitial lung disease. *Pediatr. Res.* 79, 34–41. doi: 10.1038/pr.2015.173

Gu, B. J., and Wiley, J. S. (2006). Rapid ATP-induced release of matrix metalloproteinase 9 is mediated by the P2X7 receptor. *Blood* 107, 4946–4953. doi: 10.1182/blood-2005-07-2994

Guillot, L., Epaud, R., Thouvenin, G., Jonard, L., Mohsni, A., Couderc, R., et al. (2009). New surfactant protein C gene mutations associated with diffuse lung disease. *J. Med. Genet.* 46, 490–494. doi: 10.1136/jmg.2009.066829

Gunasekara, L., Schürch, S., Schoel, W. M., Nag, K., Leonenko, Z., Haufs, M., et al. (2005). Pulmonary surfactant function is abolished by an elevated proportion of cholesterol. *Biochim. Biophys. Acta Mol. Cell Biol. Lipids* 1737, 27–35. doi: 10.1016/j.bbalip.2005.09.002

Gunasekara, L. C., Pratt, R. M., Schoel, W. M., Gosche, S., Prenner, E. J., and Amrein, M. W. (2010). Methyl-β-cyclodextrin restores the structure and function of pulmonary surfactant films impaired by cholesterol. *Biochim. Biophys. Acta Mol. Cell Biol. Lipids* 1798, 986–994. doi: 10.1016/J.BBAMEM.2009.12.003

Hamvas, A. (2010). Evaluation and management of inherited disorders of surfactant metabolism. *Chin. Med. J.* 123, 2943–2947.

Hamvas, A., Nogee, L. M., White, F., Schuler, P., Hackett, B. P., Huddleston, C. B., et al. (2004). Progressive lung disease and surfactant dysfunction with a deletion in surfactant protein C gene. *Am. J. Respir. Cell Mol. Biol.* 30, 771–776. doi: 10.1165/rcmb.2003-0323oc

Hasan, D., Blankman, P., and Nieman, G. F. (2017). Purinergic signalling links mechanical breath profile and alveolar mechanics with the pro-inflammatory innate immune response causing ventilation-induced lung injury. *Puriner. Signal.* 13, 363–386. doi: 10.1007/s11302-017-9564-9565

Hayasaka, I., Cho, K., Akimoto, T., Ikeda, M., Uzuki, Y., Yamada, M., et al. (2018). Genetic basis for childhood interstitial lung disease among Japanese infants and children. *Pediatr. Res.* 83, 477–483. doi: 10.1038/pr.2017.217

Henderson, L. B., Melton, K., Wert, S., Couriel, J., Bush, A., Ashworth, M., et al. (2013). Large ABCA3 and SFTPC deletions resulting in lung disease. *Ann. Am. Thorac. Soc.* 10, 602–607.

Hepping, N., Griese, M., Lohse, P., Garbe, W., and Lange, L. (2013). Successful treatment of neonatal respiratory failure caused by a novel surfactant protein C p.Cys121Gly mutation with hydroxychloroquine. *J. Perinatol.* 33:492. doi: 10.1038/jp.2012.131

Hevroni, A., Goldman, A., and Springer, C. (2015). Infant pulmonary function testing in chronic pneumonitis of infancy due to surfactant protein C mutation. *Pediatr. Pulmonol.* 50, E17–E23.

Hinz, B. (2012). Mechanical aspects of lung fibrosis: a spotlight on the myofibroblast. *Proc. Am. Thorac. Soc.* 9, 137–147. doi: 10.1513/pats.201202-017AW

Hinz, B., and Suki, B. (2016). Does breathing amplify fibrosis? *Am. J. Respir. Crit. Care Med.* 194, 9–11. doi: 10.1164/rccm.201601-0149ED

Hoenerhoff, M. J., Starost, M. F., and Ward, J. M. (2006). Eosinophilic crystalline pneumonia as a major cause of death in 129S4/SvJae mice. *Vet. Pathol.* 43, 682–688. doi: 10.1354/vp.43-5-682

Idiopathic Pulmonary Fibrosis Clinical Research Network, Raghu, G., Anstrom, K. J., King, T. E., Lasky, J. A., and Martinez, F. J. (2012). Prednisone, azathioprine, and N-acetylcysteine for pulmonary fibrosis. *N. Engl. J. Med.* 366, 1968–1977. doi: 10.1056/NEJMoa1113354

Jain, M. K., and Ridker, P. M. (2005). Anti-inflammatory effects of statins: clinical evidence and basic mechanisms. *Nat. Rev. Drug Discov.* 4, 977–987. doi: 10.1038/nrd1901

Jin, H., Ciechanowicz, A. K., Kaplan, A. R., Wang, L., Zhang, P. X., Lu, Y. C., et al. (2018). Surfactant protein C dampens inflammation by decreasing JAK/STAT activation during lung repair. *Am. J. Physiol. Lung. Cell Mol. Physiol.* 314, L882–L892. doi: 10.1152/ajplung.00418.2017

Johansson, J. (2001). Membrane properties and amyloid fibril formation of lung surfactant protein C. *Biochem. Soc. Trans.* 29, 601–606. doi: 10.1042/bst0290601

Johansson, J., Weaver, T. E., and Tjernberg, L. O. (2004). Proteolytic generation and aggregation of peptides from transmembrane regions: lung surfactant protein C and amyloid β-peptide. *Cell. Mol. Life Sci. CMLS* 61, 326–335. doi: 10.1007/s00018-003-3274-3276

Jolley, C. D., Dietschy, J. M., and Turley, S. D. (1999). Genetic differences in cholesterol absorption in 129/Sv and C57BL/6 mice: effect on cholesterol responsiveness. *Am. J. Physiolo. Gastrointest. Liver Physiol.* 276, G1117–G1124. doi: 10.1152/ajpgi.1999.276.5.g1117

Justice, M. J., Petrusca, D. N., Rogozea, A. L., Williams, J. A., Schweitzer, K. S., Petrache, I., et al. (2014). Effects of lipid interactions on model vesicle engulfment by alveolar macrophages. *Biophys. J.* 106, 598–609. doi: 10.1016/J.BPJ.2013.12.036

Karlmark, K. R., Weiskirchen, R., Zimmermann, H. W., Gassler, N., Ginhoux, F., Weber, C., et al. (2009). Hepatic recruitment of the inflammatory Gr1+ monocyte subset upon liver injury promotes hepatic fibrosis. *Hepatology* 50, 261–274. doi: 10.1002/hep.22950

Katzen, J., Venosa, A., Tomer, Y., Kopp, M., Morely, M., Diwadkar, A., et al. (2019). Interstitial lung disease related surfactant protein-C mutations alter the transcriptome and progenitor cell function of alveolar epithelial cells in mice. *Eur. Respirat. J.* 54, A1291–A1291. doi: 10.1183/13993003.congress-2019.PA1291

Keating, E., Rahman, L., Francis, J., Petersen, A., Possmayer, F., Veldhuizen, R., et al. (2007). Effect of cholesterol on the biophysical and physiological properties of a clinical pulmonary surfactant. *Biophys. J.* 93, 1391–1401. doi: 10.1529/BIOPHYSJ.106.099762

Knudsen, L., and Ochs, M. (2018). The micromechanics of lung alveoli: structure and function of surfactant and tissue components. *Histochem. Cell Biol.* 150, 661–676. doi: 10.1007/s00418-018-1747-1749

Knudsen, L., Ruppert, C., and Ochs, M. (2017). Tissue remodelling in pulmonary fibrosis. *Cell Tissue Res.* 367, 607–626. doi: 10.1007/s00441-016-2543-2542

Kolb, M., Margetts, P. J., Anthony, D. C., Pitossi, F., and Gauldie, J. (2001). Transient expression of IL-1beta induces acute lung injury and chronic repair leading to pulmonary fibrosis. *J. Clin. Invest.* 107, 1529–1536. doi: 10.1172/JCI12568

Kollisch-Singule, M., Emr, B., Jain, S. V., Andrews, P., Satalin, J., Liu, J., et al. (2015). The effects of airway pressure release ventilation on respiratory mechanics in extrapulmonary lung injury. *Intens. Care Med. Exper.* 3:71. doi: 10.1186/s40635-015-0071-70

Kook, S., Wang, P., Young, L. R., Schwake, M., Saftig, P., Weng, X., et al. (2016). Impaired lysosomal integral membrane protein 2-dependent peroxiredoxin 6 delivery to lamellar bodies accounts for altered alveolar phospholipid content in adaptor protein-3-deficient pearl mice. *J. Biol. Chem.* 291, 8414–8427. doi: 10.1074/jbc.M116.720201

Korfei, M., Ruppert, C., Mahavadi, P., Henneke, I., Markart, P., Koch, M., et al. (2008). Epithelial endoplasmic reticulum stress and apoptosis in sporadic idiopathic pulmonary fibrosis. *Am. J. Respir. Crit. Care Med.* 178, 838–846. doi: 10.1164/rccm.200802-313OC

Korfhagen, T. R., Glasser, S. W., Wert, S. E., Bruno, M. D., Daugherty, C. C., McNeish, J. D., et al. (1990). Cis-acting sequences from a human surfactant protein gene confer pulmonary-specific gene expression in transgenic mice. *Proc. Natl. Acad. Sci. U.S.A.* 87, 6122–6126. doi: 10.1073/pnas.87.16.6122

Kreuter, M., Costabel, U., Richeldi, L., Cottin, V., Wijsenbeek, M., Bonella, F., et al. (2018). Statin therapy and outcomes in trials of nintedanib in idiopathic pulmonary fibrosis. *Respiration* 95, 317–326. doi: 10.1159/000486286

Kroner, C., Reu, S., Teusch, V., Schams, A., Grimmelt, A.-C., Barker, M., et al. (2015). Genotype alone does not predict the clinical course of SFTPC deficiency in paediatric patients. *Eur. Respir. J.* 46, 197–206. doi: 10.1183/09031936.00129414

Kuse, N., Abe, S., Hayashi, H., Kamio, K., Saito, Y., Azuma, A., et al. (2013). Familial interstitial pneumonia in an adolescent boy with surfactant protein C gene (Y104H) mutation. *Sarcoidos. Vasculit. Diffuse Lung Dis.* 30, 73–77.

Lawson, W., Grant, S., Ambrosini, V., Womble, K., Dawson, E., Lane, K., et al. (2004). Genetic mutations in surfactant protein C are a rare cause of sporadic cases of IPF. *Thorax* 59, 977–980. doi: 10.1136/thx.2004.026336

Lawson, W. E., Cheng, D.-S., Degryse, A. L., Tanjore, H., Polosukhin, V. V., Xu, X. C., et al. (2011). Endoplasmic reticulum stress enhances fibrotic remodeling in the lungs. *Proc. Natl. Acad. Sci. U.S.A.* 108, 10562–10567. doi: 10.1073/pnas.1107559108

Lawson, W. E., Polosukhin, V. V., Stathopoulos, G. T., Zoia, O., Han, W., Lane, K. B., et al. (2005). Increased and prolonged pulmonary fibrosis in surfactant protein C-deficient mice following intratracheal bleomycin. *Am. J. Pathol.* 167, 1267–1277. doi: 10.1016/s0002-9440(10)61214-x

Lederer, D., and Martinez, F. J. (2018). Idiopathic pulmonary fibrosis. *New Engl. J. Med.* 379, 795–798.

Leicester, K. L., Olynyk, J. K., Brunt, E. M., Britton, R. S., and Bacon, B. R. (2004). CD14-positive hepatic monocytes/macrophages increase in hereditary hemochromatosis. *Liver Intern.?* 24, 446–451. doi: 10.1111/j.1478-3231.2004.0943.x

Leonenko, Z., Gill, S., Baoukina, S., Monticelli, L., Doehner, J., Gunasekara, L., et al. (2007). An elevated level of cholesterol impairs self-assembly of pulmonary surfactant into a functional film. *Biophys. J.* 93, 674–683. doi: 10.1529/biophysj.107.106310

Liao, J. K., and Laufs, U. (2004). Pleiotropic effects of statins. *Annu. Rev. Pharmacol. Toxicol.* 45, 89–118. doi: 10.1146/annurev.pharmtox.45.120403.095748

Lin, S. L., Castaño, A. P., Nowlin, B. T., Lupher, M. L., and Duffield, J. S. (2009). Bone marrow Ly6Chigh monocytes are selectively recruited to injured kidney and differentiate into functionally distinct populations. *J. Immunol.* 183, 6733–6743. doi: 10.4049/jimmunol.0901473

Liptzin, D. R., Patel, T., and Deterding, R. R. (2015). Chronic ventilation in infants with surfactant protein C mutations: an alternative to lung transplantation. *Am. J. Respir. Crit. Care Med.* 191, 1338–1340. doi: 10.1164/rccm.201411-1955LE

Litao, M. K. S., Hayes, D., Chiwane, S., Nogee, L. M., and Kurland, G. (2017). A novel surfactant protein C gene mutation associated with progressive respiratory failure in infancy. *Pediatr. Pulmonol.* 52, 57–68. doi: 10.1002/ppul.23493

Liu, T., Sano, K., Ogiwara, N., and Kobayashi, N. (2016). A novel surfactant protein C L55F mutation associated with interstitial lung disease alters subcellular localization of proSP-C in A549 cells. *Pediatr. Res.* 79, 27–33. doi: 10.1038/pr.2015.178

Lopez-Rodriguez, E., Boden, C., Echaide, M., Perez-Gil, J., Kolb, M., Gauldie, J., et al. (2016). Surfactant dysfunction during overexpression of TGF-β1 precedes profibrotic lung remodeling in vivo. *Am. J. Physiol. Lung. Cell Mol. Physiol.* 310, L1260–L1271. doi: 10.1152/ajplung.00065.2016

Lopez-Rodriguez, E., Gay-Jordi, G., Mucci, A., Lachmann, N., and Serrano-Mollar, A. (2017). Lung surfactant metabolism: early in life, early in disease and target in cell therapy. *Cell Tissue Res.* 367, 721–735. doi: 10.1007/s00441-016-2520-9

Lukovic, D., Cruz, A., Gonzalez-Horta, A., Almlen, A., Curstedt, T., Mingarro, I., et al. (2012). Interfacial behavior of recombinant forms of human pulmonary surfactant protein SP-C. *Langmuir* 28, 7811–7825. doi: 10.1021/la301134v

Lutz, D., Gazdhar, A., Lopez-Rodriguez, E., Ruppert, C., Mahavadi, P., Günther, A., et al. (2015). Alveolar derecruitment and collapse induration as crucial mechanisms in lung injury and fibrosis. *Am. J. Respir. Cell Mol. Biol.* 52, 232–243. doi: 10.1165/rcmb.2014-0078oc

Lv, Z., Wang, Y., Liu, Y.-J., Mao, Y.-F., Dong, W.-W., Ding, Z.-N., et al. (2018). NLRP3 inflammasome activation contributes to mechanical stretch-induced endothelial-mesenchymal transition and pulmonary fibrosis. *Crit. Care Med.* 46, e49–e58. doi: 10.1097/CCM.0000000000002799

Madala, S. K., Maxfield, M. D., Davidson, C. R., Schmidt, S. M., Garry, D., Ikegami, M., et al. (2011). Rapamycin regulates bleomycin-induced lung damage in SP-C-deficient mice. *Pulmon. Med.* 2011, 1–12. doi: 10.1155/2011/653524

Mai, C., Verleden, S. E., McDonough, J. E., Willems, S., de Wever, W., Coolen, J., et al. (2016). Thin-section CT features of idiopathic pulmonary fibrosis correlated with micro-CT and histologic analysis. *Radiology* 283, 252–263. doi: 10.1148/radiol.2016152362

Mainali, L., Raguz, M., O'Brien, W. J., and Subczynski, W. K. (2013). Properties of membranes derived from the total lipids extracted from the human lens cortex and nucleus. *Biochim. Biophys. Acta* 1828, 1432–1440. doi: 10.1016/j.bbamem.2013.02.006

Maitra, G., Inchley, K., Novick, R. J., Veldhuizen, R. A. W., Lewis, J. F., and Possmayer, F. (2002). Acute lung injury and lung transplantation influence in vitro subtype conversion of pulmonary surfactant. *Am. J. Physiol. Lung. Cell Mol. Physiol.* 282, L67–L74. doi: 10.1152/ajplung.2002.282.1.L67

Manon, V., Stoyan, I., Nemanja, V., Madalina, D.-M., Lazaro-Emilio, A., Thibault, B., et al. (2018). Lysosomal cholesterol hydrolysis couples efferocytosis to anti-inflammatory oxysterol production. *Circ. Res.* 122, 1369–1384. doi: 10.1161/CIRCRESAHA.117.312333

Mao, P., Li, J., Huang, Y., Wu, S., Pang, X., He, W., et al. (2017). MicroRNA-19b mediates lung epithelial-mesenchymal transition via phosphatidylinositol-3,4,5-trisphosphate 3-phosphatase in response to mechanical stretch. *Am. J. Respir. Cell Mol. Biol.* 56, 11–19. doi: 10.1165/rcmb.2015-0377OC

Mariathasan, S., Weiss, D. S., Newton, K., McBride, J., O'Rourke, K., Roose-Girma, M., et al. (2006). Cryopyrin activates the inflammasome in response to toxins and ATP. *Nature* 440, 228–232. doi: 10.1038/nature04515

Markart, P., Ruppert, C., Wygrecka, M., Schmidt, R., Korfei, M., Harbach, H., et al. (2007). Surfactant protein C mutations in sporadic forms of idiopathic interstitial pneumonias. *Eur. Respir. J.* 29, 134–137. doi: 10.1183/09031936.00034406

Mead, J., Takishima, T., and Leith, D. (1970). Stress distribution in lungs: a model of pulmonary elasticity. *J. Appl. Physiol.* 28, 596–608. doi: 10.1152/jappl.1970.28.5.596

Mechri, M., Epaud, R., Emond, S., Coulomb, A., Jaubert, F., Tarrant, A., et al. (2010). Surfactant protein C gene (SFTPC) mutation-associated lung disease: high-resolution computed tomography (HRCT) findings and its relation to histological analysis. *Pediatr. Pulmonol.* 45, 1021–1029. doi: 10.1002/ppul.21289

Menchaca, H. J., Michalek, V. N., Rohde, T. D., O'Dea, T. J., and Buchwald, H. (1998). Decreased blood oxygen diffusion in hypercholesterolemia. *Surgery* 124, 692–698. doi: 10.1067/MSY.1998.90944

Milos, S., Hiansen, J. Q., Yamashita, C., and Veldhuizen, R. (2016). The role of a high cholesterol diet on surfactant biophysics during acute lung injury. *FASEB J.* 30:1297.1. doi: 10.1096/fasebj.30.1_supplement.1297.1

Mishra, A., Chintagari, N. R., Guo, Y., Weng, T., Su, L., and Liu, L. (2011). Purinergic P2X7 receptor regulates lung surfactant secretion in a paracrine manner. *J. Cell Sci.* 124, 657–668. doi: 10.1242/jcs.066977

Molugu, T. R., and Brown, M. F. (2019). "Cholesterol effects on the physical properties of lipid membranes viewed by solid-state NMR spectroscopy," in *Cholesterol Modulation of Protein Function: Sterol Specificity and Indirect Mechanisms*, eds A. Rosenhouse-Dantsker and A. N. Bukiya (Cham: Springer International Publishing), 99–133. doi: 10.1007/978-3-030-04278-3_5

Mora, A. L., Torres-González, E., Rojas, M., Corredor, C., Ritzenthaler, J., Xu, J., et al. (2006). Activation of alveolar macrophages via the alternative pathway in herpesvirus-induced lung fibrosis. *Am. J. Respir. Cell Mol. Biol.* 35, 466–473. doi: 10.1165/rcmb.2006-0121OC

Morrow, M. R., Taneva, S., Simatos, G. A., Allwood, L. A., and Keough, K. M. W. (1993). Deuterium NMR studies of the effect of pulmonary surfactant SP-C on the 1,2-dipalmitoyl-sn-glycero-3-phosphocholine headgroup: a model for transbilayer peptides in surfactant and biological membranes. *Biochemistry* 32, 11338–11344. doi: 10.1021/bi00093a010

Mouded, M., Egea, E. E., Brown, M. J., Hanlon, S. M., Houghton, A. M. G., Tsai, L. W., et al. (2009). Epithelial cell apoptosis causes acute lung injury masquerading as emphysema. *Am. J. Respir. Cell Mol. Biol.* 41, 407–414. doi: 10.1165/rcmb.2008-0137OC

Myers, J. L., and Katzenstein, A. L. (1988). Ultrastructural evidence of alveolar epithelial injury in idiopathic bronchiolitis obliterans-organizing pneumonia. *Am. J. Pathol.* 132, 102–109.

Nakayama, M. (2018). Macrophage recognition of crystals and nanoparticles. *Front. Immunol.* 9:103. doi: 10.3389/fimmu.2018.00103

Nieman, G. F., Andrews, P., Satalin, J., Wilcox, K., Kollisch-Singule, M., Madden, M., et al. (2018). Acute lung injury: how to stabilize a broken lung. *Crit. Care* 22:136. doi: 10.1186/s13054-018-2051-2058

Nieman, G., Satalin, J., Andrews, P., Wilcox, K., Aiash, H., Baker, S., et al. (2018). Preemptive mechanical ventilation based on dynamic physiology in the alveolar microenvironment: novel considerations of time-dependent properties of the respiratory system. *J. Trauma Acute Care Surg.* 85, 1081–1091. doi: 10.1097/TA.0000000000002050

Nogee, L. M., Dunbar, A. E., Wert, S. E., Askin, F., Hamvas, A., and Whitsett, J. A. (2001). A mutation in the surfactant protein C gene associated with familial interstitial lung disease. *New Engl. J. Med.* 344, 573–579. doi: 10.1056/nejm200102223440805

Nureki, S.-I., Tomer, Y., Venosa, A., Katzen, J., Russo, S. J., Jamil, S., et al. (2018). Expression of mutant Sftpc in murine alveolar epithelia drives spontaneous lung fibrosis. *J. Clin. Invest.* 128, 4008–4024. doi: 10.1172/jci99287

Ochs, M., Nyengaard, J. R., Jung, A., Knudsen, L., Voigt, M., Wahlers, T., et al. (2004). The number of alveoli in the human lung. *Am. J. Respir. Crit. Care Med.* 169, 120–124. doi: 10.1164/rccm.200308-1107OC

Olmeda, B., Martínez-Calle, M., and Pérez-Gil, J. (2017). Pulmonary surfactant metabolism in the alveolar airspace: biogenesis, extracellular conversions, recycling. *Ann. Anat.* 209, 78–92. doi: 10.1016/j.aanat.2016.09.008

Olmeda, B., Villén, L., Cruz, A., Orellana, G., and Perez-Gil, J. (2010). Pulmonary surfactant layers accelerate O2 diffusion through the air-water interface. *Biochim. Biophys. Acta Biomemb.* 1798, 1281–1284. doi: 10.1016/J.BBAMEM.2010.03.008

Ono, S., Tanaka, T., Ishida, M., Kinoshita, A., Fukuoka, J., Takaki, M., et al. (2011). Surfactant protein C G100S mutation causes familial pulmonary fibrosis in Japanese kindred. *Eur. Respir. J.* 38, 861–869. doi: 10.1183/09031936.00143610

Orgeig, S., and Daniels, C. B. (2001). The roles of cholesterol in pulmonary surfactant: insights from comparative and evolutionary studies. *Compar. Biochem. Physiol. Part A* 129, 75–89. doi: 10.1016/s1095-6433(01)00307-5

Orgeig, S., Morrison, J. L., and Daniels, C. B. (2011). Evolution, development, and function of the pulmonary surfactant system in normal and perturbed environments. *Compr. Physiol.* 6, 363–422. doi: 10.1002/cphy.c150003

Ozyilmaz, E., Gunasti, S., Kuyucu, Y., Polat, S., Gumurdulu, D., Kuleci, S., et al. (2013). Hermansky Pudlak Syndrome and pulmonary alveolar proteinosis at the same patient: First case report in the world literature. *Sarcoidos. Vasculit. Diffuse Lung Dis.* 30, 217–220.

Park, J. S., Choi, Y. J., Kim, Y. T., Park, S., Chae, J.-H., Park, J. D., et al. (2018). Pediatric case report on an interstitial lung disease with a novel mutation of SFTPC successfully treated with lung transplantation. *J. Korean Med. Sci.* 33:e159.

Parra, E., Alcaraz, A., Cruz, A., Aguilella, V. M., and Pérez-Gil, J. (2013). Hydrophobic pulmonary surfactant proteins SP-B and SP-C induce pore formation in planar lipid membranes: evidence for proteolipid pores. *Biophys. J.* 104, 146–155. doi: 10.1016/J.BPJ.2012.11.014

Parra, E., Moleiro, L. H., López-Montero, I., Cruz, A., Monroy, F., and Pérez-Gil, J. (2011). A combined action of pulmonary surfactant proteins SP-B and SP-C modulates permeability and dynamics of phospholipid membranes. *Biochem. J.* 438, 555–564. doi: 10.1042/BJ20110681

Patel, A. S., Reigada, D., Mitchell, C. H., Bates, S. R., Margulies, S. S., and Koval, M. (2005). Paracrine stimulation of surfactant secretion by extracellular ATP in response to mechanical deformation. *Am. J. Physiol. Lung. Cell Mol. Physiol.* 289, L489–L496. doi: 10.1152/ajplung.00074.2005

Peca, D., Boldrini, R., Johannson, J., Shieh, J. T., Citti, A., Petrini, S., et al. (2015). Clinical and ultrastructural spectrum of diffuse lung disease associated with surfactant protein C mutations. *Eur. J. Hum. Genet.* 23, 1033–1041. doi: 10.1038/ejhg.2015.45

Petroulia, V., Funke, M., Zumstein, P., Berezowska, S., Ebner, L., Geiser, T., et al. (2018). Increased expiratory computed tomography density reveals possible abnormalities in radiologically preserved lung parenchyma in idiopathic pulmonary fibrosis. *Invest. Radiol.* 53, 45–51. doi: 10.1097/rli.0000000000000405

Plasencia, I., Cruz, A., Casals, C., and Pérez-Gil, J. (2001). Superficial disposition of the N-terminal region of the surfactant protein SP-C and the absence of specific SP-B-SP-C interactions in phospholipid bilayers. *Biochem. J.* 359, 651–659. doi: 10.1042/bj3590651

Plasencia, I., Rivas, L., Keough, K. M. W., Marsh, D., and Perez-Gil, J. (2004). The N-terminal segment of pulmonary surfactant lipopeptide SP-C has intrinsic propensity to interact with and perturb phospholipid bilayers. *Biochem. J.* 377, 183–193. doi: 10.1042/bj20030815

Possmayer, F., Nag, K., Rodriguez, K., Qanbar, R., and Schürch, S. (2001). Surface activity in vitro: role of surfactant proteins. *Compar. Biochem. Physiol. Part A* 129, 209–220. doi: 10.1016/S1095-6433(01)00317-318

Potter, S., Orgeig, S., Donnellan, S., and Daniels, C. B. (2007). Purifying selection drives the evolution of surfactant protein C (SP-C) independently of body temperature regulation in mammals. *Compar. Biochem. Physiol. Part A* 2, 165–176. doi: 10.1016/J.CBD.2007.02.003

Puttur, F., Gregory, L. G., and Lloyd, C. M. (2019). Airway macrophages as the guardians of tissue repair in the lung. *Immunol. Cell Biol.* 97, 246–257. doi: 10.1111/imcb.12235

Qu, L., Xue, H., Yuan, P., Zhou, L., Yao, T., Huang, Y., et al. (2009). Adenosine 5'-triphosphate stimulates the increase of TGF-beta1 in rat mesangial cells under high-glucose conditions via reactive oxygen species and ERK1/2. *Acta Pharmacol. Sin.* 30, 1601–1606. doi: 10.1038/aps.2009.155

Raghu, G., Weycker, D., Edelsberg, J., Bradford, W. Z., and Oster, G. (2006). Incidence and prevalence of idiopathic pulmonary fibrosis. *Am. J. Respir. Crit. Care Med.* 174, 810–816.

Raguz, M., Widomska, J., Dillon, J., Gaillard, E. R., and Subczynski, W. K. (2008). Characterization of lipid domains in reconstituted porcine lens membranes using EPR spin-labeling approaches. *Biochim. Biophys. Acta Biomemb.* 1778, 1079–1090. doi: 10.1016/J.BBAMEM.2008.01.024

Ramji, D. P., and Davies, T. S. (2015). Cytokines in atherosclerosis: Key players in all stages of disease and promising therapeutic targets. *Cytokine Growth. Factor. Rev.* 26, 673–685. doi: 10.1016/j.cytogfr.2015.04.003

Ramm, G. A., Nair, V. G., Bridle, K. R., Shepherd, R. W., and Crawford, D. H. (1998). Contribution of hepatic parenchymal and nonparenchymal cells to hepatic fibrogenesis in biliary atresia. *Am. J. Pathol.* 153, 527–535. doi: 10.1016/S0002-9440(10)65595-65592

Riteau, N., Gasse, P., Fauconnier, L., Gombault, A., Couegnat, M., Fick, L., et al. (2010). Extracellular ATP is a danger signal activating P2X 7 receptor in lung inflammation and fibrosis. *Am. J. Respir. Crit. Care Med.* 182, 774–783. doi: 10.1164/rccm.201003-0359OC

Robert, S., Gicquel, T., Victoni, T., Valença, S., Barreto, E., Bailly-Maître, B., et al. (2016). Involvement of matrix metalloproteinases (MMPs) and inflammasome pathway in molecular mechanisms of fibrosis. *Biosci. Rep.* 36:e00360. doi: 10. 1042/BSR20160107

Roldan, N., Nyholm, T. K. M., Slotte, J. P., Pérez-Gil, J., and García-Álvarez, B. (2016). Effect of lung surfactant protein SP-C and SP-C-promoted membrane fragmentation on cholesterol dynamics. *Biophys. J.* 111, 1703–1713. doi: 10. 1016/j.bpj.2016.09.016

Roldan, N., Pérez-Gil, J., Morrow, M. R., and García-Álvarez, B. (2017). Divide & conquer: surfactant protein SP-C and cholesterol modulate phase segregation in lung surfactant. *Biophys. J.* 113, 847–859. doi: 10.1016/j.bpj.2017. 06.059

Romero, F., Shah, D., Duong, M., Penn, R. B., Fessler, M. B., Madenspacher, J., et al. (2014). A pneumocyte-macrophage paracrine lipid axis drives the lung toward fibrosis. *Am. J. Respir. Cell Mol. Biol.* 53, 74–86. doi: 10.1165/rcmb.2014-0343OC

Rosen, D. M., and Waltz, D. A. (2005). Hydroxychloroquine and surfactant protein C deficiency. *N. Engl. J. Med.* 352, 207–208. doi: 10.1056/NEJM200501133520223

Rühl, N., Lopez-Rodriguez, E., Albert, K., Smith, B. J., Weaver, T. E., Ochs, M., et al. (2019). Surfactant protein B deficiency induced high surface tension: relationship between alveolar micromechanics, alveolar fluid properties and alveolar epithelial cell injury. *Intern. J. Mol. Sci.* 20:243. doi: 10.3390/ijms20174243

Ruwisch, J., Sehlmeyer, K., Roldan, N., Garcia-Alvarez, B., Perez-Gil, J., Weaver, T. E., et al. (2020). Air space distension precedes spontaneous fibrotic remodeling and impaired cholesterol metabolism in the absence of surfactant protein C. *Am. J. Respir. Cell Mol. Biol.* 62, 466–478. doi: 10.1165/rcmb.2019-0358OC

Saito, A., Horie, M., and Nagase, T. (2018). TGF-β signaling in lung health and disease. *Intern. J. Mol. Sci.* 19:2460. doi: 10.3390/ijms19082460

Saito, K., Tanaka, N., Ikari, J., Suzuki, M., Anazawa, R., Abe, M., et al. (2019). Comprehensive lipid profiling of bleomycin-induced lung injury. *J. Appl. Toxicol.* 39, 658–671. doi: 10.1002/jat.3758

Salerno, T., Peca, D., Menchini, L., Schiavino, A., Boldrini, R., Esposito, F., et al. (2016). Surfactant Protein C-associated interstitial lung disease; three different phenotypes of the same SFTPC mutation. *Itali. J. Pediatr.* 42:23.

Schmid-Kotsas, A., Gross, H. J., Menke, A., Weidenbach, H., Adler, G., Siech, M., et al. (1999). Lipopolysaccharide-activated macrophages stimulate the synthesis of collagen type I and C-fibronectin in cultured pancreatic stellate cells. *Am. J. Pathol.* 155, 1749–1758. doi: 10.1016/S0002-9440(10)65490-65499

Schmidt, R., Ruppert, C., Markart, P., Lübke, N., Ermert, L., Weissmann, N., et al. (2004). Changes in pulmonary surfactant function and composition in bleomycin-induced pneumonitis and fibrosis. *Toxicol. Appl. Pharmacol.* 195, 218–231. doi: 10.1016/j.taap.2003.11.011

Setoguchi, Y., Ikeda, T., and Fukuchi, Y. (2006). Clinical features and genetic analysis of surfactant protein C in adult-onset familial interstitial pneumonia. *Respirology* 11(Suppl.), S41–S45. doi: 10.1111/j.1440-1843.2006.00807.x

Sheppard, D. (2015). Epithelial-mesenchymal interactions in fibrosis and repair: transforming growth factor-β activation by epithelial cells and fibroblasts. *Ann. Am. Thorac. Soc.* 12, S21–S23. doi: 10.1513/AnnalsATS.201406-245MG

Sisson, T. H., Mendez, M., Choi, K., Subbotina, N., Courey, A., Cunningham, A., et al. (2010). Targeted injury of type II alveolar epithelial cells induces pulmonary fibrosis. *Am. J. Respir. Crit. Care Med.* 181, 254–263.

Smigiel, K. S., and Parks, W. C. (2018). Macrophages, wound healing, and fibrosis: recent insights. *Curr. Rheumatol. Rep.* 20:725. doi: 10.1007/s11926-018-0725-725

Smith, B. J., Bartolak-Suki, E., Suki, B., Roy, G. S., Hamlington, K. L., Charlebois, C. M., et al. (2017). Linking ventilator injury-induced leak across the blood-gas barrier to derangements in murine lung function. *Front. Physiol.* 8:466. doi: 10.3389/fphys.2017.00466

Smith, B. J., Grant, K. A., and Bates, J. H. T. (2013). Linking the development of ventilator-induced injury to mechanical function in the lung. *Ann. Biomed. Eng.* 41, 527–536. doi: 10.1007/s10439-012-0693-692

Snijder, J., Peraza, J., Padilla, M., Capaccione, K., and Salvatore, M. M. (2019). Pulmonary fibrosis: a disease of alveolar collapse and collagen deposition. *Expert Rev. Respir. Med.* 13, 615–619. doi: 10.1080/17476348.2019.1623028

So, A., de Smedt, T., Revaz, S., and Tschopp, J. (2007). A pilot study of IL-1 inhibition by anakinra in acute gout. *Arthrit. Res. Ther.* 9, R28–R28. doi: 10.1186/ar2143

Soraisham, A. S., Tierney, A. J., and Amin, H. J. (2006). Neonatal respiratory failure associated with mutation in the surfactant protein C gene. *J. Perinatol.* 26, 67–70. doi: 10.1038/sj.jp.7211417

Stevens, P. A., Pettenazzo, A., Brasch, F., Mulugeta, S., Baritussio, A., Ochs, M., et al. (2005). Nonspecific interstitial pneumonia, alveolar proteinosis, and abnormal proprotein trafficking resulting from a spontaneous mutation in the surfactant protein C gene. *Pediatr. Res.* 57:89. doi: 10.1203/01.pdr.0000147567. 02473.5a

Swanson, K. V., Deng, M., and Ting, J. P.-Y. (2019). The NLRP3 inflammasome: molecular activation and regulation to therapeutics. *Nat. Rev. Immunol.* 19, 477–489. doi: 10.1038/s41577-019-0165-160

Tabuchi, A., Nickles, H. T., Kim, M., Semple, J. W., Koch, E., Brochard, L., et al. (2016). Acute lung injury causes asynchronous alveolar ventilation that can be corrected by individual sighs. *Am. J. Respir. Crit. Care Med.* 193, 396–406. doi: 10.1164/rccm.201505-0901OC

Terèelj, M., Salobir, B., Simcic, S., Wraber, B., Zupancic, M., and Rylander, R. (2009). Chitotriosidase activity in sarcoidosis and some other pulmonary diseases. *Scand. J. Clin. Lab. Invest.* 69, 575–578. doi: 10.1080/00365510902829362

Thomas, A. Q., Lane, K., Phillips, J., Prince, M., Markin, C., Speer, M., et al. (2002). Heterozygosity for a surfactant protein c gene mutation associated with usual interstitial pneumonitis and cellular nonspecific interstitial pneumonitis in one kindred. *Am. J. Respir. Crit. Care Med.* 165, 1322–1328. doi: 10.1164/rccm. 200112-123OC

Thomassen, M. J., Barna, B. P., Malur, A. G., Bonfield, T. L., Farver, C. F., Malur, A., et al. (2007). ABCG1 is deficient in alveolar macrophages of GM-CSF knockout mice and patients with pulmonary alveolar proteinosis. *J. Lipid Res.* 48, 2762–2768. doi: 10.1194/jlr.P700022-JLR200

Thompson, R. W., Pesce, J. T., Ramalingam, T., Wilson, M. S., White, S., Cheever, A. W., et al. (2008). Cationic amino acid transporter-2 regulates immunity by modulating arginase activity. *PLoS Pathog.* 4:e1000023. doi: 10.1371/journal. ppat.1000023

Thouvenin, G., Taam, R. A., Flamein, F., Guillot, L., le Bourgeois, M., Reix, P., et al. (2010). Characteristics of disorders associated with genetic mutations of surfactant protein C. *Arch. Dis. Childhood* 95, 449–454. doi: 10.1136/adc.2009. 171553

Todd, N. W., Atamas, S. P., Luzina, I. G., and Galvin, J. R. (2015). Permanent alveolar collapse is the predominant mechanism in idiopathic pulmonary fibrosis. *Expert Rev. Respir. Med.* 9, 411–418. doi: 10.1586/17476348.2015. 1067609

Torday, J., and Rehan, V. (2011). Neutral lipid trafficking regulates alveolar type II cell surfactant phospholipid and surfactant protein expression. *Exper. Lung Res.* 37, 376–386. doi: 10.3109/01902148.2011.580903

Tredano, M., Griese, M., Brasch, F., Schumacher, S., Blic, J., de Marque, S., et al. (2004). Mutation of SFTPC in infantile pulmonary alveolar proteinosis with or without fibrosing lung disease. *Am. J. Med. Genet. Part A* 126A, 18–26. doi: 10.1002/ajmg.a.20670

Turcu, S., Ashton, E., Jenkins, L., Gupta, A., and Mok, Q. (2013). Genetic testing in children with surfactant dysfunction. *Arch. Dis. Child.* 98, 490–495. doi: 10.1136/archdischild-2012-303166

Turley, S. D., Andersen, J. M., and Dietschy, J. M. (1981). Rates of sterol synthesis and uptake in the major organs of the rat in vivo. *J. Lipid. Res.* 22, 551–569.

van Hoorn, J., Brouwers, A., Griese, M., and Kramer, B. (2014). Successful weaning from mechanical ventilation in a patient with surfactant protein C deficiency presenting with severe neonatal respiratory distress. *BMJ Case Rep.* 2014:203053. doi: 10.1136/bcr-2013-203053

van Meer, G., Voelker, D. R., and Feigenson, G. W. (2008). Membrane lipids: where they are and how they behave. *Nat. Rev. Mol. Cell Biol.* 9, 112–124. doi: 10.1038/nrm2330

van Moorsel, C. H. M., van Oosterhout, M. F. M., Barlo, N. P., de Jong, P. A., van der Vis, J. J., Ruven, H. J. T., et al. (2010). Surfactant protein c mutations are the basis of a significant portion of adult familial pulmonary fibrosis in a dutch cohort. *Am. J. Respir. Crit. Care Med.* 182, 1419–1425. doi: 10.1164/rccm.200906-0953oc

Vazquez De Anda, G. F., Gommers, D., Verbrugge, S. J. C., de Jaegere, A., and Lachmann, B. (2000). Mechanical ventilation with high positive end-expiratory pressure and small driving pressure amplitude is as effective as high-frequency oscillatory ventilation to preserve the function of exogenous surfactant in lung-lavaged rats. *Crit. Care Med.* 28, 2921–2925. doi: 10.1097/00003246-200008000-00039

Veldhuizen, R. A., Ito, Y., Marcou, J., Yao, L. J., McCaig, L., and Lewis, J. F. (1997). Effects of lung injury on pulmonary surfactant aggregate conversion in vivo and in vitro. *Am. J. Physiol.* 272, L872–L878. doi: 10.1152/ajplung.1997.272.5.L872

Veldhuizen, R. A., Marcou, J., Yao, L. J., McCaig, L., Ito, Y., and Lewis, J. F. (1996). Alveolar surfactant aggregate conversion in ventilated normal and injured rabbits. *Am. J. Physiol.* 270, L152–L158. doi: 10.1152/ajplung.1996.270.1.L152

Venosa, A., Katzen, J., Tomer, Y., Kopp, M., Jamil, S., Russo, S. J., et al. (2019). Epithelial expression of an interstitial lung disease-associated mutation in surfactant protein-c modulates recruitment and activation of key myeloid cell populations in mice. *J. Immunol.* 202, 2760–2771. doi: 10.4049/jimmunol.1900039

Vilaysane, A., Chun, J., Seamone, M. E., Wang, W., Chin, R., Hirota, S., et al. (2010). The NLRP3 inflammasome promotes renal inflammation and contributes to CKD. *J. Am. Soc. Nephrol.* 21, 1732–1744. doi: 10.1681/ASN.2010020143

Vockeroth, D., Gunasekara, L., Amrein, M., Possmayer, F., Lewis, J. F., and Veldhuizen, R. A. W. (2009). Role of cholesterol in the biophysical dysfunction of surfactant in ventilator-induced lung injury. *Am. J. Physiol. Lung Cell. Mol. Physiol.* 298, L117–L125. doi: 10.1152/ajplung.00218.2009

Voyno-Yasenetskaya, T. A., Dobbs, L. G., and Williams, M. C. (1991). Regulation of ATP-dependent surfactant secretion and activation of second-messenger systems in alveolar type II cells. *Am. J. Physiol. Lung Cell. Mol. Physiol.* 261, 105–109. doi: 10.1152/ajpheart.1991.261.4.105

Vyshedskiy, A., Alhashem, R. M., Paciej, R., Ebril, M., Rudman, I., Fredberg, J. J., et al. (2009). Mechanism of inspiratory and expiratory crackles. *Chest* 135, 156–164. doi: 10.1378/chest.07-1562

Wambach, J. A., Yang, P., Wegner, D. J., An, P., Hackett, B. P., Cole, F. S., et al. (2010). Surfactant Protein-C promoter variants associated with neonatal respiratory distress syndrome reduce transcription. *Pediatr. Res.* 68:216. doi: 10.1203/pdr.0b013e3181eb5d68

Wang, C.-M., Chang, Y.-Y., and Sun, S. H. (2003). Activation of P2X7 purinoceptor-stimulated TGF-beta 1 mRNA expression involves PKC/MAPK signalling pathway in a rat brain-derived type-2 astrocyte cell line, RBA-2. *Cell. Signal.* 15, 1129–1137. doi: 10.1016/s0898-6568(03)00112-118

Wang, L., Cai, P., Galla, H.-J., He, H., Flach, C. R., and Mendelsohn, R. (2005). Monolayer-multilayer transitions in a lung surfactant model: IR reflection-absorption spectroscopy and atomic force microscopy. *Eur. Biophys. J.* 34, 243–254. doi: 10.1007/s00249-004-0446-448

Weibel, E. R., and Gil, J. (1968). Electron microscopic demonstration of an extracellular duplex lining layer of alveoli. *Respir. Physiol.* 4, 42–57. doi: 10.1016/0034-5687(68)90006-90006

Wennberg, C. L., van der Spoel, D., and Hub, J. S. (2012). Large influence of cholesterol on solute partitioning into lipid membranes. *J. Am. Chem. Soc.* 134, 5351–5361. doi: 10.1021/ja211929h

Widomska, J., Subczynski, W. K., Mainali, L., and Raguz, M. (2017). Cholesterol bilayer domains in the eye lens health: a review. *Cell Biochem. Biophys.* 75, 387–398. doi: 10.1007/s12013-017-0812-817

Wree, A., McGeough, M. D., Peña, C. A., Schlattjan, M., Li, H., Inzaugarat, M. E., et al. (2014). NLRP3 inflammasome activation is required for fibrosis development in NAFLD. *J. Mol. Med.* 92, 1069–1082. doi: 10.1007/s00109-014-1170-1171

Wynn, T. A., and Barron, L. (2010). Macrophages: master regulators of inflammation and fibrosis. *Semin. Liver Dis.* 30, 245–257. doi: 10.1055/s-0030-1255354

Wynn, T. A., Chawla, A., and Pollard, J. W. (2013). Macrophage biology in development, homeostasis and disease. *Nature* 496, 445–455. doi: 10.1038/nature12034

Xing, Z., Tremblay, G. M., Sime, P. J., and Gauldie, J. (1997). Overexpression of granulocyte-macrophage colony-stimulating factor induces pulmonary granulation tissue formation and fibrosis by induction of transforming growth factor-??1 and myofibroblast accumulation. *Am. J. Pathol.* 150, 59–66.

Xu, J.-F., Washko, G. R., Nakahira, K., Hatabu, H., Patel, A. S., Fernandez, I. E., et al. (2012). Statins and pulmonary fibrosis: the potential role of NLRP3 inflammasome activation. *Am. J. Respir. Crit. Care Med.* 185, 547–556. doi: 10.1164/rccm.201108-1574OC

Yao, X., Gordon, E. M., Figueroa, D. M., Barochia, A. V., and Levine, S. J. (2016). Emerging Roles of Apolipoprotein E and apolipoprotein A-I in the pathogenesis and treatment of lung disease. *Am. J. Respir. Cell Mol. Biol.* 55, 159–169. doi: 10.1165/rcmb.2016-0060TR

Zhang, Y., Lee, T. C., Guillemin, B., Yu, M. C., and Rom, W. N. (1993). Enhanced IL-1 beta and tumor necrosis factor-alpha release and messenger RNA expression in macrophages from idiopathic pulmonary fibrosis or after asbestos exposure. *J. Immunol.* 150, 4188–4196.

Zhou, Y., Huang, X., Hecker, L., Kurundkar, D., Kurundkar, A., Liu, H., et al. (2013). Inhibition of mechanosensitive signaling in myofibroblasts ameliorates experimental pulmonary fibrosis. *J. Clin. Invest.* 123, 1096–1108. doi: 10.1172/JCI66700

Zocher, F., van der Spoel, D., Pohl, P., and Hub, J. S. (2013). Local partition coefficients govern solute permeability of cholesterol-containing membranes. *Biophys. J.* 105, 2760–2770. doi: 10.1016/J.BPJ.2013.11.003

Zuniga-Hertz, J. P., and Patel, H. H. (2019). The evolution of cholesterol-rich membrane in oxygen adaption: the respiratory system as a model. *Front. Physiol.* 10:1340. doi: 10.3389/fphys.2019.01340

Zuo, Y. Y., Veldhuizen, R. A. W., Neumann, A. W., Petersen, N. O., and Possmayer, F. (2008). Current perspectives in pulmonary surfactant–inhibition, enhancement and evaluation. *Biochim. Biophys. Acta* 1778, 1947–1977. doi: 10.1016/j.bbamem.2008.03.021

7

The Development of Integrin Alpha-8 Deficient Lungs Shows Reduced and Altered Branching and a Correction of the Phenotype During Alveolarization

Tiziana P. Cremona[1], *Andrea Hartner*[2] *and Johannes C. Schittny*[1]*

[1] *Institute of Anatomy, Department of Preclinical Medicine, Faculty of Medicine, University of Bern, Bern, Switzerland,*
[2] *Department of Pediatrics and Adolescent Medicine, University Hospital of Erlangen-Nürnberg, Erlangen, Germany*

Correspondence:
Johannes C. Schittny
schittny@ana.unibe.ch

Lung development involves epithelial–mesenchymal interactions and integrins represent one of the key elements. These extracellular matrix receptors form hetero-dimers of alpha and beta subunits. The integrin α8β1 is highly expressed in mouse tissues, including lung. It forms a cellular receptor for fibronectin, vitronectin, osteopontin, nephronectin, and tenascin-C. This study aims to investigate the role of the integrin α8-subunit (α8) during lung development. Wild type and α8-deficient lungs were explanted at embryonic days 11.5/12.5. After 24–73 h in culture α8-deficient lung explants displayed reduced growth, reduced branching, enlarged endbuds, altered branching patterns, and faster spontaneous contractions of the airways as compared to wild type. Postnatally, a stereological investigation revealed that lung volume, alveolar surface area, and the length of the free septal edge were significantly reduced in α8-deficient lungs at postnatal days P4 and P7. An increased formation of new septa in α8-deficient lungs rescued the phenotype. At day P90 α8-deficient lungs were comparable to wild type. We conclude that α8β1 takes not only part in the control of branching, but also possesses a morphogenic effect on the pattern and size of the future airways. Furthermore, we conclude that the phenotype observed at day P4 is caused by reduced branching and is rescued by a pronounced formation of the new septa throughout alveolarization. More studies are needed to understand the mechanism responsible for the formation of new septa in the absence of α8β1 in order to be of potential therapeutic benefit for patients suffering from structural lung diseases.

Keywords: integrin alpha 8, lung development, branching morphology, alveolarization, transgenic mice, integrin

---

Abbreviations: α8, α8 integrin subunit; E, embryonal; P, postnatal; WT, wild type; KO, α8 deficient mice or lungs; KO+ α8 deficient mice or lungs with phenotype; KO−, α8 deficient mice or lungs without phenotype.

INTRODUCTION

Lung Development

The lungs are the main organ of respiration present in human, mice, and higher vertebrates. They provide a large internal surface area where the inspired air and the capillary blood get in close contact to each other to allow an efficient exchange of gases. To achieve this goal, during lung development, six important and overlapping stages occur: organogenesis, pseudoglandular stage, canalicular stage, saccular stage, alveolarization, and microvascular maturation. Successful development and function of the lung also involves the biochemical development of the surfactant system required for the stability and immune defense of the large respiratory surface area (Schittny, 2017).

During the pseudoglandular and canalicular stage, large parts of the pulmonary airways are formed prenatally by branching morphogenesis. In humans, monkeys, dogs and others, the bronchial tree is formed by a repetitive dichotomous branching of the future airways whereas in rodents, branching follows a monopodial pattern (Woods and Schittny, 2016).

Mostly postnatally in rodents and human the gas exchange surface of the lungs is enlarged during alveolarization; new septa are lifted off of pre-existing ones subdividing the most distal airspaces (Mund et al., 2008; Schittny et al., 2008). Alveolarization is a process, which does not finish during early childhood but continues until young adulthood (for a review see Schittny, 2017, 2018). Throughout lung postnatal development of rodents the size of the alveoli first decreases and later increases (Mund et al., 2008; Tschanz et al., 2014). Therefore, the alveolar surface area, the number of alveoli, and the total length of free septal edge does not increase in parallel with the increase of the lung volume.

Integrins

Cellular and extracellular signaling networks orchestrate lung development. In the past the extracellular matrix was mainly viewed as the structural element of tissue. In the last two decades it became obvious that the extracellular matrix represents a dynamic and functional active zone that contributes to the establishment of cellular phenotypes. The contact to specific extracellular matrix proteins precisely modulates differentiation, migration, proliferation, and programmed cell death (Streuli, 1999). Extracellular matrix proteins like elastin, collagens, laminins and tenascin-C contribute to pre and postnatal development. These proteins are recognized by specific receptors such as integrins, α-dystroglycan and other collagen receptors (Arnaout et al., 2005). Integrins are a large family of heterodimeric transmembrane glycoproteins containing a single α and a single β subunit non-covalently linked. The expression, distribution, and role of the different integrins present on airway epithelial cells have been characterized *in vivo* and *in vitro* (Coraux et al., 1998; Sheppard, 2003).

α8β1 Integrin

The integrin α8 subunit exclusively associates with the integrin β1 subunit to form receptors for fibronectin, vitronectin, nephronectin, osteopontin, and tenascin-C (Muller et al., 1995; Schnapp et al., 1995a,b; Brandenberger et al., 2001). In the lung the presence of α8β1 appears prenatally diffusely in the mesenchyme except for cells surrounding the branching and growing ends of the future airways. Postnatally, α8 keeps its diffuse mesenchymal distribution, but co-localizes with fibronectin and also with alpha smooth muscle actin (Chiquet-Ehrismann and Tucker, 2011). It has been shown that integrin α8β1 mediates signals from the extracellular matrix to alveolar myofibroblasts and contributes to secondary septation (Wagner et al., 2003).

α8β1 Integrin Knock Out Mice

In 1997 Müller and coworkers created an integrin α8-deficient mouse line by inactivating the gene encoding the α8 subunit by gene targeting (Muller et al., 1997). They demonstrated that α8β1 plays a crucial role in epithelial-mesenchymal interactions during kidney morphogenesis. This explains renal agenesis or dysgenesis at birth in homozygote mice. The penetration of this phenotype varies between two normal kidneys and no kidneys at all. Further investigations were necessary to discover that they have inner ear defects (Littlewood and Muller, 2000), and in the lung, anomalies in airway division and fusion of the medial and caudal lung lobes (Benjamin et al., 2009). The spatiotemporal expression pattern in lung development has been studied (Wagner et al., 2003) but detailed morphometric studies during prenatal and postnatal lung development have never been done.

Aim of the Study

The aim of this study is to investigate the role of the integrin α8 subunit during lung development. We hypothesized that the α8 subunit plays an essential role in two important mechanisms: branching morphogenesis and alveolarization. To test these hypotheses, we have performed lung organ culture and morphometric studies during prenatal and postnatal lung development. We observed reduced branching, an altered branching pattern, and a higher frequency of spontaneous contractions of the future airways during prenatal development of α8 deficient lungs resulting in a reduced lung volume, surface area, and length of the free septal edge at postnatal day 4. A tremendous amount of septa are formed to rescue the prenatal phenotype of α8-deficient mice until adulthood. We conclude that integrin α8β1 takes part in the control of branching morphogenesis and that during alveolarization an incompletely developed lung may be rescued by an increased alveolarization.

MATERIALS AND METHODS

Animals

The α8-deficient mouse strain, kindly gift from Dr. Müller, was used (Muller et al., 1997). Wild type (WT) 129/Sv mice were used as age matched controls. 12.5 days old fetuses were obtained from heterozygote and the 11.5 days old ones from homozygote breeding (**Table 1**). Postnatal lungs were obtained from homozygote breading. All animal studies were approved by and conducted in accordance with the Veterinary Service of the

TABLE 1 | Summary of lung organ experiments.

	Number of explants			Penetration of branching phenotype
	KO+	KO−	WT	
Experiment 1 (E12.5)	6	3	20	66%
Experiment 2 (E11.5)	5	2	3	57%
Experiment 3 (E11.5)	6	2	4	75%
Total	17	7	27	71%

The number of used explants and the penetration of phenotype is given. KO+, explants with reduced branching, KO−, explants showing similar numbers of branches as the wild type (WT) explants.

Canton of Bern and the Canton of Basel, Switzerland and the Swiss Federal Agency for Environment, Forest and Landscape.

Lung Organ Culture

Fetal mouse lungs were obtained at day E11.5 or E12.5 under sterile conditions and cultured as described previously (Schittny et al., 2000; Roth-Kleiner et al., 2004). Depending on the size of the lungs they were either explanted as entire lungs (E11.5) or their lobes were separated (E12.5) in sterile phosphate buffered saline (127 mM NaCl, 10 mM Na_2HPO_4, pH 7.4). In both cases, the explants were cultured individually at the air-culture medium interface on a floating filter (TSTP Isopore filter, 13 mm diameter, 3 μm pore size; Millipore, Bedford, MA, United States) in a 24 well plate (Falcon-Becton Dickinson, Lincoln Park, NJ, United States) at 37°C in 5% CO_2/air. Lungs obtained at E11.5 were explanted undissected. The medium, Dulbecco's modified eagle medium(GibcoBRL-Life Technologies, Basel, Switzerland), was enriched with 10% fetal calf serum (GibcoBRL), 5 μg/ml bovine insulin (Sigma Chemicals Company, St. Louis, MO, United States), 2 mM glutamine (Sigma), 75 μg/ml Streptomycin (Sigma), and 100 μg/ml Penicillin (Sigma). Three explants were transferred onto each filter and the filters were placed in a well containing 350 μl medium. The distance between the three explants was large enough to ensure the tissues did not touch during growth. The explants were fed daily by adding 200 μl of fresh medium per well. Images of the explants were taken twice daily using an inverted microscope (Diaphot-TMD, Nikon, Tokyo, Japan).

Quantitative Evaluations of Organ Cultures

As a measure for branching, the number of terminal endbuds was counted on micrographs as shown in **Figure 1**. The growth (volume%) was estimated by area measurement of the projected organ pieces by point counting. The growth was calculated by dividing the measured area by the area of the explant at the start of the experiment and multiplying this result by 100. We may take these numbers as an estimation of the volume percentage of the growth, because the quotient of the diameter and the thickness of an individual explant was constant, especially as compared between different explants at one time point, but also between explants at different time points (Schittny et al., 2000; Roth-Kleiner et al., 2004). The α8-deficient lung explants were grouped according to their difference to WT explants. If after 48 h in culture the difference between α8-deficient and WT explants was less than 15%, the explants were defined as α8-deficient explants without phenotype (KO−) all other α8-deficient explants were defined as showing a phenotype (KO+).

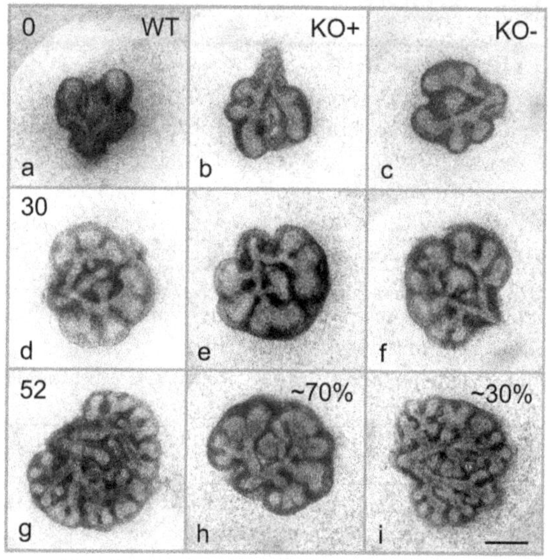

FIGURE 1 | Effects of α8 deficiency on branching morphogenesis. Representative micrographs of lung organ culture from WT and α8 deficient (KO) lung explants. Images were taken at the start of the organ culture E11.5 (**a–c**, time 0), 30 (**d–f**), and 52 h (**g–i**) after the start of the organ culture. Note that 70% of KO lungs present a phenotype (KO+) and 30% are comparable with WT (KO−). Scale bar, 0.5 mm.

Morphology

Lungs were prepared as previously published (Luyet et al., 2002; Mund et al., 2008; Tschanz et al., 2014). Briefly, at postnatal days P4, P7, P10, and P90 the pulmonary blood vessels of five animals per group and day were perfused with phosphate buffered saline (PBS = 10 mM sodium phosphate, containing 127 mM sodium chloride, pH 7.4), containing 5 units/ml heparin, 10 mg/ml procaine and 10 mM EDTA (Fluka Chemie AG, Buchs, Switzerland), and the air space filled with PBS, containing 4% freshly prepared paraformaldehyde (Merck, Darmstadt, Germany) at a constant pressure of 20 cm water column. At this pressure, the lung reaches roughly its total lung capacity (TLC). In order to prevent a recoiling of the lung, the pressure was maintained during fixation of 1 h. After fixation, the five lobes were separated and their volumes were measured by water displacement (Scherle, 1970). The total lung volume was calculated from the five lobar volumes. The specific lung volume was defined as lung volume over body weight (Weibel, 1970). Lungs were embedded in paraffin (Histosec, Merck, Darmstadt, Germany) at 60°C after three washes in PBS, followed by a graded series of ethanol and by three changes of Histoclear (Life Science International, Frankfurt, Germany). Under all conditions no recoil of the lungs was observed. A total of 3.5–5 μm sections were cut, transferred onto silanized (aminopropyl-trimethoxy-silane) micro slides, air dried over night at 37°C, dewaxed in Histoclear and stained with hematoxylin-eosin.

Stereology

Stereological measurements were done as previously published by our group (Mund et al., 2008; Schittny et al., 2008; Tschanz et al., 2014) and in compliance with standards for quantitative assessment of lung structure of the American Thoracic Society and the European Respiratory Society (Hsia et al., 2010). Briefly, 40–50 images per animal were taken at a magnification of ×250 on 10–12 sections of its left lung. Sampling of the sections and the images were done according to a systematic random sampling scheme (Cruz-Orive and Weibel, 1981). The sections were taken at equal distances to each other covering the entire length of the lung. The start of this series of sections was determent randomly. Five left lungs per day and group were analyzed. It was shown that the left lung represents a valid sample for the entire lung (Zeltner et al., 1990; Barre et al., 2016). The volume of the five lobes was measured by water displacement (Scherle, 1970) (see above). Volume densities were estimated by point counting. The lung parenchyma was defined as airspaces and septal tissue, excluding bronchi, bronchioli, and blood vessels >20 μm in diameter. Intersection counting was used to estimate the septal (alveolar) surface area density. The length density of the free septal edges was estimated by counting the number of cut free septal edges (tips of the cut septa) in a reference area on 2D paraffin sections. The total length of the free septal edge represents the total length of all alveolar entrance rings. (Mund et al., 2008; Schittny et al., 2008; Roth-Kleiner et al., 2014; Mund and Schittny, 2020). The totals of the parenchymal volume, the septal surface area, and the length of the free septal edge were calculated by multiplying their densities by the total parenchymal lung volume (Weibel, 1984; Howard and Reed, 2005). All calculations were done separately for each animal and each time point. In order to calculate the extent of newly formed alveolar septa, the length density was mathematically corrected for its change due to the growth of the volume of the lung parenchyma. An enlargement of the lung without the addition of new septa will lead to a decrease of the length density of the free edges by a factor of $\sqrt[3]{(V_x/V_0)^2}$ (where V_x represents the parenchymal lung volume at the time point X and V_0 the volume at the start of the growth). We use this correction because volume increases by a factor of x^3 and length only by a factor of x^1. We corrected the stereologically estimated length densities for its decrease due to isometric growth of the lung parenchyma by multiplying by the factor of $\sqrt[3]{(V_x/V_0)^2}$ (thereby V_0 was set to the mean value of the parenchymal lung volume at postnatal day 4). During isometric growth of the lung the resulting "growth corrected length density" remains constant and shows an increase or a decrease, if new septa are formed or if septa are degraded, respectively. We calculated the formation of new alveolar septa during lung development and compared it between controls and α8-deficient mice by following the increase of the "growth corrected length densities" between postnatal days 4 and 90. In Tschanz et al. (2014) we discuss the method described above in more details and compared the number of alveoli with the length of the free septal edge throughout lung development.

Statistical Analysis

Statistical analysis was done using 2-way ANOVA and Bonferroni post-test. Significance was defined as $P < 0.05$ and "highly significant" as $P < 0.001$ (Altman, 1991). Microsoft Excel (Office 2010, Microsoft Corporation, Redmond, WA, United States) and Prism (version 5.04, GraphPad Software Inc.) were used to calculate the statistics.

RESULTS

Integrin α8-Deficiency Reduces Branching Morphogenesis

To assess the role of the integrin α8 subunit during branching morphogenesis, we collect explants from wild type (WT) and α8 deficient mice (KO) at embryonic day E11.5–E12.5 and cultured them for up to 3 days (**Table 1**). Explants were imaged twice a day (**Figure 1**). Day E11.5 (embryonic stage) represented the earliest day, where we could start the lung organ culture. We included day E12.5 (pseudoglandular stage) in order to extend the time interval of observation. We did not observe any significant difference between days E11.5 and E12.5 (data of E12.5 not shown).

At time 0, WT and KO explants appeared comparable (**Figures 1a–c**). After 30 h of organ culture most, but not all of the KO explants showed a small reduction of branches as compared to WT explants (**Figures 1d–f**). A marked reduction of airway branching was evident in KO explants after 43 h of organ culture (**Figures 1g–i**, shown for 52 h). The deficiency, as verified by quantification, consists of diverse defects in branching and bud formation. Interestingly, only ~70% of the KO explants (**Figure 1h**) showed a pronounced phenotype (KO+) with reduced branching, the remaining ~30% (**Figure 1i**) showed the same number of branches (KO−) as WT (**Figure 1g**). New branching formation was quantified for each explant at different time points and significant differences were detected between WT and KO+ explants after 43 h of lung culture. No difference was observed between WT and KO− (**Figure 2A**). In addition, we asked whether α8 deficiency has a direct effect on the lung growth. Lung size was estimated by measuring the area of the projected organ at indicated time points and statistical differences were observed between WT and KO+ groups especially after 24, 42, and 54 h of organ culture (**Figure 2B**). These data suggest that loss of integrin α8β1 alters not only the branching morphogenesis but also the overall growth of the lung explant.

Integrin α8-Deficiency Shows Altered Branching Patterns

Experiments were performed to evaluate whether the lack of α8 integrin affects branching pattern during pulmonary development. Lungs from WT and KO obtained at E11.5–E12.5 were cultured and imaged at different time points (**Figure 3**). All WT lungs showed a normal pattern of branching over time (**Figure 3a**). Deficiency of α8, regardless of the penetrance of the phenotype caused an altered branching pattern (**Figures 3b–d**). Abnormal branching patterns were observed inside the lobes and

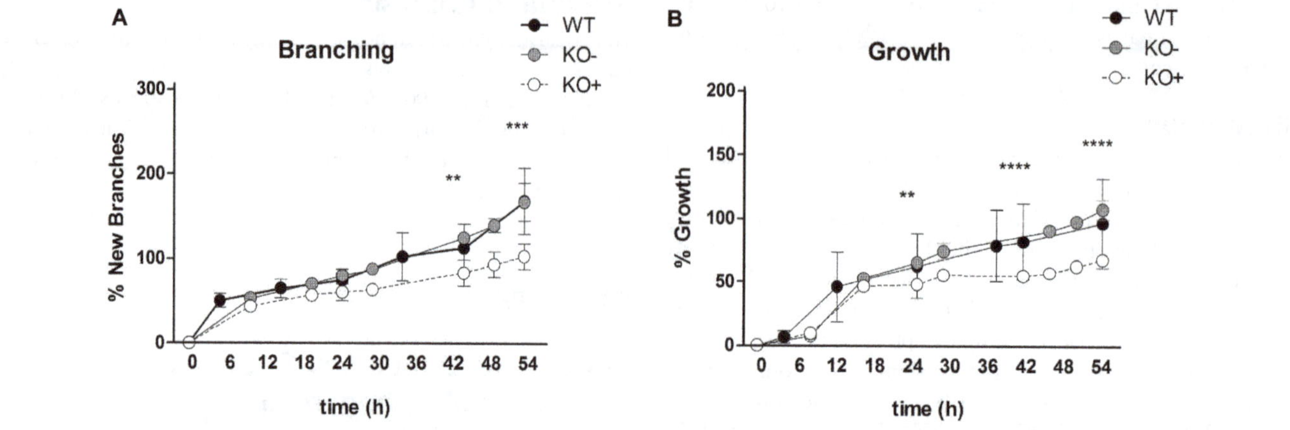

FIGURE 2 | Quantification of new branch formation and lung growth. The percentage of new branching was assessed by counting the terminal endbuds at indicated time points from E11.5 explants **(A)**. The percentage of the lung growth was estimated by measuring the area of the projected organ by point counting **(B)**. The lung explants were clustered into three groups: wild type (black, WT), α8 deficient explants without phenotype (gray circles, KO−), α8 deficient explants with phenotype (open circles, KO+). Data were analyzed by 2-way ANOVA and Bonferroni post-test, $^{**}P = 0.01$, $^{***}P = 0.001$, and $^{****}P = 0.0001$.

interestingly, none of the fives lobes was more affected than the others (**Figures 3b–d** irregularities are encircle).

Integrin α8-Deficiency Affects Lung Spontaneous Contraction and Bud Morphology

It is known that contractions of the future airways contribute to a normal airway differentiation and branching (Schittny et al., 2000) and α8β1 is expressed in contractile interstitial cells (CICs) (Levine et al., 2000). To determine whether the lack of α8 affects this ability to contract, we analyzed and counted the number of contractions per minutes after 53 and 73 h in culture of E11.5 and E12.5 explants (**Figure 4A**). We found that contractions increased with time in WT and KO independently of the presence of the phenotype. Interestingly KO showed a significantly higher frequency of contractions after 73 h of organ culture. Furthermore, we studied whether the size of terminal endbuds was affected by α8-deficiency. Photographs taken at the day of explant (0) and after 24, 43, and 52 h in culture were quantified (**Figure 4B**). The size of endbuds was similar between WT and KO−, but interestingly KO+ showed larger endbuds than WT.

Anatomical Differences Between WT and α8 Deficient Mice

The pulmonary phenotype of α8-deficient mice is characterized by a fusion of the medial and caudal lobe, as a consequence of mesenchymal and mesothelial cell anomalies and defective saccular airway branching (Benjamin et al., 2009). We found the same phenotype as Benjamin et al. (Benjamin et al., 2009) (**Figure 5A**) in the KO lungs where fusion is evident when compared to WT (**Figure 5B**). In addition, WT lungs clearly presented a fissure, which was completely missing in KO lungs (**Figures 5C,D**).

Integrin α8 Deficiency Induces Prominent Formation of New Septa With a Consequent Rescue of the Phenotype

We asked whether the phenotype observed in KO organ cultures could lead to a characteristic phenotype postnatally (**Figures 6, 7**). We investigated the impact of α8 integrin deficiency during alveolarization. Lung sections were compared between WT and KO littermates at postnatal day 4, 7, 10, and

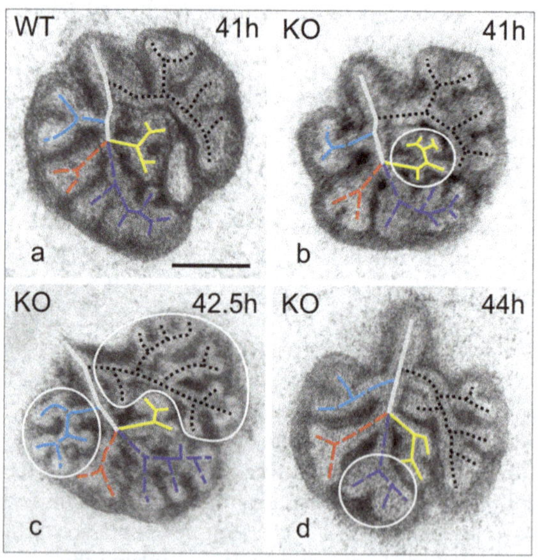

FIGURE 3 | Map of branching patterns in WT and α8KO explant cultures of E11.5 lungs. Representative WT lung **(a)**. KO lungs regardless of the phenotype (KO+ or KO−) 41–44 h after the explant **(b–d)**. Irregularities are encircled. Black dotted line indicates branching in the left lung; in blue, cranial lobe of right lung; in red, middle lobe; purple caudal lobe; yellow, accessory lobe. Bar 0.5 mm.

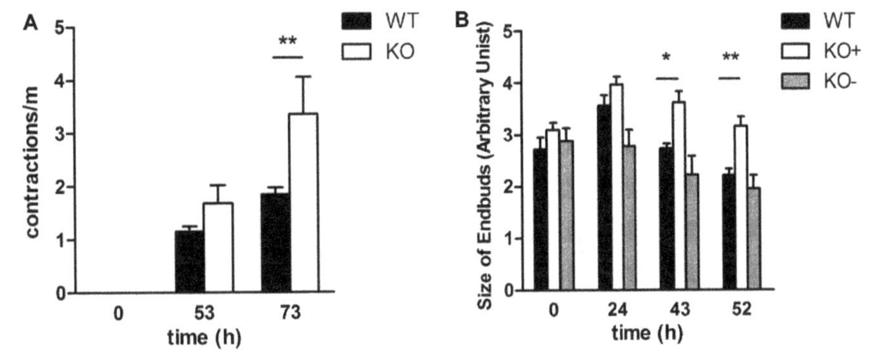

FIGURE 4 | Spontaneous contractions and size of terminal buds in E11.5 explant cultures over time. **(A)**. Contractions were measured in WT and KO explants at starting point E11.5 and after 53 and 73 h of organ culture **(B)** The size of the endbuds was determined by measuring projected surface area at the start of the culture of WT, KO−, KO+ E11.5 (time 0) explants, as well as after 24, 43, and 52 h of cultivation. Data were analyzed by 2-way ANOVA and Bonferroni post-test, $^{*}P = 0.05$ and $^{**}P = 0.01$

90. Absolute lung volume and total surface area was significantly reduced in KO lungs as compared to age-matched WT at postnatal day 4 (P4) (**Figures 6A,B**).

During the phase of alveolarization, the increase of structural complexity of the lung parenchyma may be view from two different points of view: we look either to the formation of new alveoli or to the formation of new alveolar septa. Both parameters are well suited to study postnatal rodent lung development (for a comparison see Schittny et al., 2008; Tschanz et al., 2014). We focused on the formation of new alveolar septa and estimated the total length of the free septal edge. This parameter represent the total length of all septa, measured at their upper free (not connected to anything) edge. In a first approximation, it is equal to the total length of the alveolar entrance rings. A significant reduction of this parameter was detected in KO lungs at P4 and P7 (**Figure 6C**). Interestingly, we found that the phenotype observed at an early stage, P4, did not persist until adulthood (P90): lung volume, total surface area and total length of free septal edge were comparable between WT and KO lungs (**Figures 6A–C**). These findings may be explained by the results of the stereological estimations showing that a significantly larger amount of new septa is formed in KO animals as compared to WT between postnatal days P4 and P90 (**Figure 6D**). In all KO lungs we observed the same postnatal phenotype and rescue. Therefore, postnatally the penetration of the phenotype was complete.

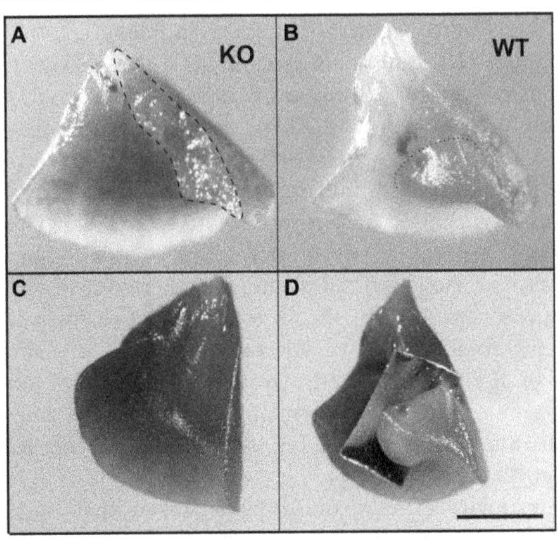

FIGURE 5 | Anomalous lung lobation in KO young adult as compared to WT. **(A)** Caudal lobe from KO lung with incomplete separation between the middle and the caudal lobe of the right lung. **(B)** Caudal lobe from WT. **(C)** KO caudal lobe from KO with incomplete or missing fissure **(C)** which is present in WT lungs (**D**, an aluminum foil demonstrates where the fissure is running). Dashed line represents area of incomplete separation **(A)**; dotted line indicates fissure in WT **(B)**. Scale bar is 2 mm.

DISCUSSION

Phenotypes and Its Penetration

In the present study, we demonstrate that integrin α8β1 is essential for the proper development of the lung and its absence causes many defects during prenatal and postnatal development. During prenatal lung development of α8 KO mice, defects include reduced and irregular branching morphogenesis, a higher frequency of spontaneous contractions of the future airways and anomalous lobation. However, in the α8 KO animals, we observed only ~70% of penetrance of the prenatal branching phenotype. Similar results were found previously (Muller et al., 1997) in the kidney of α8 KO mice, which are born with different kidney phenotypes. The presence of variable phenotypes is partially explain as a consequence of the two genetic background (129 and C57Bl/6) present in those mice. It is possible that the presence or the absence of genetic modifier locus controls specifics phenotypes. We assume that not only the two genetic backgrounds modulate the penetrance but also a compensatory effect by other integrins during the different steps in lung development. Based on kidney studies it has been hypothesized that α5 and αV could compensate the function of α8, but it was not the case due to the

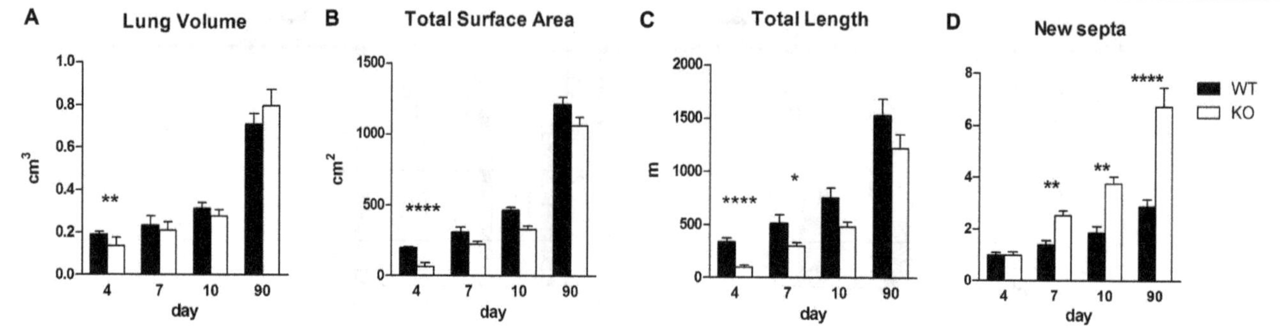

FIGURE 6 | Stereological measurements in WT and KO postnatal lungs. Stereological analysis of lung volume (cm^3) **(A)**, total surface area (cm^2) **(B)**, total length of the free septal edge (m) **(C)** and formation of new septa (expressed as multiples of the septa present at day 4) **(D)** in lungs of WT and KO mice at indicated time points. Data were analyzed by 2-way ANOVA and Bonferroni post-test, $^*P < 0.05$, $^{**}P < 0.01$, and $^{****}P < 0.0001$; N per group, 5.

negative results obtained (Haas et al., 2003). Moreover, collagens I and III were detected in the glomeruli of α8 KO mice leading to the assumption that compensation for α8 function could implicate interactions between collagens with collagen receptors. We speculate that similar mechanisms involved in the renal phenotypes are also responsible for the lung phenotype, which we observe.

During postnatal development, an increased formation of new septa was observed resulting in a nearly normal lung in adult KO mice (day 90). In opposite to the prenatal phenotype we observed a complete penetration of the postnatal phenotype. Previous studies (Wagner et al., 2003; Benjamin et al., 2009) have shown cellular function and spatiotemporal expression of α8β1 in the developing lung. However, the specific prenatal and postnatal defects, which were observed in this study, have not been described until now.

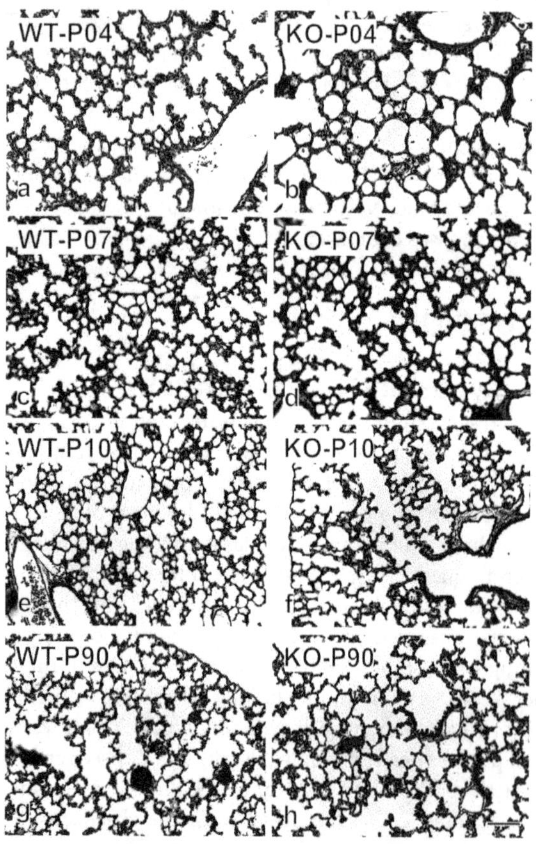

FIGURE 7 | Histological appearance of WT and KO lung throughout lung development. Examples of the original images used for the stereological estimations are shown on postnatal days 4 **(a,b)**, 7 **(c,d)**, 10 **(e,f)**, and 90 **(g,h)**. Already by eye, a significant difference is visible between WT and KO on P4. Later the difference disappears gradually. Bar, 100 μm.

Branching Morphogenesis

Branching morphogenesis is a complex phenomenon regulated by signaling factors that requires epithelial and mesenchymal interactions to form an epithelial bud (Iber and Menshykau, 2013). Only rare variations are seen in lungs of WT mice proving that branching is not random but a very well controlled mechanism (Metzger and Krasnow, 1999). We observed that α8 KO lungs with a phenotype (KO+) showed fewer branches and reduced growth compared to WT and KO without phenotype (KO−, **Figures 1, 2**) in lung organ cultures. In addition, all KO lung explants showed an irregularly altered branching pattern (**Figure 3**). Any culture system has it limits if it is compared to a live animal. However, the phenotype detected in lung organ culture was confirmed by the observation that at postnatal day 4 the lung volume, the total alveolar surface area, and the total length of the free septal edge were reduced in live animals. These results represent a confirmation, because at this time point alveolarization did not start yet (see section "Alveolarization" and **Figures 6A–C**).

Interestingly, former studies have shown that tenascin-c (TNC) represents a ligand for α8 integrin (Schnapp et al., 1995b). In addition, previous research in our laboratory (Roth-Kleiner et al., 2004) has demonstrated that TNC deficiency leads to a reduction of branching but showed normal overall growth of the explants and normal branching patterns in deficient mice. Branching and branching patterns are governed by a dynamic process of epithelial–mesenchymal interactions (Morrisey et al., 2013). Because tenascin-C as well as α8 integrin deficiency shows similar phenotypes, it may be concluded that both are involved in the epithelial–mesenchymal interactions during lung development. Typically α8 integrin and TNC-mRNA is expressed by mesenchymal cells, but the TNC-protein was found along the epithelial basement membranes (Zhao and Young, 1995). Therefore, we hypothesized that TNC signals to the epithelial and mesenchymal cells and influences their adherence to their substratum (Chiquet-Ehrismann and Tucker, 2011) and that α8 recognizes TNC (Schnapp et al., 1995b) and closes at least one loop of interactions.

Spontaneous Contractions of the Future Airways

During gestation, spontaneous contractions of the future airways have been described (Schittny et al., 2000). The responsible players of those contractions are airway smooth muscles. They contribute to normal lung development and fetal lung growth (Schittny et al., 2000). Murine and rat lung development studies have shown that primitive lung mesenchymal cells retain a generic capacity to differentiate into airway smooth muscle cells, and these cells follow the emergence of the definitive lung bud (Jesudason et al., 2005). In our study, we also noticed spontaneous contractions of the future airways in WT, KO−, and KO+. Independently from the phenotype, KO lungs showed a significantly increased number of contractions per minute (**Figure 4A**) and this correlates with an increase of the size of the endbuds (**Figure 4B**). We propose that absence of the α8 subunit could lead to signals, which activate myofibroblasts or reduce an inhibitor pathway with the result of faster contractions.

Alveolarization

Alveolarization is a complex process coordinated by multiple interactions between extracellular matrix, fibroblasts, epithelial cells, and microvasculature. Deficiencies in one of these elements have consequences on the entire alveolar development. Interestingly, at postnatal day 4, α8 deficient mice showed a significant reduction in lung volume compared with WT (**Figure 6**). Because at day 4, alveolarization did not yet start, this phenotype is exclusively caused by branching morphogenesis. However, at day 90 KO lungs were comparable to WT (**Figures 6, 7**). Therefore when mice are considered to be adults WT and KO do not show any significant difference. The same holds true for the total surface and total free septal length. The latter represents a measure for alveolarization. Based on morphological measurements we found that KO mice start with one fourth of length of the free septal edge at P4 (**Figure 6C**) and in order to become equal to WT, KO mice compensate with a massive input of new septa (**Figure 6D**). Therefore, the prenatal phenotype of the α8 deficient mice is rescued by an increased alveolarization during postnatal life.

It may be speculated about the size of the acini during the rescue of the α8-phenotype between days 4 and 90. It is likely that in the KO+ mice branching is as well reduces as the number of acini. Because the number of acini is most likely constant in postnatal mouse lung development (Barre et al., 2014, 2016), we hypothesize that KO+ mice possess a smaller number of acini which show a larger volume as compared to wildtype mice. A similar – at the end unanswered question – arise during compensatory growth after pneumonectomy: The remaining lung is able to regrow to its original size and alveolar surface (Hsia et al., 1994; Hsia and Johnson, 2006; Butler et al., 2012). If our data, that the number of acini stays constant after the saccular stage (Barre et al., 2016), are right, the only other known option will be to increase the size of the acini.

Tenascin-C is not only contributing to branching morphogenesis, but also to alveolarization. It involved in hyperoxia- (Olave et al., 2016) and steroid-induced (Roth-Kleiner et al., 2014) abnormal lung development. Furthermore, tenascin-C deficient mice show in both phases of alveolarization (classic and continued) a deceleration and acceleration of alveolarization (Mund et al., 2008; Mund and Schittny, 2020). Therefore, even if tenascin-C is a ligand of α8 integrins they exhibit different phenotypes during pulmonary alveolarization.

Conclusion

Taken together our results indicate that α8β1 integrin plays several roles in distinct phases of lung development. During prenatal lung development, regular spatio-temporal presence of α8β1 is essential for the normal pattern of branching. Most likely α8 has a direct effect on branching and on the branching pattern, but in addition an indirect effect by the alteration of the spontaneous contractions of the future airways. From these observations, we conclude that α8β1 is crucial for lung development at different time points even though the mechanism responsible for the rescue of the lung phenotype is still unknown. But the fact that a rescue takes place during alveolarization shows the enormous potential of the lung to correct early impairments of lung development. We assume that during the development chronic disease (such as emphysema, COPD and fibrosis) the lung is overwhelm by inflammation and activation of specific pathways, which do not consent the correction of septa loss.

Although numerous elements in the process of alveolarization have been determined, more studies are needed in order to clarify the complex interrelationships that are operative during normal lung development.

Our findings strongly suggest the necessity of further studies in order to determine how to improve the mechanism able to correct impairment in the lung and which is the point of no return when this mechanism is not anymore able to correct it. Switzerland and the Swiss Federal Agency for Environment, Forest and Landscape.

AUTHOR CONTRIBUTIONS

TC analyzed the data and drafted the manuscript. AH obtained the postnatal lungs and did the required breeding of the mice. JS conceived and designed the study, performed the lung organ cultures including the videotaping and analysis of the data. In addition, he did of parts of the breading of the mice, the stereological estimations of postnatal lung development including analysis of data, and contributed to writing. All authors contributed to the article and approved the submitted version.

ACKNOWLEDGMENTS

We thank Mrs. Marianne Hofstetter and Mrs. Bettina de Breuyn for expert technical assistance, and Ulrich Müller and Amanda Littlewood-Events for providing the mice for the study of the prenatal lung development.

REFERENCES

Altman, D. G. (1991). *Practical Statistics for Medical Research*. London: Chapman & Hall.

Arnaout, M. A., Mahalingam, B., and Xiong, J. P. (2005). Integrin structure, allostery, and bidirectional signaling. *Annu. Rev. Cell Dev. Biol.* 21, 381–410. doi: 10.1146/annurev.cellbio.21.090704.151217

Barre, S. F., Haberthur, D., Cremona, T. P., Stampanoni, M., and Schittny, J. C. (2016). The total number of acini remains constant throughout postnatal rat lung development. *Am. J. Physiol. Lung Cell Mol. Physiol.* 311, L1082–L1089.

Barre, S. F., Haberthur, D., Stampanoni, M., and Schittny, J. C. (2014). Efficient estimation of the total number of acini in adult rat lung. *Physiol. Rep.* 2:e12063. doi: 10.14814/phy2.12063

Benjamin, J. T., Gaston, D. C., Halloran, B. A., Schnapp, L. M., Zent, R., and Prince, L. S. (2009). The role of integrin alpha8beta1 in fetal lung morphogenesis and injury. *Dev. Biol.* 335, 407–417. doi: 10.1016/j.ydbio.2009.09.021

Brandenberger, R., Schmidt, A., Linton, J., Wang, D., Backus, C., Denda, S., et al. (2001). Identification and characterization of a novel extracellular matrix protein nephronectin that is associated with integrin alpha8beta1 in the embryonic kidney. *J. Cell Biol.* 154, 447–458. doi: 10.1083/jcb.200103069

Butler, J. P., Loring, S. H., Patz, S., Tsuda, A., Yablonskiy, D. A., and Mentzer, S. J. (2012). Evidence for adult lung growth in humans. *N. Engl. J. Med.* 367, 244–247. doi: 10.1056/nejmoa1203983

Chiquet-Ehrismann, R., and Tucker, R. P. (2011). Tenascins and the importance of adhesion modulation. *Cold Spring Harb. Perspect. Biol.* 3:a004960. doi: 10.1101/cshperspect.a004960

Coraux, C., Delplanque, A., Hinnrasky, J., Peault, B., Puchelle, E., and Gaillard, D. (1998). Distribution of integrins during human fetal lung development. *J. Histochem. Cytochem.* 46, 803–810. doi: 10.1177/002215549804600703

Cruz-Orive, L. M., and Weibel, E. R. (1981). Sampling designs for stereology. *J. Microsc.* 122, 235–257. doi: 10.1111/j.1365-2818.1981.tb01265.x

Haas, C. S., Amann, K., Schittny, J., Blaser, B., Muller, U., and Hartner, A. (2003). Glomerular and renal vascular structural changes in alpha8 Integrin-deficient mice. *J. Am. Soc. Nephrol.* 14, 2288–2296. doi: 10.1097/01.asn.0000082999.46030.fe

Howard, C. V., and Reed, M. G. (2005). *Unbiased Stereology. Three-Dimensional Measurement in Microscopy*. Abingdon: BIOS Scientific Publishers.

Hsia, C. C., Herazo, L. F., Fryder-Doffey, F., and Weibel, E. R. (1994). Compensatory lung growth occurs in adult dogs after right pneumonectomy. *J. Clin. Invest.* 94, 405–412. doi: 10.1172/jci117337

Hsia, C. C., Hyde, D. M., Ochs, M., Weibel, E. R., and Structure, A. E. (2010). An official research policy statement of the American thoracic society/european respiratory society: standards for quantitative assessment of lung structure. *Am. J. Respir. Crit. Care Med.* 181, 394–418. doi: 10.1164/rccm.200809-1522st

Hsia, C. C. W., and Johnson, R. L. (2006). Further examination of alveolar septal adaptation to left pneumonectomy in the adult lung. *Respir. Physiol. Neurobiol.* 151, 167–177. doi: 10.1016/j.resp.2006.01.013

Iber, D., and Menshykau, D. (2013). The control of branching morphogenesis. *Open Biol.* 3:130088.

Jesudason, E. C., Smith, N. P., Connell, M. G., Spiller, D. G., White, M. R., Fernig, D. G., et al. (2005). Developing rat lung has a sided pacemaker region for morphogenesis-related airway peristalsis. *Am. J. Respir. Cell Mol. Biol.* 32, 118–127. doi: 10.1165/rcmb.2004-0304oc

Levine, D., Rockey, D. C., Milner, T. A., Breuss, J. M., Fallon, J. T., and Schnapp, L. M. (2000). Expression of the integrin alpha8beta1 during pulmonary and hepatic fibrosis. *Am. J. Pathol.* 156, 1927–1935. doi: 10.1016/s0002-9440(10)65066-3

Littlewood, E. A., and Muller, U. (2000). Stereocilia defects in the sensory hair cells of the inner ear in mice deficient in integrin alpha8beta1. *Nat. Genet.* 24, 424–428. doi: 10.1038/74286

Luyet, C., Burri, P. H., and Schittny, J. C. (2002). Suppression of cell proliferation and programmed cell death by dexamethasone during postnatal lung development. *Am. J. Physiol. Lung Cell Mol. Physiol.* 282, L477–L483.

Metzger, R. J., and Krasnow, M. A. (1999). Genetic control of branching morphogenesis. *Science* 284, 1635–1639. doi: 10.1126/science.284.5420.1635

Morrisey, E. E., Cardoso, W. V., Lane, R. H., Rabinovitch, M., Abman, S. H., Ai, X., et al. (2013). Molecular determinants of lung development. *Ann. Am. Thorac. Soc.* 10, S12–S16.

Muller, U., Bossy, B., Venstrom, K., and Reichardt, L. F. (1995). Integrin alpha 8 beta 1 promotes attachment, cell spreading, and neurite outgrowth on fibronectin. *Mol. Biol. Cell* 6, 433–448. doi: 10.1091/mbc.6.4.433

Muller, U., Wang, D., Denda, S., Meneses, J. J., Pedersen, R. A., and Reichardt, L. F. (1997). Integrin alpha8beta1 is critically important for epithelial-mesenchymal interactions during kidney morphogenesis. *Cell* 88, 603–613. doi: 10.1016/s0092-8674(00)81903-0

Mund, S. I., and Schittny, J. C. (2020). Tenascin-C deficiency impairs alveolarization and microvascular maturation during postnatal lung development. *J. Appl. Physiol.* 128, 1287–1298. doi: 10.1152/japplphysiol.00258.2019

Mund, S. I., Stampanoni, M., and Schittny, J. C. (2008). Developmental alveolarization of the mouse lung. *Dev. Dyn.* 237, 2108–2116. doi: 10.1002/dvdy.21633

Olave, N., Lal, C. V., Halloran, B., Pandit, K., Cuna, A. C., Faye-Petersen, O. M., et al. (2016). Regulation of alveolar septation by microRNA-489. *Am. J. Physiol. Lung Cell Mol. Physiol.* 310, L476–L487.

Roth-Kleiner, M., Berger, T. M., Gremlich, S., Tschanz, S. A., Mund, S. I., Post, M., et al. (2014). Neonatal steroids induce a down-regulation of tenascin-C and elastin and cause a deceleration of the first phase and an acceleration of the second phase of lung alveolarization. *Histochem. Cell Biol.* 141, 75–84. doi: 10.1007/s00418-013-1132-7

Roth-Kleiner, M., Hirsch, E., and Schittny, J. C. (2004). Fetal lungs of tenascin-C-deficient mice grow well, but branch poorly in organ culture. *Am. J. Respir. Cell Mol. Biol.* 30, 360–366. doi: 10.1165/rcmb.2002-0266oc

Scherle, W. (1970). A simple method for volumetry of organs in quantitative stereology. *Mikroskopie* 26, 57–60.

Schittny, J. C. (2017). Development of the lung. *Cell Tissue Res.* 367, 427–444.

Schittny, J. C. (2018). How high resolution 3-dimensional imaging changes our understanding of postnatal lung development. *Histochem. Cell Biol.* 150, 677–691. doi: 10.1007/s00418-018-1749-7

Schittny, J. C., Miserocchi, G., and Sparrow, M. P. (2000). Spontaneous peristaltic airway contractions propel lung liquid through the bronchial tree of intact and fetal lung explants. *Am. J. Respir. Cell Mol. Biol.* 23, 11–18. doi: 10.1165/ajrcmb.23.1.3926

Schittny, J. C., Mund, S. I., and Stampanoni, M. (2008). Evidence and structural mechanism for late lung alveolarization. *Am. J. Physiol. Lung Cell Mol. Physiol.* 294, L246–L254.

Schnapp, L. M., Breuss, J. M., Ramos, D. M., Sheppard, D., and Pytela, R. (1995a). Sequence and tissue distribution of the human integrin alpha 8 subunit: a beta 1-associated alpha subunit expressed in smooth muscle cells. *J. Cell Sci.* 108, 537–544.

Schnapp, L. M., Hatch, N., Ramos, D. M., Klimanskaya, I. V., Sheppard, D., and Pytela, R. (1995b). The human integrin alpha 8 beta 1 functions as a receptor for tenascin, fibronectin, and vitronectin. *J. Biol. Chem.* 270, 23196–23202. doi: 10.1074/jbc.270.39.23196

Sheppard, D. (2003). Functions of pulmonary epithelial integrins: from development to disease. *Physiol. Rev.* 83, 673–686. doi: 10.1152/physrev.00033.2002

Streuli, C. (1999). Extracellular matrix remodelling and cellular differentiation. *Curr. Opin. Cell Biol.* 11, 634–640. doi: 10.1016/s0955-0674(99)00026-5

Tschanz, S. A., Salm, L. A., Roth-Kleiner, M., Barre, S. F., Burri, P. H., and Schittny, J. C. (2014). Rat lungs show a biphasic formation of new alveoli during postnatal development. *J. Appl. Physiol.* 117, 89–95. doi: 10.1152/japplphysiol.01355.2013

Wagner, T. E., Frevert, C. W., Herzog, E. L., and Schnapp, L. M. (2003). Expression of the integrin subunit alpha8 in murine lung development. *J. Histochem. Cytochem.* 51, 1307–1315. doi: 10.1177/002215540305101008

Weibel, E. R. (1970). Morphometric estimation of pulmonary diffusion capacity. I. Model and method. *Respir. Physiol.* 11, 54–75. doi: 10.1016/0034-5687(70)90102-7

Weibel, E. R. (1984). "Morphometric and stereological methods in respiratory physiology including fixation techniques," in *Techniques in Respiratory Physiology Part I*, ed. A. B. Otis (Amsterdam: Elsevier Scientific Publishers), 1–35.

Woods, J. C., and Schittny, J. C. (2016). "Lung structure at preterm and term birth," in *Fetal Lung Development - Clinical Correlates & Future Technologies*, eds A. H. Jobe, J. A. Whitsett, and S. H. Abman (New York, NY: Cambridge University Press), 126–140. doi: 10.1017/cbo9781139680349.008

Zeltner, T. B., Bertacchini, M., Messerli, A., and Burri, P. H. (1990). Morphometric estimation of regional differences in the rat lung. *Exp. Lung Res.* 16, 145–158. doi: 10.3109/01902149009087879

Zhao, Y., and Young, S. L. (1995). Tenascin in rat lung development: in situ localization and cellular sources. *Am. J. Physiol.* 269, L482–L491.

8

Quantifying Regional Lung Deformation Using Four-Dimensional Computed Tomography: A Comparison of Conventional and Oscillatory Ventilation

Jacob Herrmann[1,2,3], Sarah E. Gerard[1], Wei Shao[4], Monica L. Hawley[3], Joseph M. Reinhardt[1,5], Gary E. Christensen[4,6], Eric A. Hoffman[1,5,7] and David W. Kaczka[1,2,3,5]*

[1] Roy J. Carver Department of Biomedical Engineering, University of Iowa, Iowa City, IA, United States, [2] Department of Anesthesia, University of Iowa, Iowa City, IA, United States, [3] OscillaVent, Inc., Iowa City, IA, United States, [4] Department of Electrical and Computer Engineering, University of Iowa, Iowa City, IA, United States, [5] Department of Radiology, University of Iowa, Iowa City, IA, United States, [6] Department of Radiation Oncology, University of Iowa, Iowa City, IA, United States, [7] Department of Internal Medicine, University of Iowa, Iowa City, IA, United States

***Correspondence:**
David W. Kaczka
david-kaczka@uiowa.edu*

Mechanical ventilation strategies that reduce the heterogeneity of regional lung stress and strain may reduce the risk of ventilator-induced lung injury (VILI). In this study, we used registration of four-dimensional computed tomographic (4DCT) images to assess regional lung aeration and deformation in 10 pigs under baseline conditions and following acute lung injury induced with oleic acid. CT images were obtained via dynamic axial imaging (Siemens SOMATOM Force) during conventional pressure-controlled mechanical ventilation (CMV), as well as high-frequency and multi-frequency oscillatory ventilation modalities (HFOV and MFOV, respectively). Our results demonstrate that oscillatory modalities reduce intratidal strain throughout the lung in comparison to conventional ventilation, as well as the spatial gradients of dynamic strain along the dorsal-ventral axis. Harmonic distortion of parenchymal deformation was observed during HFOV with a single discrete sinusoid delivered at the airway opening, suggesting inherent mechanical nonlinearity of the lung tissues. MFOV may therefore provide improved lung-protective ventilation by reducing strain magnitudes and spatial gradients of strain compared to either CMV or HFOV.

Keywords: mechanical ventilation, ventilator-induced lung injury, respiratory mechanics, high-frequency oscillatory ventilation, multi-frequency oscillatory ventilation, computed tomography, image registration

INTRODUCTION

Ventilator-induced lung injury (VILI) may inadvertently occur in critically ill patients receiving mechanical ventilation, due to the harmful stresses and strains associated with gas flows driven under positive pressure (Slutsky and Ranieri, 2013). Patients with injured, inflamed, and/or edematous lungs, such as those with the acute respiratory distress syndrome (ARDS), are especially at risk for VILI due to increased ventilation heterogeneity (Carrasco Loza et al., 2015). Maintaining normal levels of arterial oxygen and carbon dioxide tensions in patients with ARDS may be extremely difficult using conventional mechanical ventilation (CMV), since increasing the tidal volume or driving pressure to compensate for gas exchange deficiencies may be detrimental to the mechanically over-burdened lung (Acute Respiratory Distress Syndrome Network, 2000; Amato et al., 2015; Gattinoni et al., 2016a). The goal of lung-protective ventilation is to provide life-sustaining gas exchange without exacerbating existing injury within vulnerable parenchymal tissues.

In some instances, high-frequency oscillatory ventilation (HFOV) has been proposed as a rescue treatment for refractory hypoxemia in ARDS, given its theoretically ideal qualities for lung-protection: small tidal volumes that mitigate the risk of dynamic strain injury (i.e., volutrauma), and high mean airway pressures that prevent cyclic recruitment/derecruitment (i.e., atelectrauma) (Sklar et al., 2017). Despite an extensive history of scientific and clinical research over several decades, optimal strategies for HFOV initiation and management remain a subject of controversy (Malhotra and Drazen, 2013; Kneyber and Markhorst, 2016; Nguyen et al., 2016). As it is currently delivered, HFOV may not be an appropriate ventilatory modality in many patients with ARDS for several reasons. First, the use of high mean airway pressures may result in hemodynamic compromise due to impaired venous return and low cardiac output (Meade et al., 2017). In addition, high strain rates within the lung tissues during HFOV may also contribute to VILI, by increasing the mechanical power dissipated across the parenchyma (Gattinoni et al., 2016b; Protti et al., 2016; Herrmann et al., 2019b). Finally, high frequency oscillatory flows are distributed in a heterogeneous and frequency-dependent manner, predisposing overventilated regions to excess mechanical strain, and underventilated regions to derecruitment and atelectasis (Amini and Kaczka, 2013; Herrmann et al., 2016).

Multi-frequency oscillatory ventilation (MFOV) has thus also been proposed as an alternative modality for lung-protective ventilation, by delivering multiple frequencies of oscillatory flow and pressure simultaneously (Kaczka et al., 2015; Herrmann et al., 2019b). MFOV has been shown to improve gas exchange and mechanical function compared to traditional "single-frequency" HFOV (Kaczka et al., 2015; Herrmann et al., 2018). Its postulated mechanism of benefit relies on the frequency-dependence of ventilation distribution and gas transport during conventional and oscillatory modes of ventilation (Herrmann et al., 2018), which can be exploited by using flow waveforms with enhanced harmonic content. Given such frequency-dependence of gas flow throughout the airway tree, mechanically disparate regions of an injured lung may thus selectively filter out "less desirable" frequency components of a broadband oscillatory waveform delivered at the airway opening. The corresponding homogenization of intrapulmonary gas transport with MFOV may then contribute to enhanced gas exchange, and simultaneously distribute the mechanical burden of ventilation more uniformly throughout the lung. Nonetheless, specific experimental evidence to support such a mechanism is lacking, and it remains to be seen whether MFOV improves the regional distribution of parenchymal strain throughout the lung compared to CMV or traditional HFOV.

The purpose of this study was to characterize the distribution of regional intratidal lung deformation during conventional and oscillatory modes of ventilation in pigs under baseline conditions and following acute lung injury with oleic acid. We hypothesized that such variations would be less heterogeneous during MFOV, compared to CMV or traditional single-frequency HFOV. Specifically, we quantified intratidal variations in dynamic regional lung aeration, volumetric strain, and volumetric strain rate during CMV, HFOV, and MFOV using frequency-selective four-dimensional computed tomographic (4DCT) image reconstruction (Herrmann et al., 2017) and registration (Zhao et al., 2016).

MATERIALS AND METHODS

Animal Preparation

All experimental procedures were approved by the University of Iowa Institute for Animal Care and Use Committee (Protocol Number 5061428). Ten healthy pigs were used in this study, weighing between 9 and 13 kg. Following intramuscular injection of 2.2 mg kg^{-1} telazol, 1.1 mg kg^{-1} ketamine, and 1.1 mg kg^{-1} xylazine, general anesthesia was induced during spontaneous breathing with inhaled isoflurane delivered via nosecone. Each pig was then intubated with a cuffed endotracheal tube (4.5–5.5 mm inner diameter), and mechanically ventilated (Uni-Vent Eagle Model 754, ZOLL Medical Corporation, Chelmsford, MA). Capnography, peripheral oxygen saturation (S_pO_2), and electrocardiogram waveforms were obtained using a Philips patient monitor equipped with the M3001A measurement module (Philips Healthcare, Andover, MA). Surgical incision into the neck was performed to allow cannulation of the internal jugular vein and carotid artery, as well as relocation of the endotracheal tube into an incision in the trachea just below the larynx. Endotracheal tubes were manually shortened (to final length 12–15 cm depending on tube diameter) prior to tracheostomy, to reduce apparatus deadspace. Anesthesia was maintained using an intravenous infusion of propofol (7–9 mg kg^{-1} hr^{-1}), and muscular relaxation was achieved using intermittent intravenous boluses of either rocuronium (1–2 mg kg^{-1}) or pancuronium (0.01–0.15 mg kg^{-1}).

Lung injury was induced by slow infusion of 0.08 cm^3 kg^{-1} oleic acid into the internal jugular vein over 15 min. Maturation of injury required ~90 min, and was confirmed by a ratio of arterial oxygen tension to inspired oxygen fraction ($P_aO_2 : F_iO_2$) <300 mmHg during ventilation with 5 cmH$_2$O of positive end-expiratory pressure (PEEP). Additional oleic acid (0.04 cm^3 kg^{-1}) was administered if $P_aO_2 : F_iO_2$ remained >300 mmHg 90 min after the initial dose. If necessary, normal systemic arterial blood pressure (systolic/diastolic $\geq$ 90/60 mmHg) was maintained with intravenous crystalloid solutions and intermittent doses of phenylephrine (1–2 μg kg^{-1}).

Experimental Protocol

All measurements and ventilation modalities were performed under baseline conditions and following lung injury. Each subject was mechanically ventilated with CMV, HFOV, and MFOV in random order over 30-min intervals, using a FabianHFO hybrid oscillator/ventilator (Acutronic Medical Systems AG, Switzerland). Mean airway pressure ($\overline{P}_{aw}$) was set to 12 cmH_2O for all modalities. During baseline conditions, F_iO_2 was set to 40%, but was increased to maintain $S_pO_2 \geq 90\%$ following lung injury. Pressure-controlled CMV was delivered at rates between 20 and 32 min^{-1} (0.33 to 0.53 Hz), with inspiratory:expiratory ratio of 1:2. Single-frequency HFOV was delivered at 5 Hz, while MFOV was delivered using a combination of 5, 10, 15, and 20 Hz superimposed sinusoids with uniform flow amplitudes (Kaczka et al., 2015). Example ventilator waveforms are provided in **Supplementary Figures S-1, S-2, S-3**. Sampling frequency for recorded ventilator waveforms was 200 Hz. Ventilator driving pressure or pressure amplitudes were adjusted to obtain arterial CO_2 tension (P_aCO_2) in the target range of 30–60 mmHg. Each 30-min experimental interval was followed by an arterial blood gas analysis and 4DCT scan sequence, without interrupting mechanical ventilation (Herrmann et al., 2017). Between each experimental ventilation interval, a 15-min wash-out period of CMV and a 30-s recruitment maneuver to 35 cmH_2O of airway pressure were used to restore a control mechanical and physiological state. After completion of the experimental protocol, subjects were euthanized with an intravenous solution of pentobarbital sodium and phenytoin sodium (1 mL + 0.2 mL kg^{-1}).

Assessment of Gas Exchange and Mechanics

Oxygenation was assessed using the oxygenation index (OI), defined as (Ortiz et al., 1987):

$$OI = \frac{\overline{P}_{aw} \cdot F_iO_2}{P_aO_2} \tag{1}$$

The efficiency of CO_2 elimination during each modality was assessed using a ventilatory cost function (V_C), defined as (Kaczka et al., 2015):

$$V_C = \frac{V_{rms}^2 \cdot P_aCO_2}{Wt} \tag{2}$$

where V_{rms} is the root mean-square of the volume waveform $V(t)$ delivered to the airway opening:

$$V_{rms} = \sqrt{\frac{1}{T}\int_0^T \left[V(t) - \overline{V}\right]^2 dt}. \tag{3}$$

T denotes the time duration over which the integration in Equation (3) is performed (i.e., one breath for CMV or one second during HFOV/MFOV), and $\overline{V}$ is the mean of the volume waveform over the interval 0 to T.[1] Peak-to-peak range of volume (V_{pp}) was computed as the difference between the largest and smallest values of time-varying volume:

$$V_{pp} = \max_t V(t) - \min_t V(t). \tag{4}$$

[1]The use of V_{rms} enables comparison between single-frequency modalities, which are typically described by a single tidal volume, and MFOV, which is described by a distinct volume amplitude at each frequency (Kaczka et al., 2015).

Dynamic respiratory system elastance (E_{rs}) during pressure-controlled CMV was computed as the quotient of driving pressure (ΔP_{aw}) and tidal volume:

$$E_{rs} = \Delta P_{aw} \cdot V_{pp}^{-1} \tag{5}$$

where:

$$\Delta P_{aw} = \max_t P_{aw}(t) - \min_t P_{aw}(t). \tag{6}$$

Measurements of respiratory impedance (Z_{rs}) were obtained under baseline conditions and after maturation of lung injury. A pseudorandom waveform consisting of nine sinusoids ranging in frequency from 0.078 to 8.9 Hz was generated by a digital-to-analog converter (NI USB-6356, National Instruments, Austin, TX), low-pass filtered at 12 Hz (858L8B-2, Frequency Devices, Haverhill, MA), and used as the input driving signal to a custom servo-controlled pneumatic pressure oscillator (Kaczka and Lutchen, 2004). Airway pressure was measured with a transducer placed at the proximal end of the endotracheal tube (Celesco LCVR-0050, Canoga Park, CA), while flow was measured using a screen pneumotach (4700A, Hans Rudolph, Shawnee, KS) coupled to a differential pressure transducer (Celesco LCVR-0002, Canoga Park, CA). The airway pressure and flow signals were sampled at 40 Hz over ~90 s during the application of forced oscillations, allowing for three repetitions of the 25.6-s periodic control signal. Each Z_{rs} spectrum and its corresponding coherence function (γ^2) was computed using the Welch periodogram technique (Welch, 1967), with rectangular windowing and 80% overlap. The complex values of Z_{rs} were evaluated only at the nine frequencies used in the control signal (Suki and Lutchen, 1992). Corresponding resistance R_{rs} and reactance X_{rs} spectra were defined by the real and imaginary parts of Z_{rs}, respectively. The resonant frequency f_{res} was estimated from the zero-crossing of X_{rs} using spline interpolation. Each Z_{rs} spectrum was then characterized by a 4-element constant-phase model consisting of parameters for Newtonian airway and chest wall resistance (R), airway inertance (I_{aw}), tissue hysteresivity (η), and tissue elastance (H):

$$\hat{Z}_{rs}(f) = R + j2\pi f I_{aw} + \frac{(\eta - j)H}{(2\pi f)^{\alpha}} \tag{7}$$

where $\hat{Z}_{rs}$ denotes the model-predicted Z_{rs} and $\alpha = \left(\frac{2}{\pi}\right)\tan^{-1}\left(\frac{1}{\eta}\right)$. Model parameters were estimated by constrained nonlinear gradient descent technique (MATLAB, Natick, MA).

Image Acquisition and Processing

CT scans were acquired using a Siemens SOMATOM Force (Siemens Healthineers, Germany) in an axial scanning mode, with 5.76 cm of axial coverage and 0.6 mm slice thickness. Subjects were continuously scanned at 80 kVp tube voltage and 150 mA tube current, with 250 ms scanner rotation period. Each scan lasted a total duration of 30 s, resulting in a radiation exposure of 345 mGy and generating a continuous set of projection images. The 4DCT image sequences were

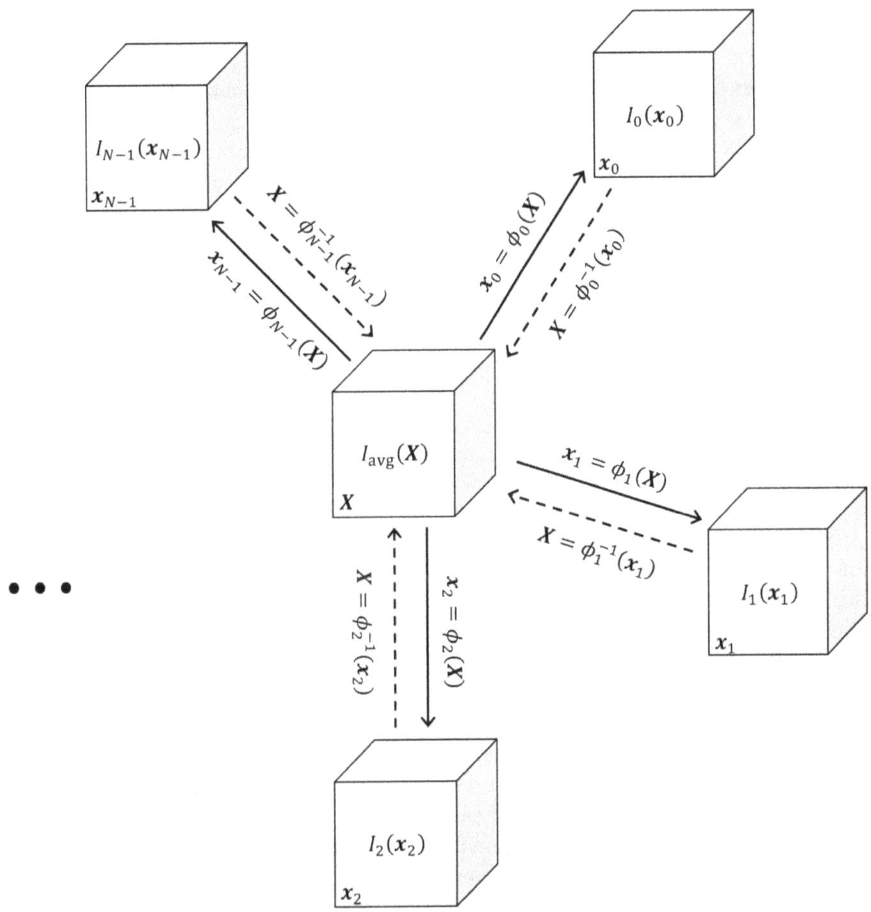

FIGURE 1 | Schematic illustrating the jointly estimated 3D transformations $\phi_n(\mathbf{X}) = \mathbf{x}_n$ mapping between all images in the periodic 4DCT image sequence $I_n(\mathbf{x}_n)$ and the target average image $I_{avg}(\mathbf{X})$. Solid black arrows indicate the transformation from the target reference frame $\mathbf{X}$ to the general reference frame $\mathbf{x}_n$. Dashed black arrows indicate the inverse transformation. Gray arrows represent the periodic sequence of N ventilatory phases indexed from 0 to $N-1$. Any $I_n(\mathbf{x}_n)$ may be deformed to achieve structural alignment with any other $I_m(\mathbf{x}_m)$ by applying a sequence of two transformations $\mathbf{x}_n = \phi_n(\phi_m^{-1}(\mathbf{x}_m))$, warping $\mathbf{x}_m$ through $\mathbf{X}$.

reconstructed by retrospective binning of x-ray projection data according to mechanical ventilation phase using a frequency-selective reconstruction algorithm (Herrmann et al., 2017), yielding between 13 and 21 volumetric images per 4DCT sequence with isotropic 0.6 mm spatial resolution. The corresponding temporal sampling frequencies for 21-phase image sequences were 7 Hz during CMV with fundamental 0.33 Hz, and 105 Hz during HFOV or MFOV with fundamental 5 Hz. Each sequence was periodic in the temporal (i.e., ventilation phase) dimension, such that the choice of "initial" image in the sequence was arbitrary. Each volumetric image in the temporal sequence was labeled $I_n(\mathbf{x}_n)$, where n indexes the number of images in the sequence 0 through $N-1$, and $\mathbf{x}_n$ is a vector representing 3-dimensional spatial position. Voxels corresponding to spatial positions within the lungs were identified by a fully automated segmentation algorithm using a deep convolutional neural network (Gerard et al., 2018, 2020), generating a distinct lung mask $M_n(\mathbf{x}_n)$ for each image phase. The neural network was trained using manually segmented lungs in CT images obtained from multiple datasets of experimental lung injury models, including a subset of images from the current study.

The periodic motion of respiratory structures was estimated using a deformable 4D image registration technique. This procedure produced N 3-dimensional transformation functions denoted as $\phi_n(\mathbf{X}) = \mathbf{x}_n$, where $\mathbf{X}$ is a vector representing 3-dimensional spatial position within the reference frame of a phase-averaged image $I_{avg}(\mathbf{X})$, and $\mathbf{x}_n$ represents spatial position in image $I_n(\mathbf{x}_n)$. Image $I_{avg}(\mathbf{X})$ was used as the target for groupwise image registration of the images $I_n(\mathbf{x}_n)$, $n = 0 \ldots N-1$. Thus, $\phi_n(\mathbf{X}) = \mathbf{x}_n$ is a spatial mapping from the coordinate system of $I_{avg}(\mathbf{X})$ to that of $I_n(\mathbf{x}_n)$, such that a deformed image $I_{n\rightarrow avg}(\mathbf{X})$ was generated with respiratory structures aligned to the target image as:

$$I_{n\rightarrow avg}(\mathbf{X}) = I_n(\phi_n(\mathbf{X})) \tag{8}$$

Figure 1 shows a schematic of the transformations mapping between all images in the periodic sequence and $I_{avg}(\mathbf{X})$.

The transformations $\phi_n(\mathbf{X})$ were coupled together using 4-dimensional cubic B-splines and jointly estimated to ensure smoothness across both spatial and temporal dimensions (Metz et al., 2011). The parameters of the transformation function were iteratively adjusted using the Elastix library (Klein et al., 2010) to minimize the sum of squared tissue volume differences (SSTVD) between each $I_{n\to\text{avg}}(\mathbf{X})$ and $I_{\text{avg}}(\mathbf{X})$, such that each deformed image preserved the volume of tissue contained within each voxel (Gorbunova et al., 2008; Yin et al., 2009; Zhao et al., 2016). Thus, changes in CT voxel density due to variations in fractional gas content were adjusted using this similarity cost function. Following registration, $\phi_n(\mathbf{X})$ and its inverse mapping $\phi_n^{-1}(\mathbf{x}_n)$ were used to align images between arbitrary phases. Deformed images were denoted as $I_{n\to m}(\mathbf{x}_m)$, indicating the nth image deformed into the mth spatial reference frame:

$$I_{n\to m}(\mathbf{x}_m) = I_n\left(\phi_n\left(\phi_m^{-1}(\mathbf{x}_m)\right)\right) \tag{9}$$

For the trivial case of $m = n$, Equation (9) simplifies to $I_{n\to n}(\mathbf{x}_n) = I_n(\mathbf{x}_n)$. Conceptually, aligning images from any two phases can be achieved by warping one spatial reference frame to another, passing through the target reference frame $\mathbf{X}$ (see **Figure 1**). Using this approach, all images were warped to align structures with a single, arbitrarily selected reference phase at $m = 0$. Phasic variations in regional aeration and strain could then be associated with the tissue contained within the region of interest at the reference phase. **Figure 2** schematizes the use of a single reference phase to align respiratory structures across several ventilatory phases, thus tracking tissue-correlated changes in aeration and regional volume. Changes in regional aeration were then assessed by the range of voxel intensity values in the deformed image:

$$\Delta I(\mathbf{x}_0) = \max_n I_{n\to 0}(\mathbf{x}_0) - \min_n I_{n\to 0}(\mathbf{x}_0) \tag{10}$$

while changes in regional volumetric strain were estimated using the Jacobian matrix ($\mathcal{J}_{n\to m}$) of transformation spatial derivatives:

$$\mathcal{J}_{n\to m}(\mathbf{x}_m) = \nabla_{\mathbf{x}_m}\left(\phi_n\left(\phi_m^{-1}(\mathbf{x}_m)\right)\right) \tag{11}$$

where $\nabla_{\mathbf{x}_m}$ is the spatial gradient operator. Note that $\mathcal{J}_{n\to m}$ is expressed in the mth spatial reference frame and describes the gradient of the "pullback" transformation $\phi_n\left(\phi_m^{-1}(\mathbf{x}_m)\right)$. This pullback transformation is interpreted as "pulling back" point $\mathbf{x}_n$ in ventilation phase n to the corresponding point $\mathbf{x}_m$ in phase m. Regional volume changes relative to the reference phase (i.e., $m = 0$) were computed by the determinant of $\mathcal{J}_{n\to m}$:

$$\frac{V_n(\mathbf{x}_0)}{V_0(\mathbf{x}_0)} = \left|\mathcal{J}_{n\to 0}(\mathbf{x}_0)\right| \tag{12}$$

where $V_n(\mathbf{x}_0)$ corresponds to the phase-varying volume of a region which, in the reference phase 0, occupies a single voxel centered at position $\mathbf{x}_0$. Accordingly, $V_0(\mathbf{x}_0)$ is everywhere equal to the volume of a single voxel δV, determined by the image spatial resolution. Thus, Equation (12) may be simplified to:

$$V_n(\mathbf{x}_0) = \delta V \cdot \left|\mathcal{J}_{n\to 0}(\mathbf{x}_0)\right| \tag{13}$$

Note that $|\mathcal{J}_{n\to 0}| < 1$ when the corresponding region deflates relative to the reference phase, $|\mathcal{J}_{n\to 0}| > 1$ when it expands, and $|\mathcal{J}_{n\to 0}| = 1$ when there is no volume change (i.e., isovolumetric deformation). **Figure 3** shows an example image sequence for each ventilation modality in one injured subject, demonstrating phase-varying aeration $I_{n\to 0}(\mathbf{x}_0)$ and volume change $V_n(\mathbf{x}_0)$ for each voxel in a sample region of interest in $\mathbf{x}_0$. Animated image sequences for one subject under baseline and injured conditions are also provided (**Supplementary Animations S-1, S-2**). Phase-varying strain (ε) for each lung region with respect to its respective minimum inflation state was defined as:

$$\varepsilon_n(\mathbf{x}_0) = \frac{V_n(\mathbf{x}_0) - \min_n V_n(\mathbf{x}_0)}{\min_n V_n(\mathbf{x}_0)} \tag{14}$$

Changes in regional volumetric strain were assessed by the range of $\varepsilon_n(\mathbf{x}_0)$:

$$\Delta\varepsilon(\mathbf{x}_0) = \max_n \varepsilon_n(\mathbf{x}_0) - \min_n \varepsilon_n(\mathbf{x}_0) \tag{15}$$

Since the minimum value of $\varepsilon_n(\mathbf{x}_0)$ is zero by definition, Equation (15) may be reduced to:

$$\Delta\varepsilon(\mathbf{x}_0) = \max_n \varepsilon_n(\mathbf{x}_0) \tag{16}$$

Similarly, regional volumetric strain rate ($\dot{\varepsilon}$) was computed by the temporal rate of change in $\varepsilon_n(\mathbf{x})$ using the forward difference scheme:

$$\dot{\varepsilon}_n(\mathbf{x}_0) = \frac{\varepsilon_{(n+1)\bmod N}(\mathbf{x}_0) - \varepsilon_n(\mathbf{x}_0)}{\delta t} \tag{17}$$

where δt is the time difference between adjacent phases. The modulo operator is used to indicate the periodicity of ventilatory phase. The value of δt is computed from the ventilatory fundamental frequency (f_0) and the number of images in the 4DCT sequence (N):

$$\delta t = \frac{1}{f_0 N} \tag{18}$$

Finally, changes in regional volumetric strain rate were assessed by the range of $\dot{\varepsilon}_n(\mathbf{x}_0)$:

$$\Delta\dot{\varepsilon}(\mathbf{x}_0) = \max_n \dot{\varepsilon}_n(\mathbf{x}_0) - \min_n \dot{\varepsilon}_n(\mathbf{x}_0) \tag{19}$$

Note that $\dot{\varepsilon}_n(\mathbf{x}_0)$ generally will be positive during inflation of a specified lung region, and negative during the corresponding deflation. Thus, $\Delta\dot{\varepsilon}(\mathbf{x}_0)$ will reflect the sum of the fastest inflation and deflation rates of the region.

Voxels within 6.0 mm of the image boundaries along the rostral-caudal axis were excluded from the mask for the purposes of image analysis, due to potential registration artifacts caused by motion of lung tissue into or out of the axial field of view. Regional aeration (ΔI), strain ($\Delta\varepsilon$), and strain rate ($\Delta\dot{\varepsilon}$) were compared across subjects, lung conditions, and ventilation modalities by their mean value throughout the lung mask,

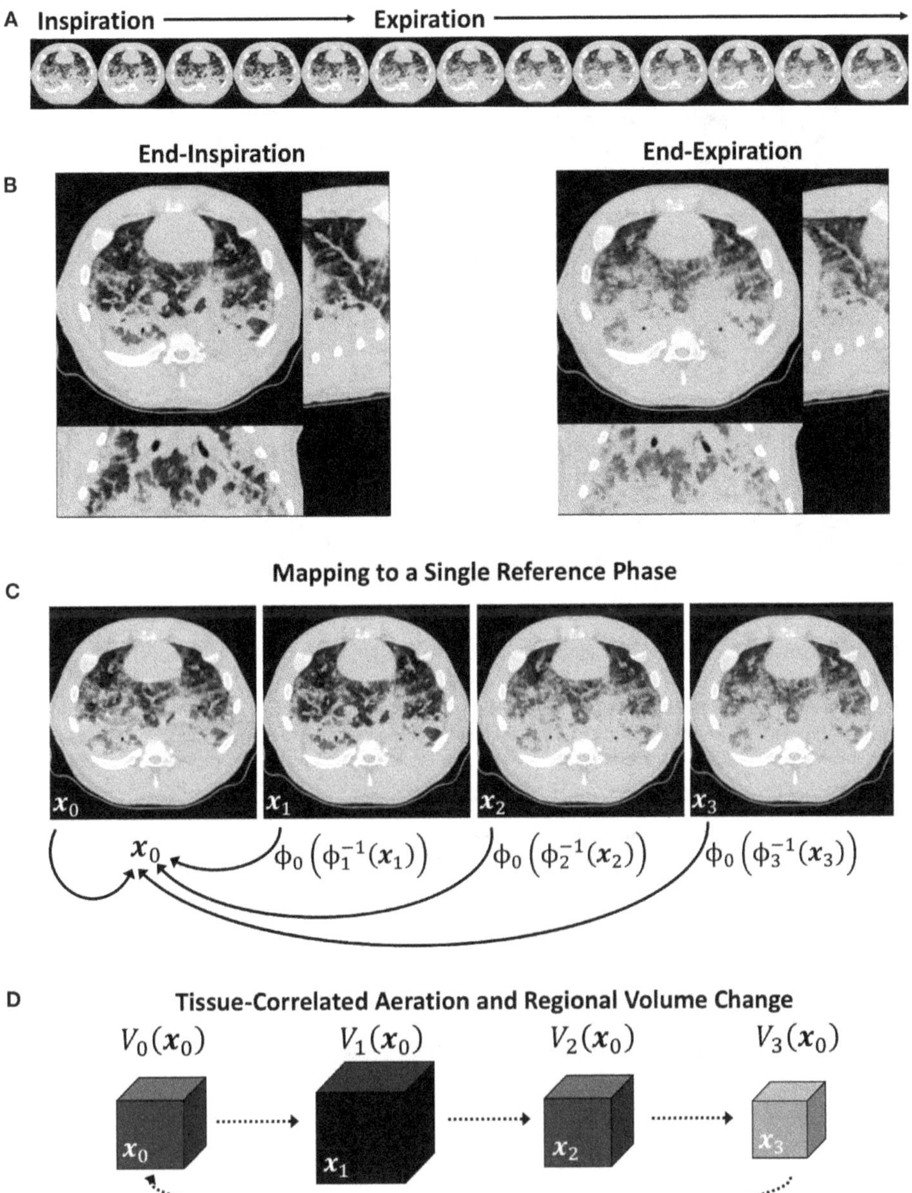

FIGURE 2 | Schematic of a periodic 4DCT image sequence during conventional mechanical ventilation **(A)**, with inspiratory and expiratory phases **(B)**. Image registration is used to map each image in the sequence to a single reference phase **(C)**, after which intratidal variations in aeration and regional volume may be associated to specific regions of lung tissue **(D)**.

coefficient of variation, and spatial gradients in the right-left, dorsal-ventral, and rostral-caudal directions. Spatial gradients for each variable were determined from the slopes computed by linear regression with respect to position along each of the principal anatomic axes. Spatial gradients were examined unnormalized and normalized by the spatial mean, in each case comparing both signed values of the gradient (i.e., positive and negative) and gradient magnitude (i.e., absolute value).

Given the harmonic nature of MFOV, the individual frequency components of I_n, ε_n, and $\dot{\varepsilon}_n$ were assessed using the Discrete Fourier Transform (DFT), to relate these periodic time-varying properties at each spatial position into harmonic amplitude and phase components. The regional heterogeneity of volumetric strain ($\Delta\varepsilon$) was assessed using octree and supervoxel decomposition, each of which recursively subdivide regions-of-interest (ROIs) within the lung mask. Both decomposition methods were initialized with a single ROI containing the entire lung mask. At each recursive step, the designated ROI was subdivided into multiple new ROIs if the standard deviation of the contained voxel intensity was greater than a fixed

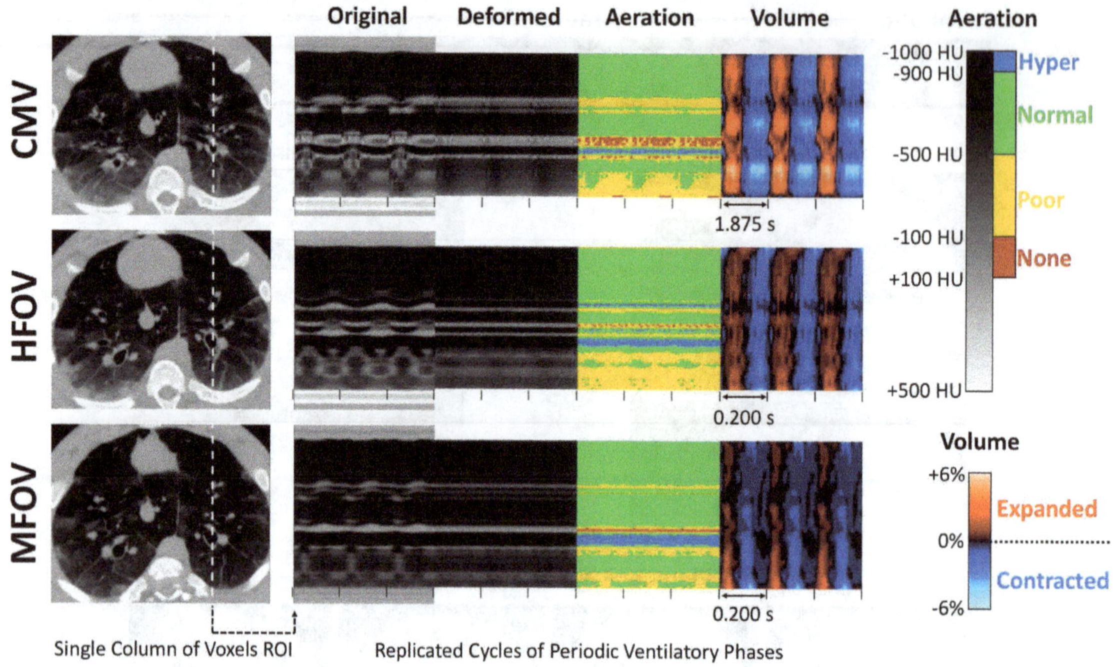

FIGURE 3 | Four-dimensional image registration was used to deform images such that respiratory structures were aligned to a single reference phase. After registration, regional aeration and volume change throughout the lung were assessed by the variations in deformed image voxel value and determinant of the Jacobian matrix of the deformation. This technique was applied during conventional mechanical ventilation (CMV), high-frequency oscillatory ventilation (HFOV), and multi-frequency oscillatory ventilation (MFOV). Ventilatory cycle duration is indicated by spacing between tick marks. In this example, each ventilatory cycle corresponds to a sequence of images representing 21 distinct ventilatory phases. Note that multiple cycles of each ventilation waveform are shown for clarity, however all cycles are identical replicates. See also **Supplementary Animations S-1, S-2**.

threshold, set to a standard deviation of mean-normalized $\Delta\varepsilon \geq 0.3$.[2] Octree decomposition, a three-dimensional extension of quadtree decomposition, was used to partition each ROI into eight octants according to bisecting coronal, sagittal, and transverse planes (Perchiazzi et al., 2014). Supervoxel decomposition was used to partition each ROI into two new ROIs by a weighted k-means clustering of voxels according to intensity similarity and spatial proximity (Conze et al., 2017). Recursive subdivision was continued until all ROIs either contained below-threshold values of standard deviation, or were <0.2% of the lung mask. Regional heterogeneity of $\Delta\varepsilon$ was then quantified by the mean ROI volume ($\overline{V}_{\text{ROI}}$) as a fraction of the lung mask.

Statistics

Non-parametric Kruskal-Wallis rank sum tests were performed for each outcome, testing for main effects of lung condition (i.e., baseline, injured) and ventilation modality (i.e., CMV, HFOV, MFOV) at the 0.05 significance level. The effect of ventilation modality was tested separately under baseline and injured conditions. For outcomes with a significant main effect of ventilation modality, differences among modalities were identified by a Dunn *post hoc* comparison with adjustment for rank ties and further adjustment by the Benjamini-Hochberg procedure for reduced false discovery rate. A web-based tool was used for statistical calculations (Vasavada, 2016).

RESULTS

Figure 4 shows a summary of the respiratory impedance spectra Z_{rs} across all subjects measured under baseline and injured conditions, while **Table 1** provides a summary of the constant phase model applied to Z_{rs}. Under baseline conditions, average model-based tissue elastance H was 121 $\text{cmH}_2\text{O L}^{-1}$ at 1 rad s^{-1} (0.16 Hz) with a coefficient of variation of 0.31. The increase in H after oleic acid injury was highly variable, resulting in a mean of 435 $\text{cmH}_2\text{O L}^{-1}$ at 1 rad s^{-1} with a coefficient of variation of 0.94. By comparison, measurement of dynamic elastance (E_{rs}) during CMV (Equation 5) was 148.9 ± 26.9 $\text{cmH}_2\text{O L}^{-1}$ and 257.5 ± 64.2 $\text{cmH}_2\text{O L}^{-1}$ under baseline and injured conditions, respectively. Resonant frequency (f_{res}) increased after lung injury, in some cases above the measurement range allowed by the sampling parameters. **Table 2** contains a summary of all significant effects identified by non-parametric Kruskal-Wallis tests, as well as *post hoc* comparisons as appropriate. These results are described further in the context of specific figures below.

[2]This threshold value was empirically chosen to be lower than the values of the regional strain coefficient of variation observed across all subjects, to ensure that the recursive subdivision would not be terminated trivially at the level of the entire lung mask, yet high enough to avoid termination at the level of individual voxels. The same threshold was used for all normalized images.

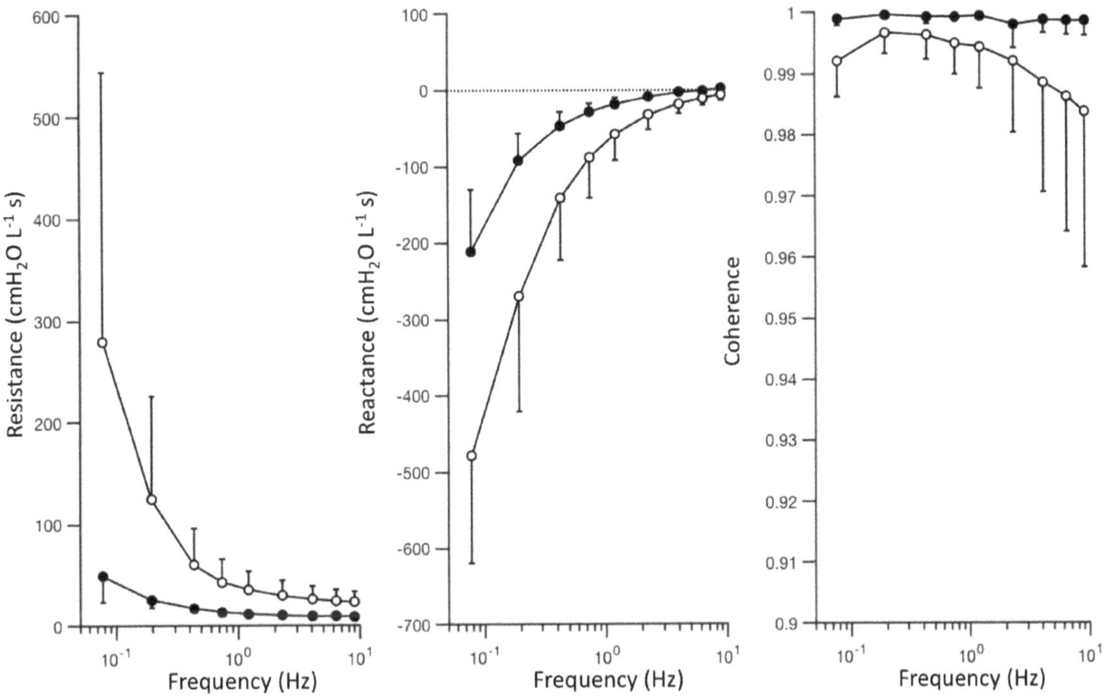

FIGURE 4 | Respiratory impedance measured under baseline (black) and injured (white) conditions, represented by the mean value (circles) and standard deviation (error bars) at each frequency, across subjects. The complex-valued impedance spectrum is represented by its real part or in-phase component (i.e., resistance), and its imaginary part or out-of-phase component (i.e., reactance). Coherence provides an estimate of signal quality and linearity of the measured relationship between pressure and flow oscillations.

TABLE 1 | Respiratory system mechanics.

Condition	$\bar{P}_{aw}$§	R	I_{aw}	η	H	f_{res}†	E_{rs}‡
Baseline	11.5 ± 0.8	8.9 ± 3.2	0.11 ± 0.03	0.17 ± 9.93	121 ± 38	6.7 ± 1.7	149 ± 27
Injured	12.6 ± 2.9	22.4 ± 13.5	0.13 ± 0.08	0.27 ± 0.04	435 ± 407	9.2 ± 1.3	258 ± 64

§$\bar{P}_{aw}$ during respiratory impedance measurements. †f_{res} interpolation was possible only for nine subjects under baseline conditions and five subjects under injured conditions, due to resonance in other cases occurring above the 12 Hz low-pass filter cutoff frequency. ‡E_{rs} measurements obtained during conventional mechanical ventilation by Equation (5). $\bar{P}_{aw}$, mean airway pressure (cmH_2O); R, Newtonian airway and chest wall resistance ($cmH_2O\ L^{-1}\ s$); I_{aw}, airway inertance ($cmH_2O\ L^{-1}\ s^2$); η, tissue hysteresivity; H, tissue elastance ($cmH_2O\ L^{-1}$ at 1 rad s^{-1}); f_{res}, resonant frequency (Hz); E_{rs}, dynamic respiratory system elastance ($cmH_2O\ L^{-1}$).

Figure 5 shows gas exchange outcomes related to mechanical ventilation, including oxygenation index ($OI = P_aO_2^{-1} \cdot F_iO_2 \cdot \overline{P}_{aw}$) and ventilatory cost function ($V_C = P_aCO_2 \cdot V_{rms}^2 \cdot Wt^{-1}$). A significant main effect of lung condition (baseline vs. injured) was found for P_aO_2, $P_aO_2 \cdot F_iO_2^{-1}$, OI, and P_aCO_2 ($p < 0.001$). A significant main effect of ventilation modality was found in ΔP_{aw}, $V_{pp} \cdot Wt^{-1}$, $V_{rms} \cdot Wt^{-1}$, and V_C ($p < 0.001$) for both lung conditions, as well as in OI for the injured condition ($p < 0.05$). In particular, median OI increased by 300% for injured subjects compared to baseline ($p < 0.001$), but was 48% lower for injured subjects during MFOV compared to CMV ($p < 0.05$). MFOV and HFOV were associated with lower median V_C for both baseline and injured conditions compared to CMV (HFOV 84% lower than CMV, $p < 0.01$; MFOV 93% lower than CMV, $p < 0.001$). Pairwise comparison of V_C for MFOV against HFOV also achieved a statistically significant difference, with 60% lower median V_C for MFOV compared to HFOV ($p < 0.05$). Median $V_{rms} \cdot Wt^{-1}$ was 41% lower for MFOV vs. HFOV ($p = 0.0505$ baseline; $p < 0.05$ injured) and 75% lower for MFOV vs. CMV ($p < 0.001$).

Figure 6 shows registration-based estimates of regional ventilation, as intratidal changes in voxel aeration (ΔI), volumetric strain ($\Delta\varepsilon$), and volumetric strain rate ($\Delta\dot{\varepsilon}$). A significant main effect of condition (baseline vs. injured) was found for ΔI spatial mean ($p < 0.001$), $\Delta\varepsilon$ coefficient of variation ($p < 0.001$) and $\Delta\dot{\varepsilon}$ coefficient of variation ($p < 0.01$). A significant main effect of ventilation modality was found for the spatial means of all three variables—ΔI, $\Delta\varepsilon$, and $\Delta\dot{\varepsilon}$–in both baseline and injured lung conditions ($p < 0.001$). In particular, MFOV and HFOV both produced smaller ΔI, smaller $\Delta\varepsilon$, and larger $\Delta\dot{\varepsilon}$ compared to CMV under baseline and injured conditions ($p < 0.05$). For the injured condition, MFOV resulted

TABLE 2 | Statistically significant effects determined by Kruskal-Wallis rank sum test for main effects of lung condition (i.e., baseline, injured) and ventilation modality (i.e., CMV, HFOV, MFOV).

		Baseline				**Injured**			
	Condition main effect	**Ventilation main effect**	**CMV vs. HFOV**	**CMV vs. MFOV**	**HFOV vs. MFOV**	**Ventilation main effect**	**CMV vs. HFOV**	**CMV vs. MFOV**	**HFOV vs. MFOV**
P_aO_2	♦♦♦								
$P_aO_2 \cdot F_iO_2^{-1}$	♦♦♦								
OI	♦♦♦					♦		♦	
P_aCO_2	♦♦♦								
ΔP_{aw}		♦♦♦	♦	♦♦♦	♦♦	♦♦♦	♦♦	♦♦♦	
$V_{pp} \cdot Wt^{-1}$		♦♦♦	♦♦	♦♦♦		♦♦♦	♦♦	♦♦♦	
$V_{rms} \cdot Wt^{-1}$		♦♦♦	♦♦	♦♦♦		♦♦♦	♦	♦♦♦	♦
V_C		♦♦♦	♦♦	♦♦♦	♦	♦♦♦	♦♦	♦♦♦	♦
ΔI Mean	♦♦♦	♦♦♦	♦♦	♦♦		♦♦♦	♦♦♦	♦♦♦	♦♦♦
ΔI Coef. Var.									
ΔI Right-Left		♦	♦						
ΔI Dorsal-Ventral		♦♦♦ ○○○	♦♦ ○	♦♦♦ ○○○					
ΔI Caudal-Rostral		♦♦♦ ○○○	♦♦♦ ○○○	♦♦♦ ○○○		♦♦ ○○○	♦♦ ○○	♦♦ ○○○	
$\|\Delta I\|$ Right-Left	♦♦♦ ○○○					♦		♦	
$\|\Delta I\|$ Dorsal-Ventral		♦♦♦ ○○	♦♦♦ ○○	♦♦♦ ○		♦♦ ○		♦♦ ○	
$\|\Delta I\|$ Caudal-Rostral						♦	♦	♦	
$\Delta\varepsilon$ Mean		♦♦♦	♦♦	♦♦♦		♦♦♦	♦	♦♦♦	♦
$\Delta\varepsilon$ Coef. Var.	♦♦♦								
$\Delta\varepsilon$ Right-Left	♦♦ ○○								
$\Delta\varepsilon$ Dorsal-Ventral	♦♦♦ ○○○	♦♦♦ ○		♦♦♦ ○	♦ ○				
$\Delta\varepsilon$ Caudal-Rostral	♦♦♦ ○○○	♦♦	♦♦	♦♦					
$\|\Delta\varepsilon\|$ Right-Left	♦ ○	♦	♦			♦		♦	
$\|\Delta\varepsilon\|$ Dorsal-Ventral		♦♦		♦♦		♦		♦	
$\|\Delta\varepsilon\|$ Caudal-Rostral		♦	♦	♦					
$\Delta\dot{\varepsilon}$ Mean		♦♦♦	♦♦♦	♦♦♦		♦♦♦	♦♦♦	●●	
$\Delta\dot{\varepsilon}$ Coef. Var.	♦♦								
$\Delta\dot{\varepsilon}$ Right-Left	♦ ○○								
$\Delta\dot{\varepsilon}$ Dorsal-Ventral	♦ ○	♦♦ ○○		♦♦ ○○	♦	♦	♦	♦	
$\Delta\dot{\varepsilon}$ Caudal-Rostral		♦ ○○○	♦ ○○	♦ ○○		♦ ○○		♦ ○○	
$\|\Delta\dot{\varepsilon}\|$ Right-Left		♦♦	♦♦	♦♦					
$\|\Delta\dot{\varepsilon}\|$ Dorsal-Ventral	♦	♦		♦	♦	♦	♦	♦	
$\|\Delta\dot{\varepsilon}\|$ Caudal-Rostral						♦		♦	
$\overline{V}_{ROI}$ Supervoxel									
$\overline{V}_{ROI}$ Octree	♦♦♦								

Post-hoc comparisons for ventilation modality performed using the Dunn method with Benjamini-Hochberg adjustment. (♦$p < 0.05$, ♦♦$p < 0.01$, ♦♦♦$p < 0.001$). Symbols distinguish unnormalized (♦) and mean-normalized (○) spatial gradients. P_aO_2, arterial oxygen tension; F_iO_2, fractional inspired oxygen; OI, oxygenation index; ΔP_{aw}, pressure amplitude; V_{pp}, peak-peak volume; Wt, body weight; V_{rms}, root-mean-square volume; V_C, ventilatory cost function; P_aCO_2, arterial carbon dioxide tension; ΔI, range of CT value; $\Delta\varepsilon$, range of volumetric strain; $\Delta\dot{\varepsilon}$, range of volumetric strain rate; $\overline{V}_{ROI}$, mean cluster volume; $|\cdots|$, absolute value of enclosed argument.

in significantly lower ΔI and $\Delta\varepsilon$ compared to HFOV ($p < 0.05$), but no difference for $\Delta\dot{\varepsilon}$ ($p = 0.20$).

Figure 7 shows unnormalized spatial gradients of ΔI, $\Delta\varepsilon$, and $\Delta\dot{\varepsilon}$ in the right-left, dorsal-ventral, and caudal-rostral axes. The largest spatial gradient magnitudes observed occurred along the dorsal-ventral axis. In particular, the injured lung condition was associated with significantly more positive dorsal-ventral gradients of $\Delta\varepsilon$ ($p < 0.001$) and $\Delta\dot{\varepsilon}$ ($p < 0.05$). Ventilation modality had a significant effect on all dorsal-ventral gradients under baseline conditions (ΔI, $p < 0.001$; $\Delta\varepsilon$, $p < 0.001$; $\Delta\dot{\varepsilon}$, $p < 0.01$), with MFOV producing the least negative dorsal-ventral gradients of ΔI and $\Delta\varepsilon$, but the most positive dorsal-ventral gradients of $\Delta\dot{\varepsilon}$. Although modality was not a significant predictor of variability in the actual value (positive or negative) of any dorsal-ventral gradient for injured subjects, it was a significant main effect for the *magnitudes* of all dorsal-ventral gradients (ΔI, $p < 0.001$; $\Delta\varepsilon$, $p < 0.01$; $\Delta\dot{\varepsilon}$, $p < 0.05$). In general HFOV and MFOV reduced the dorsal-ventral gradient magnitudes of ΔI and $\Delta\varepsilon$ under both baseline and injured conditions, while increasing the corresponding

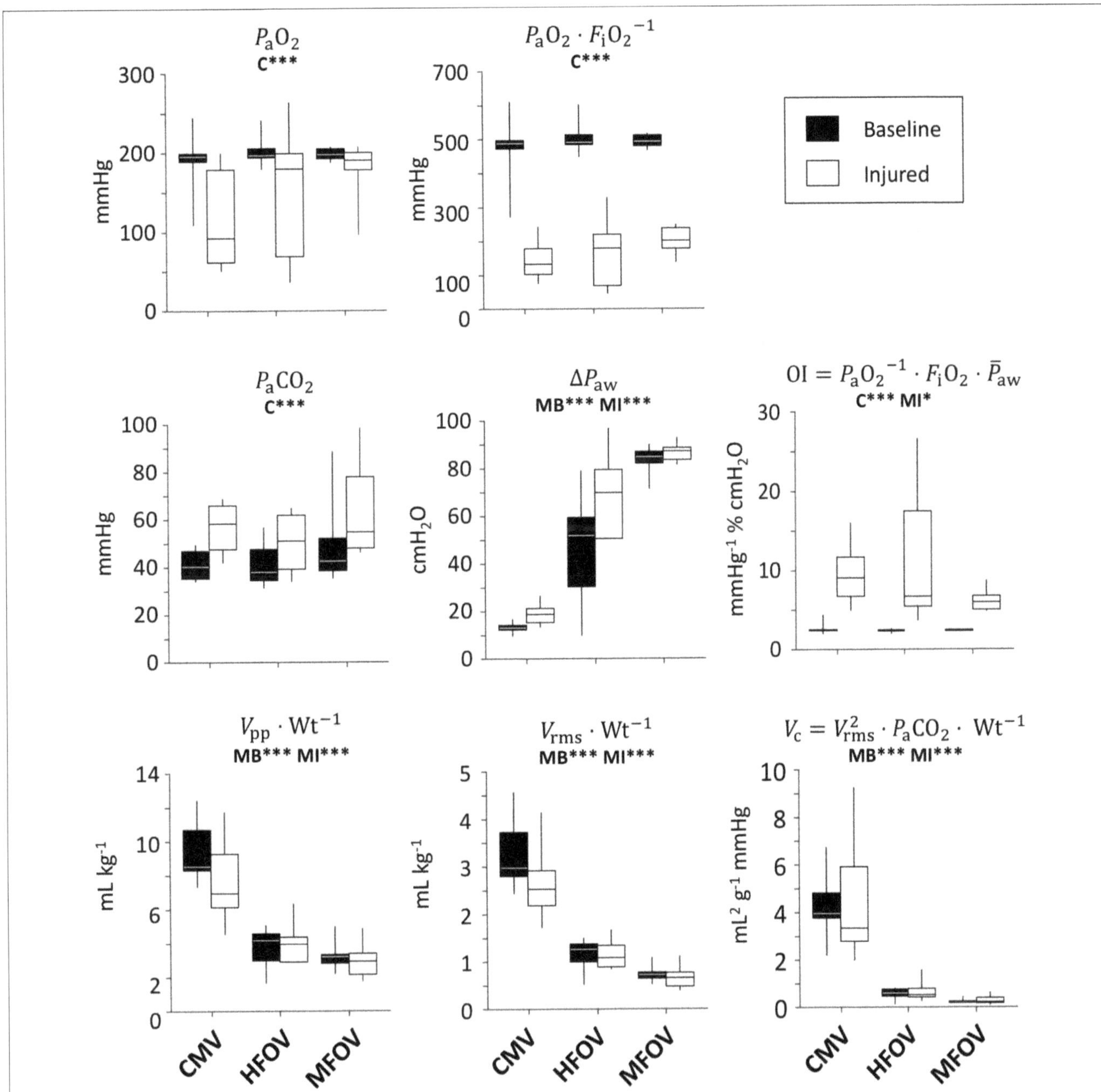

FIGURE 5 | Gas exchange outcomes, represented by box plots showing minimum, maximum, and quartiles across subjects under baseline (black) and injured (white) conditions, during conventional mechanical ventilation (CMV), high-frequency oscillatory ventilation (HFOV), and multi-frequency oscillatory ventilation (MFOV). Asterisks indicate significance levels (*$p < 0.05$, ***$p < 0.001$) for main effects (C = lung condition, MB = modality for baseline condition, MI = modality for injured condition). See **Table 2** for additional clarification. P_aO_2 = arterial oxygen tension; F_iO_2 = fractional inspired oxygen; P_aCO_2 = arterial carbon dioxide tension; ΔP_{aw} = airway pressure amplitude; V_{pp} = peak-to-peak volume range; Wt = body weight; V_{rms} = root-mean-square volume.

$\Delta\dot{\varepsilon}$ gradient. **Figure 8** shows corresponding mean-normalized spatial gradients. In general, normalizing each spatial gradients by the respective spatial mean accounted for much of the variability observed in the unnormalized spatial gradients (**Figure 7**) with respect to varying ventilation modality. This is also evidenced by the loss of significant differences between ventilation modalities for the corresponding spatial gradients as indicated in **Table 2**.

Figure 9 shows an example of regions-of-interest defined by recursive supervoxel and octree decomposition performed on mean-normalized $\Delta\varepsilon$ in one subject. Clustered regions are illustrated using contours and filled regions in two-dimensional

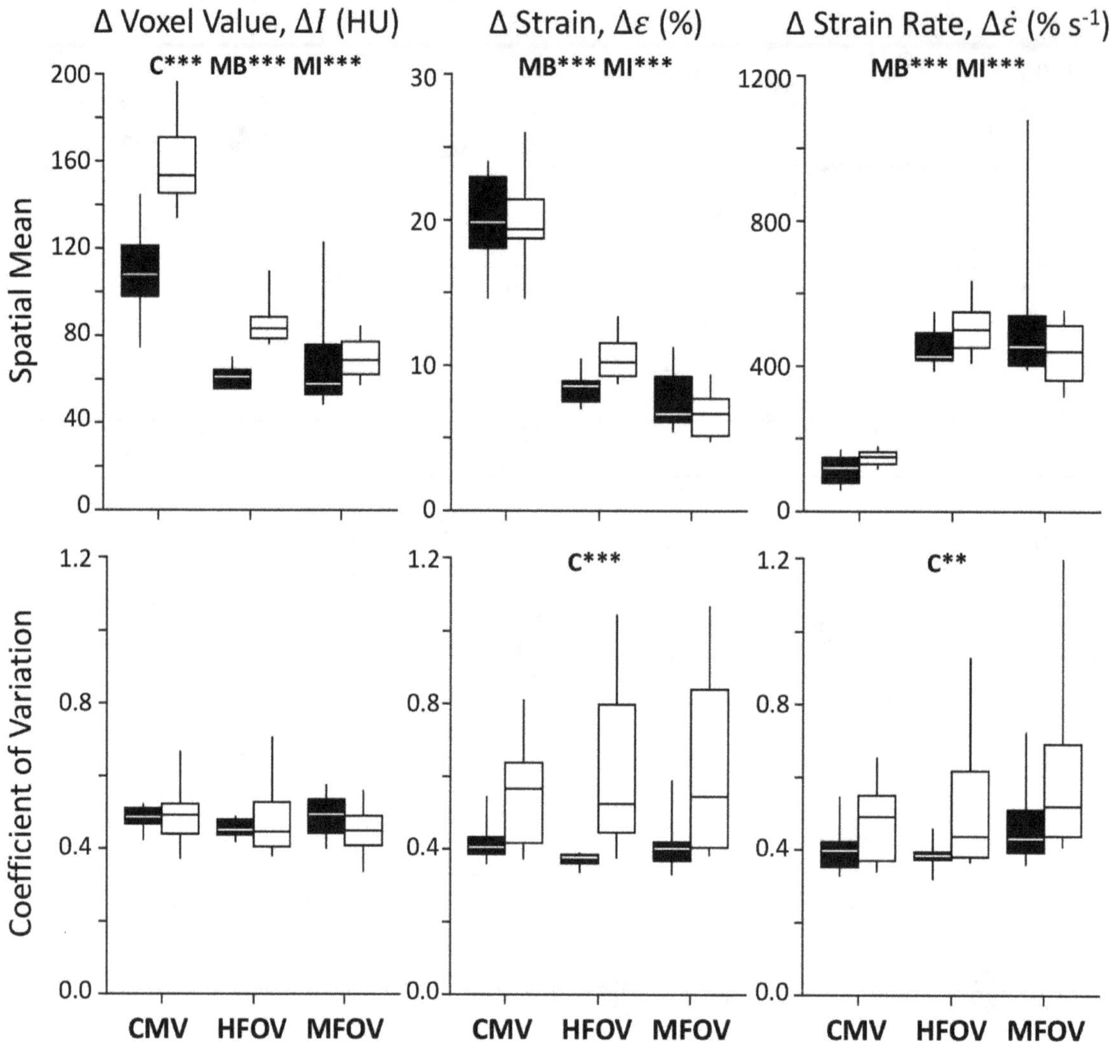

FIGURE 6 | Summary of image registration-based regional ventilation measures for intratidal changes in aeration (ΔI), volumetric strain ($\Delta\varepsilon$), and volumetric strain rate ($\Delta\dot{\varepsilon}$). Mean and coefficient of variation throughout the lung mask are shown for each variable, represented by box plots showing minimum, maximum, and quartiles across subjects under baseline (black) and injured (white) conditions, during conventional mechanical ventilation (CMV), high-frequency oscillatory ventilation (HFOV), and multi-frequency oscillatory ventilation (MFOV). Asterisks indicate significance levels ($^{**}p < 0.01$, $^{***}p < 0.001$) for main effects (C = lung condition, MB = modality for baseline condition, MI = modality for injured condition). See **Table 2** for additional clarification.

views of a slice, as well as translucent surface renderings in three-dimensional projections. Note that supervoxel decomposition produces larger contiguous ROIs, despite using the same decision criteria for recursive cluster subdivision. **Figure 9** also provides a summary of mean cluster size ($\overline{V}_{ROI}$) across subjects, condition, and ventilation modality. A significant effect of lung condition was found for the octree technique ($p < 0.001$), with 32% smaller median $\overline{V}_{ROI}$ in injured lungs.

Figure 10 shows example distributions of strain amplitude and phase at the first four harmonics for CMV, HFOV, or MFOV, computed using the discrete Fourier transform of time-varying Jacobian determinants in aligned images. **Figure 11** provides a summary of the harmonic strain amplitudes during HFOV and MFOV across all subjects, correlated with corresponding amplitudes of the ventilator volume waveform $V(t)$. The oscillatory waveforms were a 5 Hz sinusoid (HFOV) and a combination of 5, 10, 15, and 20 Hz sinusoids with uniform flow amplitudes (MFOV). The relative amplitude distributions in the flow waveforms delivered by the ventilator were largely preserved throughout the lung, according to the registration-based metrics ($r^2 = 0.78$). However, harmonic distortion measurements during HFOV indicated nearly 20% of the spectral power in regional strain was concentrated in the higher-order harmonics of the 5 Hz waveform (i.e., 10, 15, 20 Hz), whereas the ventilator volume waveform exhibited only 5% harmonic distortion (Zhang et al., 1995; Amini et al., 2017).

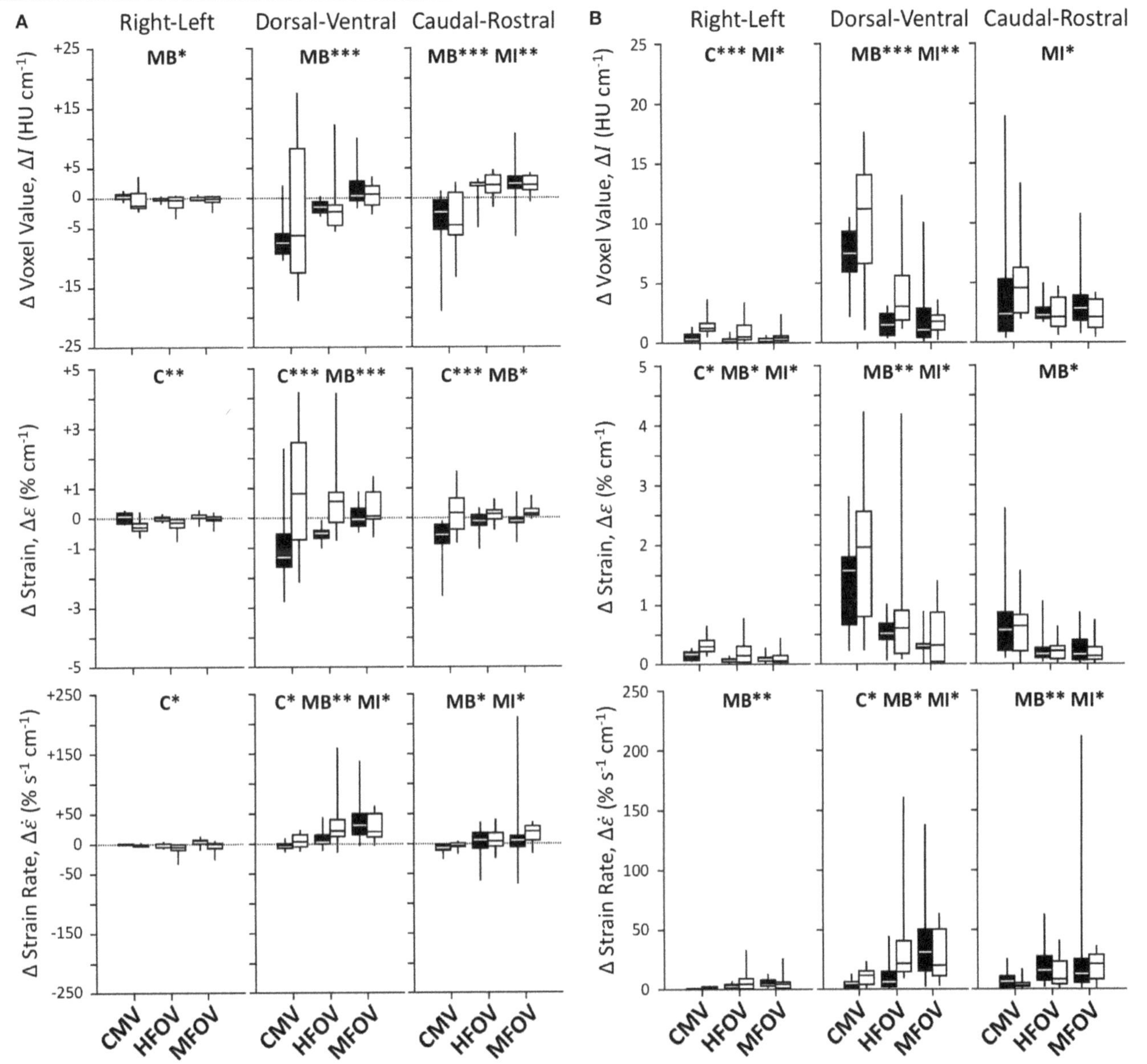

FIGURE 7 | Unnormalized spatial gradient values **(A)** and magnitudes **(B)** for image registration-based regional ventilation measures of intratidal changes in aeration (ΔI), volumetric strain ($\Delta\varepsilon$), and volumetric strain rate ($\Delta\dot{\varepsilon}$). Linear spatial gradients in each of the three principal anatomic directions throughout the lung mask are shown for each variable, represented by box plots showing minimum, maximum, and quartiles across subjects under baseline (black) and injured (white) conditions, during conventional mechanical ventilation (CMV), high-frequency oscillatory ventilation (HFOV), and multi-frequency oscillatory ventilation (MFOV). Asterisks indicate significance levels ($^*p < 0.05$, $^{**}p < 0.01$, $^{***}p < 0.001$) for main effects (C = lung condition, MB = modality for baseline condition, MI = modality for injured condition). See **Table 2** for additional clarification.

DISCUSSION

In this study, we demonstrated that oscillatory ventilation improves the average regional lung strain, as well as the spatial gradients of lung strain, compared to a conventional pressure-controlled modality in pigs with heterogeneous lung injury. This study revealed a mechanism by which enhanced harmonic content in MFOV waveforms may improve gas exchange compared to either CMV or single-frequency HFOV waveforms.

The increase in respiratory system elastance following lung injury (i.e., 183% increase in E_{rs} and 355% increase in H) is consistent with substantial lung derecruitment and/or surfactant dysfunction. Consequently, increased driving pressure was required to maintain eucapnia at comparable respiratory rates. Despite similar $V_{pp} \cdot Wt^{-1}$ and ventilatory cost function (V_C), the driving pressure (ΔP_{aw}) after lung injury increased to 18.7 cmH_2O, compared to 13.0 cmH_2O at baseline (**Figure 5**). Increased ΔP_{aw} during CMV after injury exceeded the 15 cmH_2O threshold identified by Amato et al. (2015), above

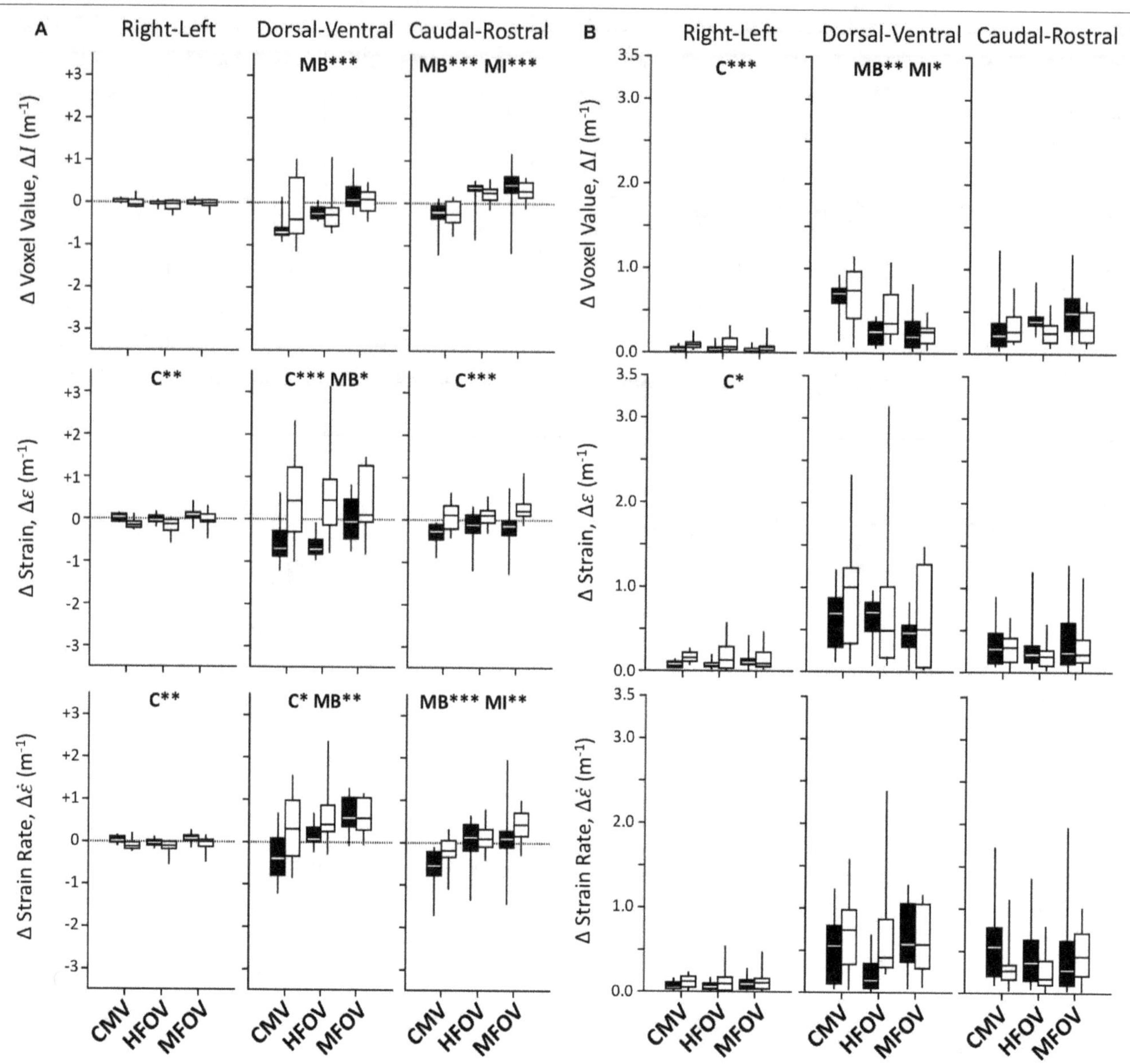

FIGURE 8 | Mean-normalized spatial gradient values **(A)** and magnitudes **(B)** for image registration-based regional ventilation measures of intratidal changes in aeration (ΔI), volumetric strain ($\Delta\varepsilon$), and volumetric strain rate ($\Delta\dot{\varepsilon}$). Linear spatial gradients in each of the three principal anatomic directions throughout the lung mask are shown for each variable, represented by box plots showing minimum, maximum, and quartiles across subjects under baseline (black) and injured (white) conditions, during conventional mechanical ventilation (CMV), high-frequency oscillatory ventilation (HFOV), and multi-frequency oscillatory ventilation (MFOV). Asterisks indicate significance levels ($^*p < 0.05$, $^{**}p < 0.01$, $^{***}p < 0.001$) for main effects (C = lung condition, MB = modality for baseline condition, MI = modality for injured condition). See **Table 2** for additional clarification.

which the mortality odds ratio was greater than unity in patients with ARDS. The use of $\Delta P_{aw} > 15$ cmH_2O suggests substantial potential for VILI despite average measured $V_{pp} \cdot Wt^{-1}$ of 7.5 mL kg^{-1} (**Figure 5**). However, such heuristics are only applicable during CMV, for which P_{aw} fluctuations are well-correlated with lung strain. During oscillatory modes of ventilation, ΔP_{aw} as computed from Equation (6) does not represent elastic pressures distending peripheral alveoli, but also includes substantial pressure losses due to resistive and inertial loads imposed by the endotracheal tube and conducting airways, especially with increasing frequency. The fact that ΔP_{aw} was greater during MFOV than HFOV indicates that larger pressure amplitudes were required to overcome the increased resistive and inertial losses at frequencies up to 20 Hz compared to 5 Hz, but does not indicate that these larger airway pressures were transmitted to distal alveoli (Pillow et al., 2002). We found that the spatial mean of strain throughout the entire lung during CMV was unchanged after injury, despite increased ΔP_{aw} and

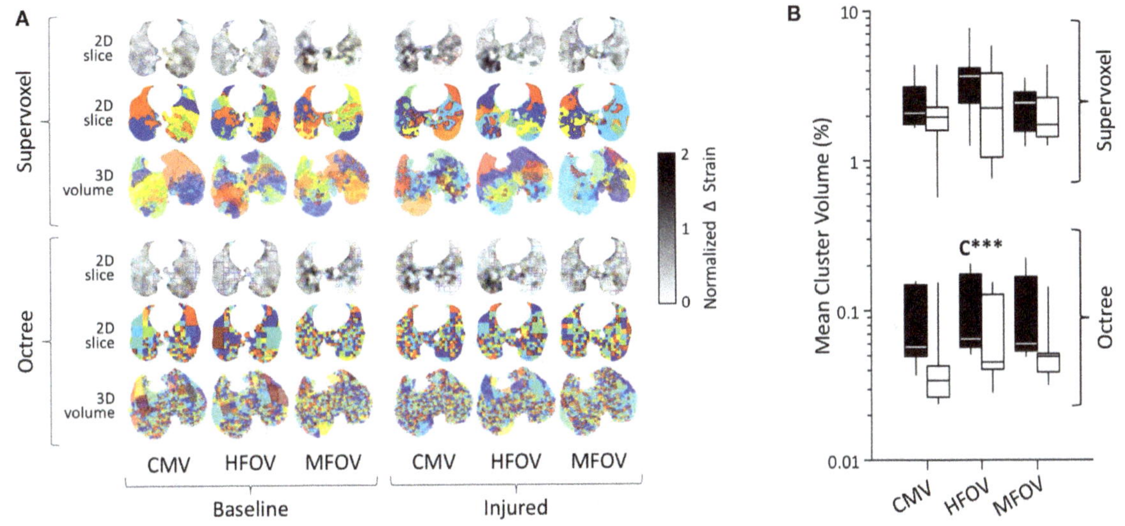

FIGURE 9 | Regional patchiness of intratidal variations in volumetric strain ($\Delta\varepsilon$) during conventional mechanical ventilation (CMV), high-frequency oscillatory ventilation (HFOV), and multi-frequency oscillatory ventilation (MFOV). Regional patchiness was assessed by the size, number, and distribution of regions-of-interest or clusters (randomized colors) obtained by recursive supervoxel or octree decomposition. Examples from a representative subject **(A)**, and cluster volumes as a fraction of the lung mask **(B)** represented by box plots showing minimum, maximum, and quartiles across subjects under baseline (black) and injured (white) conditions. Asterisks indicate significance levels (***$p < 0.001$) for main effects (C = lung condition).

ΔI spatial mean (**Figure 6**). Some evidence to reconcile this discrepancy is apparent in the greatly increased coefficient of variation for $\Delta\varepsilon$ (**Figure 6**). Upon closer examination of the regional strain distributions in injured lungs, $\Delta\varepsilon$ was nearly zero in consolidated regions of the lung with $I >$-100 HU. By contrast, $\Delta\varepsilon$ was increased by 25% in normally aerated regions (i.e., -900 HU $< I < -500$ HU) relative to the average throughout the entire lung mask. Thus, the increased ΔP_{aw} required to deliver similar $V_{pp} \cdot \mathrm{Wt}^{-1}$ (**Figure 5**) resulted in concentrated strains within the recruited lung. This finding is consistent with the concept of the "baby lung," which describes reduced functional recruited volume in ARDS (Gattinoni and Pesenti, 2005; Gattinoni et al., 2016a).

Spatial gradients of intratidal strain also provide some insight into the redistribution of mechanical flows after lung injury. As expected, the magnitudes of right-left gradients were small relative to those of the dorsal-ventral and caudal-rostral gradients (**Figure 7**). Most noticeably, lung injury was associated with dramatic changes in dorsal-ventral $\Delta\varepsilon$ gradients. Ventilation in healthy subjects during CMV tended to distribute toward the dorsal and caudal lung regions. However, varying degrees of lung injury resulted in consolidation or derecruitment of the dependent lung, such that dorsal-ventral $\Delta\varepsilon$ gradients were reduced (or even reversed) depending on the extent of edema, particularly for CMV and HFOV. Interestingly, intratidal changes in aeration tended to preserve the dorsal-ventral ΔI gradient before and after injury, despite the positive shift observed in dorsal-ventral $\Delta\varepsilon$ gradients. It should be noted that actual spatial distributions of ΔI and $\Delta\varepsilon$ are likely not well-described by linear functions of spatial position following lung injury, and may even be non-monotonic (Johnson et al., 2017). For example, negative dorsal-ventral gradients may be possible in the recruited lung, but counteracted by zero ventilation in the derecruited dependent lung such that the resulting overall linear gradient may be negative, zero, or even positive. Nonetheless compared to either CMV of HFOV, MFOV reduced the magnitude of spatial gradients in ventilation regardless of the lung condition. Other strategies for improving ventilation distribution and eliminating large dorsal-ventral gradients include prone position ventilation (Scholten et al., 2017; Xin et al., 2018), which was not used in this study. Prone posture serves to eliminate large-scale gravitational gradients in lung expansion (Hoffman, 1985), but would not be expected to affect the local, region-to-region mechanical differences which MFOV targets. Finally, both HFOV and MFOV were associated with more positive caudal-rostral ΔI gradients compared to CMV, regardless of injured condition ($p < 0.001$). CMV-associated findings indicate that in contrast to oscillatory modalities, CMV preferentially ventilates the basal regions of the lungs, consistent with a previous positron emission tomography study (Venegas et al., 1993).

Much of the variability in spatial gradient magnitudes across different ventilation modalities was due to changes in the spatial means. By contrast, the normalized gradients (i.e., the spatial gradients divided by the spatial mean) exhibited fewer significant differences across modalities (**Figure 8**, **Table 2**). This finding indicates that, at least for the particular frequencies and waveforms used in this study, the *relative* spatial gradients were not substantially altered by modality. This may be due in part to the predominance of the 5 Hz component in both HFOV and MFOV waveforms, which was below the resonant frequency in almost every case (**Table 1**), and therefore

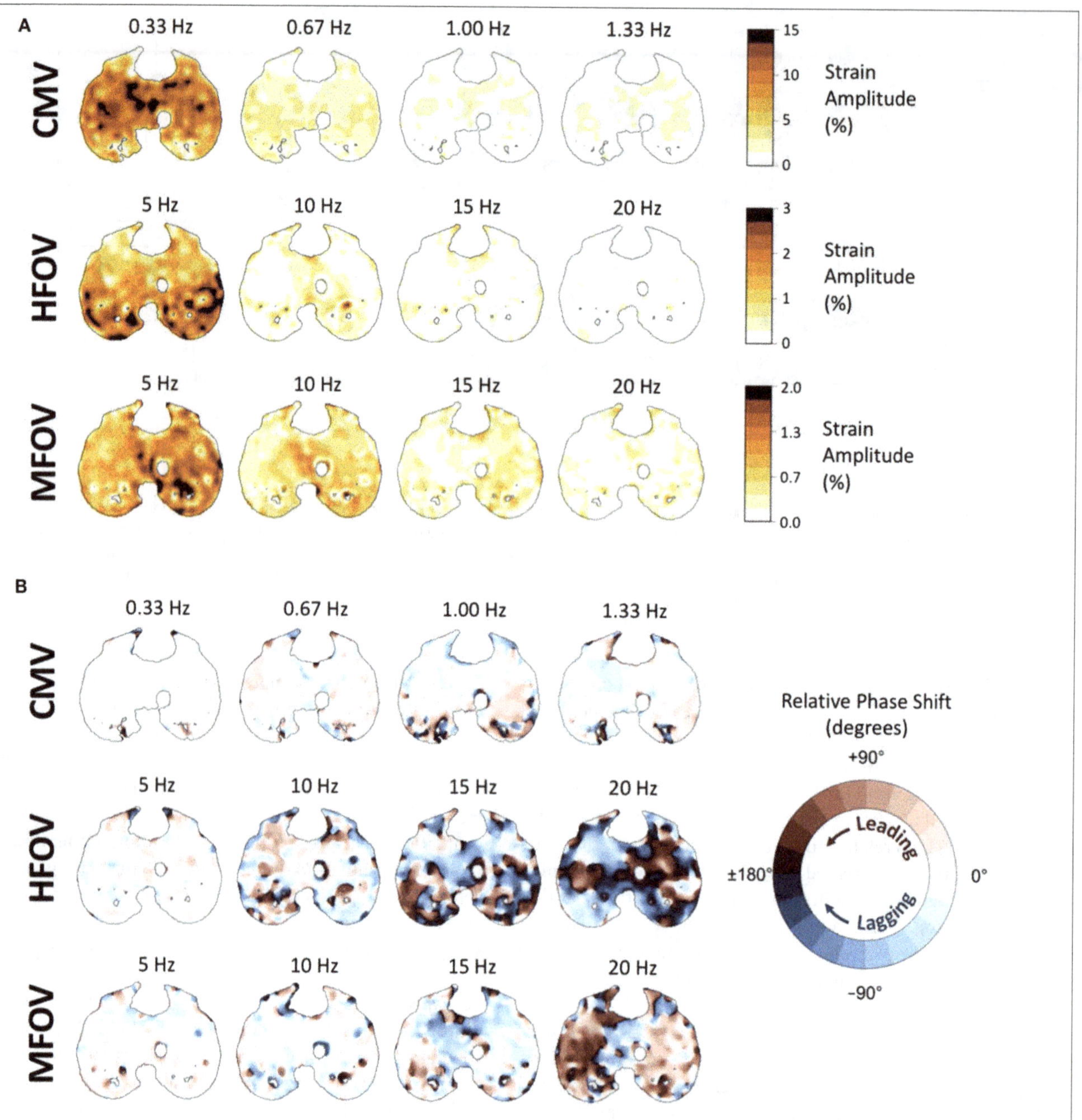

FIGURE 10 | Frequency-domain representations of tissue-correlated regional strain amplitude **(A)** and phase variations **(B)** in one subject during conventional mechanical ventilation (CMV), high-frequency oscillatory ventilation (HFOV), and multi-frequency oscillatory ventilation (MFOV). For each ventilation modality, strain amplitudes and phases were obtained from the discrete Fourier transform of time-varying Jacobian determinants within each voxel, using transformations mapped to a single reference image. In each cross-section of the reference image, voxel color in **(A)** indicates the strain amplitude at that frequency, corresponding to the amplitude of volumetric strain relative to the minimum volume of that particular voxel. Voxel color in **(B)** indicates the amount of phase shift (leading or lagging) relative to the median phase of all lung voxels at the specified frequency.

below a threshold frequency for developing regional ventilation heterogeneity due to resonant amplification (Herrmann et al., 2019a). Our results then indicate that broadband MFOV waveforms, while producing the same *relative* ventilation heterogeneity as HFOV, still reduce the average strain and magnitude of strain gradients that are associated with risk for VILI.

Based on our supervoxel and octree analysis, regional strain heterogeneity did not differ greatly across ventilation modality, although the injured lungs did require smaller sizes to describe the spatial clustering of $\Delta\varepsilon$ compared to the baseline conditions (**Figure 9**). Lung injury may thus result in increased small-scale strain heterogeneity (Kaczka et al., 2011; Perchiazzi et al., 2014). It should be noted that our estimates of regional strain

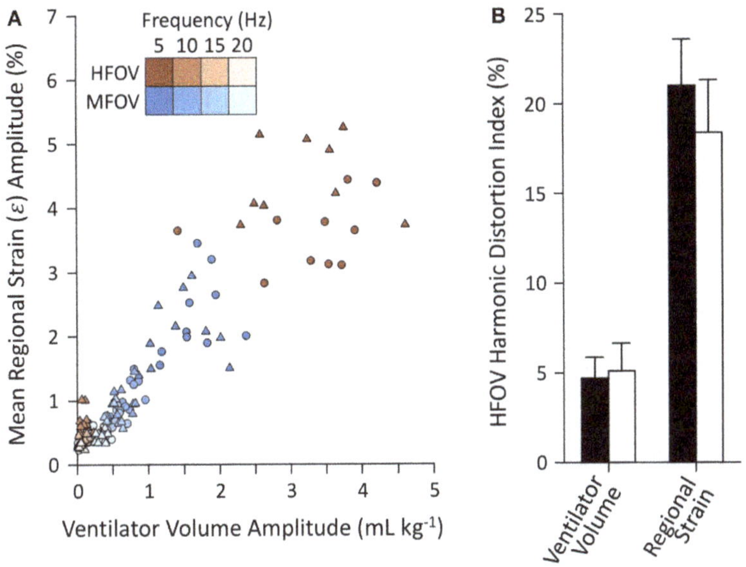

FIGURE 11 | Harmonic amplitudes **(A)** from imaging-based regional strain measurements and corresponding amplitudes from the ventilator volume waveform measured at the airway opening under baseline (circles) and injured (triangles) conditions. Harmonic distortion index **(B)** mean and standard deviation for each set of measurements, grouped by baseline (black) and injured (white) lung conditions.

derived from image registration are inherently smooth due to the use of B-splines to define the spatiotemporal deformations. The discrepancy between the supervoxel- and octree-based results may also be due in part to the discrete anatomic structure of lungs, which consist of an assumed continuum of spongy parenchymal tissues penetrated by branching networks of airways and vessels. Airways and vessels are not expected to undergo large volumetric strains during mechanical ventilation, and therefore give rise to irregularities in the spatial field of $\Delta\varepsilon$. Such irregularities may be approximately contoured by supervoxel boundaries, which are not rigidly constrained. By contrast, octree decomposition is strictly planar, and therefore may require greater degrees of recursive subdivision to isolate such irregular spatial distributions of $\Delta\varepsilon$ (Perchiazzi et al., 2014). The supervoxel decomposition incorporates spatial proximity as well as image intensity, such that reducing the spatial proximity weighting may facilitate the identification of larger clusters albeit with irregular boundaries. Therefore, it is possible that our findings would be altered if smaller airways and blood vessels were further segmented from the lung parenchyma prior to cluster analysis, or if a different spatial proximity weighting was used for the supervoxel decomposition.

Separation of the harmonic content of regional ventilation illustrates a potential influence of nonlinear mechanics during HFOV at 5 Hz (**Figure 11**). For example, image registration resulted in estimation of $\dot{\varepsilon}$ amplitudes at 10, 15, and 20 Hz of roughly one third those at 5 Hz, despite the ventilator waveform consisting of only 5 Hz oscillation (**Supplementary Figure S-4**). By contrast, $\dot{\varepsilon}$ amplitudes during MFOV approximated the input distribution of uniform amplitude flow at all four harmonics (**Supplementary Figure S-4**). Intrapulmonary harmonic distortion of distributed flows during HFOV (with only a single frequency) may result from the use of larger-amplitude flows exacerbating inherent mechanical nonlinearities, but may also result from the complex interaction of mechanically-interdependent lung tissues (Suki and Bates, 1991; Suki et al., 1991). During MFOV, the use of small-amplitude flows may contribute to relatively linear mechanical behavior of the lung tissues. It is also possible that the observed nonlinearity may be due in part to imaging artifact and errors in image registration resulting in misidentified high-frequency, small-amplitude motion. Assuming that our registration results are accurate however, the $\dot{\varepsilon}$ amplitudes measured at the higher harmonics during HFOV are surprisingly large, almost comparable to those intentionally delivered during MFOV. It is plausible that the mechanisms by which MFOV may enhance gas transport already occur, at least to some extent, within the lung periphery during HFOV. However, MFOV may induce these higher harmonics directly, without incurring the overhead of generating high flow rates at the fundamental frequency. The consequences of such overhead may include, for example, increased spatial gradients of strain and strain rate due to gravitational dependence (**Figure 7**).

Limitations

MFOV may improve ventilation distribution and the efficiency gas exchange efficacy (Kaczka et al., 2015; Herrmann et al., 2018, 2019b). However, given the technical limitations of the mechanical ventilator as well as our dynamic CT image reconstruction technique which assumed strict periodicity of motion (Herrmann et al., 2017), the MFOV waveform used in this study comprised only harmonic components of the fundamental frequency. Cardiogenic motion was not synchronized with respiratory motion and therefore presents a source of artifact in the reconstructed 4DCT images of respiratory motion, depending on the relative periodicity between the ventilator frequency and the heart rate. Such artifact may manifest as rapid oscillations in CT density (Herrmann et al., 2017), which may influence registration-based estimates of strain rate, especially in regions adjacent to the mediastinum.

In addition, the interpretation of regional strain in the proximity of recruitment/derecruitment is challenging for several reasons. Standard image registration techniques (e.g., using a similarity cost function defined as the sum of squared intensity differences) assume a uniform intensity transform to predict voxel-wise correspondence, but cannot account for local changes in intensity associated with changing gas fraction. Consequently, these approaches may result in the prediction of non-physical deformations, such as contraction of nonaerated lung regions. The sum of squared tissue volume differences (SSTVD) similarity cost function used in this study addresses this problem using a non-uniform intensity transform that accounts for local variations in CT intensity that are due to changing proportions of gas-to-tissue content in each lung region during breathing or ventilation (Zhao et al., 2016). Another challenge to registration of injured lungs is the lack of contrast or structural landmarks in consolidated regions, which renders validation of estimated voxel-wise correspondence nearly impossible, especially when large changes in recruitment occur between two images. In this study, high temporal resolution imaging (7–105 Hz) was used to minimize the time between adjacent ventilation phases, which resulted in small deformations and small changes in recruitment between adjacent images being registered. Linear elastic regularization produces plausible predictions of voxel-wise correspondence in regions with little contrast, assuming the lung parenchyma deforms as a linear elastic material. An important limitation of most registration techniques is the assumption of smoothly varying deformation, which may not accurately reflect discontinuous motion at distinct structural boundaries between aerated and nonaerated lung tissue. Due to the limited spatial resolution in this study (0.6 mm), each voxel may contain up to dozens of alveoli. Thus, it is difficult, if not impossible, to distinguish the underlying cause of observed changes in aeration (Cereda et al., 2019). For example, the same change in aeration of a single voxel may represent uniform deflation of its alveoli, complete derecruitment of only a portion of alveoli, or any combination thereof. Thus, prediction of recruitment/derecruitment on the basis of voxel aeration is speculative.

Finally, while our study focused on regional distributions of aeration, strain, and strain rate as the primary indicators of ventilation and VILI, the exact relationship between these mechanical variables and VILI is difficult to ascertain. VILI is a complicated process associated with a diverse range of mechanical stimuli (Hussein et al., 2013; Carrasco Loza et al., 2015; Güldner et al., 2016; Smith et al., 2017; Tonetti et al., 2017). So-called "mechanical power" (i.e., the rate of energy dissipation across parenchymal tissues) may provide a better prediction of VILI compared to either strain or strain rate alone (Gattinoni et al., 2016b; Serpa Neto et al., 2018). However, measurement of regional mechanical power is not practical, given the requirement of regional gas pressure within the lung for its estimation. Alternatively, VILI may also be assessed using fluoro-deoxyglucose (FDG) uptake (Wellman et al., 2014), serum or alveolar inflammatory cytokines (Liu et al., 2013), protein content in bronchoalveolar lavage fluid (Smith et al., 2017), and histopathology. All of these quantitative measurements of lung injury require extensive durations of mechanical ventilation prior to measurement, some of which may only be obtained *post mortem*.

Conclusion

In an oleic acid model of porcine ARDS, high-frequency and multi-frequency oscillatory ventilation resulted in improved gas exchange efficiency and reduced regional lung strain compared to conventional mechanical ventilation. MFOV also reduced spatial gradients in lung strain compared to CMV or HFOV, resulting in a more uniform overall distribution of lung strain. By contrast, mean-normalized spatial gradients exhibited less dependence on ventilation modality, indicating that the use of higher harmonic frequencies in MFOV does not substantially alter *relative* ventilation heterogeneity. Thus, the reduced spatial strain gradients observed with MFOV, compared to HFOV or CMV, may be explained by reductions in the *average* parenchymal strain. In summary, MFOV supports gas exchange with reduced lung strain, and may provide additional benefit over HFOV by reducing ventilation heterogeneity associated with spatial gradients in absolute strain, and by reducing the strain associated with conventional ventilation or single-frequency oscillation.

AUTHOR CONTRIBUTIONS

JH and DK conceived the study, collected the data, and wrote the manuscript. JH, SG, WS, MH, JR, GC, EH, and DK analyzed the data and revised the manuscript.

FUNDING

This work was supported by the Office of the Assistant Secretary of Defense for Health Affairs, through the Peer Reviewed Medical Research Program under Award No. W81XWH-16-1-0434. Opinions, interpretations, conclusions, and recommendations are those of the authors and are not necessarily endorsed by the Department of Defense. This study was also supported by the Department of Anesthesia at the University of Iowa Hospital and Clinics, and by National Institutes of Health awards R41 HL140640, R01 CA166703, and R01 HL142625. This work utilized a CT scanner that was purchased with funding from National Institutes of Health Shared Instrumentation Grant 1S10OD018526. This research was supported in part through high-performance computing resources provided by The University of Iowa, Iowa City, Iowa.

ACKNOWLEDGMENTS

Andrea Fonseca da Cruz, Bakir Hajdarevic, Eli Schmidt, Chelsea Sloan, and Kelly M. Stark assisted with performing the experimental protocol. Melissa Saylor, Jarron Atha, and

Shayna Hogue assisted with computed tomographic imaging. Ahmed Halaweish, Mathew K. Fuld, and Siemens Healthineers (Forchheim, Germany) provided technical assistance for image reconstruction. Andrea Fonseca da Cruz, Eli Schmidt, Charles A. Mascardo, and Ethan L. Chen assisted with manual image segmentation. ZOLL Medical Corporation generously loaned a portable ventilator for use in animal experiments. The authors are deeply grateful for all of their contributions to this investigation.

REFERENCES

Acute Respiratory Distress Syndrome Network (2000). Ventilation with lower tidal volumes as compared with traditional tidal volumes for acute lung injury and the acute respiratory distress syndrome. The Acute Respiratory Distress Syndrome Network. *N. Engl. J. Med.* 342, 1301–1308. doi: 10.1056/NEJM200005043421801

Amato, M. B., Meade, M. O., Slutsky, A. S., Brochard, L., Costa, E. L., Schoenfeld, D. A., et al. (2015). Driving pressure and survival in the acute respiratory distress syndrome. *N. Engl. J. Med.* 372, 747–755. doi: 10.1056/NEJMsa1410639

Amini, R., Herrmann, J., and Kaczka, D. W. (2017). Intratidal overdistention and derecruitment in the injured lung: a simulation study. *IEEE Trans. Biomed. Eng.* 64, 681–689. doi: 10.1109/TBME.2016.2572678

Amini, R., and Kaczka, D. W. (2013). Impact of ventilation frequency and parenchymal stiffness on flow and pressure distribution in a canine lung model. *Ann. Biomed. Eng.* 41, 2699–2711. doi: 10.1007/s10439-013-0866-7

Carrasco Loza, R., Villamizar Rodríguez, G., and Medel Fernández, N. (2015). Ventilator-induced lung injury (VILI) in acute respiratory distress syndrome (ARDS): volutrauma and molecular effects. *Open Respir. Med. J.* 9, 112–119. doi: 10.2174/1874306401509010112

Cereda, M., Xin, Y., Goffi, A., Herrmann, J., Kaczka, D. W., Kavanagh, B. P., et al. (2019). Imaging the injured lung: Mechanisms of action and clinical use. *Anesthesiology.* 131, 716–749. doi: 10.1097/ALN.0000000000002583

Conze, P. H., Noblet, V., Rousseau, F., Heitz, F., de Blasi, V., Memeo, R., et al. (2017). Scale-adaptive supervoxel-based random forests for liver tumor segmentation in dynamic contrast-enhanced CT scans. *Int. J. Comput. Assist. Radiol. Surg.* 12, 223–233. doi: 10.1007/s11548-016-1493-1

Gattinoni, L., Marini, J. J., Pesenti, A., Quintel, M., Mancebo, J., and Brochard, L. (2016a). The "baby lung" became an adult. *Intensive Care Med.* 42, 663–673. doi: 10.1007/s00134-015-4200-8

Gattinoni, L., and Pesenti, A. (2005). The concept of "baby lung". *Intensive Care Med.* 31, 776–784. doi: 10.1007/s00134-005-2627-z

Gattinoni, L., Tonetti, T., Cressoni, M., Cadringher, P., Herrmann, P., Moerer, O., et al. (2016b). Ventilator-related causes of lung injury: the mechanical power. *Intensive Care Med.* 42, 1567–1575. doi: 10.1007/s00134-016-4505-2

Gerard, S. E., Herrmann, J., Kaczka, D. W., Musch, G., Fernandez-Bustamante, A., and Reinhardt, J. M. (2020). Multi-resolution convolutional neural networks for fully automated segmentation of acutely injured lungs in multiple species. *Med. Image Anal.* 60:101592. doi: 10.1016/j.media.2019.101592

Gerard, S. E., Herrmann, J., Kaczka, D. W., and Reinhardt, J. M. (2018). "Transfer learning for segmentation of injured lungs using coarse-to-fine convolutional neural networks," in *Image Analysis for Moving Organ, Breast, and Thoracic Images* (Granada: Springer International Publishing), 191–201.

Gorbunova, V., Lol, P., Ashraf, H., Dirksen, A., Nielsen, M., and de Bruijne, M. (2008). Weight preserving image registration for monitoring disease progression in lung CT. *Med. Image Comput. Comput. Interv.* 11, 863–870. doi: 10.1007/978-3-540-85990-1_104

Güldner, A., Braune, A., Ball, L., Silva, P. L., Samary, C., Insorsi, A., et al. (2016). Comparative effects of volutrauma and atelectrauma on lung inflammation in experimental acute respiratory distress syndrome. *Crit. Care Med.* 44, 1–12. doi: 10.1097/CCM.0000000000001721

Herrmann, J., Hoffman, E. A., and Kaczka, D. W. (2017). Frequency-selective computed tomography: applications during periodic thoracic motion. *IEEE Trans. Med. Imaging* 36, 1722–1732. doi: 10.1109/TMI.2017.2694887

Herrmann, J., Lilitwat, W., Tawhai, M. H., and Kaczka, D. W. (2019a). High-frequency oscillatory ventilation and ventilator-induced lung injury: size does matter. *Crit. Care Med.* 48, e66–e73. doi: 10.1097/CCM.00000000000 04073

Herrmann, J., Tawhai, M. H., and Kaczka, D. W. (2016). Regional gas transport in the heterogeneous lung during oscillatory ventilation. *J. Appl. Physiol.* 121, 1306–1318. doi: 10.1152/japplphysiol.00097.2016

Herrmann, J., Tawhai, M. H., and Kaczka, D. W. (2018). Parenchymal strain heterogeneity during oscillatory ventilation: why two frequencies are better than one. *J. Appl. Physiol.* 124, 653–663. doi: 10.1152/japplphysiol.00615.2017

Herrmann, J., Tawhai, M. H., and Kaczka, D. W. (2019b). Strain, strain rate, and mechanical power: an optimization comparison for oscillatory ventilation. *Int. j. Numer. Method. Biomed. Eng.* 35:e3238. doi: 10.1002/cnm.3238

Hoffman, E. A. (1985). Effect of body orientation on regional lung expansion: a computed tomographic approach. *J. Appl. Physiol.* 59, 468–480. doi: 10.1152/jappl.1985.59.2.468

Hussein, O., Walters, B., Stroetz, R., Valencia, P., McCall, D., and Hubmayr, R. D. (2013). Biophysical determinants of alveolar epithelial plasma membrane wounding associated with mechanical ventilation. *Am. J. Physiol. Lung Cell. Mol. Physiol.* 305, L478–L484. doi: 10.1152/ajplung.00437.2012

Johnson, N. J., Luks, A. M., and Glenny, R. W. (2017). Gas exchange in the prone posture. *Respir. Care* 62, 1097–1110. doi: 10.4187/respcare.05512

Kaczka, D. W., Cao, K., Christensen, G. E., Bates, J. H., and Simon, B. A. (2011). Analysis of regional mechanics in canine lung injury using forced oscillations and 3D image registration. *Ann. Biomed. Eng.* 39, 1112–1124. doi: 10.1007/s10439-010-0214-0

Kaczka, D. W., Herrmann, J., Zonneveld, C. E., Tingay, D. G., Lavizzari, A., Noble, P. B., et al. (2015). Multifrequency oscillatory ventilation in the premature lung: effects on gas exchange, mechanics, and ventilation distribution. *Anesthesiology* 123, 1394–1403. doi: 10.1097/ALN.0000000000000898

Kaczka, D. W., and Lutchen, K. R. (2004). Servo-controlled pneumatic pressure oscillator for respiratory impedance measurements and high-frequency ventilation. *Ann. Biomed. Eng.* 32, 596–608. doi: 10.1023/b:abme.0000019179.87974.7d

Klein, S., Staring, M., Murphy, K., Viergever, M. A., and Pluim, J. P. (2010). Elastix: a toolbox for intensity-based medical image registration. *IEEE Trans. Med. Imaging* 29, 196–205. doi: 10.1109/TMI.2009.2035616

Kneyber, M. C. J., and Markhorst, D. G. (2016). Do we really know how to use high-frequency oscillatory ventilation in critically ill children? *Am. J. Respir. Crit. Care Med.* 193, 1067–1068. doi: 10.1164/rccm.201512-2418LE

Liu, S., Yi, Y., Wang, M., Chen, Q., Huang, Y., Liu, L., et al. (2013). Higher frequency ventilation attenuates lung injury during high-frequency oscillatory ventilation in sheep models of acute respiratory distress syndrome. *Anesthesiology* 119, 398–411. doi: 10.1097/ALN.0b013e31829419a6

Malhotra, A., and Drazen, J. M. (2013). High-frequency oscillatory ventilation on shaky ground. *N. Engl. J. Med.* 368, 863–865. doi: 10.1056/NEJMe1300103

Meade, M. O., Young, D., Hanna, S., Zhou, Q., Bachman, T. E., Bollen, C., et al. (2017). Severity of hypoxemia and effect of high-frequency oscillatory ventilation in acute respiratory distress syndrome. *Am. J. Respir. Crit. Care Med.* 196, 727–733. doi: 10.1164/rccm.201609-1938OC

Metz, C. T., Klein, S., Schaap, M., van Walsum, T., and Niessen, W. J. (2011). Nonrigid registration of dynamic medical imaging data using nD+t B-splines and a groupwise optimization approach. *Med. Image Anal.* 15, 238–249. doi: 10.1016/j.media.2010.10.003

Nguyen, A. P., Schmidt, U. H., and MacIntyre, N. R. (2016). Should high-frequency ventilation in the adult be abandoned? *Respir. Care* 61, 791–800. doi: 10.4187/respcare.04584

Ortiz, R. M., Cilley, R. E., and Bartlett, R. H. (1987). Extracorporeal membrane oxygenation in pediatric respiratory failure. *Pediatr. Clin. North Am.* 34, 39–46. doi: 10.1016/S0031-3955(16)36179-X

Perchiazzi, G., Rylander, C., Derosa, S., Pellegrini, M., Pitagora, L., Polieri, D., et al. (2014). Regional distribution of lung compliance by image analysis of computed tomograms. *Respir. Physiol. Neurobiol.* 201, 60–70. doi: 10.1016/j.resp.2014.07.001

Pillow, J. J., Sly, P. D., Hantos, Z., and Bates, J. H. (2002). Dependence of intrapulmonary pressure amplitudes on respiratory mechanics during high-frequency oscillatory ventilation in preterm lambs. *Pediatr. Res.* 52, 538–544. doi: 10.1203/00006450-200210000-00013

Protti, A., Maraffi, T., Milesi, M., Votta, E., Santini, A., Pugni, P., et al. (2016). Role of strain rate in the pathogenesis of ventilator-induced lung edema. *Crit. Care Med.* 44, e838–e845. doi: 10.1097/CCM.0000000000001718

Scholten, E. L., Beitler, J. R., Prisk, G. K., and Malhotra, A. (2017). Treatment of ARDS with prone positioning. *Chest* 151, 215–224. doi: 10.1016/j.chest.2016.06.032

Serpa Neto, A., Deliberato, R. O., Johnson, A. E. W., Bos, L. D., Amorim, P., Pereira, S. M., et al. (2018). Mechanical power of ventilation is associated with mortality in critically ill patients: An analysis of patients in two observational cohorts. *Intensive Care Med.* 44, 1914–1922. doi: 10.1007/s00134-018-5375-6

Sklar, M. C., Fan, E., and Goligher, E. C. (2017). High-frequency oscillatory ventilation in adults with ARDS: past, present, and future. *Chest* 152, 1306–1317. doi: 10.1016/j.chest.2017.06.025

Slutsky, A. S., and Ranieri, V. M. (2013). Ventilator-induced lung injury. *N. Engl. J. Med.* 369, 2126–2136. doi: 10.1056/NEJMra1208707

Smith, B. J., Bartolak-Suki, E., Suki, B., Roy, G. S., Hamlington, K. L., Charlebois, C. M., et al. (2017). Linking ventilator injury-induced leak across the blood-gas barrier to derangements in murine lung function. *Front. Physiol.* 8:466. doi: 10.3389/fphys.2017.00466

Suki, B., and Bates, J. H. (1991). A nonlinear viscoelastic model of lung tissue mechanics. *J. Appl. Physiol.* 71, 826–833. doi: 10.1152/jappl.1991.71.3.826

Suki, B., Hantos, Z., Daróczy, B., Alkaysi, G., and Nagy, S. (1991). Nonlinearity and harmonic distortion of dog lungs measured by low-frequency forced oscillations. *J. Appl. Physiol.* 71, 69–75. doi: 10.1152/jappl.1991.71.1.69

Suki, B., and Lutchen, K. R. (1992). Pseudorandom signals to estimate apparent transfer and coherence functions of nonlinear systems: applications to respiratory mechanics. *IEEE Trans. Biomed. Eng.* 39, 1142–1151. doi: 10.1109/10.168693

Tonetti, T., Vasques, F., Rapetti, F., Maiolo, G., Collino, F., Romitti, F., et al. (2017). Driving pressure and mechanical power: new targets for VILI prevention. *Ann. Transl. Med.* 5:286. doi: 10.21037/atm.2017.07.08

Vasavada, N. (2016). Kruskal-Wallis rank sum test calculator. Available online at: https://astatsa.com/KruskalWallisTest/ (accessed September 18, 2019).

Venegas, J. G., Tsuzaki, K., Fox, B. J., Simon, B. A., and Hales, C. A. (1993). Regional coupling between chest wall and lung expansion during HFV: a positron imaging study. *J. Appl. Physiol.* 74, 2242–2252. doi: 10.1152/jappl.1993.74.5.2242

Welch, P. (1967). The use of fast Fourier transform for the estimation of power spectra: a method based on time averaging over short, modified periodograms. *IEEE Trans Audio Electroacoust* 15, 70–73. doi: 10.1109/TAU.1967.1161901

Wellman, T. J., Winkler, T., Costa, E. L., Musch, G., Harris, R. S., Zheng, H., et al. (2014). Effect of local tidal lung strain on inflammation in normal and lipopolysaccharide-exposed sheep. *Crit. Care Med.* 42, e491–500. doi: 10.1097/CCM.0000000000000346

Xin, Y., Cereda, M., Hamedani, H., Pourfathi, M., Siddiqui, S., Meeder, N., et al. (2018). Unstable inflation causing injury insight from prone position and paired computed tomography scans. *Am. J. Respir. Crit. Care Med.* 198, 197–207. doi: 10.1164/rccm.201708-1728OC

Yin, Y., Hoffman, E. A., and Lin, C.-L. (2009). Mass preserving nonrigid registration of CT lung images using cubic B-spline. *Med. Phys.* 36, 4213–4222. doi: 10.1118/1.3193526

Zhang, Q., Suki, B., and Lutchen, K. R. (1995). Harmonic distortion from nonlinear systems with broadband inputs: applications to lung mechanics. *Ann. Biomed. Eng.* 23, 672–681. doi: 10.1007/bf02584464

Zhao, B., Christensen, G. E., Hyun Song, J., Pan, Y., Gerard, S. E., Reinhardt, J. M., et al. (2016). "Tissue-volume preserving deformable image registration for 4DCT pulmonary images," in *IEEE Conference on Computer Vision and Pattern Recognition Workshops (CVPRW)* (Las Vegas, NV), 41–49.

NOMENCLATURE

4DCT	Four-dimensional computed tomography
ARDS	Acute respiratory distress syndrome
CMV	Conventional mechanical ventilation
CO_2	Carbon dioxide
E_{rs}	Dynamic respiratory system elastance
FDG	Fluorodeoxyglucose
f	Frequency
f_0	Fundamental frequency
f_{res}	Resonant frequency
F_iO_2	Fraction of oxygen in inspired gas
HFOV	High-frequency oscillatory ventilation
H	Tissue elastance
I_{aw}	Airway inertance
I	Volumetric CT density image
I_{avg}	Target image for registration, representing the average of deformed images
$I_{n\to m}$	Result of deforming the nth image into the mth spatial reference frame
ΔI	Intratidal range of CT density
$J_{n\to m}$	Jacobian matrix of the transformation from the nth to mth spatial reference frames
j	Unit imaginary number, i.e., $j = \sqrt{-1}$
k	Frequency index
MFOV	Multi-frequency oscillatory ventilation
M	Lung segmentation mask
m	Image index, corresponding to phase of periodic ventilation cycle
n	Image index, corresponding to phase of periodic ventilation cycle
N	Number of images in periodic sequence
OI	Oxygenation index
P	Pressure
P_{aw}	Pressure at the airway opening
$\overline{P}_{aw}$	Mean airway pressure
ΔP_{aw}	Intratidal range of airway pressure
P_aCO_2	Partial pressure of carbon dioxide in arterial blood
P_aO_2	Partial pressure of oxygen in arterial blood
PEEP	Positive end-expiratory pressure
ROI	Region of interest
R	Airway resistance
SFOV	Single-frequency oscillatory ventilation
SSTVD	Sum of squared tissue volume differences
t	Time
δt	Time step between adjacent image phases
T	Time duration of the ventilatory cycle
VILI	Ventilator-induced lung injury
V	Volume
$\overline{V}$	Time-averaged volume over the ventilatory cycle
V_{pp}	Peak-to-peak volume
V_{rms}	Root-mean-square volume
$\overline{V}_{ROI}$	Mean cluster size after recursive octree or supervoxel decomposition
δV	Volume of a single voxel
V_C	Ventilatory cost function
Wt	Body weight
x_n	Vector of 3-dimensional spatial coordinates in nth image reference frame
X	Vector of 3-dimensional spatial coordinates in target image reference frame
X_{rs}	Respiratory system reactance
Z_{rs}	Respiratory system mechanical impedance
$\hat{Z}_{rs}$	Model-predicted respiratory system mechanical impedance
α	Exponent of frequency in constant phase model
ε	Volumetric strain
$\Delta\varepsilon$	Intratidal range of volumetric strain
$\dot{\varepsilon}$	Volumetric strain rate
$\Delta\dot{\varepsilon}$	Intratidal range of volumetric strain rate
γ^2	Coherence spectrum
η	Tissue hysteresivity
π	Number of radians in a semicircle
ϕ	4-dimensional transformation mapping image sequence to target average image
∇_x	Spatial gradient operator

9

Mechanical Ventilation Lessons Learned from Alveolar Micromechanics

Michaela Kollisch-Singule[1], Joshua Satalin[2], Sarah J. Blair[2], Penny L. Andrews[3], Louis A. Gatto[2,4], Gary F. Nieman[2] and Nader M. Habashi[3]*

Department of Pediatric Surgery, Arkansas Children's Hospital, Little Rock, AR, United States, [2] Department of Surgery, SUNY Upstate Medical University, Syracuse,[1] NY, United States, [3] Department of Critical Care, R Adams Cowley Shock Trauma Center, University of Maryland Medical Center, Baltimore, MD, United States, [4] Department of Biological Sciences, SUNY Cortland, Cortland, NY, United States

***Correspondence:**
Joshua Satalin
SatalinJ@upstate.edu

Morbidity and mortality associated with lung injury remains disappointingly unchanged over the last two decades, in part due to the current reliance on lung macro-parameters set on the ventilator instead of considering the micro-environment and the response of the alveoli and alveolar ducts to ventilator adjustments. The response of alveoli and alveolar ducts to mechanical ventilation modes cannot be predicted with current bedside methods of assessment including lung compliance, oxygenation, and pressure-volume curves. Alveolar tidal volumes (Vt) are less determined by the Vt set on the mechanical ventilator and more dependent on the number of recruited alveoli available to accommodate that Vt and their heterogeneous mechanical properties, such that high lung Vt can lead to a low alveolar Vt and low Vt can lead to high alveolar Vt. The degree of alveolar heterogeneity that exists cannot be predicted based on lung calculations that average the individual alveolar Vt and compliance. Finally, the importance of time in promoting alveolar stability, specifically the inspiratory and expiratory times set on the ventilator, are currently under-appreciated. In order to improve outcomes related to lung injury, the respiratory physiology of the individual patient, specifically at the level of the alveolus, must be targeted. With experimental data, this review highlights some of the known mechanical ventilation adjustments that are helpful or harmful at the level of the alveolus.

Keywords: alveolar stability, alveolar heterogeneity, lung injury, *in vivo* microscopy, micromechanics

INTRODUCTION

Acute lung injury is caused by a pathologic tetrad of alveolar instability, endothelial leakage, alveolar edema, and surfactant dysfunction (Nieman et al., 2018). Atelectrauma and associated repetitive opening and collapse of the injured alveoli results in alveolar instability (Schiller et al., 2001). An increase in pulmonary capillary permeability (Matthay et al., 2012) combined with damage to the alveolar-capillary barrier leads to alveolar edema (Budinger and Sznajder, 2006). This edema and repetitive opening and collapse of unstable alveoli alters surfactant function and abundance, resulting in increased surface tension (Greene et al., 1999; Warriner et al., 2002), and promotion of alveolar epithelial injury (Ruhl et al., 2019). Finally, tissue injury activates pro-inflammatory signaling, leading to biotrauma (Tremblay et al., 1997). Although mechanical ventilation can be necessary to support the injured lung in order to promote gas exchange, it can itself be injurious by exacerbating atelectrauma and recruitment/derecruitment ultimately leading to the acute respiratory distress syndrome (ARDS) (Gajic et al., 2004; Albert, 2012).

Despite decades of research into protective mechanical ventilation strategies, mortality rates associated with ARDS have remained disappointing with mortality rates ranging from 34.9 to 46.1% (Bellani et al., 2016) despite the use of protective non-injurious ventilation (Villar et al., 2011). When a patient is placed on the mechanical ventilator, the ventilator settings are modified to accommodate the physiology of the lung [tidal volumes (Vt), compliance, pressure-volume curves, oxygen saturation, etc...], while taking into account the patient's underlying volume status and cardiac physiology (Vieillard-Baron et al., 2016). Regional microscale responses [in the alveoli, conducting airway, and interstitium] are not predictable from the macroscale inputs of the mechanical ventilator (Kollisch-Singule et al., 2014a). Therefore, the universal application of generic mechanical ventilator settings to all patients without considering patient-specific differences in the underlying micromechanics may not benefit the lung and even cause further injury. Personalizing mechanical ventilation in order to link the macro-parameters set on the mechanical ventilator to the dynamic changes that occur at the level of the alveolus will be important to attenuate the pathophysiology of lung injury: alveolar instability, endothelial leakage, alveolar edema, and surfactant dysfunction (Kollisch-Singule et al., 2018; Nieman et al., 2018). Herein, we review the current literature investigating the response of the lung micro-anatomy: the alveoli and alveolar ducts, to varying mechanical ventilation settings.

ALVEOLAR RECRUITMENT

The majority of what is known about alveolar micromechanics is based on *in vivo* and *in vitro* models (Tschumperlin et al., 2000; Perlman and Bhattacharya, 2007; Mertens et al., 2009) incorporating methods of histology, electron microscopy, *in vivo* microscopy, optical coherence tomography, computed tomography, synchrotron imaging, electrical impedance tomography, inhaled polarized gases, and computer-based theoretical models (Broche et al., 2017; Grune et al., 2019), but there are no direct methods of assessing alveolar micromechanics, particularly the response to mechanical ventilation strategies (Roan and Waters, 2011).

At the level of the lung, it is well-recognized that even relatively high pressures are not harmful to the lung when applied tonically (as static strain) but becomes harmful when applied dynamically (as dynamic strain or with large driving pressures) (Protti et al., 2013; Amato et al., 2015; Jain et al., 2017). This does correlate with alveoli in that cyclic stretching and higher amplitude deformation of alveolar epithelial cells leads to greater cell damage whereas static or lower amplitude deformations do not (Tschumperlin et al., 2000). An individual alveolus requires a certain pressure to re-open (critical opening pressure) and also have a pressure where it will collapse (critical closing pressure) (Albert et al., 2009) which is less than the opening pressure. This suggests that, in order for a recruited alveolus to remain open, the system must have a certain minimum airway pressure that is greater than the alveolar closing pressure, but does not need to be as high as the opening pressure (Bates and Irvin, 2002). Therefore, the application of positive end expiratory pressure (PEEP) at or above the alveolar closing pressure offers a static level of pressure to prevent alveolar derecruitment (Bates and Irvin, 2002).

In vivo microscopy has been used to directly monitor the alveolar recruitment patterns in response to lung injury and varying levels of PEEP (Kollisch-Singule et al., 2014a, 2016). Such studies have demonstrated that higher levels of PEEP lead to increased alveolar recruitment and surface area with particular benefit derived from mechanical ventilation strategies that offer a higher mean airway pressure (Paw) (Kollisch-Singule et al., 2014a), which allows for improved intratidal recruitment without causing alveolar overdistension (Smith et al., 2015). The distension that occurs at the level of the alveolus and alveolar duct in response to the stress of the mechanical ventilator is the micro-strain and has been calculated as:

$$\text{microstrain} = \Delta L_P / L_{Pe}$$

where ΔL_P is the change in perimeter length between inspiration and expiration and L_{Pe} is the original perimeter length at expiration (Kollisch-Singule et al., 2014a). Using this calculation, it was shown that alveoli and alveolar ducts are both exposed to less micro-strain with higher levels of PEEP and P_{aw} (Kollisch-Singule et al., 2014a,b).

Although PEEP is critical to stabilizing both the alveoli and alveolar ducts (Kollisch-Singule et al., 2014a,b), it may cause impaired minute ventilation and subsequent hypercapnia (Acute Respiratory Distress Syndrome Network et al., 2000), and also may lead to a point when PEEP increases do not lead to any additional stability. This is the so-called 'best PEEP,' however there is no consensus over what 'best' PEEP is. The 'best PEEP' should be dependent on the underlying alveolar compliance, alveolar closing pressures, and time (Bates and Irvin, 2002; Albert et al., 2009), but the majority of PEEP titration strategies do not provide a micromechanical basis (Chiumello et al., 2014; Pintado et al., 2017; Writing Group for the Alveolar Recruitment for Acute Respiratory Distress Syndrome Trial Investigators et al., 2017; Beitler et al., 2019). Alveolar stabilization may occur at varying levels of PEEP depending on the degree and type of underlying injury (Carvalho et al., 2008). In one murine model of direct lung injury, the 'best PEEP' leading to alveolar stability was found to be 9 cmH2O (Andrews et al., 2015), whereas in another it was at 16 cmH2O (Kollisch-Singule et al., 2014a). In a rabbit model of lung injury utilizing synchrotron imaging to estimate the response of the terminal airway to varying levels of PEEP, Broche et al. (2017) found that increasing PEEP led to improved lung aeration and that terminal airway derecruitment increased markedly for PEEP less than 6 cmH_2O. The study also revealed that, although recruitment/derecruitment was attenuated with increasing PEEP, it was still present at PEEP levels as high as 12 cmH2O (Broche et al., 2017). Although creative methods have been used to determine the best PEEP of the lung using bedside measurements, these strategies do not account for the variability or physiology of the alveoli and alveolar ducts (Chiumello et al., 2014; Pintado et al., 2017; Writing Group for the Alveolar Recruitment for Acute Respiratory Distress Syndrome Trial Investigators et al., 2017; Beitler et al., 2019). For instance, using *in vivo* microscopy, alveolar recruitment and derecruitment were compared against the inflection points of the pressure-volume curves and overall found to have a poor correlation, with the exception of the deflation limb upper inflection point, which was found to be related to the derecruitment pressure (Dirocco et al., 2007).

In a porcine model of acute lung injury, a recruitment maneuver was performed followed by stepwise decreases in PEEP with CT scans at end-inspiration and end-expiration, as well as calculation of respiratory system elastance, stress index, and percentage of volume-dependent elastance (Carvalho et al., 2008). The method of injury (pulmonary injury by lavage versus extrapulmonary lung injury with systemically administered oleic acid) changed the pulmonary mechanics such that the extrapulmonary lung injury revealed greater stability at higher PEEP (Carvalho et al., 2008), consistent with prior studies comparing the etiology of lung injury to PEEP-responsiveness (Gattinoni et al., 1998). The stress index and percentage of volume-dependent elastance were meant to be used as surrogates for alveolar hyperinflation but were found to be useful only in the non-injured lungs, as there was no significant change to either when PEEP was reduced in the injured lungs (Carvalho et al., 2008). In the injured lung, recruitment and overdistension were found to occur simultaneously, with higher PEEP leading to recruitment of dependent lung regions but hyperinflation of non-dependent regions (Carvalho et al., 2008). The study determined that the PEEP that generated the lowest respiratory system elastance provided the best balance between lung recruitment and hyperinflation (Carvalho et al., 2008). But the study also served to demonstrate that strict reliance on pressure-volume curves may fail in the injured lung when there is co-existence of hyperinflation and collapse (Carvalho et al., 2008).

Oxygenation has also been found to be a poor marker of alveolar stability (Cereda et al., 2016b). In a murine model of direct lung injury and ventilator induced lung injury, strain (but not oxygenation) was found to predict propagation of lung injury (Cereda et al., 2016b). In a murine model of lung injury, alveolar stability was achieved at 9 cmH_2O with further increases in PEEP not leading to an increase in microscopic stability despite an improvement in oxygenation (Andrews et al., 2015). In another *in vivo* study, increases in PEEP from 5 to 10 cmH_2O led to only a transient increase in oxygenation despite a marked improvement in stability with increasing PEEP (Halter et al., 2003). This has been demonstrated in other studies in which repeated recruitment maneuvers are necessary to maintain oxygen saturation (Fujino et al., 2001) with higher PEEP at the conclusion of the recruitment maneuver being crucial to maintaining open alveoli and sustained improvements in oxygenation (Rimensberger et al., 1999).

ALVEOLAR TIDAL VOLUME

The low tidal volume (LVt) ventilation strategy has been embraced as a standard method of minimizing lung injury in patients with ARDS (Acute Respiratory Distress Syndrome Network et al., 2000), yet LVt has not demonstrated a persistent reduction in ARDS-associated mortality (Meade et al., 2008; Villar et al., 2011). This is likely because this strategy does not account for variability in patient disease, individual pulmonary mechanics, nor the alveolar micro-environment (Kollisch-Singule et al., 2018). A subsequent retrospective analysis of the LVt data (Acute Respiratory Distress Syndrome Network et al., 2000) revealed that the change in mortality was due to differences in driving pressure, or the pressure differential between inspiration and expiration (Amato et al., 2015). This study therefore demonstrated that when ventilator settings are adjusted to the lung compliance, an individual patient measurement, lung injury as measured by mortality may be attenuated (Amato et al., 2015). Even LVt can generate altered stress distribution in diseased state conditions such as emphysema (De Ryk et al., 2007) whereby stress concentrates in the injured alveoli, both at the perimeter of the weakened regions as well as the septal junction points (De Ryk et al., 2007).

LVt ventilation strategies in and of themselves do not lead to alveolar stabilization where alveolar stability is assessed by low *alveolar* volume change (Schiller et al., 2001; Kollisch-Singule et al., 2014a). The number of open and homogenous alveoli upon which a Vt is distributed is a greater determinant of alveolar stability and resulting alveolar Vt than the Vt set at the level of the mechanical ventilator (Kollisch-Singule et al., 2014a, 2016). Thus, factors that increase the number and openness of alveoli, such as increased P_{aw}, lead to alveolar stabilization (Halter et al., 2003).

In a murine model of direct lung injury, LVt (6 $mL{\cdot}kg^{-1}$) was set at the level of the mechanical ventilator but the alveolar Vt (dynamic change in alveolar cross-sectional area between inspiration and expiration) varied considerably (Kollisch-Singule et al., 2014a). The alveolar Vt was less dependent on the set Vt on the ventilator but more on the Paw (Kollisch-Singule et al., 2014a). High alveolar Vt was observed when P_{aw} was low, even though the lung Vt was held constant at 6 $mL{\cdot}kg{-}^{1}$ (Kollisch-Singule et al., 2014a). Alveolar Vt and micro-strain decreased only once PEEP was set at 10 cmH_2O or greater, as the associated alveolar recruitment allowed for additional surface area for the same Vt to be distributed across evenly (Kollisch-Singule et al., 2014a). This study demonstrated that even the LVt strategy may be deleterious when not applied to an open lung, but also revealed that higher Vt of up to 11 $mL{\cdot}kg^{-1}$ set on the ventilator can be associated with low alveolar Vt and micro-strain when combined with higher P_{aw} and a concomitant increase in alveolar recruitment (Kollisch-Singule et al., 2014a).

These findings are supported by a confocal study by Namati et al. (2008) in which alveolar size was found to increase as airway pressure increases, with a stabilization in alveolar number at ~25 cmH_2O. Following this, subsequent increases in pressure above 30 cmH_2O led not to additional alveolar strain, but to alveolar recruitment, with an increase in alveolar number but a decrease in alveolar size as measured by chord length (Namati et al., 2008). One hypothesis for this is that a separate population of daughter alveoli are recruited during times of increased pressure in order to re-distribute stress amongst the alveoli (Namati et al., 2008). In another alveolar study in which alveoli were exposed to inflation pressures as high as 40 cmH_2O, the alveoli were not observed to overdistend but rather to increase in number (Dirocco et al., 2007). This data must be interpreted with caution as 40 cmH_2O may be a supraphysiologic pressure for a mouse (Zosky et al., 2008), however, pressures in excess of 40 cmH_2O have not demonstrated structural lung parenchymal damage (Soutiere and Mitzner, 2004), and the lung mechanics ultimately returned to baseline, even after being stressed to 40 cmH2O (Zosky et al., 2008). Zosky et al. (2008) found that mice have a standard sigmoid pressure-volume curve up to 20 cmH_2O but that subsequent inflation to 40 cmH_2O led to a significant elevation in the slope of the pressure-volume curve, and a double sigmoidal pattern. One possibility for this finding is that there is a second population of alveoli that are not recruited until a pressure above 20 cmH_2O is reached (Soutiere and Mitzner, 2004) but begin to recruit at higher pressures, consistent with the findings of Dirocco et al. (2007) and Namati et al. (2008). This newly recruited second population of alveoli then inflate smoothly during subsequent inhalations, leading to an overall improvement in compliance and an increase in tidal volume (Zosky et al., 2008). The findings of these studies demonstrating more alveolar recruitment and less overdistension were corroborated by a large animal model in which the majority of lung volume change was secondary to recruitment/derecruitment, but not due to alveolar distension (Carney et al., 1999).

ALVEOLAR RECRUITMENT OVER TIME

The other component to mechanical ventilation that is seldom discussed but remains of critical importance for alveolar micromechanics is that of time. Alveolar opening and closing pressures are in part determined by both time and lung volume history (Bates and Irvin, 2002), as well as the open/closed status of the neighboring alveoli (Broche et al., 2017). In an *in vivo* study, alveolar recruitment was monitored over a 40 s recruitment maneuver (Albert et al., 2009). Despite keeping the recruitment pressure static, alveoli continued to recruit over the 40 s duration, suggesting that not only pressure but the time over which the pressure is held is vital to both alveolar recruitment and stability (Albert et al., 2009). Recruitment maneuvers, or pressure spurts over a short of time, in the absence of a sufficient PEEP allows for potential collapse of the alveoli that had just been recruited (Halter et al., 2003). In another *in vivo* study of alveolar responses to mechanical ventilation, brief increases in pressure with Vt failed to induce sustained alveolar recruitment, supporting the importance of the inspiratory time on alveolar opening (Kollisch-Singule et al., 2014a). Although medium to high PEEP attenuates some degree of alveolar collapse at end expiration, extended expiratory times led to alveolar derecruitment (Kollisch-Singule et al., 2014a). Taken together, the inspiratory to expiratory ratio plays an important role in alveolar stability with brief inspiratory times and extended expiratory times leading to increased alveolar micro-strain with wide amplitude swings between inspiration and expiration (Kollisch-Singule et al., 2014a).

The development of alveolar instability is not immediate and is dependent on the time alveoli are exposed to injurious mechanical ventilation settings (Pavone L.A. et al., 2007). In a murine model, alveoli that are initially exposed to injurious mechanical ventilation settings in the form of low PEEP with a high driving pressure did not immediately reveal instability (Pavone L.A. et al., 2007). Progressive injury, measured in the form of recruitment/derecruitment, took up to 30 min to manifest, with progressive injury demonstrated over time (Pavone L.A. et al., 2007).

The importance of time is not limited to the alveoli. The alveolar ducts in the setting of low PEEP with an extended expiratory time and brief inspiratory time can be injuriously distended with increased micro-strain (Kollisch-Singule et al., 2014b). Alveolar collapse in proximity to an airway can lead to heterogeneous parenchymal tethering which can impact airway stability and peribronchial stress (Ryans et al., 2019). This parenchymal heterogeneity can drive further injury, however, higher mean airway pressures, a function of both pressure and time, also have a stabilizing effect on the parenchyma (Roy et al., 2013; Ryans et al., 2019).

Yamaguchi et al. (2017) demonstrated in an *in vitro* model of non-uniform bifurcating airways that flow will divert to the airways of lower resistance. Variation in airway width affects both hydraulic and capillary pressures and therefore has a greater divergence pattern as compared with variations in airway length, which affects hydraulic resistance alone (Yamaguchi et al., 2017). The study demonstrated that a 15% change in width between two airways can lead to a 100-fold change in relative velocity through the airways when combined with high surface tension, but that lower surface tension has a protective effect on asymmetric reopening (Yamaguchi et al., 2017).

In a mathematical model of a heterogeneous airway network, Stewart and Jensen (2015) found that the air finger, which mimics the pressure delivered by the mechanical ventilator, halts its progression through the airway network at specific points. These points of stagnation occur where the ductal opening pressure is greater than the delivery pressure, and the airway network will not open until either the airway pressure or the time of this applied pressure is increased, which triggers further recruitment (Stewart and Jensen, 2015). Full recruitment of the airway network was found to be dependent on the airway pressure, the time a given pressure was applied, and airway heterogeneity (Stewart and Jensen, 2015).

ALVEOLAR EDEMA

One of the primary physiologic factors leading to ARDS is the accumulation of alveolar edema, which impairs gas exchange, deactivates surfactant, and leads to heterogeneous mechanical ventilation and ultimately a higher mortality (Greene et al., 1999; Warriner et al., 2002). Stress is concentrated between healthy

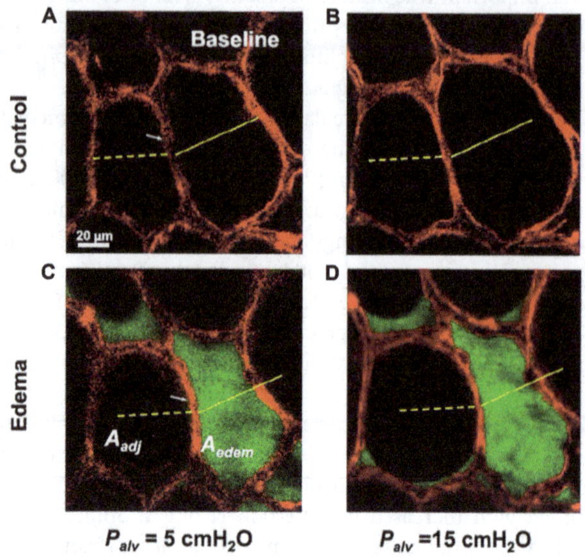

FIGURE 1 | Confocal microscopy is utilized to determine the effect a single liquid-filled alveolus has on a neighboring alveolus with changes in PEEP (black: air, red: alveolar epithelium). **(A)** The alveolar diameters at baseline at a PEEP of 5 cmH_2O **(B)** increase with a PEEP increase to 15 cmH_2O. **(C)** Introduction of edema (green: albumin) to the alveolus leads to a decrease in diameter of the liquid-filled alveolus but alters the trans-septal pressures such that the neighboring alveolus increases in diameter to accommodate. **(D)** The fluid-filled alveolus maintains its ability to expand with PEEP increases, suggesting the individual alveolar compliance is unchanged, whereas the neighboring alveolus loses compliance (Perlman et al., 2011). *Published with permission*.

and edematous alveoli (Wu et al., 2017). This stress level is proportional to the surface tension and can be exacerbated by mechanical ventilation (Wu et al., 2017).

In a study by Perlman et al. (2011) confocal microscopy was utilized to determine the effect of a single liquid-filled alveolus on neighboring alveoli when exposed to varying pressures. In that study, the edematous alveolus decreased in size at a PEEP of 5 cmH_2O but maintained its ability to increase in size in response to rising pressure, suggesting the individual alveolar compliance is unchanged (Perlman et al., 2011). But the presence of edema changed the *trans*-septal pressures such that the septum bowed toward the fluid-filled alveolus, mandating that the neighboring alveoli increased in size to accommodate, with a concomitant loss in compliance by approximately 24% (**Figure 1**) (Perlman et al., 2011). This phenomenon is well-supported by simulation models of injured and healthy alveoli which reveal that the recruitment maneuvers and pressures necessary to stabilize injured alveoli may lead to overdistension of the neighboring alveoli (Schirrmann et al., 2010).

Alveolar edema is also heterogeneous with alveolar flooding of the dependent regions of the lung and less flooding of the non-dependent regions (Wu et al., 2014). In an isolated perfused lung model with induced alveolar flooding, the permeability of the alveolar-capillary barrier increased over the study duration (Wu et al., 2014). Ventilation in all forms was found to be injurious, particularly with higher tidal volume, PEEP, and surface tension (Wu et al., 2014). This study therefore highlights the importance of protecting the alveoli and alveolar ducts from edema with protective mechanical ventilation before the injury has a chance to occur (Nieman et al., 2018).

In another isolated perfusion lung model of both local and global alveolar edema, the impact of surface tension and accelerated deflation on alveolar edema clearance was studied (Wu et al., 2017). In lungs with local edema alone, and thus a relatively normal surface tension, accelerated deflation led to release of fluid from flooded alveoli, allowing for redistribution of the fluid, and a decrease in flooding heterogeneity (Wu et al., 2017). In lungs with global edema, accelerated deflation also led to release of fluid from flooded alveoli, but the fluid redistributed to neighboring alveoli due to the higher surface tension, with no improvement in flooding heterogeneity (Wu et al., 2017). The importance of accelerated deflation on mucous clearance has similarly been described in a porcine lung model and represents a ventilator setting that may alter the lung micro-environment (Mahajan et al., 2019).

ALVEOLAR HETEROGENEITY

An injured lung induces heterogeneity at the level of the terminal airways which concentrates regional stress secondary to atelectasis, edema, and alterations in alveolar surface tension (Greene et al., 1999; Mertens et al., 2009; Schirrmann et al., 2010). This regional stress can concentrate alveolar strain to up to quadruple that of global strain (Rausch et al., 2011), propagating additional alveolar injury, apoptosis (Tschumperlin and Margulies, 1998), inflammation (Albaiceta and Blanch, 2011), and even membrane rupture (Vlahakis and Hubmayr, 2005). Given the degree of heterogeneity that manifests both at the regional and at the microscopic level in the injured lung, a given Vt will not distribute evenly but will rather preferentially distribute to the regions of increased alveolar compliance (Cressoni et al., 2014; Zhao et al., 2014).

Lung inhomogeneity is correlated with not only the severity of ARDS but also with patient mortality (Cressoni et al., 2014). The degree of lung inhomogeneity in a patient with ARDS can be quantified using computerized tomography scans and determining regions of stress-risers where there is an inferred regional amplification of forces (**Figure 2**) (Cressoni et al., 2014). Theoretically, when lungs are healthy and homogenously inflated, a delivered pressure will distribute across an open set of alveoli and the load-bearing elements will be exposed to the same degree of stress, such that the stretch elements will uniformly expand (Roan and Waters, 2011). In reality, stress is concentrated in regions of inhomogeneity where an open alveolus is adjacent to a collapsed or fluid-filled alveolus (Mead et al., 1970). Cressoni et al. (2014) calculated this stress multiplication factor to be an average of 1.9, concluding that these regions of increased stress are exposed to nearly double the applied transpulmonary pressure (**Figure 2**).

For the majority of patients, lung inhomogeneity decreases with increasing airway pressures but this is not true in all patients in which PEEP, lung inhomogeneity, and lung recruitability

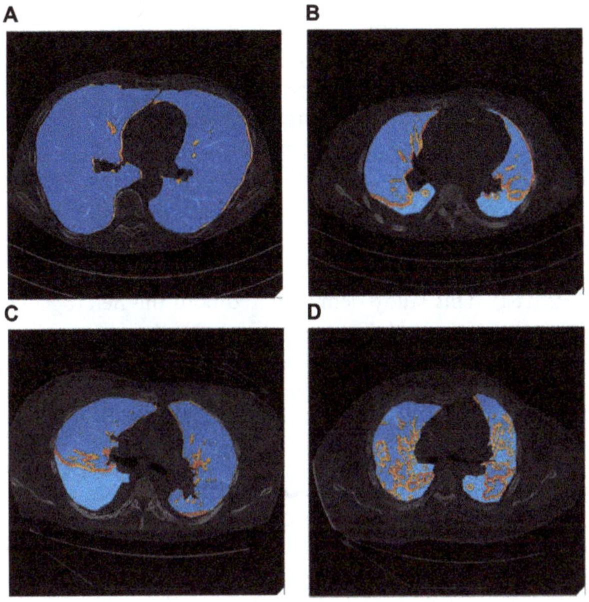

FIGURE 2 | Lung inhomogeneity can be visualized grossly on CT scan as evident in these false-color images in which stress-raisers are color mapped (blue = regions of mild stress-raisers, orange = regions of moderate stress-raisers, red = regions of severe stress-raisers). Blue intensity differences are due to overlapping between the underlying CT scanning images and the false-color map of lung inhomogeneities. **(A)** Represents a control subject with healthy lungs taken at end-inspiration. **(B)** a patient with mild ARDS, **(C)** a patient with moderate ARDS, **(D)** a patient with severe ARDS, all taken during the expiratory phase with a PEEP of 5 cmH_2O. The regions of stress-risers expose the neighboring alveoli to nearly double the applied transpulmonary pressure (Cressoni et al., 2014). *Published with permission.*

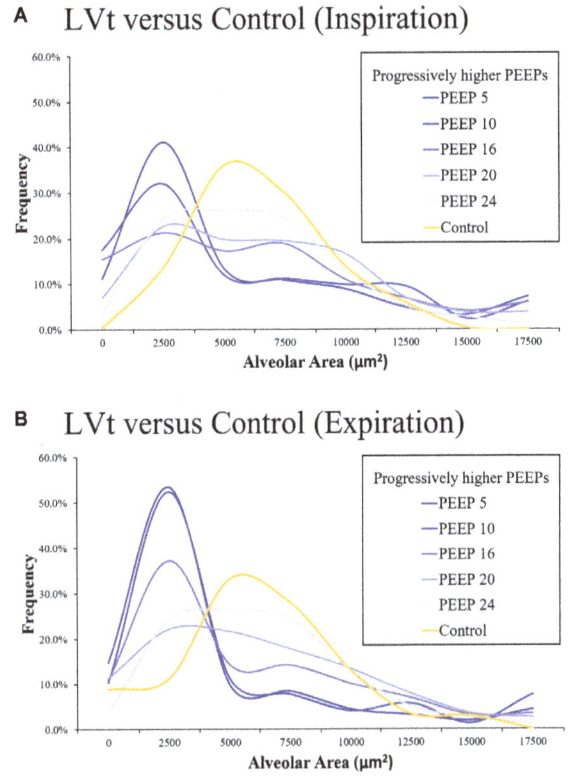

FIGURE 3 | Using *in vivo* microscopy, injured alveoli were ventilated with low tidal volume (LTVV) and evaluated by their response to increasing levels of PEEP and compared against a Control set of alveoli in a healthy, uninjured lung (orange). The distribution of alveolar cross-sectional areas was interpreted with the use of a histogram, with bin sizes selected to be 2500 μm^2. There is a rightward skew in the injured alveolar cross-sectional areas with a predominant population of small, collapsed alveoli that is more prominent at expiration than inspiration both at inspiration **(A)** and expiration **(B)**. With increasing PEEP, there is a decrease in the skewness and a more normal distribution of alveoli. Even at a PEEP of 24 cmH_2O, the population of injured alveoli never achieve the same normal distribution as the Control group. With increasing PEEP, it becomes apparent that there are two populations of alveoli: those that remain collapsed despite increases in pressure and those that are responsive to pressure increases, achieving an average alveolar cross-sectional area similar to the Control group (Kollisch-Singule et al., 2016). *Published and color scheme modified with permission, License 4703140582126.*

were not related (Cressoni et al., 2014). This is consistent with other studies which have demonstrated that the best PEEP is not always the highest PEEP (Kollisch-Singule et al., 2014a), particularly when patients are stratified according to whether the ARDS is pulmonary or extrapulmonary in origin (Gattinoni et al., 1998), and has prompted searches for an algorithm to calculate the best PEEP for an individual patient (Chiumello et al., 2014). These scaled PEEP maneuvers, however, do not consider the heterogeneity within the subunits of the lung where regional specific tissue elastance, edema, and atelectasis will have different responses to the macro-parameter changes that are set on the ventilator (Chiumello et al., 2014; Pintado et al., 2017; Writing Group for the Alveolar Recruitment for Acute Respiratory Distress Syndrome Trial Investigators et al., 2017; Beitler et al., 2019).

On a microscopic level using *in vivo* microscopy, injured alveoli were evaluated by their response to increasing levels of PEEP (Kollisch-Singule et al., 2016). Increases in alveolar homogeneity were observed with higher set PEEP and P_{aw}, and particularly in the setting of an inverted inspiratory to expiratory ratio (**Figure 3**) (Kollisch-Singule et al., 2016). Re-establishing alveolar homogeneity becomes more difficult as alveoli become more injured (Kollisch-Singule et al., 2016). Even with PEEP levels set as high as 24 cmH_2O, the population of injured alveoli never achieved the same normal distribution of alveolar sizes as compared with a Control group of healthy alveoli (Kollisch-Singule et al., 2016). With increasing PEEP, it became apparent that there were two distinct populations of alveoli: those that were responsive to PEEP with a mean cross-sectional area similar to that of the Control group and a group of non-responders with an average cross-sectional area markedly less than that of the Control group (**Figure 3**) (Kollisch-Singule et al., 2016). This may be one reason why trials that set an arbitrarily higher PEEP do not routinely demonstrate a lower mortality than those patients set with lower PEEP, as the setting adjustments did not target the underlying alveolar pathophysiology (Mercat et al., 2008).

High-frequency oscillatory ventilation (HFOV) is a ventilation mode that should be considered lung-protective with increased mean airway pressures and small tidal volumes promoting recruitment while minimizing lung injury and ventilation-to-perfusion mismatching (Kaczka et al., 2015; Herrmann et al., 2020), but it is generally applied with a single frequency, and has failed to demonstrate improved outcomes over conventional modes (Ferguson et al., 2013; Young et al., 2013). HFOV, like all ventilator modes, relies on inference to predict how changes in pressure, frequency, and flow lead to changes in the alveoli and alveolar ducts (Herrmann et al., 2020). Using a computational model of the human lung, Herrmann et al. (2020) demonstrated that HFOV applied to all lung sizes, but especially larger lung sizes, resulted in regional heterogeneity, and that increasing frequency led to increasing flow heterogeneity. This study therefore demonstrated that increasing frequency in order to lower tidal volume may propagate lung injury by promoting ventilation heterogeneity (Herrmann et al., 2020). Furthermore, these results highlight the importance of considering the individual patient pathology, with each set of lungs benefiting from a different frequency and change in pressure (Herrmann et al., 2020).

One ventilation strategy that has been developed to account for underlying heterogeneity is that of multi-frequency oscillatory ventilation (MFOV) (Kaczka et al., 2015). Herrmann et al. (2018) demonstrated that the use of two frequencies led to reduced acinar strain heterogeneity as compared with the use of either isolated frequency. Kaczka et al. (2015) elevated this idea by proposing MFOV as a method of applying several frequencies simultaneously, thereby taking into account the regional heterogeneity that exists in the premature and injured lung, and minimizing underventilation of one region and overventilation of another. Using a preterm lamb model, MFOV resulted in a more uniform distribution of gas flow to the alveoli with a lower distending pressure, improved oxygenation index, and reduced respiratory system elastance, as compared with traditional single frequency oscillatory ventilation (Kaczka et al., 2015).

In a murine model of lung injury induced by surfactant wash-out and moderate tidal volumes (Vt 12 $mL{\cdot}kg^{-1}$, PEEP 3 cmH_2O), the lung parenchyma was analyzed with CT (Cereda et al., 2016b). This study demonstrated that ventilator induced lung injury propagated from the induced regions of lung injury concentrically outward (Cereda et al., 2016b). This suggests the alveoli neighboring the injured tissue are subjected to increased strain and subsequent injury from recruitment/derecruitment (Mertens et al., 2009; Cereda et al., 2016b). In a parallel group of rats that received no lung injury but injurious mechanical ventilation by way of large tidal volumes and ZEEP (Vt 30 $mL{\cdot}kg^{-1}$, PEEP 0 cmH_2O), the ventilator induced lung injury was found to begin in the periphery and spread centrally (Cereda et al., 2016b). This heterogeneous injury pattern is likely due to dependent alveoli/alveolar ducts undergoing recruitment/derecruitment (Cereda et al., 2016b).

In a murine model of surfactant depletion, atelectasis was found to occur primarily in dependent regions of the lung but demonstrated that ventilator induced injury occurred in the non-dependent/non-atelectatic regions (Tsuchida et al., 2006), likely because tidal volumes were distributed to the regions of increased compliance (Gattinoni and Pesenti, 2005). Another murine study of healthy lungs mechanically ventilated with Vt 10 $mL{\cdot}kg^{-1}$ and ZEEP plus recruitment maneuvers used CT and MRI imaging to determine regional lung variations in response to mechanical ventilation (Cereda et al., 2016a). Ventilation with ZEEP led to heterogeneity of and an increase in regional fractional ventilation as measured by MRI, yet did not demonstrate macroscopic atelectasis on CT scan (Cereda et al., 2016a). This study demonstrated both the heterogeneous effect mechanical ventilation may have on the lung and also that subtle alterations in the micro-environment may not manifest on a macro-scale (Cereda et al., 2016a).

SUMMARY AND CONCLUSION

Investigating the response of alveoli to parameters set on the mechanical ventilator may help to determine protective mechanical ventilation strategies that are also broadly protective at the microscopic level and take the physiology of the various underlying micro-environments into account. The mechanical ventilation modes and settings that appreciate alveolar stability will ultimately be the ones that minimize ventilator induced lung injury and limit the mortality of ARDS. When considering alveolar micromechanics in the acutely injured lung, alveolar instability may be directly related to alveolar heterogeneity and high alveolar Vt.

Alveolar Vt are not determined by the Vt set on the mechanical ventilator but by the number of recruited alveoli available to accommodate that Vt and their heterogeneous mechanical properties. Thus, LVt set on the ventilator can lead to high alveolar Vt when imposed on a partially collapsed lung, but a high Vt set on the ventilator can lead to low alveolar Vt when expressed over a recruited lung with open, homogenous alveoli. In parallel, the pressure that alveoli are exposed to may not be as important as the duration of time those alveoli are exposed to a given pressure. A higher pressure when applied in only brief spurts may not improve long-term alveolar recruitment but may conversely cause harm with large amplitude pressure swings leading to increased strain. But a low pressure exposed over an extended period of time may be insufficient to open alveoli with high opening pressures (Albert et al., 2009). Thus, medium to higher pressures over an extended duration of time may be crucial to achieving alveolar stability. Finally, heterogeneity may be present on several size scales within the lungs, regions of the lung, alveolar subunits, and even the individual alveolar constituents.

CT scans can show regional atelectasis, edema and changes in tissue density to suggest unstable inflation (Cereda et al., 2016a, 2017; Xin et al., 2018) but is not specific enough to detect the immediate response of the alveoli and alveolar ducts to changes in mechanical ventilation (Cereda et al., 2016a, 2019). Electrical impedance tomography has demonstrated usefulness as a potential bedside tool to demonstrate changes in regional ventilation but may not be sensitive enough to detect subtle changes (Kaczka et al., 2015). Oxygenation has been demonstrated to be a poor marker of alveolar instability (Halter et al., 2003; Andrews et al., 2015). Pressure-volume curves have also been shown to be a suboptimal indicator of alveolar recruitment and derecruitment (Dirocco et al., 2007). The ventilator calculates the respiratory system compliance [Vt/(P_{Plat}-PEEP)] but does not partition out lung and chest wall compliance (Hess, 2014) where the lung compliance is impacted by alveolar stability (Pavone L. et al., 2007; Knudsen et al., 2018). The lung compliance as a single value may not account for the regional and alveolar heterogeneity associated with the injured lung (Kollisch-Singule et al., 2016), with discordant alveolar compliance even in adjacent alveoli (Perlman et al., 2011; Broche et al., 2017). Thus, many of the bedside maneuvers clinicians have available to guide mechanical ventilation alterations are poor mirrors of alveolar health and stability. With experimental data, this review highlights some of the known mechanical ventilation adjustments that are helpful or harmful at the level of the alveolus.

AUTHOR CONTRIBUTIONS

MK-S drafted the manuscript. JS, SB, PA, LG, GN, and NH critically revised the manuscript. All authors read and approved the final manuscript.

REFERENCES

Acute Respiratory Distress Syndrome Network, Brower, R. G., Matthay, M. A., Morris, A., Schoenfeld, D., Thompson, B. T., et al. (2000). Ventilation with lower tidal volumes as compared with traditional tidal volumes for acute lung injury and the acute respiratory distress syndrome. *N. Engl. J. Med.* 342, 1301–1308. doi: 10.1056/nejm200005043421801

Albaiceta, G. M., and Blanch, L. (2011). Beyond volutrauma in ARDS: the critical role of lung tissue deformation. *Crit. Care* 15:304. doi: 10.1186/cc10052

Albert, R. K. (2012). The role of ventilation-induced surfactant dysfunction and atelectasis in causing acute respiratory distress syndrome. *Am. J. Respir. Crit. Care Med.* 185, 702–708. doi: 10.1164/rccm.201109-1667pp

Albert, S. P., Dirocco, J., Allen, G. B., Bates, J. H., Lafollette, R., Kubiak, B. D., et al. (2009). The role of time and pressure on alveolar recruitment. *J. Appl. Physiol.* 106, 757–765. doi: 10.1152/japplphysiol.90735.2008

Amato, M. B., Meade, M. O., Slutsky, A. S., Brochard, L., Costa, E. L., Schoenfeld, D. A., et al. (2015). Driving pressure and survival in the acute respiratory distress syndrome. *N. Engl. J. Med.* 372, 747–755.

Andrews, P. L., Sadowitz, B., Kollisch-Singule, M., Satalin, J., Roy, S., Snyder, K., et al. (2015). Alveolar instability (atelectrauma) is not identified by arterial oxygenation predisposing the development of an occult ventilator-induced lung injury. *Intensive Care Med. Exp.* 3:54.

Bates, J. H., and Irvin, C. G. (2002). Time dependence of recruitment and derecruitment in the lung: a theoretical model. *J. Appl. Physiol.* 93, 705–713. doi: 10.1152/japplphysiol.01274.2001

Beitler, J. R., Sarge, T., Banner-Goodspeed, V. M., Gong, M. N., Cook, D., Novack, V., et al. (2019). Effect of titrating positive end-expiratory pressure (PEEP) with an esophageal pressure-guided strategy vs an empirical high peep-Fio2 strategy on death and days free from mechanical ventilation among patients with acute respiratory distress syndrome: a randomized clinical trial. *JAMA* 321, 846–857.

Bellani, G., Laffey, J. G., Pham, T., Fan, E., Investigators, L. S., and The, E. T. G. (2016). The LUNG SAFE study: a presentation of the prevalence of ARDS according to the berlin definition! *Crit. Care* 20:268.

Broche, L., Perchiazzi, G., Porra, L., Tannoia, A., Pellegrini, M., Derosa, S., et al. (2017). Dynamic mechanical interactions between neighboring airspaces determine cyclic opening and closure in injured lung. *Crit. Care Med.* 45, 687–694. doi: 10.1097/ccm.0000000000002234

Budinger, G. R., and Sznajder, J. I. (2006). The alveolar-epithelial barrier: a target for potential therapy. *Clin. Chest. Med.* 27, 655–669. doi: 10.1016/j.ccm.2006.06.007

Carney, D. E., Bredenberg, C. E., Schiller, H. J., Picone, A. L., Mccann, U. G., Gatto, L. A., et al. (1999). The mechanism of lung volume change during mechanical ventilation. *Am. J. Respir. Crit. Care Med.* 160, 1697–1702.

Carvalho, A. R., Spieth, P. M., Pelosi, P., Vidal Melo, M. F., Koch, T., Jandre, F. C., et al. (2008). Ability of dynamic airway pressure curve profile and elastance for positive end-expiratory pressure titration. *Intensive Care Med.* 34, 2291–2299. doi: 10.1007/s00134-008-1301-7

Cereda, M., Xin, Y., Goffi, A., Herrmann, J., Kaczka, D. W., Kavanagh, B. P., et al. (2019). Imaging the injured lung: mechanisms of action and clinical use. *Anesthesiology* 131, 716–749. doi: 10.1097/aln.0000000000002583

Cereda, M., Xin, Y., Hamedani, H., Bellani, G., Kadlecek, S., Clapp, J., et al. (2017). Tidal changes on CT and progression of ARDS. *Thorax* 72, 981–989. doi: 10.1136/thoraxjnl-2016-209833

Cereda, M., Xin, Y., Hamedani, H., Clapp, J., Kadlecek, S., Meeder, N., et al. (2016a). Mild loss of lung aeration augments stretch in healthy lung regions. *J. Appl. Physiol.* 120, 444–454. doi: 10.1152/japplphysiol.00734.2015

Cereda, M., Xin, Y., Meeder, N., Zeng, J., Jiang, Y., Hamedani, H., et al. (2016b). Visualizing the propagation of acute lung injury. *Anesthesiology* 124, 121–131.

Chiumello, D., Cressoni, M., Carlesso, E., Caspani, M. L., Marino, A., Gallazzi, E., et al. (2014). Bedside selection of positive end-expiratory pressure in mild, moderate, and severe acute respiratory distress syndrome. *Crit. Care Med.* 42, 252–264. doi: 10.1097/ccm.0b013e3182a6384f

Cressoni, M., Cadringher, P., Chiurazzi, C., Amini, M., Gallazzi, E., Marino, A., et al. (2014). Lung inhomogeneity in patients with acute respiratory distress syndrome. *Am. J. Respir. Crit. Care Med.* 189, 149–158.

De Ryk, J., Thiesse, J., Namati, E., and Mclennan, G. (2007). Stress distribution in a three dimensional, geometric alveolar sac under normal and emphysematous conditions. *Int. J. Chron. Obstruct. Pulmon. Dis.* 2, 81–91. doi: 10.2147/copd.2007.2.1.81

Dirocco, J. D., Carney, D. E., and Nieman, G. F. (2007). Correlation between alveolar recruitment/derecruitment and inflection points on the pressure-volume curve. *Intensive Care Med.* 33, 1204–1211. doi: 10.1007/s00134-007-0629-8

Ferguson, N. D., Cook, D. J., Guyatt, G. H., Mehta, S., Hand, L., Austin, P., et al. (2013). High-frequency oscillation in early acute respiratory distress syndrome. *N. Engl. J. Med.* 368, 795–805.

Fujino, Y., Goddon, S., Dolhnikoff, M., Hess, D., Amato, M. B., and Kacmarek, R. M. (2001). Repetitive high-pressure recruitment maneuvers required to maximally recruit lung in a sheep model of acute respiratory distress syndrome. *Crit. Care Med.* 29, 1579–1586. doi: 10.1097/00003246-200108000-00014

Gajic, O., Dara, S. I., Mendez, J. L., Adesanya, A. O., Festic, E., Caples, S. M., et al. (2004). Ventilator-associated lung injury in patients without acute lung injury at the onset of mechanical ventilation. *Crit. Care Med.* 32, 1817–1824. doi: 10.1097/01.ccm.0000133019.52531.30

Gattinoni, L., Pelosi, P., Suter, P. M., Pedoto, A., Vercesi, P., and Lissoni, A. (1998). Acute respiratory distress syndrome caused by pulmonary and extrapulmonary disease. Different syndromes? *Am. J. Respir. Crit. Care Med.* 158, 3–11. doi: 10.1164/ajrccm.158.1.9708031

Gattinoni, L., and Pesenti, A. (2005). The concept of baby lung. *Intensive Care Med.* 31, 776–784. doi: 10.1007/s00134-005-2627-z

Greene, K. E., Wright, J. R., Steinberg, K. P., Ruzinski, J. T., Caldwell, E., Wong, W. B., et al. (1999). Serial changes in surfactant-associated proteins in lung and serum before and after onset of ARDS. *Am. J. Respir. Crit. Care Med.* 160, 1843–1850. doi: 10.1164/ajrccm.160.6.9901117

Grune, J., Tabuchi, A., and Kuebler, W. M. (2019). Alveolar dynamics during mechanical ventilation in the healthy and injured lung. *Intensive Care Med. Exp.* 7:34.

Halter, J. M., Steinberg, J. M., Schiller, H. J., Dasilva, M., Gatto, L. A., Landas, S., et al. (2003). Positive end-expiratory pressure after a recruitment maneuver prevents both alveolar collapse and recruitment/derecruitment. *Am. J. Respir. Crit. Care Med.* 167, 1620–1626. doi: 10.1164/rccm.200205-435oc

Herrmann, J., Lilitwat, W., Tawhai, M. H., and Kaczka, D. W. (2020). High-frequency oscillatory ventilation and ventilator-induced lung injury: size does matter. *Crit. Care Med.* 48, e66–e73. doi: 10.1097/ccm.0000000000004073

Herrmann, J., Tawhai, M. H., and Kaczka, D. W. (2018). Parenchymal strain heterogeneity during oscillatory ventilation: why two frequencies are better than one. *J. Appl. Physiol.* 124, 653–663. doi: 10.1152/japplphysiol.00615.2017

Hess, D. R. (2014). Respiratory mechanics in mechanically ventilated patients. *Respir. Care* 59, 1773–1794. doi: 10.4187/respcare.03410

Jain, S. V., Kollisch-Singule, M., Satalin, J., Searles, Q., Dombert, L., Abdel-Razek, O., et al. (2017). The role of high airway pressure and dynamic strain on ventilator-induced lung injury in a heterogeneous acute lung injury model. *Intensive Care Med. Exp.* 5:25.

Kaczka, D. W., Herrmann, J., Zonneveld, C. E., Tingay, D. G., Lavizzari, A., Noble, P. B., et al. (2015). Multifrequency oscillatory ventilation in the premature lung: effects on gas exchange. mechanics, and ventilation distribution. *Anesthesiology* 123, 1394–1403. doi: 10.1097/aln.0000000000000898

Knudsen, L., Lopez-Rodriguez, E., Berndt, L., Steffen, L., Ruppert, C., Bates, J. H. T., et al. (2018). Alveolar micromechanics in bleomycin-induced lung injury. *Am. J. Respir. Cell Mol. Biol.* 59, 757–769. doi: 10.1165/rcmb.2018-0044oc

Kollisch-Singule, M., Emr, B., Smith, B., Roy, S., Jain, S., Satalin, J., et al. (2014a). Mechanical breath profile of airway pressure release ventilation: the effect on alveolar recruitment and microstrain in acute lung injury. *JAMA Surg.* 149, 1138–1145.

Kollisch-Singule, M., Emr, B., Smith, B., Ruiz, C., Roy, S., Meng, Q., et al. (2014b). Airway pressure release ventilation reduces conducting airway micro-strain in lung injury. *J. Am. Coll. Surg.* 219, 968–976. doi: 10.1016/j.jamcollsurg.2014.09.011

Kollisch-Singule, M., Jain, S., Andrews, P., Smith, B. J., Hamlington-Smith, K. L., Roy, S., et al. (2016). Effect of airway pressure release ventilation on dynamic alveolar heterogeneity. *JAMA Surg.* 151, 64–72.

Kollisch-Singule, M. C., Jain, S. V., Andrews, P. L., Satalin, J., Gatto, L. A., Villar, J., et al. (2018). Looking beyond macroventilatory parameters and rethinking ventilator-induced lung injury. *J. Appl. Physiol.* 124, 1214–1218. doi: 10.1152/japplphysiol.00412.2017

Mahajan, M., Distefano, D., Satalin, J., Andrews, P., Al-Khalisy, H., Baker, S., et al. (2019). Time-controlled adaptive ventilation (TCAV) accelerates simulated mucus clearance via increased expiratory flow rate. *Intensive Care Med. Exp.* 7:27.

Matthay, M. A., Ware, L. B., and Zimmerman, G. A. (2012). The acute respiratory distress syndrome. *J. Clin. Invest.* 122, 2731–2740.

Mead, J., Takishima, T., and Leith, D. (1970). Stress distribution in lungs: a model of pulmonary elasticity. *J. Appl. Physiol.* 28, 596–608. doi: 10.1152/jappl.1970.28.5.596

Meade, M. O., Cook, D. J., Guyatt, G. H., Slutsky, A. S., Arabi, Y. M., Cooper, D. J., et al. (2008). Ventilation strategy using low tidal volumes, recruitment maneuvers, and high positive end-expiratory pressure for acute lung injury and acute respiratory distress syndrome: a randomized controlled trial. *JAMA* 299, 637–645.

Mercat, A., Richard, J. C., Vielle, B., Jaber, S., Osman, D., Diehl, J. L., et al. (2008). Positive end-expiratory pressure setting in adults with acute lung injury and acute respiratory distress syndrome: a randomized controlled trial. *JAMA* 299, 646–655.

Mertens, M., Tabuchi, A., Meissner, S., Krueger, A., Schirrmann, K., Kertzscher, U., et al. (2009). Alveolar dynamics in acute lung injury: heterogeneous distension rather than cyclic opening and collapse. *Crit. Care Med.* 37, 2604–2611. doi: 10.1097/ccm.0b013e3181a5544d

Namati, E., Thiesse, J., De Ryk, J., and Mclennan, G. (2008). Alveolar dynamics during respiration: are the pores of Kohn a pathway to recruitment? *Am. J. Respir. Cell Mol. Biol.* 38, 572–578. doi: 10.1165/rcmb.2007-0120oc

Nieman, G. F., Andrews, P., Satalin, J., Wilcox, K., Kollisch-Singule, M., Madden, M., et al. (2018). Acute lung injury: how to stabilize a broken lung. *Crit. Care* 22:136.

Pavone, L., Albert, S., Dirocco, J., Gatto, L., and Nieman, G. (2007). Alveolar instability caused by mechanical ventilation initially damages the nondependent normal lung. *Crit. Care* 11:R104.

Pavone, L. A., Albert, S., Carney, D., Gatto, L. A., Halter, J. M., and Nieman, G. F. (2007). Injurious mechanical ventilation in the normal lung causes a progressive pathologic change in dynamic alveolar mechanics. *Crit. Care* 11:R64.

Perlman, C. E., and Bhattacharya, J. (2007). Alveolar expansion imaged by optical sectioning microscopy. *J. Appl. Physiol.* 103, 1037–1044. doi: 10.1152/japplphysiol.00160.2007

Perlman, C. E., Lederer, D. J., and Bhattacharya, J. (2011). Micromechanics of alveolar edema. *Am. J. Respir. Cell Mol. Biol.* 44, 34–39. doi: 10.1165/rcmb.2009-0005oc

Pintado, M. C., De Pablo, R., Trascasa, M., Milicua, J. M., and Sanchez-Garcia, M. (2017). Compliance-guided versus FiO2-driven positive-end expiratory pressure in patients with moderate or severe acute respiratory distress syndrome according to the Berlin definition. *Med. Intensiva* 41, 277–284. doi: 10.1016/j.medin.2016.08.009

Protti, A., Andreis, D. T., Monti, M., Santini, A., Sparacino, C. C., Langer, T., et al. (2013). Lung stress and strain during mechanical ventilation: any difference between statics and dynamics?. *Crit. Care Med.* 41, 1046–1055. doi: 10.1097/CCM.0b013e31827417a6

Rausch, S. M., Haberthur, D., Stampanoni, M., Schittny, J. C., and Wall, W. A. (2011). Local strain distribution in real three-dimensional alveolar geometries. *Ann. Biomed. Eng.* 39, 2835–2843. doi: 10.1007/s10439-011-0328-z

Rimensberger, P. C., Cox, P. N., Frndova, H., and Bryan, A. C. (1999). The open lung during small tidal volume ventilation: concepts of recruitment and optimal positive end-expiratory pressure. *Crit. Care Med.* 27, 1946–1952. doi: 10.1097/00003246-199909000-00038

Roan, E., and Waters, C. M. (2011). What do we know about mechanical strain in lung alveoli? *Am. J. Physiol. Lung Cell Mol. Physiol.* 301, L625–L635.

Roy, S., Habashi, N., Sadowitz, B., Andrews, P., Ge, L., Wang, G., et al. (2013). Early airway pressure release ventilation prevents ards-a novel preventive approach to lung injury. *Shock* 39, 28–38.

Ruhl, N., Lopez-Rodriguez, E., Albert, K., Smith, B. J., Weaver, T. E., Ochs, M., et al. (2019). Surfactant protein B deficiency induced high surface tension: relationship between alveolar micromechanics, alveolar fluid properties and alveolar epithelial cell injury. *Int. J. Mol. Sci.* 20:E4243.

Ryans, J. M., Fujioka, H., and Gaver, D. P. (2019). Microscale to mesoscale analysis of parenchymal tethering: the effect of heterogeneous alveolar pressures on the pulmonary mechanics of compliant airways. *J. Appl. Physiol.* 126, 1204–1213. doi: 10.1152/japplphysiol.00178.2018

Schiller, H. J., Mccann, U. G. II, Carney, D. E., Gatto, L. A., Steinberg, J. M., and Nieman, G. F. (2001). Altered alveolar mechanics in the acutely injured lung. *Crit. Care Med.* 29, 1049–1055. doi: 10.1097/00003246-200105000-00036

Schirrmann, K., Mertens, M., Kertzscher, U., Kuebler, W. M., and Affeld, K. (2010). Theoretical modeling of the interaction between alveoli during inflation and deflation in normal and diseased lungs. *J. Biomech.* 43, 1202–1207. doi: 10.1016/j.jbiomech.2009.11.025

Smith, B. J., Lundblad, L. K., Kollisch-Singule, M., Satalin, J., Nieman, G., Habashi, N., et al. (2015). Predicting the response of the injured lung to the mechanical breath profile. *J. Appl. Physiol.* 118, 932–940. doi: 10.1152/japplphysiol.00902.2014

Soutiere, S. E., and Mitzner, W. (2004). On defining total lung capacity in the mouse. *J. Appl. Physiol.* 96, 1658–1664. doi: 10.1152/japplphysiol.01098.2003

Stewart, P. S., and Jensen, O. E. (2015). Patterns of recruitment and injury in a heterogeneous airway network model. *J. R. Soc. Interf.* 12:20150523. doi: 10.1098/rsif.2015.0523

Tremblay, L., Valenza, F., Ribeiro, S. P., Li, J., and Slutsky, A. S. (1997). Injurious ventilatory strategies increase cytokines and c-fos m-RNA expression in an isolated rat lung model. *J. Clin. Invest.* 99, 944–952. doi: 10.1172/jci119259

Tschumperlin, D. J., and Margulies, S. S. (1998). Equibiaxial deformation-induced injury of alveolar epithelial cells in vitro. *Am. J. Physiol.* 275, L1173–L1183.

Tschumperlin, D. J., Oswari, J., and Margulies, A. S. (2000). Deformation-induced injury of alveolar epithelial cells. Effect of frequency, duration, and amplitude. *Am. J. Respir. Crit. Care Med.* 162, 357–362. doi: 10.1164/ajrccm.162.2.9807003

Tsuchida, S., Engelberts, D., Peltekova, V., Hopkins, N., Frndova, H., Babyn, P., et al. (2006). Atelectasis causes alveolar injury in nonatelectatic lung regions. *Am. J. Respir. Crit. Care Med.* 174, 279–289. doi: 10.1164/rccm.200506-1006oc

Vieillard-Baron, A., Matthay, M., Teboul, J. L., Bein, T., Schultz, M., Magder, S., et al. (2016). Experts' opinion on management of hemodynamics in ARDS patients: focus on the effects of mechanical ventilation. *Intensive Care Med.* 42, 739–749. doi: 10.1007/s00134-016-4326-3

Villar, J., Blanco, J., Anon, J. M., Santos-Bouza, A., Blanch, L., Ambros, A., et al. (2011). The ALIEN study: incidence and outcome of acute respiratory distress syndrome in the era of lung protective ventilation. *Intensive Care Med.* 37, 1932–1941. doi: 10.1007/s00134-011-2380-4

Vlahakis, N. E., and Hubmayr, R. D. (2005). Cellular stress failure in ventilator-injured lungs. *Am. J. Respir. Crit. Care Med.* 171, 1328–1342. doi: 10.1164/rccm.200408-1036so

Warriner, H. E., Ding, J., Waring, A. J., and Zasadzinski, J. A. (2002). A concentration-dependent mechanism by which serum albumin inactivates replacement lung surfactants. *Biophys. J.* 82, 835–842. doi: 10.1016/s0006-3495(02)75445-3

Writing Group for the Alveolar Recruitment for Acute Respiratory Distress Syndrome Trial Investigators, Cavalcanti, A. B., Suzumura, E. A., Laranjeira, L. N., Paisani, D. M., Damiani, L. P., et al. (2017). Effect of lung recruitment and titrated positive end-expiratory pressure (PEEP) vs low PEEP on mortality in patients with acute respiratory distress syndrome: a randomized clinical trial. *JAMA* 318, 1335–1345.

Wu, Y., Kharge, A. B., and Perlman, C. E. (2014). Lung ventilation injures areas with discrete alveolar flooding, in a surface tension-dependent fashion. *J. Appl. Physiol.* 117, 788–796. doi: 10.1152/japplphysiol.00569.2014

Wu, Y., Nguyen, T. L., and Perlman, C. E. (2017). Accelerated deflation promotes homogeneous airspace liquid distribution in the edematous lung. *J. Appl. Physiol.* 122, 739–751. doi: 10.1152/japplphysiol.00526.2016

Xin, Y., Cereda, M., Hamedani, H., Pourfathi, M., Siddiqui, S., Meeder, N., et al. (2018). Unstable inflation causing injury: insight from prone position and paired CT scans. *Am. J. Respir. Crit. Care Med.* 198, 197–207. doi: 10.1164/rccm.201708-1728oc

Yamaguchi, E., Nolan, L. P., and Gaver, D. P. (2017). Microscale distribution and dynamic surface tension of pulmonary surfactant normalize the recruitment of asymmetric bifurcating airways. *J. Appl. Physiol.* 122, 1167–1178. doi: 10.1152/japplphysiol.00543.2016

Young, D., Lamb, S. E., Shah, S., Mackenzie, I., Tunnicliffe, W., Lall, R., et al. (2013). High-frequency oscillation for acute respiratory distress syndrome. *N. Engl. J. Med.* 368, 806–813.

Zhao, Z., Pulletz, S., Frerichs, I., Muller-Lisse, U., and Moller, K. (2014). The EIT-based global inhomogeneity index is highly correlated with regional lung opening in patients with acute respiratory distress syndrome. *BMC Res. Notes* 7:82. doi: 10.1186/1756-0500-7-82

Zosky, G. R., Janosi, T. Z., Adamicza, A., Bozanich, E. M., Cannizzaro, V., Larcombe, A. N., et al. (2008). The bimodal quasi-static and dynamic elastance of the murine lung. *J. Appl. Physiol.* 105, 685–692. doi: 10.1152/japplphysiol.90328.2008

10

Hidden Microatelectases Increase Vulnerability to Ventilation-Induced Lung Injury

*Karolin Albert[1], Jeanne-Marie Krischer[1], Alexander Pfaffenroth[1], Sabrina Wilde[2,3], Elena Lopez-Rodriguez[1,3,4], Armin Braun[2,3], Bradford J. Smith[5] and Lars Knudsen[1,3]**

[1] Institute of Functional and Applied Anatomy, Hannover Medical School, Hanover, Germany, [2] Fraunhofer Institute for Toxicology and Experimental Medicine, Hanover, Germany, [3] Biomedical Research in Endstage and Obstructive Lung Disease Hannover (BREATH), German Center for Lung Research, Hanover, Germany, [4] Institute for Functional Anatomy, Charité, Berlin, Germany, [5] Department of Bioengineering, College of Engineering, Design and Computing, University of Colorado Denver, Anschutz Medical Campus, Aurora, CO, United States

***Correspondence:**
Lars Knudsen
Knudsen.lars@mh-hannover.de

Mechanical ventilation of lungs suffering from microatelectases may trigger the development of acute lung injury (ALI). Direct lung injury by bleomycin results in surfactant dysfunction and microatelectases at day 1 while tissue elastance and oxygenation remain normal. Computational simulations of alveolar micromechanics 1-day post-bleomycin predict persisting microatelectases throughout the respiratory cycle and increased alveolar strain during low positive end-expiratory pressure (PEEP) ventilation. As such, we hypothesize that mechanical ventilation in presence of microatelectases, which occur at low but not at higher PEEP, aggravates and unmasks ALI in the bleomycin injury model. Rats were randomized and challenged with bleomycin (B) or not (H = healthy). One day after bleomycin instillation the animals were ventilated for 3 h with PEEP 1 (PEEP1) or 5 cmH_2O (PEEP5) and a tidal volume of 10 ml/kg bodyweight. Tissue elastance was repetitively measured after a recruitment maneuver to investigate the degree of distal airspace instability. The right lung was subjected to bronchoalveolar lavage (BAL), the left lung was fixed for design-based stereology at light- and electron microscopic level. Prior to mechanical ventilation, lung tissue elastance did not differ. During mechanical ventilation tissue elastance increased in bleomycin-injured lungs ventilated with PEEP = 1 cmH_2O but remained stable in all other groups. Measurements at the conclusion of ventilation showed the largest time-dependent increase in tissue elastance after recruitment in B/PEEP1, indicating increased instability of distal airspaces. These lung mechanical findings correlated with BAL measurements including elevated BAL neutrophilic granulocytes as well as BAL protein and albumin in B/PEEP1. Moreover, the increased septal wall thickness and volume of peri-bronchiolar-vascular connective tissue in B/PEEP1 suggested aggravation of interstitial edema by ventilation in presence of microatelectases. At the electron microscopic level, the largest surface area of injured alveolar epithelial was observed in bleomycin-challenged lungs after PEEP = 1 cmH_2O ventilation. After bleomycin treatment cellular markers of endoplasmic reticulum stress (p-Perk and p-EIF-2α) were positive within the septal wall and ventilation with PEEP = 1 cmH_2O ventilation increased the surface area stained positively for p-EIF-2α. In conclusion, hidden microatelectases are linked with an increased pulmonary vulnerability for mechanical ventilation characterized by an aggravation of epithelial injury.

Keywords: microatelectases, alveolar interdependence, ventilation-induced lung injury, surfactant, blood-gas barrier

INTRODUCTION

The clinical picture encompassing refractory blood deoxygenation, decrease in respiratory system's compliance and bilateral infiltrates in conventional chest X-ray has been described originally as acute respiratory distress syndrome (ARDS) by Ashbaugh et al. (1967). For those patients suffering from ARDS, mechanical ventilation represents the decisive lifesaving therapeutic intervention. On the other hand, mechanical ventilation has also been identified to be an independent trigger for the progression of acute lung injury (ALI) through a process referred to as ventilator-induced lung injury (VILI) (Slutsky and Ranieri, 2013) and a substantial fraction of ARDS patients develop the complete picture of the ARDS during mechanical ventilation (Nieman et al., 2015). Moreover, mechanical ventilation in presence of surfactant abnormalities plays a central role in the development of an ARDS/ ALI (Albert, 2012; Rühl et al., 2019).

The underlying pathomechanisms involve abnormalities in alveolar micromechanics. Alveolar micromechanics can be defined as the dynamic changes of alveoli in size and shape during a respiratory cycle (Knudsen and Ochs, 2018). In healthy lungs the alveolar airspaces are stabilized by connective tissue elements located within the inter-alveolar septal walls as well as the intra-alveolar surfactant layer at the gas-liquid interface which reduces surface tension during expiration (Wilson and Bachofen, 1982; Knudsen and Ochs, 2018). In presence of a functional surfactant system the stresses are balanced and roughly homogenously distributed within the lung (Mead, 1961; Mead et al., 1970). During a respiratory cycle the strains and stresses acting on the inter-alveolar septa (e.g., the blood-gas barrier) are therefore minimized (Knudsen and Ochs, 2018). Direct or indirect lung injury results in inflammation, edema formation, and surfactant dysfunction that cause severe organ dysfunction. These pathologies introduce heterogeneous ventilation and abnormal alveolar micromechanics. Surfactant dysfunction results in intra-tidal alveolar recruitment and derecruitment (Schiller et al., 2001), an abnormality which, in presence of high surface tension, injures the epithelium and is therefore named atelectrauma (Slutsky and Ranieri, 2013; Cressoni et al., 2017; Rühl et al., 2019). The inter-alveolar walls of those alveoli which remain open are subject to increased strain and overdistension. This volutrauma further injures the very thin and delicate blood-gas barrier by rupturing the endothelial or alveolar epithelial cells (Dreyfuss and Saumon, 1998; Vlahakis et al., 2002; Cong et al., 2017). A more insidious mechanism of volutrauma results from the concept of alveolar interdependence (Mead et al., 1970; Makiyama et al., 2014). In this situation, microatelectases act as stress concentrators that impose tethering forces on surrounding inter-alveolar septal walls so that these areas of lung parenchyma are prone to overdistension and therefore volutrauma (Albert, 2012; Albert et al., 2019).

Ruptures of the plasma membrane of alveolar epithelial cells increase cytoplasmic Ca^{2+} levels which are responsible for activation of the cellular integrated stress response (ISR) (Dolinay et al., 2017, 2018). Stretch-induced ISR is initiated by Ca^{2+} dependent auto-phosphorylation of protein kinase RNA-like endoplasmic reticulum kinase (Perk). Phosphorylated Perk (p-Perk) moreover phosphorylates eukaryotic translation initiating factor 2α (EIF-2α), a step critical to switch off the protein biosynthesis machinery of the cell (Harding et al., 2000). If the ISR lingers on then cell death is initiated by selective expression of CCAAT/Enhancer binding Protein homologous Protein (CHOP) (Günther et al., 2012; Dolinay et al., 2018).

Intratracheal instillation of bleomycin is a common animal model of dose-dependent direct acute lung injury and fibrosis (Bonniaud et al., 2018). We have previously characterized the alveolar micromechanics of this model in detail during disease progression. The first abnormality observed after 24 h was a slight surfactant dysfunction linked with pathological alterations in alveolar micromechanics (Lutz et al., 2015; Steffen et al., 2017; Knudsen et al., 2018) where a decrease in airway opening pressure below 5 cmH_2O on expiration resulted in a derecruitment of alveoli. At a light microscopic level, further pathologies including edema formation or inflammation were virtually absent (Lutz et al., 2015; Knudsen et al., 2018). Moreover, at this very early stage of injury the lung mechanical properties, including organ scale tissue elastance within a range of PEEP levels from 1 to 5 cmH_2O as well as oxygen saturation, did not significantly differ from healthy subjects. Due to the fact that pressures needed to recruit alveoli were much higher than those needed to prevent their decruitment, computational simulations of alveolar micromechanics suggested that in this model there was only little intra-tidal alveolar recruitment and derecruitment during ventilation with PEEPs between 0 and 15 cmH_2O and a tidal volume of 10 ml/kg bodyweight (Knudsen et al., 2018). Instead, ventilation with PEEP below 5 cmH_2O was associated with permanent alveolar derecruitment (=microatelectases) combined with increased tidal alveolar volume changes indicating an increased dynamic alveolar strain. In addition, the open alveoli were characterized by lower individual elastance, a phenomenon explainable by outward tethering forces imposed by nearby derecruited alveoli. Based on these observations, we considered the bleomycin-injured lung to be at risk for VILI when PEEP is below 5 cmH_2O due to the presence of microatelectases. Since neither tissue elastance nor blood oxygenation differed from healthy controls there were no clinical signs of ALI at the organ scale. The microatelectases were therefore considered to be hidden.

In order to investigate the hypothesis whether these hidden microatelectases are linked with an increased susceptibility to VILI, bleomycin challenged lungs were ventilated with a PEEP of 1 (=microatelectases present) or 5 cmH_2O (=microatelectases absent) and compared to healthy controls. After a period of 3 h of mechanical ventilation ALI was unmasked in bleomycin challenged lungs if ventilated with PEEP of 1 but not 5 cmH_2O based on tissue elastance measurements, alveolar edema, ultrastructural signs of injury of alveolar epithelial cells and markers of ISR.

MATERIALS AND METHODS

Subjects and Study Design

The animal experiments were approved by the Niedersächsisches Landesamt für Verbraucherschutz und Lebensmittelsicherheit (LAVES, Oldenburg, Lower Saxony, Germany, approval number 17/2068) which house the German equivalent of an institutional animal care and use committee, according to the European Animal Welfare Regulations. In total 50 male Fisher 344/DuCrl rats (Charles River, Sulzfeld, Germany) aged 11 to 13 weeks with body weights ranging between 208 and 250 g were randomly assigned to a healthy group (H; n = 23) and a bleomycin-injured group (B; n = 27). The bleomycin group received intratracheal instillation of 4.5 U/kg bodyweight of bleomycin dissolved in 0.9% NaCl solution. One day later animals were further randomized to the subgroups which were either not ventilated (groups H/No ventil, n = 9, and B/No ventil, n = 8) or ventilated with PEEP = 1 cmH_2O (groups H/PEEP1, n = 7, and B/PEEP1, n = 9) or PEEP = 5 cmH_2O (groups H/PEEP5, n = 7, and B/PEEP5, n = 10). The animals were anesthetized by intraperitoneal injection of Ketamine (80 mg/kg bodyweight) combined with Xylazine (5 mg/kg bodyweight) and tracheotomized. Those animals assigned to "no ventilation" were directly subjected to bronchoalveolar lavage, and instillation fixation or vascular perfusion fixation as outlined below. Those animals assigned to ventilation groups were ventilated with room air, initially with PEEP = 3 cmH_2O, tidal volume = 10 ml/kg bodyweight and an inspiratory-to-expiratory ratio of 1:2. The respiratory rate was 90/min. The choice of these parameters was geared to previous studies applying similar volumes per minute and kg bodyweight during mechanical ventilation (Allen et al., 2005). The baseline lung mechanical properties were measured using derecruitability tests administered with a *newFlexiVent-System* (SCIREQ®, Montreal). These derecruitability tests included 2 deep inflations consisting of a continuous ramp of airway opening pressure from 3 to 30 cmH_2O over 3 s and an end-inspiratory plateau at 30 cmH_2O for 3 s. The deep inflations, or recruitment maneuvers, were followed by 10 repetitive forced oscillation perturbations (FOT) over a period of 4.5 minutes with the first FOT performed 2 seconds after the recruitment. The impedance spectra measured by FOT over a frequency range between 1 and 20.5 Hz were fit to the constant-phase model in order to calculate tissue elastance H (Hantos et al., 1992). The first tissue elastance value of this derecruitability test was referred to as H1 and reflected lung mechanical properties at the highest degree of recruitment. The mean of the last three measurements of the tissue elastance was referred to as Hs and reflected steady state conditions between 3.5 and 4.5 min after recruitment. The increase of tissue elastance over time after recruitment maneuver has been linked with progressive derecruitment of distal airspaces and was calculated as $\Delta H = Hs - H1$. After assessments of baseline lung mechanical properties, the PEEP was set to either 1 cmH_2O (PEEP1 groups) or 5 cmH_2O (PEEP5 groups). Anesthesia was maintained by inhalation narcosis using 1% isoflurane in room air combined with subcutaneous injection of 2 mg/kg bodyweight butorphanol (Torbugesic®). The tidal volume, inspiratory-to-expiratory ratio and respiratory rate remained unchanged. Derecruitability tests were performed every 60 min as described above with a PEEP, and FOT onset pressure, set according to the ventilation pattern (1 or 5 cmH_2O). After 3 h of mechanical ventilation a final derecruitability test was conducted at PEEP = 3 cmH_2O. Since the PEEP value has an impact on the lung mechanical properties (Knudsen et al., 2018) the measurements before and after the 3 h period of either PEEP = 1 or 5 cmH_2O ventilation could be compared between study groups so that differences in tissue elastance reflected the degree of lung injury. Monitoring of animals during mechanical ventilation was based on transcutaneous pulse oximetry using a rodent oximeter (MouseOx Plus, Rat Foot Sensor, Starr Life Sciences Corp., United States) and the oxygen saturation as well as heart rate was documented every 30 min. In addition the pressure in the ventilator cylinder (Pcycl) of the flexiVent system and airway opening at the expiratory limb (Pao) was recorded continuously in n = 3 animals per experimental group to describe the time course of the peak inspiratory pressure (PIP) during mechanical ventilation.

BAL and Tissue Processing

After ventilation, all rats were euthanized with Ketamine (80 mg/kg bodyweight) combined with Xylazine (5 mg/kg bodyweight, Rompun®) and the opening of the abdominal aorta. Except for 1–2 lungs per study group all were subjected to BAL and instillation fixation. For this purpose, the right lungs received three repetitions of a 4 ml bronchoalveolar lavage (BAL) using 0.9% sodium chloride (NaCl). Left lungs were fixed by instillation fixation (1.5% Paraformaldehyde, 1.5% Glutaraldehyde, 0.15 M HEPES buffer) at a hydrostatic instillation pressure of 25 cmH_2O. The lung volumes of fixed lungs were determined before a systematic uniform sampling for light and electron microscopic assessments was performed based on established methods (Tschanz et al., 2014). This sampling process resulted in 5–6 slices sampled for analyses at light microscopical level and at least 6 tissue blocks sampled for analyses at electron microscopic level. Samples were embedded in Technovit 8100

(Kulzer GmbH, Wehrheim, Germany) or epoxy resin (Epon®, Polyscience, Hirschberg an der Bergstraße, Germany) for light and electron microscopy, respectively (Mühlfeld et al., 2013). Within each study group the remaining lungs (n = 1–2) were fixed by vascular perfusion fixation at an end-inspiratory hold during PEEP = 1 cmH_2O ventilation using 0.1% glutaraldehyde and 4% paraformaldehyde in 0.2 M Hepes buffer solution. This "fixation from behind" allows assessment of the air-filled lung and therefore the effects of high surface tension on lung structure, e.g., the occurrence of microatelectases or intra-alveolar edema formation, are maintained. This fixative has also been used for immunolabeling since it maintains antigenicity and molecular identity of cells (Hsia et al., 2010). Perfusion fixed lungs were sampled for Technovit embedding and structural investigations as well as O.C.T. (optical cutting temperature) embedding for cryosections and immunolabeling of cellular stress markers.

BAL Analyses

For protein and cellular analysis, the BAL components were separated by centrifugation. The protein concentration inside the BAL fluid was analyzed by a protein assay (Pierce™ BCA Protein Assay, Fisher Scientific, Hampton, VA, United States) based on the manufacturer's instructions. Albumin concentration in the BAL was measured via ELISA (Rat Albumin ELISA Kit, Bethyl Laboratories, Montgomery). The BAL samples were diluted 1:1000 and compared to the standard curve according to the manufacturer's protocol. For cellular analysis, the BAL cells were separated from the rest of the BAL via centrifugation. Cytospin slides (Thermo Shandon Cytospin 3, Marshall Scientific, Hampton VA, United States) were prepared with 50.000 cells per BAL diluted in 100 μl phosphate buffer (PBS). Lymphocytes, macrophages and neutrophilic granulocytes were differentiated after staining the Cytospins with DiffQuik. Using Visiopharm® Software a systematic uniform area sampling was performed and at least 100 to 200 cells were categorized and counted using a primary magnification of 40×. Furthermore, we assessed the concentration of IL-6 within the BAL using an ELISA Kit (DuoSet® ELISA Rat IL-6, R&D Systems, Minneapolis, MI, United States). We utilized 96 well-plates and photometric measurements for cytokine concentration. Calculations were made with Magellan Software.

Design-Based Stereology

For stereology, lungs fixed by airway instillation were used. Initially we performed a volumetry based on the Archimedes principle for the whole left lung to obtain the volume of the reference space, the lung volume, for further structural assessments (Scherle, 1970). Embedded tissue for light microscopic analyses was cut into 1.5 μm sections by a microtome (Leica RM 2165, Leica Biosystems, Wetzlar, Germany). Afterward, a toluidine blue staining was performed. The slides for light microscopy were scanned (AxioScanZ.1) and 10% of the area of each slide was randomly sampled with the use of Visiopharm® Software to obtain between 60 and 200 representative fields of view per lung. The pictures were examined by using the STEPanizer stereology tool (Tschanz et al., 2011) or the newCAST Visiopharm software. Following a cascade sampling design (Ochs, 2006) non-parenchyma (nonpar) was initially differentiated from parenchyma (par) and volume fractions of these compartments (V_V(par/lung) and V_V(nonpar/lung)) within the lung were determined by point counting. Parenchyma was defined as regions of the lung that contribute to diffusive gas exchange so that this compartment included alveolar and ductal airspaces as well as interalveolar septal walls. Non-parenchyma included the conducting airways (bronchi and bronchioles), larger vessels (excluding capillaries and corner vessels within the septa) and the peri-bronchiolar-vascular connective tissue. In a second step the components within the non-parenchyma and parenchyma were further differentiated by means of point-counting. Taking the non-parenchyma compartment as reference space, the volume fractions within non-parenchyma of conducting airways (V_V(airway/nonpar)), larger vessels (V_V(ves/nonpar)) and peri-bronchiolar-vascular connective tissue (V_V(pbvtis/nonpar)) were determined. Within parenchyma, alveolar (V_V(alv/par)) and ductal airspaces (V_V(duct/par)) as well as interalveolar septa (V_V(sep/par)) were distinguished. Volume fractions were, in general, calculated by dividing the number of test points falling on the structure of interest (e.g., non-parenchyma) and the test points hitting the reference space (e.g., the total lung volume). Volume fractions were converted to absolute volumes of the structures of interest per lung by multiplication with the volume of the reference space. In addition, the surface area density of alveolar walls within the lung parenchyma (S_V(alv/par)) was determined by intersection counting based on established methods (Knudsen et al., 2010). The surface density was converted into a total surface area per lung (S(alv,par)) by multiplication with the reference volume, in this case the volume of lung parenchyma (V(par,lung)). For all structures of interest between 100 and 200 counting events per lung were generated since this has been shown to result in a sufficiently high precision of stereological estimators (Gundersen and Jensen, 1987). The mean arithmetic thickness of interalveolar septal walls (t(sep)) was calculated as a volume-to-surface ratio (Mühlfeld and Ochs, 2013).

Electron microscopy (FEI Morgagni transmission electron microscope, Eindhoven, The Netherlands) was used to investigate the health of the alveolar epithelium based on ultrastructural criteria (Dreyfuss and Saumon, 1998; Fehrenbach et al., 1999; Lutz et al., 2015; Rühl et al., 2019). The samples for electron microscopy were embedded in epoxy resin and cut into 80 nm sections (Ultracut S, Leica Reichert, Wetzlar, Germany). Six sections per lung were analyzed and 100 to 200 fields of view per lung were imaged within a systematic uniform area sampling process (Tschanz et al., 2014). Test lines were superimposed on each image and intersections of the test line with the epithelial basal lamina were counted. At each intersection, the covering epithelial cell was categorized as alveolar epithelial type I (AEI) or type II (AE2) cell. Based on ultrastructural criteria, the corresponding epithelial cell was further categorized as being either "intact" or "injured." The criteria for an injured epithelial cell were as follows: clearing and swelling of the cytoplasmic ground substance (in relation to the other cells in the septum), blebbing and fragmentation of cells, or denudation of the epithelial basal lamina. The surface densities of the basal lamina covered by the differently categorized epithelial cells were then calculated. By multiplication of the surface densities with the reference volume, in this case the total volume of interalveolar septa (V(sep,par)), absolute surface areas of the basal lamina covered by intact (S(AE1_intact,par); S(AE2_intact,par)) or injured AE1 or AE2 cells (S(AE1_injure,par); S(AE2_injure,par) could be determined (Lutz et al., 2015; Rühl et al., 2019). The light and electron microscopic images used for design-based stereology in this study are available on https://zenodo.org (Albert et al., 2020, DOI: 10.5281/zenodo.3738928).

Immunohistochemistry and Immunofluorescence of Cellular Stress Markers

Cryosections with a thickness of 5 μm were cut for immunohistochemistry of cellular stress markers (p-Perk and p-EIF-2α). Sections were pre-treated for 7 min at 37°C with 0.01% trypsin in 0.1% CaCl and repetitively washed with phosphate buffer (PBS). Endogenous peroxidases were blocked with 0.06% hydrogen peroxide in PBS. Primary antibodies (Rabbit anti p-EIF-2α, Cell Signaling Technologies #3398; Rabbit anti p-Perk, Cell Signaling Technologies #3179) were diluted 1:200 in PBS and used for incubation at 4°C in a moist chamber overnight. Staining with an isotype control antibody (Rabbit mAb, IgG, Cell Signaling Technologies, #3900) were used as a negative control according to the manufacturer's recommendations. Biotinylated mouse-anti-rabbit antibody was used as the secondary antibody. For detection, a streptavidin - HRP -DAB reaction system was applied and the color development observed. Counterstaining was carried out by means of hematoxylin. For quantification of the percentage of the alveolar surface area covered by p-EIF-2α positive cells a systematic uniform area sampling was performed on four sections per group to obtain at least 200 pictures. Test-lines were randomly projected on the fields of view and intersections of the test lines with brown or not brown colored surfaces were counted. The surface fraction of brown colored surface after p-EIF-2α (S_S(pEIF2α/sep)) staining was calculated as the ratios of intersections with brown surfaces and all surfaces.

Statistics

Statistical analysis of the data was done using *GraphPad Prism Version 7* (GraphPad Software, San Diego, CA, United States). A two-way ANOVA was used to take the influencing factors "pre-treatment" (Bleo) and "ventilation pattern" (vent: no ventilation vs. PEEP 1 vs. PEEP 5) or "duration of ventilation" as well as their interaction into account. In case of significant differences based on the two-way ANOVA the Bonferroni *post hoc* test for multiple comparisons and adjustment of the p-level was added. Correlation analyses were performed using Pearson's test. In general, *p* values below 0.05 were considered as statistically significant. The raw data measured during mechanical ventilation while performing the FOT perturbations were fit to the constant phase model. If the coefficient of determination of the model fit to the raw data (impedance spectra) was below 0.9 the data were excluded from further consideration.

RESULTS

Effects of Mechanical Ventilation on Lung Function and Mechanics

During mechanical ventilation oxygen saturation (SO_2) was measured as a functional parameter. No significant differences could be detected between the study groups both at the beginning and at the end of the 3 h period of mechanical ventilation. Initially, the mean and standard deviation of SO_2 were 98.8% (0.3%), 98.8% (0.6%), 98.8% (1.3%), and 98.6% (1.5%) for H/PEEP1, H/PEEP5, B/PEEP1 and B/PEEP5, respectively. At the end of the mechanical ventilation SO_2 data were 98.7% (0.72%), 97.3% (1.6%), 96.2% (2.5%), and 97.7% (1.3%) for H/PEEP1, H/PEEP5, B/PEEP1, and B/PEEP5, respectively.

Continuous recording of the airway opening pressure (Pao) describes the time course of the peak inspiratory pressure (PIP) during mechanical ventilation. Representative examples of the recorded Pao data are illustrated in **Figure 1**. In general, in all recorded datasets the PIP increased between the derecruitability tests and could be reduced by a deep inflation (= recruitment manoeuvre). The increase in PIP between derecruitability tests was most pronounced in B/PEEP1. However, in none of the datasets did the peak inspiratory pressures exceed 20 cmH_2O. Derecruitability tests were performed at PEEP = 3 cmH_2O both before and after the 3-hour period of mechanical ventilation. Since the PEEP level has significant effects on tissue elastance (Knudsen et al., 2018), these measurements were necessary to obtain lung mechanical data under exactly the same conditions for comparison between study groups. The data of the 4 study groups during PEEP = 3 cmH_2O ventilation are illustrated in **Figure 2A** (baseline) and **Figure 2B** (outcome after mechanical ventilation). H1 did not show any differences between study groups and the factor "Bleo" did not affect H1 at baseline according to the two-way ANOVA. However, the tissue elastance increased during the time course of the derecruitability test in particular in the bleomycin group. Hence, the level of tissue elastance values at the end of the derecruitability test (Hs), was slightly higher in the groups having been challenged with bleomycin (groups B/PEEP1 and B/PEEP5) compared to those which were healthy (groups H/PEEP1 and H/PEEP5) before starting either PEEP = 1 or 5 cmH_2O ventilation. Accordingly, the two-way ANOVA demonstrated a significant effect of the factor "Bleo" on Hs during PEEP = 3 cmH_2O ventilation ($p < 0.01$). No differences between the groups which were randomized to either PEEP1 or PEEP5 ventilation could be detected at baseline so that the study groups entered the different ventilation protocols with comparable lung mechanical properties.

After 3 h of mechanical ventilation the tissue elastance data in the B/PEEP1 group was significantly elevated above the other groups including B/PEEP5 as is shown in **Figure 2B**. With this regard, both bleomycin challenge ($p = 0.001$) as well as the PEEP level ($p = 0.009$) had a significant effect on Hs and these two factors demonstrated a significant interaction ($p = 0.028$). The study design also allowed within-group comparison of Hs before and after the 3 h period of mechanical ventilation. Using a student's *t*-test for dependent measurements a highly

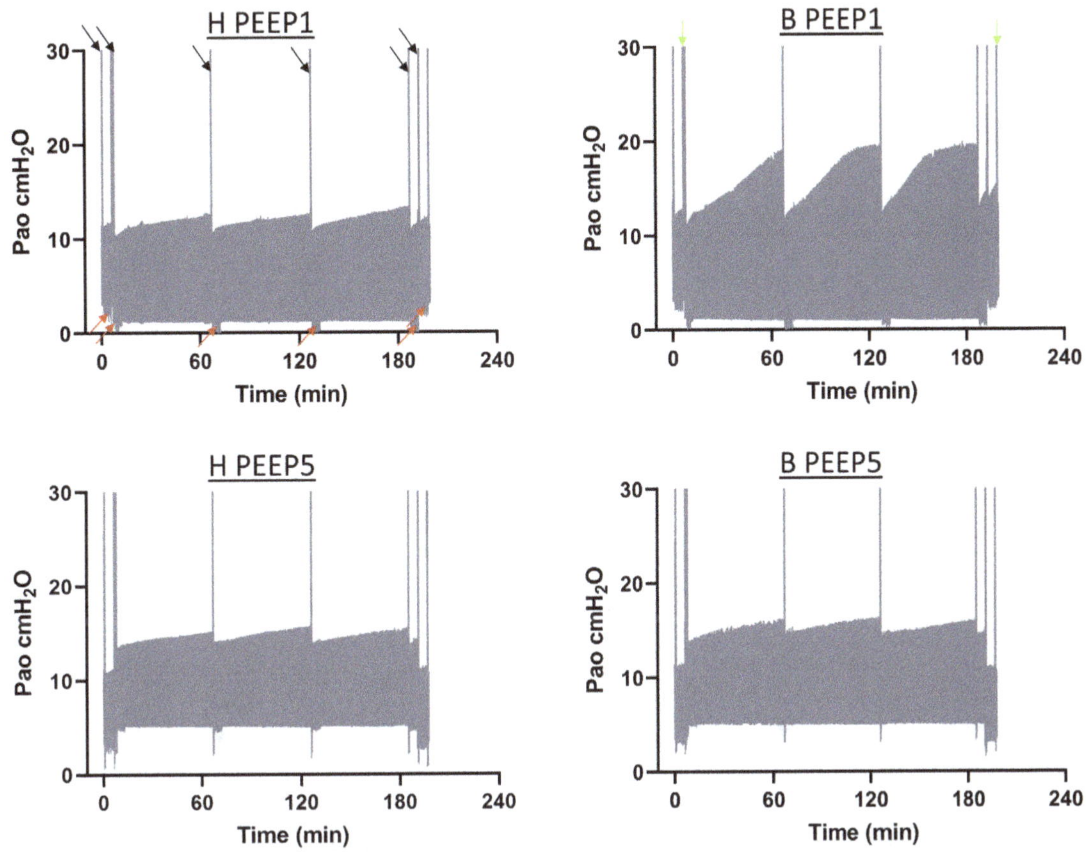

FIGURE 1 | The airway opening pressure (Pao) at the expiratory limb of the rodent ventilator were continuously recorded during the mechanical ventilation in $n = 3$ lungs per experimental group. The graphs illustrate representative examples of the range of Pao for the different study groups. The lower limit represents the PEEP level while the upper limit corresponds to the peak inspiratory pressures. The black arrows indicate pressure increases during recruitment maneuvers (=deep inflations) which were followed by repetitive measurements of tissue elastance using the forced oscillation perturbation (FOT, red arrows). The green arrows indicate recording of pressure controlled pressure volume loops with a stepwise increase of Pao up to a maximum of 30 cmH_2O (quasistatic PV-loops). Hence, the second bar is a combination of quasistatic PV-loops and deep inflations. The peak inspiratory pressures increased between the recruitment maneuvers in all study groups but did in none of the recorded datasets exceed 20 cmH_2O.

significant increase in Hs was observed in the B/PEEP1 group but not in the other three groups B/PEEP5, H/PEEP1 and H/PEEP5 (**Figure 2C**). The increase of tissue elastance during the observational period after the recruitment manoeuvre, ΔH, was significantly increased in B/PEEP1 compared to the other three groups (**Figure 2D**) indicating increased progressive stiffening in B/PEEP1 after recruitment compared to the other groups. Derecruitability tests were also performed every 60 min during mechanical ventilation with PEEP = 1 or 5 cmH_2O. **Figures 2E,F** illustrate the initial tissue elastance after recruitment manoeuvre, H1, as a function of time of mechanical ventilation during PEEP = 1 and 5 cmH_2O ventilation. Changes in the first tissue elastance measurement after recruitment manoeuvre have been shown to correlate with the degree of alveolar epithelial injury based on quantitative ultrastructural data (Smith et al., 2017; Hamlington et al., 2018). During PEEP = 1 cmH_2O ventilation the first tissue elastance after recruitment remained roughly stable in healthy lungs (H/PEEP1) but demonstrated a significant increase with time in the bleomycin challenged lungs (B/PEEP1) (**Figure 2E**, bleomycin effect $p = 0.003$, time effect $p < 0.001$, interaction < 0.001). Of note, both H/PEEP1 and B/PEEP1 started at the same level without any significant differences. On the other hand, during PEEP = 5 cmH_2O both bleomycin challenged (B/PEEP5) as well as healthy lungs (H/PEEP5) did not show a temporal increase in H1. The level of H1 differed between PEEP = 1 cmH_2O and PEEP = 5 cmH_2O ventilation in both B and H and this is the effect of the increased onset pressure the FOT started (Knudsen et al., 2018).

Taken together, during and after the 3 h period of mechanical ventilation, there is a significant increase in tissue elastance in bleomycin challenged lungs ventilated with PEEP = 1 cmH_2O. In the other study groups, tissue elastance remained comparably stable. In none of the study groups a relevant respiratory failure in terms of deoxygenation could be detected.

Effects of Mechanical Ventilation on Lung Architecture

Left lungs were instillation fixed and available for qualitative and quantitative structural assessments. Additional pairs of lungs per

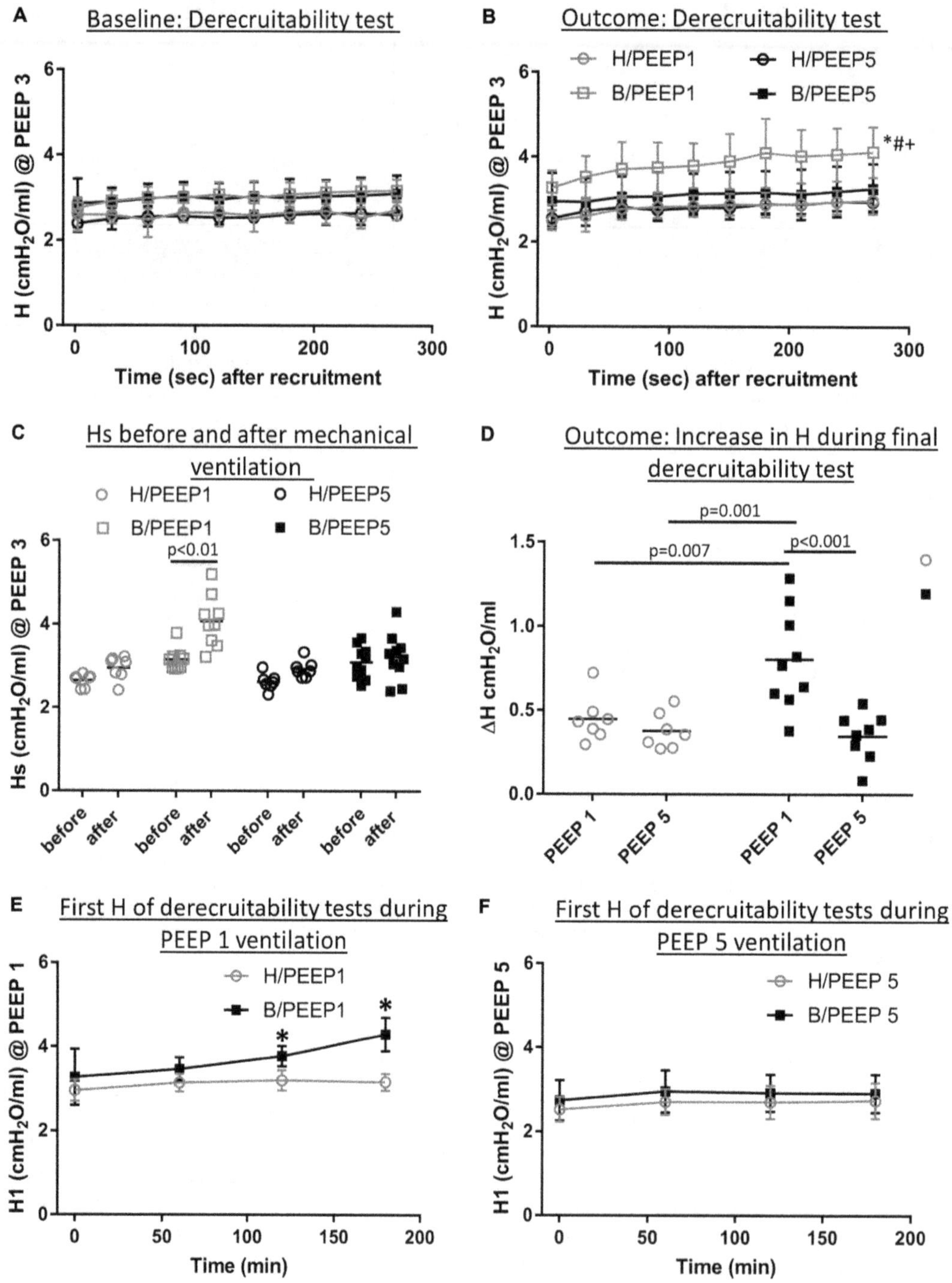

FIGURE 2 | Lung mechanical data. **(A)** Derecruitability tests at baseline: Tissue Elastance (cmH_2O/ml) was measured repetitively after first recruitment maneuver for 10 times before the onset of mechanical ventilation. H1 did not differ between study groups while Hs demonstrated significant Bleomycin effects. The data show that there was no difference present before subjects were assigned to the different ventilation protocols. Mean and standard deviation of at least seven independent measurements per group are given. **(B)** Shows derecruitability tests during PEEP = 3 cmH2O ventilation after 3 h of mechanical ventilation. Hs was significantly increased in B/PEEP1 compared to the other groups, including B/PEEP5. Mean and standard deviation of at least seven independent measurements per group are given. **(C)** Compares Hs data before and after mechanical ventilation in the different study groups. A statistical significant increase was only observed in B/PEEP1. **(D)** The increase in tissue Elastance (ΔH) was calculated from derecruitability tests after mechanical ventilation. Compared to the other groups, a significantly larger ΔH was observed in B/PEEP1. **(E)** The development of H1 is presented for H/PEEP1 and B/PEEP 1 during mechanical ventilation. Whereas H1 increased significantly ($p < 0.05$) in B/PEEP1, H1 remained stable in H/PEEP1. The same measurements are shown for H/PEEP5 and B/PEEP5 in **panel F**, where no increase can be identified in any of study groups. In **(E,F)** the mean and standard deviation of at least seven independent measurements per group are given. Statistics is based on two-way ANOVA followed by Bonferroni's *post hoc* adjustment of the *p*-value in all graphs except for C where a dependent *t*-test was used. The level of statistical significance was $p < 0.05$. Hs: tissue elastance at steady state (mean of last 3 tissue elastance measurement of derecruitability test), H1: first tissue elastance after recruitment, ΔH = Hs–H1.

study group were fixed by vascular perfusion at end-inspiration to describe microatelectases and intra-alveolar edema fluid at light microscopic level. These pathological alterations are usually not preserved in lungs fixed by airway instillation (Hsia et al., 2010; Lutz et al., 2015). Representative images of instillation fixed lungs are illustrated in **Figures 3**, **4D** while images of perfusion fixed lungs are shown in **Figure 5D**. The healthy lungs, independent of ventilation pattern, did not show any evidence of increased numbers of inflammatory cells within the airspaces or the peri-bronchiolar-vascular connective tissue compartment (**Figure 3**). The interalveolar septa were not thickened and the distal airspaces were open. The bleomycin-challenged lungs which were either not mechanically ventilated or ventilated with PEEP 5 cmH_2O looked very similar to the healthy lungs (**Figure 3**). In contrast, PEEP = 1 cmH_2O ventilation of bleomycin-challenged lungs was characterized by more inflammatory cells within the distal airspaces as well as in the peri-bronchiolar-vascular connective tissue compartment. In addition, in some areas of lung parenchyma, the interalveolar septal walls appeared to be thickened (**Figure 3**).

Instillation fixed lungs were subjected to stereological analyses at light microscopic level. These data are presented in **Table 1** and illustrated in **Figure 4**. The total lung volume (V(lung)) was not affected by bleomycin or the mechanical ventilation pattern. On the contrary, the total volume of lung parenchyma (V(par,lung)) as well as non-parenchyma (V(nonpar,lung)) per lung demonstrated significant bleomycin effects: V(par,lung) was reduced while V(nonpar,lung) was increased. Within the bleomycin-treated lungs, the Bonferroni *post hoc* comparison demonstrated significantly lower V(par,lung) in B/PEEP1 compared to B/No ventil (p = 0.047). On the other hand V(nonpar,lung) was largest in B/PEEP1 but no significant differences from B or B/PEEP5 were identified. The parenchyma was divided into the compartments of alveolar airspaces (V(alv,par)), ductal airspaces (V(duct,par)) and interalveolar septa (V(sep,par)). With regard to V(alv,par) a significant effect of the factor "bleomycin treatment" could be identified resulting in a decrease. Within the bleomycin challenged groups a significant reduction of V(alv,par) could be identified in B/PEEP1 compared to B/No ventil while no significant difference existed between B/PEEP5 and B/No ventil or B/PEEP1 (**Figure 4A**). In a further step, the alveolar surface area (S(alv,par)) within the lung was determined and this parameter was affected by both the bleomycin treatment and the mechanical ventilation pattern. S(alv,par) was reduced by bleomycin pre-treatment and mechanical ventilation resulted in an additional reduction, which was most prominent in B/PEEP1. Compared to B/No ventil, S(alv,par) was significantly reduced in B/PEEP1 (p = 0.014) but also in B/PEEP5 (p = 0.033). The arithmetic mean thickness of interalveolar septa [t(sep)] was calculated as a volume-to-surface ratio and data are illustrated in **Figure 4B**. While the bleomycin-challenge itself had a significant effect on this parameter, the Bonferroni test revealed that t(sep) was significantly higher in B/PEEP1 compared to B/PEEP5 (p = 0.022), indicating a ventilation effect on this parameter.

The different compartments of non-parenchyma were categorized into the total volumes of vessels (V(ves,nonpar)), conducting airways (V(airway,nonpar)) and peri-bronchiolo-vascular connective tissue (V(pbvtis,nonpar)). V(ves,nonpar) and V(airway,nonpar) did not show any significant differences. However, V(pbvtis,nonpar) was clearly effected by both the bleomycin-challenge and the mechanical ventilation pattern (**Figure 4C**). Prior to mechanical ventilation, bleomycin pre-treatment (group B/No ventil) resulted in a near doubling of V(pbvtiss,nonpar) compared to healthy controls (group H/No ventil). Mechanical ventilation with PEEP1 in addition to bleomycin challenge (B/PEEP1) resulted in a further increase so that V(pbvtiss,nonpar) became significantly larger compared to B/No ventil (p = 0.015) but also compared to B/PEEP5 (p = 0.003). A closer look at the peri-bronchiolo-vascular connective tissue compartment demonstrated an increased infiltration with inflammatory cells but also very prominent, enlarged lymphatic vessels in B/PEEP1 in comparison to the other study groups (**Figure 4D**). The adjacent interalveolar septa of infiltrated and thickened connective tissue cuffs around airways and vessels appeared to be thickened (**Figure 4D**). In healthy lungs, mechanical ventilation did not have any effects on the peri-bronchiolo-vascular connective tissue compartment.

Taken together, low PEEP mechanical ventilation of bleomycin pre-treated lungs resulted in an additional decrease in the volume of alveolar airspaces and surface area of alveoli. The interalveolar septa were thickest and the total volume of peri-bronchiolo-vascular connective tissue largest in B/PEEP1.

BAL Measurements

The right lungs were subjected to broncho-alveolar lavage. Altogether 12 ml of 0.9% NaCl solution were instilled per lung and between 10 and 11 ml were recovered. **Figures 5A–C** illustrates the data obtained from the BAL measurements. While the total numbers of alveolar macrophages and lymphocytes per BAL did not differ between the study groups (data not shown), the number of neutrophilic granulocytes was markedly increased and was influenced by both the bleomycin pre-treatment ($p < 0.001$) and the mechanical ventilation pattern ($p = 0.003$). No significant interaction between the factors bleomycin pre-treatment and PEEP level were observed ($p = 0.131$). Within the healthy lungs, however, the mechanical ventilation did not show statistical significant differences. In bleomycin pre-treated lungs on the other hand highest numbers of neutrophilic granulocytes were found in B/PEEP1 and this was statistically significant compared to both B/No ventil and B/PEEP5 (**Figure 5A**). Hence, PEEP 1 ventilation but not PEEP 5 ventilation resulted in an additional increase in neutrophilic granulocytes after bleomycin pre-treatment.

The levels of protein (**Figure 5B**) and albumin (**Figure 5C**) were measured within the BAL as surrogate markers for leakage of the blood-gas barrier. Bleomycin pre-treatment ($p \leq 0.001$) and PEEP level ($p < 0.001$) had significant effects on protein and albumin levels and also demonstrated relevant interactions with regard to these parameters ($p < 0.001$). Bleomycin challenge without ventilation significantly increased protein ($p < 0.001$) and albumin ($p < 0.001$) levels. Investigation of the effects of the ventilation pattern within the bleomycin challenged group showed elevated BAL protein in B/PEEP1 compared to both

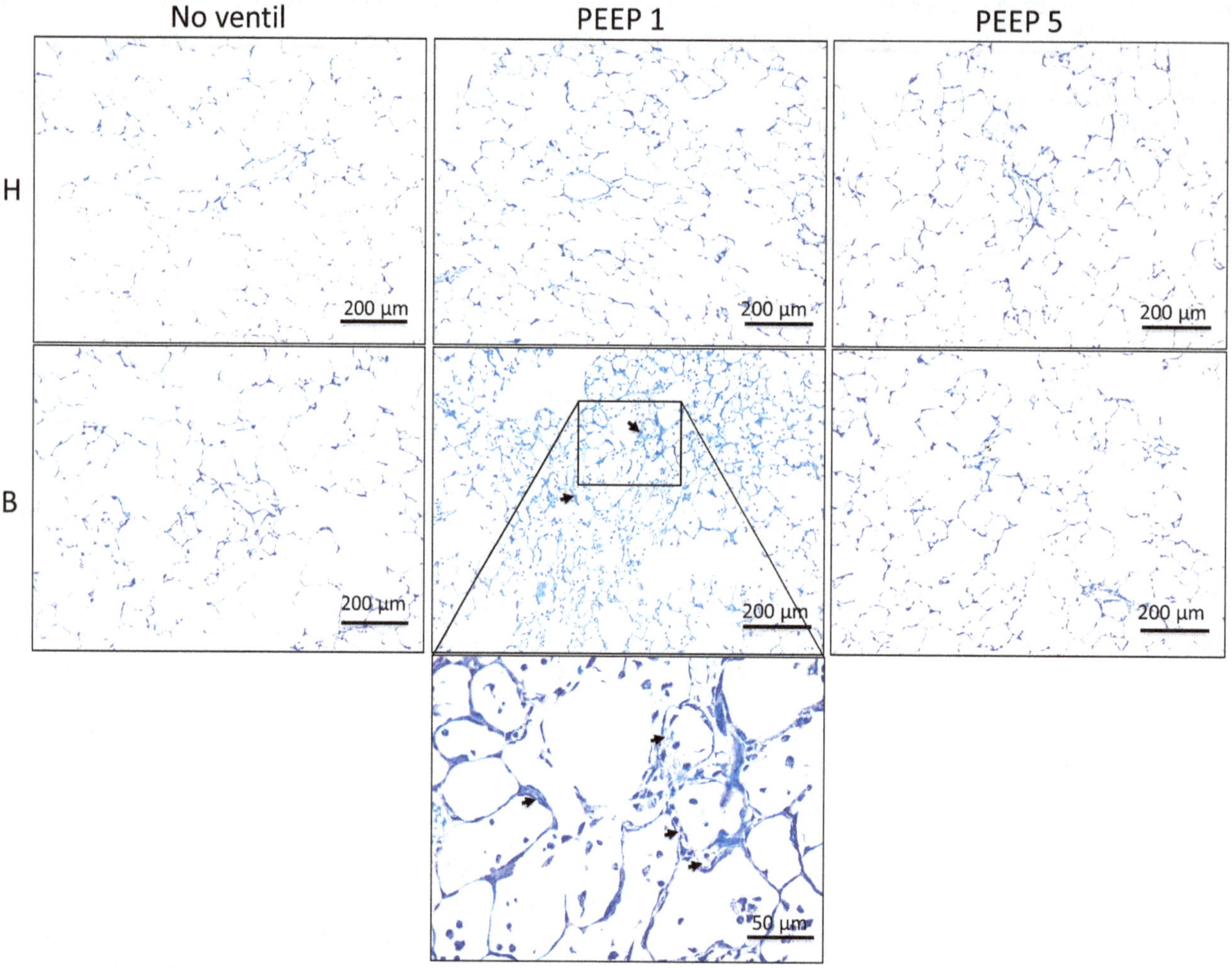

FIGURE 3 | Representative toluidine blue stained light microscopic images are shown after airway instillation fixation at low magnification. Septal walls are slim and infiltrates are missing in H with and without mechanical ventilation. Inflammatory cells and thickened inter-alveolar septal walls (arrows) can be seen in B/ PEEP1 but not in B/PEEP5.

B/No ventil ($p < 0.001$) and B/PEEP5 ($p < 0.001$). Within the healthy lungs BAL protein trended higher in H/PEEP1 compared to H ($p = 0.069$). The BAL albumin level behaved differently from the protein level (**Figure 5C**). PEEP 1 ventilation after bleomycin challenge did not result in an additional increase in albumin level so that there are no statistical differences between B and B/PEEP1. On the other hand, B/PEEP5 had significant lower albumin levels compared to B ($p < 0.001$) and B/PEEP1 ($p < 0.001$). Within initially healthy lungs, PEEP = 1 cmH_2O ventilation resulted in a significant increase in albumin levels ($p = 0.01$), a finding which could not be observed after PEEP = 5 cmH_2O ventilation. Measurements of IL-6 were performed in the BAL since this parameter has been shown to correlate with the outcome in an animal model of VILI (Szabari et al., 2019). While in healthy control, the level of IL-6 was underneath the detection level, mechanical ventilation resulted in an increase which was more pronounced in H/PEEP1 [mean = 522 (SD = 238) pg/ml] than in H/PEEP5 [mean = 179 (SD = 115) pg/ml]. Bleomycin challenge resulted in measureable IL-6 levels in BAL [mean = 123 (SD = 54) pg/ml] which increased in B/PEEP1 [mean = 779 (SD = 246) pg/ml] and B/PEEP5 [mean = 959 (SD = 739) pg/ml] groups to a similar degree.

Taken together, PEEP1 but not PEEP5 ventilation of bleomycin pre-injured lungs aggravated markers of lung injury including the number of BAL granulocytes and BAL protein level. From previous studies it is known that the volume of edema fluid one day after bleomycin-induced lung injury is increased based on electron microscopic assessments but cannot be detected at light microscopic level since the protein rich edema covering the alveolar walls is too thin and beyond light microscopic resolution (Knudsen et al., 2018). In the present study we investigated lungs at light microscopic level which were fixed during PEEP = 1 cmH_2O ventilation at an end-inspiratory arrest by vascular perfusion fixation (**Figure 5D**). The goal was to identify microatelectases and intraalveolar edema fluid. Healthy lungs, independent of mechanical ventilation did not show any signs of microatelectases or intraalveolar edema. On the other hand, all bleomycin pre-treated lungs during PEEP = 1 cmH_2O

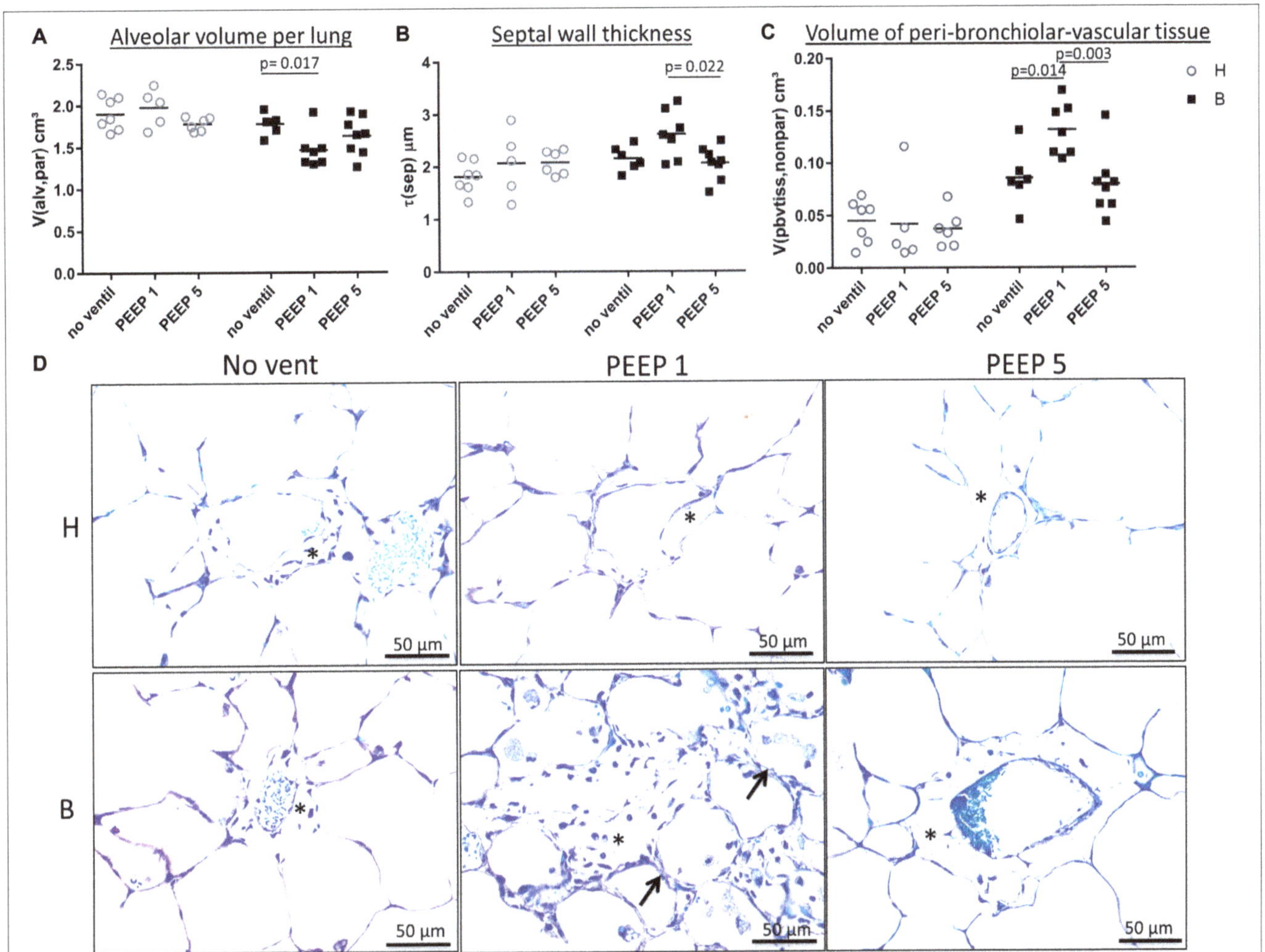

FIGURE 4 | Light microscopical stereological data and interstitial edema. **(A)** The absolute volume of alveolar airspaces (V(alv,par) was reduced in group B compared to group H. Within group B data were lowest in B/PEEP1. **(B)** Within group B a significant effect of ventilation on arithmetic mean septal wall thickness was observed resulting in an increase in B/PEEP1 compared to B/PEEP5. **(C)** Bleomycin pre-treatment resulted in an increase in the volume of peri-bronchiolar vascular connective tissue (V(pbvtis,nonpar)). Within group B a significant ventilation effect could be observed resulting in largest values in B/PEEP1 compared to both B/no ventil as well as B/PEEP5. Statistics were made with the use of two-way ANOVA and Bonferroni's multiple comparisons. **(D)** High magnification, representative light microscopic images after airway instillation fixation are shown, stained with toluidine blue. Healthy lungs show only marginal peri-bronchiolar-vascular connective tissue (asterisks), whereas B/PEEP1 reveals cellular and edema influx into the non-parenchymal connective tissue compared with all other groups, which is further confirmed by our quantitative measurements in 3C. Also, thickened septal walls were observed in B/PEEP1 (arrows).

ventilation demonstrated end-inspiratory microatelectases as a common finding. No intraalveolar edema fluid could be detected in lungs after PEEP5 ventilation or those which were not mechanically ventilated. After PEEP1 ventilation, however, there were traces of intraalveolar edema fluid visible in some regions at light microscopic level and these were in general co-located with areas of microatelectases. Hence, mechanical ventilation of bleomycin pre-injured lungs with PEEP1 but not with PEEP5 seems to aggravate intraalveolar edema fluid so that it becomes clearly detectable at light microscopic level.

Injury of the Blood-Gas Barrier

Microatelectases have been suggested to function as stress concentrators and might induce volutrauma in neighboring interalveolar septa during mechanical ventilation via alveolar interdependence. This mechanism would result in ruptures of the cellular components of the blood-gas barrier (Cong et al., 2017) followed by leakage. Accordingly, the blood-gas barrier was investigated for ultrastructural signs of injury in the present study. Representative micrographs are provided in **Figure 6**. Signs of injury of the alveolar epithelial type 1 (AE1) cells were found in all ventilated lungs and, in addition, in unventilated bleomycin treated lungs. Except for group B/PEEP1 the injury was characterized by a swelling of AE1 cells combined with a clearing of their cytoplasmic ground substance. In group B/No ventil this was the typical ultrastructural presentation of the injury of the blood-gas barrier and more severe signs of injury were hardly present, reproducing previous observations in this animal model (Lutz et al., 2015). In B/PEEP1, however, complete denudations of the epithelial basal lamina were observed quite

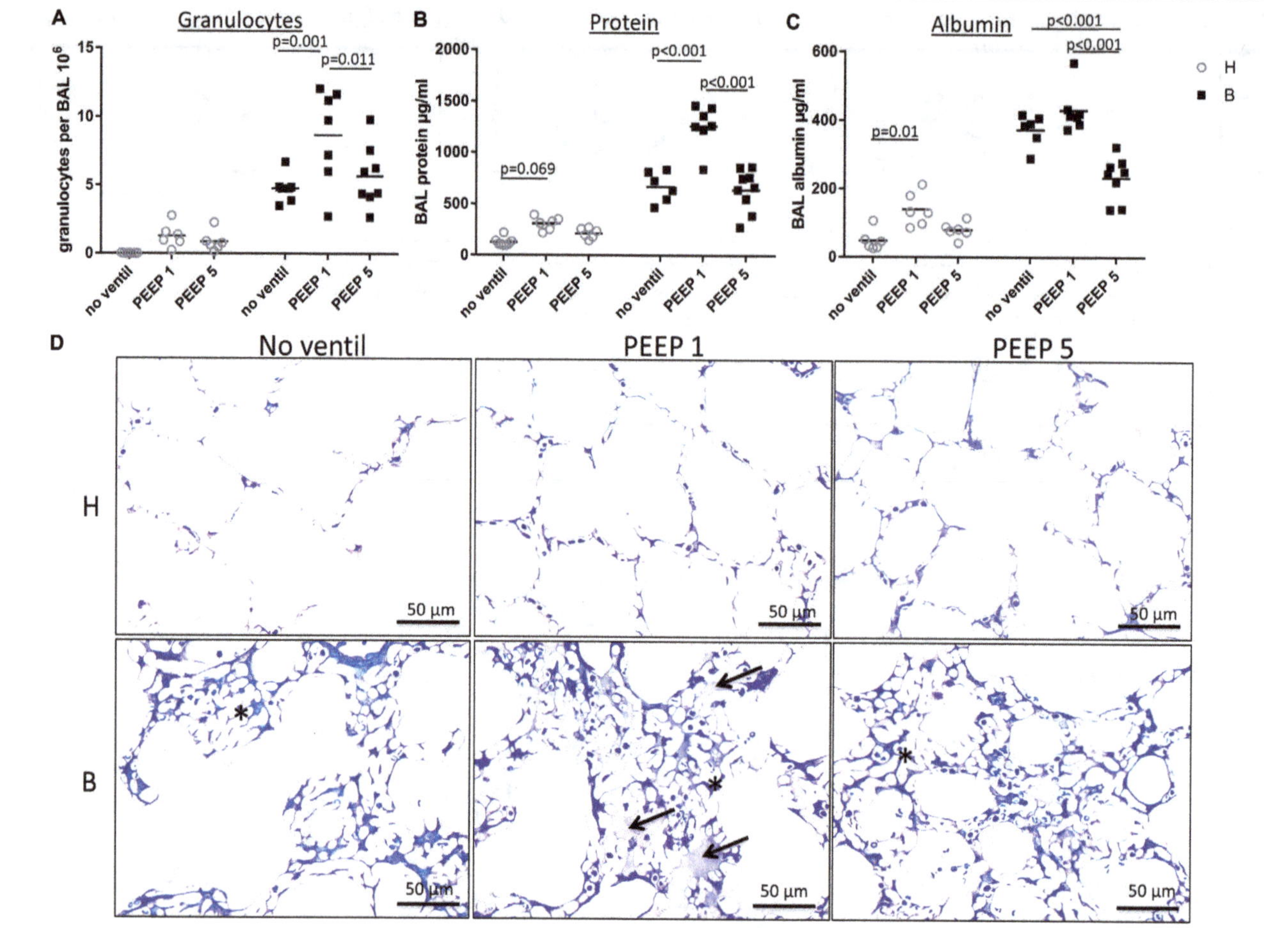

FIGURE 5 | BAL data and intra-alveolar edema. **(A)** In this figure, the amount of neutrophil granulocytes within the BAL is presented for each group and demonstrates an enormous influx of neutrophil granulocytes into the alveolar space in group B/PEEP1. This influx is statistically significantly higher compared to B/PEEP5 and B/no ventil. **(B)** The BAL protein concentration in µg/ml is shown. For group B/PEEP1, the protein content is significantly elevated versus B/PEEP5 ($p < 0.001$) and B ($p < 0.001$). Furthermore, initially healthy lungs demonstrate a trend for an increased amount of BAL protein level after ventilation with PEEP = 1 cmH_2O (H/PEEP1). **(C)** The concentrations of BAL albumin in µg/ml show a slightly different distribution than the protein measurements but highest albumin concentration can be identified in group B/PEEP1 which differs significantly from B/PEEP5 but not from B/no ventil. Of note, the albumin level is significantly lower in B/PEEP5 compared to B/no ventil. There is a significant difference between H and H/PEEP1 ($p = 0.01$). **(D)** Light microscopic images after vascular perfusion fixation at end-inspiratory pressure during PEEP = 1 cmH_2O ventilation. Sections were stained with toluidine blue. Microatelectases or alveolar edema are absent in healthy lungs. All Bleomycin-treated lungs demonstrate microatelectatic regions at end-inspiratory status (asterisk). In lungs from group B/PEEP1, alveolar edema fluid in adjacency to microatelectasis can be observed (arrows). Intraalveolar edema is hardly visible in B/PEEP5.

frequently (**Figure 6**). This was accompanied by thickening of the interalveolar septa and a divergence of the formed extracellular components such as the collagen fibrils due to interstitial fluid accumulation. The degree of injured epithelial cells was quantified by determining the total surface area of the basal lamina covered by healthy or injured AE1 cells as well as AE2 cells (**Figure 7**). Bleomycin and the ventilation pattern had both a significant effect on the surface area covered by injured AE1 cells (**Table 1**). While in bleomycin pre-injured lungs the PEEP = 1 cmH_2O ventilation resulted in an additional, although not significant ($p = 0.056$), decrease in surface area covered by intact AE1 cells (**Figure 7A**) combined with an increase in surface area covered by injured AE1 cells (**Figure 7B**), this was not the case with PEEP = 5 cmH_2O ventilation where no difference from non-ventilated bleomycin lungs were observed. In the healthy lungs, both PEEP levels resulted in a slight, although statistically not significant increase in the surface area of injured AE1 cells. In general, the effect of bleomycin and/ or mechanical ventilation on ultrastructural AE2 cell injury markers was much less pronounced compared to AE1 cells. In all study groups the ratio of injured AE2 cells to intact AE2 cells was much smaller compared to the ratio of injured AE1 cells and intact AE1 cells. Neither bleomycin nor mechanical ventilation demonstrated an effect on the surface area covered by intact AE2 cells (**Figure 7C**). On the other hand, bleomycin, but not the ventilation pattern, demonstrated an effect on the surface area covered by injured AE2 cells (**Figure 7D**). Within the group of bleomycin challenged lungs no significant differences in AE2 injury attributable to ventilation pattern were observed.

TABLE 1 | Summarized stereological data are given as mean (standard deviation).

Parameter	H			B			Two-way ANOVA		
	No ventil	PEEP1	PEEP5	No ventil	PEEP1	PEEP5	Bleo	Vent	inter
V(lung) cm^3	2.72 (0.24)	2.80 (0.29)	2.71 (0.15)	2.74 (0.17)	2.52 (0.29)	2.55 (0.27)	0.10	0.56	0.313
V(par,lung) cm^3	2.47 (0.27)	2.58 (0.28)	2.53 (0.12)	2.49 (0.15)	2.16 (0.28)*	2.29 (0.23)	0.006	0.53	0.068
V(nonpar,lung) cm^3	0.25 (0.1)	0.22 (0.1)	0.17 (0.04)	0.26 (0.05)	0.36 (0.08)	0.26 (0.1)	0.005	0.12	0.128
V(alv,par) cm^3	1.90 (0.19)	1.98 (0.22)	1.78 (0.08)	1.78 (0.12)	1.47 (0.22)*	1.63 (0.23)	<0.001	0.15	0.027
V(duct,par) cm^3	0.44 (0.08)	0.47 (0.06)	0.63 (0.07)*#	0.58 (0.07)	0.56 (0.1)	0.54 (0.09)	0.099	0.033	0.003
V(sep,par) cm^3	0.12 (0.02)	0.13 (0.04)	0.12 (0.02)	0.13 (0.01)	0.14 (0.03)	0.11 (0.02)	0.779	0.151	0.379
S(alv,par) cm^2	1299 (79)	1306 (120)	1191 (62)	1232 (81)	1066 (126)*	1089 (104)*	<0.001	0.009	0.089
τ(sep) μm	1.81 (0.3)	2.07 (0.63)	2.08 (0.24)	2.15 (0.24)	2.62 (0.46)	2.06 (0.32)#	0.022	0.062	0.169
V(airway,nonpar) mm^3	131 (74)	128 (32)	126 (28)	127 (22)	173 (63)	143 (48)	0.247	0.559	0.483
V(ves,nonpar) mm^3	58.4 (31.7)	45.3 (46.1)	20.7 (8.7)*	42.9 (8.4)	56.0 (6.8)	40.1 (22.2)	0.536	0.057	0.17
V(pbvtis,nonpar) mm^3	45.2 (20.4)	42.0 (42.0)	37.5 (17.6)	85.8 (27.3)	131.9 (25.3)*	79.9 (30.2)#	<0.001	0.041	0.058
S(AE1_intact,par) cm^2	918 (274)	792 (103)	820 (192)	421 (115)	263 (92)	504 (177)#	<0.001	0.108	0.275
S(AE1_injure,par) cm^2	60 (36)	128 (93)	201 (122)	305 (79)	455 (187)*	204 (111)#	<0.001	0.017	0.012
S(AE2_intact,par) cm^2	57.4 (39.4)	41 (24)	94.2 (47.5)	24.1 (25.6)	40.6 (31.3)	125 (180)	0.951	0.083	0.647
S(AE2_injure,par) cm^2	0 (0)	1.0 (2.3)	3.0 (3.5)	6.7 (6.0)	12.6 (8.7)	11.6 (13.2)	0.001	0.389	0.795

*A two-way ANOVA on ranks was performed to take the factors of treatment (bleomycin effects, B vs. H) and ventilation (no ventil vs. PEEP1 vs. PEEP5) as well as their interaction (inter) into consideration. Within each treatment group (B and H) an adjustment of the p-level for multiple testing using the Bonferroni post hoc test was added. Within each group (B and H) statistical significant differences of ventilation effects are indicated as follows: *$p < 0.05$ vs. no ventil; #$p < 0.05$ vs. PEEP1. H, healthy; B, bleomycin pre-treatment; Vent, ventilation pattern; V, volume; S, surface area; τ, arithmetic mean thickness; par, lung parenchyma; nonpar, non-parenchyma; alv, alveolar airspace; duct, ductal airspace; sep, interalveolar septa; airway, conducting airway; ves, blood vessel; pbvtis, peri-bronchiolar-vascular connective tissue; AE1, alveolar epithelial type 1 cell; AE2, alveolar epithelial type 2 cell.*

Taken together, mechanical ventilation of a bleomycin pre-injured lung with a low PEEP increased the surface area of epithelial basal lamina covered by of abnormal appearing AE1 cells. This behavior could not be observed during mechanical ventilation with PEEP = 5 cmH_2O.

Cellular Stress Markers of Alveolar Epithelial Cells

In vitro models of increased epithelial stretch demonstrated that the integrated stress response is activated by mechanical stress of primary alveolar epithelial cells (Dolinay et al., 2017, 2018). Therefore, we performed immunohistochemical staining of p-Perk and p-EIF-2α in four sections per experimental group. Staining with isotype control antibody (rabbit IgG) did not show any evidence of unspecific binding of the primary antibodies used against p-Perk or p-EIF-2α (**Supplementary Figure S1**). Regarding p-Perk, positive cells could occasionally be detected in healthy lungs independent of whether or not the lungs were mechanically ventilated. These positive cells were predominantly found within the septal wall. After bleomycin and mechanical ventilation, alveolar epithelial p-Perk expression demonstrated a marked increase (**Figure 8**). p-EIF-2α was not detectable in healthy lungs before or after mechanical ventilation. After bleomycin instillation, however, alveolar epithelial cells were positive for p-EIF-2α. Mechanical ventilation of bleomycin-treated lungs appeared to increase the fraction of p-EIF-2α positive cells particularly in and in close proximity to microatelectases (**Figure 9**). For quantification, the fraction of the alveolar surface area which stained positive for p-EIF-2α was determined by means of intersection counting. Since healthy lungs did not show any positive cell this investigation was only performed in bleomycin challenged experimental groups. The mean and standard deviation of the fraction of alveolar surface area covered by p-EIF-2α positive cells of $n = 4$ sections per study group were 0.23 (0.04), 0.35 (0.07), and 0.21 (0.03) for B/No ventil, B/PEEP1 and B/PEEP5, respectively. In B/PEEP1 a trend for a significantly larger surface fraction was found compared to B/No ventil ($p = 0.055$).

In summary, mechanical ventilation with PEEP1 increased the surface fraction of p-EIF-2α positive epithelial cells by trend, a finding which correlated with the occurrence of p-Perk positive epithelial cells.

Correlation Analyses

During mechanical ventilation with PEEP = 1 cmH_2O, H1 increased with time in the bleomycin pre-treated lungs while it remained stable in the healthy lung. With the goal to investigate which abnormalities in lung structure and BAL measurements were best linked with this increase in H1, correlation analyses were performed. The total volume of peri-bronchiolar-vascular connective tissue per lung (V(pbvtis,nonpar), **Figure 10A**), protein and albumin levels in BAL (**Figure 10B**), the surface area of basal lamina covered by injured alveolar epithelial cell as well the volume of alveolar airspaces (**Figure 10C**) demonstrated highly significant ($p < 0.01$) correlations with H1 measured at PEEP = 1 cmH_2O.

Hs measured at the conclusion of ventilation during PEEP = 3 cmH2O ventilation demonstrated significant correlations with

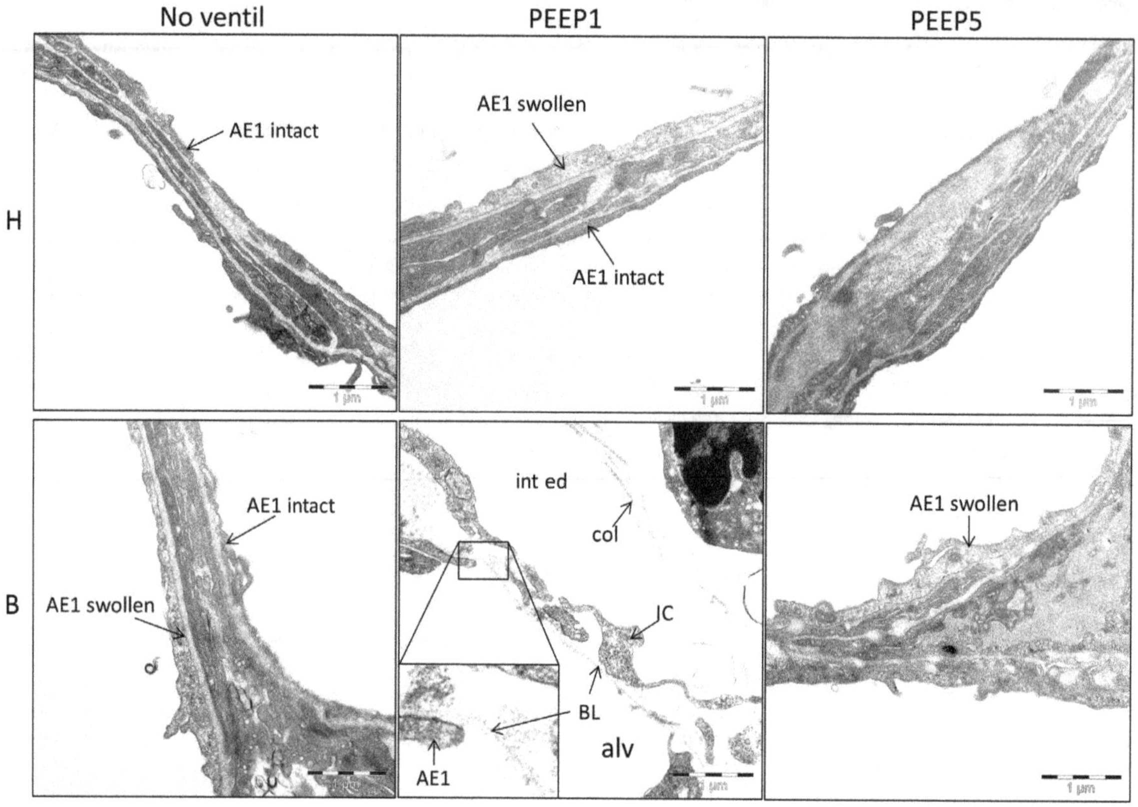

FIGURE 6 | Injury of alveolar epithelial cells. Representative electron-microscopic images are shown at primary magnification of 11,000×. There is evidence of epithelial injury, like swollen AE1 cells, in most of the experimental groups, except H/No ventil. Regarding B/PEEP1, the injury of the blood-gas barrier was severe, since complete denudations of the epithelial basal lamina (BL) was observed in particular in areas characterized by a widening of the septal walls due to interstitial fluid accumulation (int ed). col, collagen fibrils; IC, interstitial cell; alv, alveolar airspace.

arithmetic mean thickness of septal walls [t(sep), $r = 0.575$, $p < 0.01$)] and peri-bronchiolar-vascular connective tissue (V(pbvtis,par), **Figure 10D**) but also the mean volume of alveolar airspaces (V(alv,par), $r = 0.619$, $p < 0.01$). The most statistical correlation with Hs, however, could be established for BAL protein (**Figure 10E**) and albumin level ($r = 0.788$, $p < 0.01$). The increase in tissue elastance during 4.5 min of low tidal volume, PEEP = 3 cmH_2O ventilation following a recruitment manoeuvre (ΔH) demonstrated statistically significant correlations with BAL protein (**Figure 10F**) and BAL albumin ($r = 0.616$, $p < 0.01$) levels only while correlations with structural data were, at best, moderate. The BAL protein or albumin level were highly correlated to the total volume of peri-bronchiolar-vascular connective tissue as well as to the surface area of the epithelial basal lamina covered by injured epithelial type I cells (data not shown).

DISCUSSION

Abnormalities of alveolar micromechanics may not always be reflected in measurements at the organ scale such as arterial blood oxygenation or lung mechanical properties (Knudsen et al., 2018; Grune et al., 2019). On the other hand, it has been shown that abnormal alveolar micromechanics can aggravate acute lung injury during mechanical ventilation by atelectrauma and volutrauma (Knudsen and Ochs, 2018). The mechanisms of atelectrauma and volutrauma are linked with each other via alveolar interdependence. Derecruited alveoli act as stress concentrators and could increase dynamic strain and therefore micromechanical volutrauma in adjacent, open alveoli (Mead et al., 1970; Makiyama et al., 2014; Albert et al., 2019). In healthy lungs both atelectrauma (e.g., a PEEP of 0 cmH_2O) and volutrauma (e.g., high tidal volume of 30 ml/kg bodyweight) are required in combination to produce VILI in mice (Seah et al., 2011).

In the present study we tested the hypothesis whether hidden microatelectases increase VILI susceptibility during mechanical ventilation that does not harm healthy lungs. Such microatelectases have been shown to occur at end-expiratory airway pressures below 5 cmH_2O in the early stage of bleomycin-induced lung injury (Knudsen et al., 2018). We termed these microatelectases one day after bleomycin instillation as "hidden" since oxygenation and tissue elastance, which represent typically available organ scale measurements during mechanical ventilation, were virtually unchanged compared to healthy controls (Knudsen et al., 2018). During mechanical ventilation of bleomycin challenged lungs with PEEP = 1 cmH_2O the

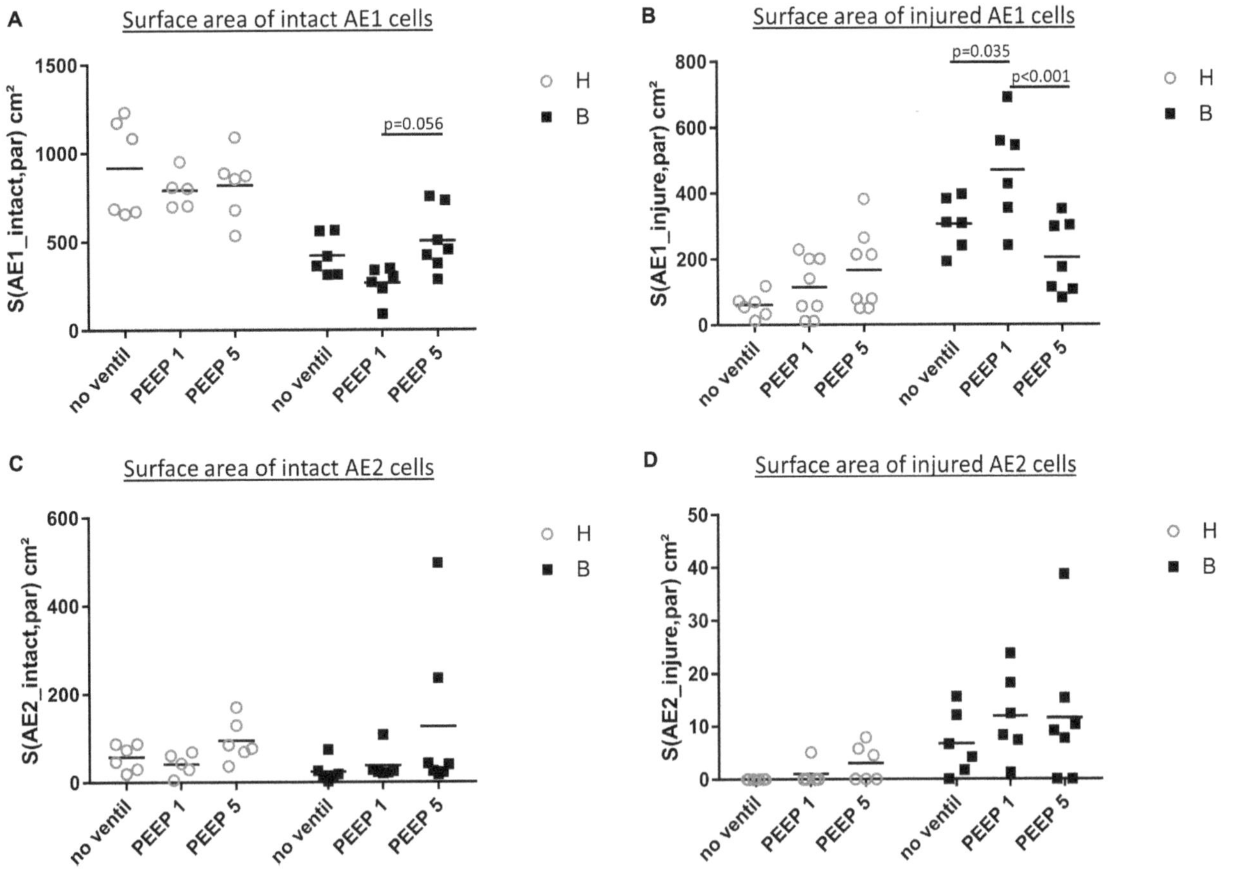

FIGURE 7 | Stereological data of alveolar epithelial injury. **(A)** The surface area of basal lamina covered by intact (healthy) AE1 cells (S(AE1_intact,par) was larger in group H compared to group B. Within group B a tendency for reduced values were found in B/PEEP1 compared to B/PEEP5. **(B)** The surface area of basal lamina covered by injured AE1 cells S(AE1_injured,par) increases in group B compared to group H. This was most pronounced in B/PEEP1 where S(AE1_injured,par) was significantly larger compared to B/no ventil or B/PEEP5. No significant effect of mechanical ventilation was found within H. The surface area of basal lamina covered by healthy **(C)** or injured AE2 cells S(AE2_intact,par) **(D)** demonstrates a Bleomycin but no ventilation effect on S(AE2_intact,par).

peak inspiratory pressure was at the very beginning within the range found in healthy lungs. However, with time the peak inspiratory pressure demonstrated a considerable and progressive increase in the bleomycin pre-treated lungs (**Figure 1**) so that the pre-existing injury became manifest at the organ level. The increase in peak inspiratory pressure could be reduced by recruitment manoeuvres and might therefore reflect the occurrence of progressive but still recruitable atelectasis during low PEEP mechanical ventilation (Allen et al., 2005).

In the current study we demonstrate that the presence of microatelectases during mechanical ventilation for 3 h is linked with increased interstitial edema (**Figures 4B,C**), pulmonary inflammation (**Figure 5A**), protein levels in BAL (**Figure 5B**), and (based on ultrastructural criteria) injury of the alveolar epithelial cells (**Figures 6, 7**). This ventilation-induced exacerbation of occult injury is reflected in organ-scale lung mechanics as shown in tissue elastance during and after the 3 h period of mechanical ventilation (**Figure 2**). During mechanical ventilation with PEEP = 1 cmH_2O in presence of microatelectases (B/PEEP1) the first tissue elastance measured 2 s after a recruitment manoeuvre (H1) is characterized by a progressive increase with ventilation time (**Figure 2E**). This behavior was not observed in the lungs where we have previously not observed any microatelectases such as H/PEEP1 and B/PEEP5. Since H1 was measured immediately after recruitment it can be considered as a parameter reflecting lung mechanical properties at highest degree of recruitment and therefore components of lung injury which are not responsive to deep inflations (Massa et al., 2008; Smith et al., 2017). The increase in H1 during PEEP = 1 cmH_2O ventilation was highly correlated with structural parameters reflecting interstitial edema such as the volume of peri-bronchiolar vascular connective tissue (**Figure 10A**).

In addition, markers reflecting pulmonary inflammation (the number of neutrophilic granulocytes per BAL) or leakage of protein into the airspace (protein and albumin levels) were highly correlated with H1 during PEEP = 1 cmH_2O ventilation. The BAL data indicate progressive, protein-rich alveolar edema formation in B/PEEP1 and this is supported by qualitative light microscopical observations in lungs fixed by vascular perfusion at end-expiratory airway opening pressure of 1 cmH_2O that show interposing alveolar edema within areas of microatelectases (**Figure 5D**). Since it has been previously shown

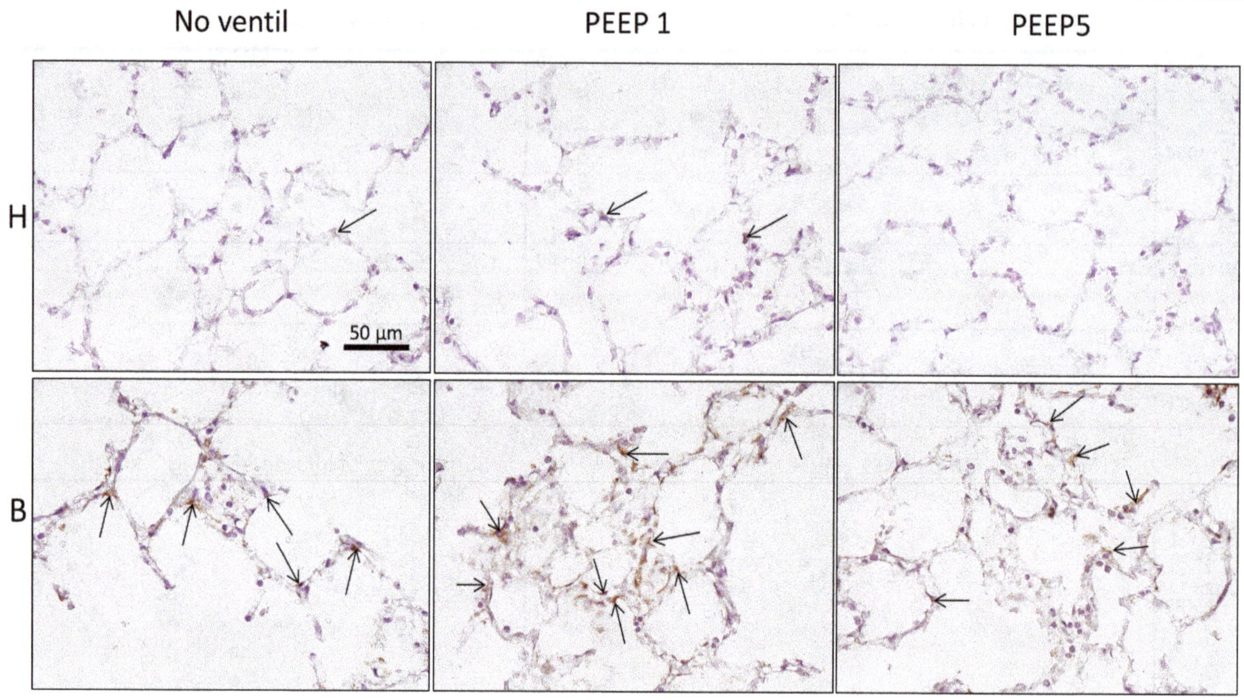

FIGURE 8 | Endoplasmic reticulum stress. p-Perk positive cells (arrows), stained by immunohistochemistry, were found in all experimental groups but most profiles of p-Perk positive cells were present in B. There was no clear effect of mechanical ventilation visible.

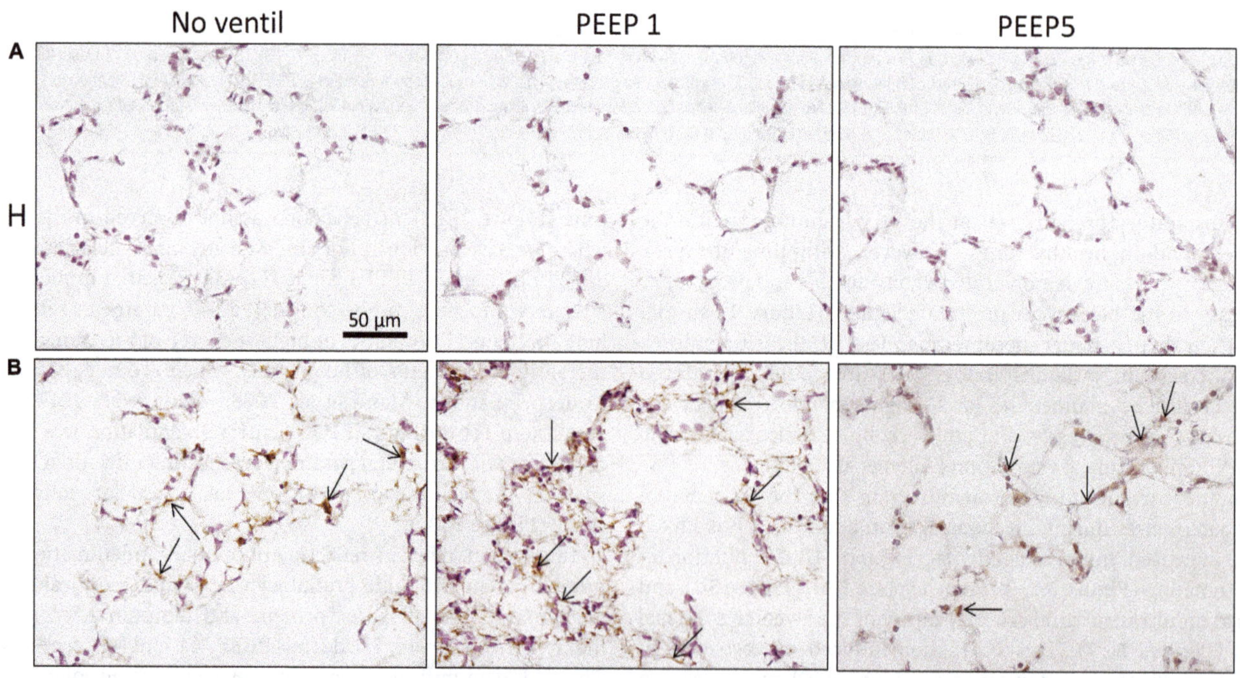

FIGURE 9 | Integrated stress response. Immunohistochemistry of p-EIF-2α is shown (arrows). While no staining was seen in H, bleomycin alone resulted in a positive labeling of cells in septal walls and this appears to be aggravated by mechanical ventilation with PEEP = 1 cmH_2O in some regions. Qualitatively, p-EIF-2α labeled cells were predominantly found in adjacency to microatelectatic regions.

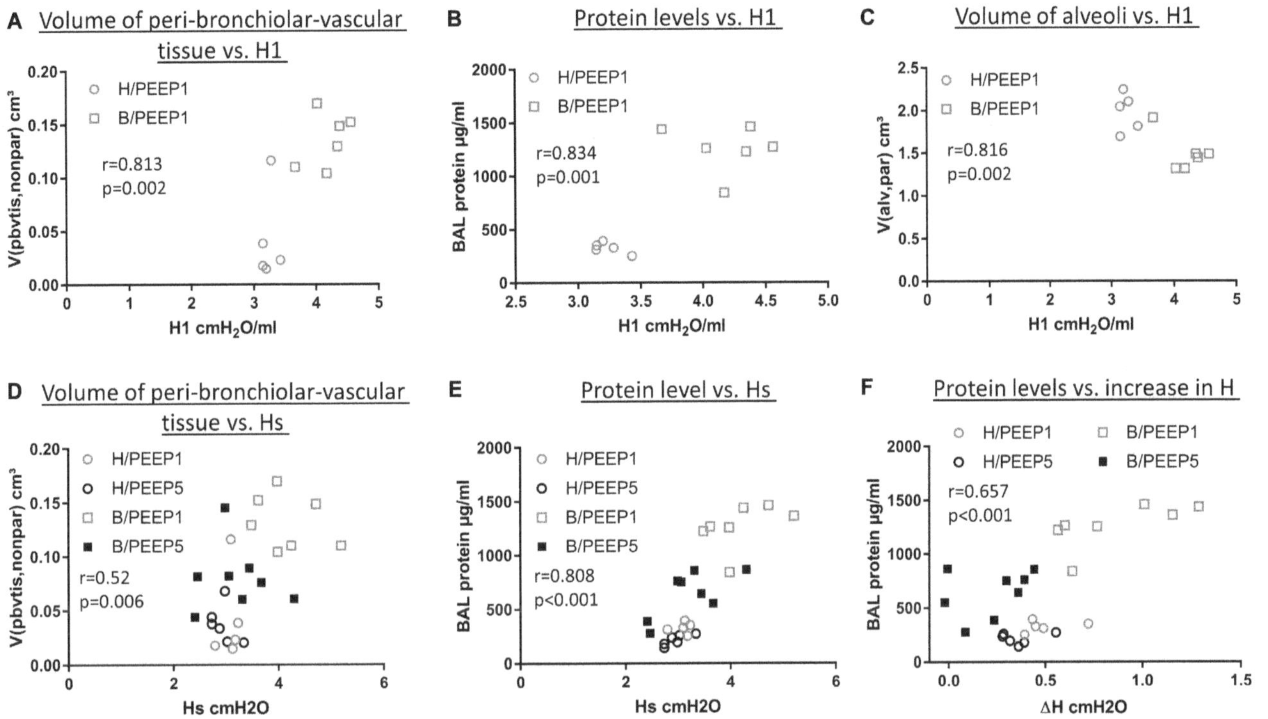

FIGURE 10 | Correlation with lung mechanical data. H1 in the last derecruitability test performed after 3 h of mechanical ventilation with PEEP = 1 cmH_2O demonstrated strong positive correlations with the volume of peri-bronchiolo-vascular connective tissue **(A)** and BAL protein content **(B)** and a negative correlation with the absolute volume of alveolar airspaces in lung parenchyma (V(alv,par)) **(C)**. Hs, referred to as the mean of the last three measurements of H during the derecruitability test at PEEP = 3 cmH_2O ventilation performed after the 3 h period of mechanical ventilation, was tested for correlation to the volume of peri-bronchiolo-vascular connective tissue (V(pbvtis,nonpar) **(D)** and BAL protein concentration **(E)** and both parameters demonstrated a strong correlation with Hs. Regarding the increase in tissue elastance during the derecruitability test at PEEP = 3 cm H_2O ventilation performed after the 3 h period of mechanical ventilation, ΔH, the BAL protein level showed the strongest correlation **(F)**. Hs: tissue elastance at steady state, H1: first tissue elastance after recruitment, ΔH = Hs–H1.

that protein-rich alveolar fluid accumulation in the context of high surface tension reduces the recruitability of distal airspaces (Rühl et al., 2019) it can be speculated that in the present study the progressive increase in H1 with time reflects reduced alveolar recruitment. This can be a consequence of altered alveolar lining fluid rheology and/ or progressive inactivation of pulmonary surfactant by plasma proteins (Seeger et al., 1993). In addition, increased dynamic strain of alveoli adjacent to microatelectases has also the potential to inactivate surfactant, e.g., by increased conversation from biophysically active large aggregates to inactive small aggregates (Veldhuizen et al., 1996; Albert, 2012). The increased dynamic alveolar strain might result in ruptures of the surfactant layer giving plasma proteins the opportunity to compete with the surfactant at the air-liquid interface ending up in a further destabilization of distal airspaces (Lopez-Rodriguez and Pérez-Gil, 2014).

Of note, the protein and albumin levels in the BAL fluid did not follow the same trend after mechanical ventilation of bleomycin challenged lungs. While PEEP = 1 cmH_2O ventilation increased the protein level (**Figure 5B**) the albumin level remained roughly stable (**Figure 5C**). The protein level (but not the albumin level) correlated with the surface area of the epithelial basal lamina covered by injured type I alveolar epithelial cells (**Figure 6B**). The increase in BAL protein in B/PEEP1 can therefore hardly be explained by leakage of albumin from the blood into the alveolar space. Based on the ultrastructural findings the endothelial cells were unaffected by the mechanical ventilation so that the barrier function on the blood side seemed to be still intact and prevented an additional leakage of albumin into the airspace. Since the protein level correlates with ultrastructural signs of injury of alveolar epithelial cells leakage of intracellular proteins into alveolar space in combination with increased inflammation appears to be an important source for protein accumulation after PEEP 1 ventilation of bleomycin pre-injured lungs.

The largest increase in tissue elastance over the observational period of 4.5 min after a recruitment manoeuvre was found in the group B/PEEP1 (ΔH, **Figure 2D**). This behavior can be the consequence of an increased time-dependent derecruitment of distal airspaces (Massa et al., 2008; Smith et al., 2012) and therefore, in the context of the present study, a result of increased alveolar instability due to surfactant inactivation. The increase in ΔH was highly correlated to the albumin and protein levels in the BAL (**Figure 10E**), an observation which is in line with previous observations in a VILI mouse model (Smith et al., 2017). As opposed to Hs, ΔH demonstrated at best moderate correlations (e.g., $r < 0.5$) to structural data and this could be a consequence of the fact that ΔH reflects the dynamic, time-dependent alterations which have their foundation in the properties of the air-liquid interface, e.g., high surface tension or redistribution of alveolar liquid which is dependent on alveolar protein content but not represented in the stereological data. Hs, e.g., the tissue elastance under steady state conditions after recruitment manoeuvre, on the other hand is dependent on both the mechanical properties of the inter-alveolar septa (Knudsen et al., 2015) and the characteristics of the air-liquid interface (Mead, 1961).

In the current study, quantitative structural data were generated in lungs which were fixed by airway instillation at a hydrostatic pressure of 25 cmH_2O. In these liquid-filled lungs the air-liquid interface has been abolished so that the effects of surface tension on lung structure, such as microatelectases or the location of intra-alveolar edema, cannot be investigated (Gil et al., 1979; Wilson and Bachofen, 1982). The fact that the volume of alveolar airspaces as well as the surface area of alveoli was significantly reduced in bleomycin injured lungs ventilated with PEEP = 1 cmH_2O (**Figure 4A** and **Table 1**) indicates that the mechanical properties of the interalveolar septa were altered due to the mechanical ventilation of lungs suffering from microatelectases, independent of the surface tension at the air-liquid interface. At the electron microscopic level we observed interstitial edema at the thick side of the blood-gas barrier where the epithelial and endothelial basal laminae are separated by interstitial tissue including collagen fibrils and fibroblasts (**Figure 6**). Here, a diverging of collagen fibrils was seen. At light microscopic level this observation was linked with an increase of the mean septal wall thickness. Hence, an interstitial edema-related stiffening of the inter-alveolar septa is assumed to occur due to a disarrangement of collagen fibrils.

The presented data suggest a causal relationship between the existence of microatelectases during mechanical ventilation and the progression of VILI, although they do not provide a definite proof. This causality is supported by theoretical considerations using spring models to simulate the distribution of septal stresses and strains within a network of elastic elements (Mead et al., 1970; Makiyama et al., 2014; Albert et al., 2019). As long as the mechanical properties of the spring elements are similar the distribution of stresses and strains, and therefore the tissue deformation, is homogenous. In presence of springs with increased stiffness e.g., due to alveolar derecruitment the stresses on surrounding elements have been calculated to be increased 16-fold (Makiyama et al., 2014). Albert and co-workers simulated the strain of alveoli adjacent to derecruited alveoli and found that in dependence of the number of derecruited alveoli (which was in that model between 1 and 7) there could be an increase in septal wall strain of 30 to 50% at resting volume (Albert et al., 2019). Those predictions were in agreement with previous physiology-based, non-linear multi-compartment model simulations of mean static and dynamic alveolar strain during mechanical ventilation in bleomycin-treated rats at PEEPs where microatelectases were observed in tissue sections (Knudsen et al., 2018). Taken together, those simulations suggest that although there is no increased strain at the organ scale there might be local increased dynamic and static strain of a cohort of alveoli due to stress concentration in a lung which suffers from microatelectases (=group of derecruited alveoli).

There are several imaging studies which support the concept of the injurious potential of microatelectases creating locally increased strain via alveolar interdependence. Using functional magnetic resonance imaging (MRI) to determine the apparent diffusion coefficient (ADC), evidence for airspace overdistension in close proximity to atelectasis due to low PEEP ventilation or surfactant removal was established (Cereda et al., 2013, 2016). The ADC correlates very well with the mean linear intercept length of acinar airspaces measured at light microscopic level (Woods et al., 2006). However, the mean linear intercept length has to be interpreted with caution in terms of alveolar pathophysiology since it depends on both the dimension of the ductal and the alveolar airspaces (Knudsen et al., 2010). The use of the mean linear intercept length or ADC as a marker for alveolar or septal wall strain is therefore not appropriate and it is difficult to conclude whether or not there is injurious septal wall strain due to atelectases from those studies. Nevertheless, in spite of normal strain at the organ level, increased regional tidal strain of distal airspaces, as measured from the distribution of a tracer by means of positron emission tomography, has been shown to correlate with the degree of neutrophilic inflammation after invasive mechanical ventilation indicating induction of regional ventilation-induced lung injury (Wellman et al., 2014). Using an *ex vivo* approach and confocal microscopy to resolve individual alveolar septa, Wu and co-workers directly analyzed the effects of alveolar interdependence during mechanical ventilation by observing the interactions between an alveolus filled with protein-rich edema and a healthy alveolus (Wu et al., 2014). Although the strain at the organ scale was considered to be harmless, injury of the healthy alveolus, as measured by leakage of tracer into alveolar airspace, was induced and correlated to surface tension in the flooded alveolus (Wu et al., 2014).

Dolinay and co-workers demonstrated in a primary alveolar epithelial cell culture model that a bi-axial strain of 25%, which corresponds to ventilation with 15 ml/kg bodyweight (Tschumperlin and Margulies, 1999), the unfolded protein response is activated in a Ca^{2+} dependent manner. These findings could be reproduced *in vivo* in a rat model ventilated with a tidal volume of 20 ml/kg bodyweight and an *ex vivo* porcine model ventilated with a tidal volume of 15 ml/kg bodyweight (Dolinay et al., 2017, 2018). The investigators suggested that a stretch-induced cytosolic increase in Ca^{2+} concentration resulted in an autophosphorylation of Perk which in a further step phosphorylated EIF-2α. By p-Perk inhibition experiments, the authors also demonstrated that this pathway was of relevance for dysfunction of the blood-gas barrier resulting in a leakage of proteins into the alveolar space. In the present study, we used immunohistochemistry to localize phosphorylated EIF-2α within lung parenchyma and observed that in the healthy lung there was hardly any staining while after bleomycin challenge, approximately 23% of the alveolar surface area was covered by positive cells. While during PEEP 5 cmH_2O this fraction remained roughly stable, PEEP = 1 cmH_2O ventilation increased that fraction up to 35%. Of note, positive cells were predominantly observed in adjacent to microatelectases so that increased static and dynamic strain of alveoli appears to be a plausible explanation for this observation. Furthermore, this observation suggests that microatelectases could be the spatiotemporal origin for spreading of the integrated stress response.

The present study has several limitations. Based on the functional data described in this study the bleomycin injured lungs did not develop a severe respiratory failure after 3 h of mechanical ventilation with PEEP = 1 cmH_2O. The transcutaneously measured oxygen saturation did not illustrate a substantial desaturation although lung mechanical properties as well as structural and BAL parameters measurably deteriorated. Hence, long term experiments expanding the duration of mechanical ventilation to allow further worsening of lung function are necessary to embed the relevance of our observations into the context of ARDS. As an alternative the PEEP could be reduced to zero (=ZEEP). This adjustment in the experimental protocol would result in an aggravation of microatelectases (Knudsen et al., 2018) and could potentially increase the vulnerability to ventilation-induced lung injury in this animal model even with shorter periods of mechanical ventilation. Moreover, in order to monitor the mechanical ventilation we used the oxygen saturation which demonstrated for all study groups under the given conditions sufficient gas exchange. However, we did not monitor arterial partial pressure of CO_2, bicarbonate and pH during mechanical ventilation which would have provided an additional assessment of ventilation adequacy. While the measured oxygen saturation at room air makes a relevant hypoventilation unlikely we cannot exclude a hyperventilation with subsequent respiratory alkalosis which as such might have had an impact on our read-out parameters. However, the volumes of ventilated air per minute were comparable between the different PEEP levels and study groups (900 ml/min/kg bodyweight). Based on ultrastructural criteria, we quantified the degree of injury of the alveolar epithelial cells in lungs fixed by airway instillation and observed that after bleomycin challenge without mechanical ventilation approximately 42% of the epithelial basal lamina was covered by cells which showed ultrastructural criteria for injury. Using exactly the same stereological approach for quantification of alveolar epithelial injury (Lutz et al., 2015) used lung tissue fixed via vascular perfusion and found one day after bleomycin instillation a surface fraction of injured alveolar epithelium of 27%. Hence, the route of fixation might have had an impact on this parameter in a way that airway instillation of the fixative e.g., via fluid-induced shear stress aggravated the ultrastructural signs of epithelial injury in the present study.

In conclusion, we could demonstrate that bleomycin-induced microatelectases, which are hard to detect using organ-scale lung mechanical and functional data, are linked with an increased susceptibility for VILI during ventilation with tidal volumes that are not injurious to the initially healthy lung. Through the mechanism of alveolar interdependence these microatelectases might elevate local septal strains (in absence of abnormal strain at the organ-scale) to cause volutrauma of adjacent open alveoli which is characterized by progressive injury of the blood-gas barrier, reduced recruitability, and increased instability of distal airspaces. The role of the activated integrated stress response in the tethering-induced expansion of microatelectases and the progression of VILI warrants further investigation.

AUTHOR CONTRIBUTIONS

KA contributed to the conception and design, acquisition of data, analysis and interpretation of data, drafting and revising of the manuscript. J-MK contributed to the conception and design, acquisition of data, analyses and interpretation of data, revising of the manuscript. AP contributed to the conception and design, analysis and interpretation of data, revising of the manuscript. SW contributed to the conception and design, acquisition, analysis and interpretation of data, revising of the manuscript. EL-R contributed to the conception and design, analysis and interpretation of data, revising of the manuscript. AB contributed to the conception and design, analysis and interpretation of data, revising of the manuscript. BS contributed to the conception and design, analysis and interpretation of data, drafting and revising of the manuscript. LK contributed to the conception and design, acquisition of data, analysis and interpretation of data, drafting and revising of the manuscript.

ACKNOWLEDGMENTS

We thank Beatrix Sczygiel, Michela Kaisler, Susanne Faßbender, and Olaf Macke for their excellent technical assistance.

REFERENCES

Albert, K., Krischer, J.-M., and Knudsen, L. (2020). *Light and Transmission Electron Microscopic Images for Quantitative Lung Morphology of Mechanichally Ventilated Rat Lungs. [Data set]*. Geneva: Zenodo, doi: 10.5281/zenodo.3738928

Albert, R. K. (2012). The role of ventilation-induced surfactant dysfunction and atelectasis in causing acute respiratory distress syndrome. *Am. J. Respir. Crit. Care Med.* 185, 702–708. doi: 10.1164/rccm.201109-1667pp

Albert, R. K., Smith, B., Perlman, C. E., and Schwartz, D. A. (2019). Is progression of pulmonary fibrosis due to ventilation-induced lung injury? *Am J Respir Crit Care Med.* 200, 140–151. doi: 10.1164/rccm.201903-0497pp

Allen, G. B., Pavone, L. A., DiRocco, J. D., Bates, J. H., and Nieman, G. F. (2005). Pulmonary impedance and alveolar instability during injurious ventilation in rats. *J. Appl. Physiol.* 99, 723–730. doi: 10.1152/japplphysiol.01339.2004

Ashbaugh, D. G., Bigelow, D. B., Petty, T. L., and Levine, B. E. (1967). Acute respiratory distress in adults. *Lancet* 2, 319–323.

Bonniaud, P., Fabre, A., Frossard, N., Guignabert, C., Inman, M., Kuebler, W. M., et al. (2018). Optimising experimental research in respiratory diseases: an ERS statement. *Eur. Respir. J.* 51:1702133. doi: 10.1183/13993003.02133-2017

Cereda, M., Emami, K., Xin, Y., Kadlecek, S., Kuzma, N. N., Mongkolwisetwara, P., et al. (2013). Imaging the interaction of atelectasis and overdistension in surfactant-depleted lungs. *Crit. Care Med.* 41, 527–535. doi: 10.1097/ccm.0b013e31826ab1f2

Cereda, M., Xin, Y., Hamedani, H., Clapp, J., Kadlecek, S., Meeder, N., et al. (2016). Mild loss of lung aeration augments stretch in healthy lung regions. *J. Appl. Physiol.* 120, 444–454. doi: 10.1152/japplphysiol.00734.2015

Cong, X., Hubmayr, R. D., Li, C., and Zhao, X. (2017). Plasma membrane wounding and repair in pulmonary diseases. *Am. J. Physiol. Lung. Cell Mol. Physiol.* 312, L371–L391.

Cressoni, M., Chiumello, D., Algieri, I., Brioni, M., Chiurazzi, C., Colombo, A., et al. (2017). Opening pressures and atelectrauma in acute respiratory distress syndrome. *Intensive Care Med.* 43, 603–611. doi: 10.1007/s00134-017-4754-8

Dolinay, T., Aonbangkhen, C., Zacharias, W., Cantu, E., Pogoriler, J., Stablow, A., et al. (2018). Protein kinase R-like endoplasmatic reticulum kinase is a mediator of stretch in ventilator-induced lung injury. *Respir. Res.* 19:157.

Dolinay, T., Himes, B. E., Shumyatcher, M., Lawrence, G. G., and Margulies, S. S. (2017). Integrated stress response mediates epithelial injury in mechanical ventilation. *Am. J. Respir. Cell Mol. Biol.* 57, 193–203. doi: 10.1165/rcmb.2016-0404oc

Dreyfuss, D., and Saumon, G. (1998). Ventilator-induced lung injury: lessons from experimental studies. *Am. J. Respir. Crit. Care Med.* 157, 294–323. doi: 10.1164/ajrccm.157.1.9604014

Fehrenbach, H., Schepelmann, D., Albes, J., Bando, T., Fischer, F., Fehrenbach, A., et al. (1999). Pulmonary ischemia/reperfusion injury: a quantitative study of structure and function in isolated heart-lungs of the rat. *Anat. Rec.* 255, 84–89. doi: 10.1002/(sici)1097-0185(19990501)255:1<84::aid-ar10>3.0.co;2-#

Gil, J., Bachofen, H., Gehr, P., and Weibel, E. (1979). Alveolar volume-surface area relation in air- and saline-filled lungs fixed by vascular perfusion. *J. Appl. Physiol.* 47, 990–1001. doi: 10.1152/jappl.1979.47.5.990

Grune, J., Tabuchi, A., and Kuebler, W. M. (2019). Alveolar dynamics during mechanical ventilation in the healthy and injured lung. *Intensive Care Med. Exp.* 7:34.

Gundersen, H., and Jensen, E. (1987). The efficiency of systematic sampling in stereology and its prediction. *J. Microsc.* 147, 229–263. doi: 10.1111/j.1365-2818.1987.tb02837.x

Günther, A., Korfei, M., Mahavadi, P., von der Beck, D., Ruppert, C., and Markart, P. (2012). Unravelling the progressive pathophysiology of idiopathic pulmonary fibrosis. *Eur. Respir. Rev.* 21, 152–160. doi: 10.1183/09059180.00001012

Hamlington, K. L., Smith, B. J., Dunn, C. M., Charlebois, C. M., Roy, G. S., and Bates, J. H. T. (2018). Linking lung function to structural damage of alveolar epithelium in ventilator-induced lung injury. *Respir. Physiol. Neurobiol.* 255, 22–29. doi: 10.1016/j.resp.2018.05.004

Hantos, Z., Daróczy, B., Suki, B., Nagy, S., and Fredberg, J. J. (1992). Input impedance and peripheral inhomogeneity of dog lungs. *J. Appl. Physiol.* 72, 168–178. doi: 10.1152/jappl.1992.72.1.168

Harding, H. P., Zhang, Y., Bertolotti, A., Zeng, H., and Ron, D. (2000). Perk is essential for translational regulation and cell survival during the unfolded protein response. *Mol. Cell.* 5, 897–904. doi: 10.1016/s1097-2765(00)80330-5

Hsia, C., Hyde, D., Ochs, M., and Weibel, E. (2010). An official research policy statement of the American Thoracic Society/European respiratory society: standards for quantitative assessment of lung structure. *Am. J. Respir. Crit. Care Med.* 181, 394–418. doi: 10.1164/rccm.200809-1522st

Knudsen, L., Atochina-Vasserman, E. N., Massa, C. B., Birkelbach, B., Guo, C. J., Scott, P., et al. (2015). The role of inducible nitric oxide synthase for interstitial remodeling of alveolar septa in surfactant protein D-deficient mice. *Am. J. Physiol. Lung. Cell Mol. Physiol.* 309, L959–L969.

Knudsen, L., Lopez-Rodriguez, E., Berndt, L., Steffen, L., Ruppert, C., Bates, J. H. T., et al. (2018). Alveolar micromechanics in bleomycin-induced lung injury. *Am. J. Respir. Cell Mol. Biol.* 59, 757–769. doi: 10.1165/rcmb.2018-0044oc

Knudsen, L., and Ochs, M. (2018). The micromechanics of lung alveoli: structure and function of surfactant and tissue components. *Histochem. Cell Biol.* 150, 661–676. doi: 10.1007/s00418-018-1747-9

Knudsen, L., Weibel, E. R., Gundersen, H. J. G., Weinstein, F. V., and Ochs, M. (2010). Assessment of air space size characteristics by intercept (chord) measurement: an accurate and efficient stereological approach. *J. Appl. Physiol.* 108, 412–421. doi: 10.1152/japplphysiol.01100.2009

Lopez-Rodriguez, E., and Pérez-Gil, J. (2014). Structure-function relationships in pulmonary surfactant membranes: from biophysics to therapy. *Biochim. Biophys. Acta* 1838, 1568–1585. doi: 10.1016/j.bbamem.2014.01.028

Lutz, D., Gazdhar, A., Lopez-Rodriguez, E., Ruppert, C., Mahavadi, P., Gunther, A., et al. (2015). Alveolar derecruitment and collapse induration as crucial mechanisms in lung injury and fibrosis. *Am. J. Respir. Cell Mol. Biol.* 52, 232–243. doi: 10.1165/rcmb.2014-0078oc

Makiyama, A. M., Gibson, L. J., Harris, R. S., and Venegas, J. G. (2014). Stress concentration around an atelectatic region: a finite element model. *Respir. Physiol. Neurobiol.* 201, 101–110. doi: 10.1016/j.resp.2014.06.017

Massa, C. B., Allen, G. B., and Bates, J. H. (2008). Modeling the dynamics of recruitment and derecruitment in mice with acute lung injury. *J. Appl. Physiol.* 105, 1813–1821. doi: 10.1152/japplphysiol.90806.2008

Mead, J. (1961). Mechanical properties of lungs. *Physiol. Rev.* 41, 281–330. doi: 10.1152/physrev.1961.41.2.281

Mead, J., Takishima, T., and Leith, D. (1970). Stress distribution in lungs: a model of pulmonary elasticity. *J. Appl. Physiol.* 28, 596–608. doi: 10.1152/jappl.1970.28.5.596

Mühlfeld, C., Knudsen, L., and Ochs, M. (2013). Stereology and morphometry of lung tissue. *Methods Mol. Biol.* 931, 367–390. doi: 10.1007/978-1-62703-056-4_18

Mühlfeld, C., and Ochs, M. (2013). Quantitative microscopy of the lung: a problem-based approach. Part 2: stereological parameters and study designs in various diseases of the respiratory tract. *Am. J. Physiol. Lung. Cell Mol. Physiol.* 305, L205–L221.

Nieman, G. F., Gatto, L. A., and Habashi, N. M. (2015). Impact of mechanical ventilation on the pathophysiology of progressive acute lung injury. *J. Appl. Physiol.* 119, 1245–1261. doi: 10.1152/japplphysiol.00659.2015

Ochs, M. (2006). A brief update on lung stereology. *J. Microsc.* 222, 188–200. doi: 10.1111/j.1365-2818.2006.01587.x

Rühl, N., Lopez-Rodriguez, E., Albert, K., Smith, B. J., Weaver, T. E., Ochs, M., et al. (2019). Surfactant protein B deficiency induced high surface tension: relationship between alveolar micromechanics, alveolar fluid properties and alveolar epithelial cell injury. *Int. J. Mol. Sci.* 20:4243. doi: 10.3390/ijms20174243

Scherle, W. (1970). A simple method for volumetry of organs in quantitative stereology. *Mikroskopie* 26, 57–60.

Schiller, H. J., McCann, U. G., Carney, D. E., Gatto, L. A., Steinberg, J. M., and Nieman, G. F. (2001). Altered alveolar mechanics in the acutely injured lung. *Crit. Care Med.* 29, 1049–1055. doi: 10.1097/00003246-200105000-00036

Seah, A. S., Grant, K. A., Aliyeva, M., Allen, G. B., and Bates, J. H. (2011). Quantifying the roles of tidal volume and PEEP in the pathogenesis of ventilator-induced lung injury. *Ann. Biomed. Eng.* 39, 1505–1516. doi: 10.1007/s10439-010-0237-6

Seeger, W., Grube, C., Günther, A., and Schmidt, R. (1993). Surfactant inhibition by plasma proteins: differential sensitivity of various surfactant preparations. *Eur. Respir. J.* 6, 971–977.

Slutsky, A. S., and Ranieri, V. M. (2013). Ventilator-induced lung injury. *N. Engl. J. Med.* 369, 2126–2136.

Smith, B. J., Bartolak-Suki, E., Suki, B., Roy, G. S., Hamlington, K. L., Charlebois, C. M., et al. (2017). Linking ventilator injury-induced leak across the blood-gas barrier to derangements in murine lung function. *Front. Physiol.* doi: 10.3389/fphys.2017.00466

Smith, B. J., Grant, K. A., and Bates, J. H. (2012). Linking the Development of Ventilator-Induced Injury to Mechanical Function in the Lung. *Ann. Biomed. Eng.* 41, 527–536. doi: 10.1007/s10439-012-0693-2

Steffen, L., Ruppert, C., Hoymann, H. G., Funke, M., Ebener, S., Kloth, C., et al. (2017). Surfactant replacement therapy reduces acute lung injury and collapse induration-related lung remodeling in the bleomycin model. *Am. J. Physiol. Lung. Cell Mol. Physiol.* 313, L313–L327.

Szabari, M. V., Takahashi, K., Feng, Y., Locascio, J. J., Chao, W., Carter, E. A., et al. (2019). Relation between respiratory mechanics, inflammation, and survival in experimental mechanical ventilation. *Am. J. Respir. Cell Mol. Biol.* 60, 179–188. doi: 10.1165/rcmb.2018-0100oc

Tschanz, S., Schneider, J. P., and Knudsen, L. (2014). Design-based stereology: planning, volumetry and sampling are crucial steps for a successful study. *Anat.* 196, 3–11. doi: 10.1016/j.aanat.2013.04.011

Tschanz, S. A., Burri, P. H., and Weibel, E. R. (2011). A simple tool for stereological assessment of digital images: the STEPanizer. *J. Microsc.* 243, 47–59. doi: 10.1111/j.1365-2818.2010.03481.x

Tschumperlin, D. J., and Margulies, S. S. (1999). Alveolar epithelial surface area-volume relationship in isolated rat lungs. *J. Appl. Physiol.* 86, 2026–2033. doi: 10.1152/jappl.1999.86.6.2026

Veldhuizen, R. A., Marcou, J., Yao, L. J., McCaig, L., Ito, Y., and Lewis, J. F. (1996). Alveolar surfactant aggregate conversion in ventilated normal and injured rabbits. *Am. J. Physiol.* 270, L152–L158.

Vlahakis, N. E., Schroeder, M. A., Pagano, R. E., and Hubmayr, R. D. (2002). Role of deformation-induced lipid trafficking in the prevention of plasma membrane stress failure. *Am. J. Respir. Crit. Care Med.* 166, 1282–1289. doi: 10.1164/rccm.200203-207oc

Wellman, T. J., Winkler, T., Costa, E. L., Musch, G., Harris, R. S., Zheng, H., et al. (2014). Effect of local tidal lung strain on inflammation in normal and lipopolysaccharide-exposed sheep*. *Crit. Care Med.* 42, e491–e500.

Wilson, T. A., and Bachofen, H. (1982). A model for mechanical structure of the alveolar duct. *J. Appl. Physiol.* 52, 1064–1070. doi: 10.1152/jappl.1982.52.4.1064

Woods, J. C., Choong, C. K., Yablonskiy, D. A., Bentley, J., Wong, J., Pierce, J. A., et al. (2006). Hyperpolarized 3He diffusion MRI and histology in pulmonary emphysema. *Magn. Reson. Med.* 56, 1293–1300.

Wu, Y., Kharge, A. B., and Perlman, C. E. (2014). Lung ventilation injures areas with discrete alveolar flooding, in a surface tension-dependent fashion. *J. Appl. Physiol.* 117, 788–796. doi: 10.1152/japplphysiol.00569.2014

11

The Contribution of Surface Tension-Dependent Alveolar Septal Stress Concentrations to Ventilation-Induced Lung Injury in the Acute Respiratory Distress Syndrome

*Carrie E. Perlman**

Department of Biomedical Engineering, Stevens Institute of Technology, Hoboken, NJ, United States

***Correspondence:**
Carrie E. Perlman
cperlman@stevens.edu*

In the acute respiratory distress syndrome (ARDS), surface tension, *T*, is likely elevated. And mechanical ventilation of ARDS patients causes ventilation-induced lung injury (VILI), which is believed to be proportional to *T*. However, the mechanisms through which elevated *T* may contribute to VILI have been under-studied. This conceptual analysis considers experimental and theoretical evidence for static and dynamic mechanical mechanisms, at the alveolar scale, through which elevated *T* exacerbates VILI; potential causes of elevated *T* in ARDS; and *T*-dependent means of reducing VILI. In the last section, possible means of reducing *T* and improving the efficacy of recruitment maneuvers during mechanical ventilation of ARDS patients are discussed.

Keywords: acute respiratory distress syndrome (ARDS), mechanical ventilation, ventilation-induced lung injury (VILI), surface tension, stress concentrations, recruitment maneuvers

INTRODUCTION

In healthy lungs, the alveoli are lined by a thin, aqueous liquid lining layer with associated surface tension, *T* (Gil et al., 1979). Surface tension acts in parallel with lung tissue elasticity to tend to collapse the lungs. The impact of *T* is lessened by alveolar epithelial type II cell secretion of pulmonary surfactant, a complex mixture of phospholipids, neutral lipids, and hydrophobic and hydrophilic proteins (Haagsman and van Golde, 1991). Surfactant reduces *T* at the alveolar interface, yet *T* varies cyclically as lung inflation decreases interfacial surfactant concentration and increases *T* (Kharge et al., 2014). Surfactant is first produced in the third trimester of gestation. In neonatal respiratory distress syndrome (NRDS), babies born severely prematurely have reduced levels of lung surfactant, thus high surface tension in their lungs, and are unable to breathe unassisted (Clements, 1997). This situation demonstrates the important contribution of *T* to lung mechanics.

In adults, a variety of pulmonary or systemic insults—e.g., pneumonia caused by a coronavirus, gastric aspiration, sepsis, or acute pancreatitis—can lead to acute respiratory distress syndrome (ARDS) (Ware, 2006; Wu et al., 2020). In ARDS, regardless of initial insult, pulmonary inflammation is present and causes an increase in alveolar–capillary barrier permeability. Barrier permeability leads first to interstitial and then to alveolar edema. The edema liquid, which contains plasma proteins, impairs gas exchange. Additionally, in ARDS, alveolar T is believed to be elevated (Günther et al., 1996; Holm et al., 1999).

Both NRDS and ARDS patients are treated by mechanical ventilation, which supports gas exchange but also causes an exacerbation of underlying lung injury—known as ventilation-induced lung injury (VILI)—and can prevent patient recovery (Jobe et al., 1983; Brower et al., 2000; Cereda et al., 2017). In NRDS, surfactant therapy, i.e., tracheal instillation of exogenous surfactant, is a successful intervention that supplements the low surfactant level of immature lungs and reduces or prevents VILI (Clements, 1997). Stemming from the success in NRDS, it is widely believed that surfactant therapy should likewise reduce VILI in ARDS. However, surfactant therapy has failed in clinical trials to reduce ARDS mortality (Brower and Fessler, 2011).

The failure of surfactant therapy for ARDS raises doubts about the connection between T and VILI, and the mechanical mechanism through which T may influence VILI is not fully understood. While there have been excellent studies of T effects on the mechanics of injured whole lungs (e.g., Bachofen et al., 1987; Gommers et al., 1993; Yamashita et al., 2008), T effects on alveolar septal micromechanics in the presence of injury or edema have been under-studied. Following below is a conceptual analysis of the influence of T on septal mechanics in injured regions, causes of elevated T in ARDS, and possible means of reducing VILI by reducing T-dependent septal stress concentrations in injured regions.

MECHANICAL MECHANISMS OF VENTILATION-INDUCED LUNG INJURY AND THE EFFECTS OF SURFACE TENSION

If mechanical properties were homogenous throughout the parenchyma of injured lungs, then elevated T would uniformly restrain the lungs and be protective. As mechanical properties throughout injured lungs are heterogeneous, however, there are stress concentrations present that are proportional to T and can be exacerbated by elevated T.

Injury Heterogeneity

Injury throughout ARDS lungs is heterogeneous in type and in spatial distribution. Types of parenchymal injury include, but are not limited to: (i) edematous alveoli flooded with proteinaceous blood plasma; (ii) hemorrhagic alveoli flooded with whole blood, including lysed red blood cells (RBCs); and (iii) collapsed alveoli (Staub et al., 1967; Henzler et al., 2011; Santos et al., 2012; de Prost et al., 2014). By microscopy of the injured lung surface, flooding and hemorrhage have been observed. By histology, all three forms of injury have been observed (Wu et al., 2017).

Spatial heterogeneity of injury is evident at scales from that of the alveolus to that of the whole lung. At the alveolar scale, histologic analysis shows that edema, hemorrhage, and collapse are all present in a heterogeneous fashion, interspersed with aerated alveoli (Staub et al., 1967; Henzler et al., 2011; Santos et al., 2012; de Prost et al., 2014). At an intermediate scale, the surfaces of lungs excised after 5 min of ventilation with a high peak inspiratory pressure (PIP) of 45 cm H_2O exhibit focal regions of injury surrounded by apparently healthy parenchyma (Dreyfuss and Saumon, 1998). And at the scale of the whole lung, computed tomography (CT) shows edema/collapse to be prevalent in the dependent lung (Gattinoni et al., 2001).

Static, *T*-Dependent Stress Concentrations Due to Injury Heterogeneity

At the alveolar scale, with the lungs held at constant volume, alveoli that are flooded are diminished in size (**Figure 1A**) (Staub et al., 1967; Perlman et al., 2011). The diminishment is attributable to the interface of the flooding liquid forming a meniscus at the alveolar mouth (**Figure 1B**) (Bachofen et al., 1993; Perlman et al., 2011; Rühl et al., 2019) and the fact that there is a pressure drop, ΔP_M, across the meniscus. Consider an alveolus that is initially aerated and surrounded by aerated neighbors; air pressure in all alveoli is P_{ALV} (**Figure 1C**, left). As air pressure is the same across all septa, septa are planar. When the central alveolus becomes flooded, air pressure above the meniscus and in surrounding alveoli remains P_{ALV}. However, according to the Laplace relation, $\Delta P_M = P_{ALV} - P_{LIQ} = 2T/R$, where P_{LIQ} is liquid pressure below the meniscus, and R is meniscus radius of the curvature, such that $P_{LIQ} < P_{ALV}$ (**Figure 1C**, right). As a result of the lower pressure within than around the flooded alveolus, the flooded alveolus decreases in size. In particular, the decrease is often due to bowing into the flooded alveolus of "intervening" septa (**Figure 1A**, arrows; **Figure 1C**, blue septa) (Staub et al., 1967; Perlman et al., 2011) separating the flooded alveolus from surrounding aerated alveoli. Intervening septal bowing is caused by pressure difference ΔP_S, equal to higher P_{ALV} in the aerated alveolus to one side minus lower P_{LIQ} in the flooded alveolus to the other side. The bowing over-extends intervening septa beyond their length when they are planar in normal, aerated lungs, making intervening septa sites of stress concentration. Further, $\Delta P_S = P_{ALV} - P_{LIQ} = \Delta P_M \sim T$. Thus, intervening septa are over-extended to a degree $\sim T$.

Alveolar derecruitment and collapse have also been attributed to elevated T (Albert et al., 2019; Kiefmann et al., 2019; Rühl et al., 2019). And diminishment of an individual alveolus tends, by pulling inward, to over-extend "radiating" septa that splay outward through the surrounding aerated parenchyma (**Figure 1C**, red septa). Thus, as supported by modeling (Mead et al., 1970; Albert et al., 2019), radiating septa are likely another site of T-dependent stress concentration. At the same time as a diminished alveolus pulls inward on radiating septa, each radiating septum transmits a higher-than-normal axial distending force, F_A, to the diminished alveolus. The ratio of the summed F_A around an alveolus to the surface area (or in a two-dimensional analog, perimeter length) of that alveolus applies an effective outward distending pressure, P_D, to the alveolus, and a

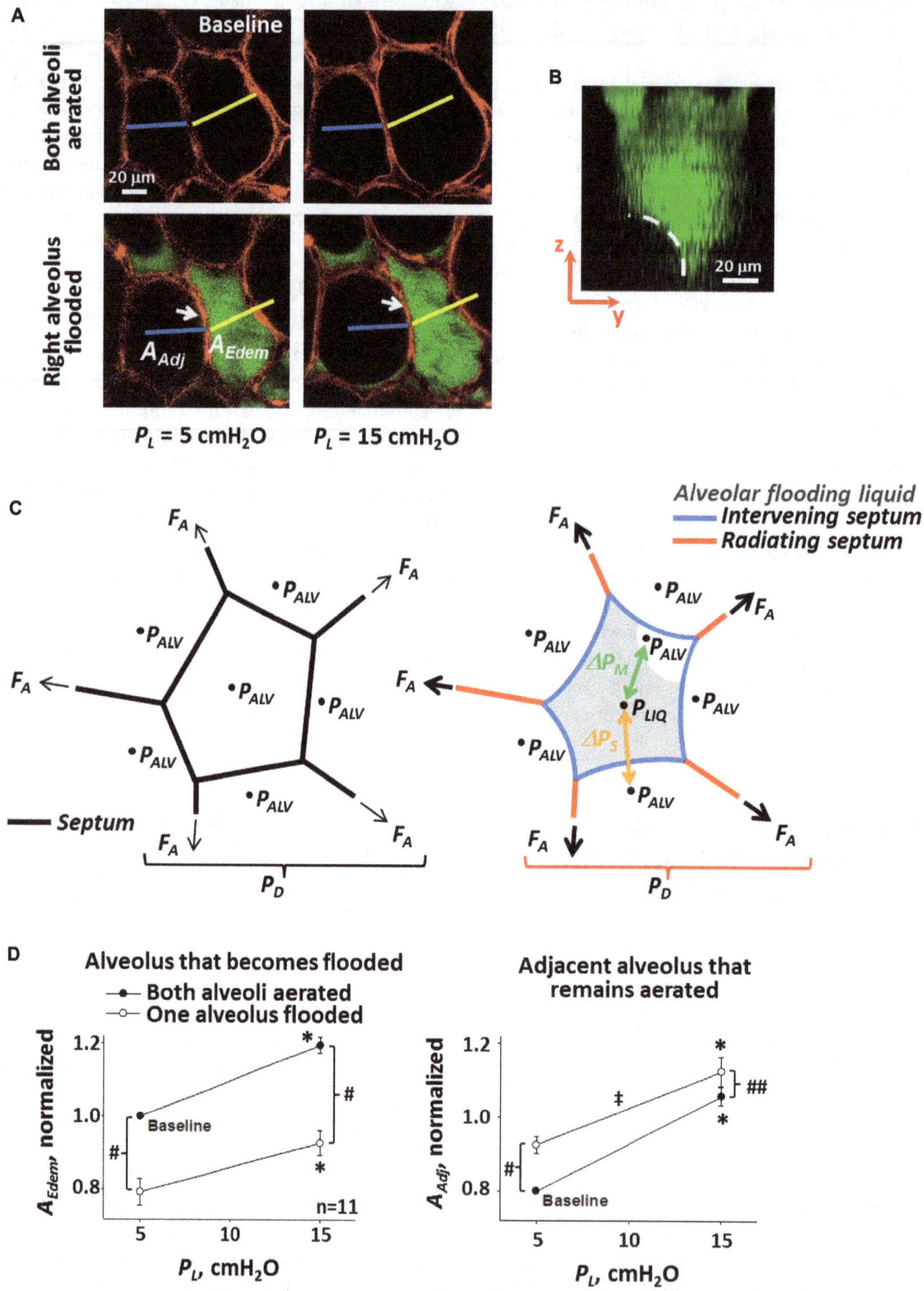

FIGURE 1 | Single alveolar edema model. **(A)** Inflation and flooding effects on alveolar geometry. Optical sections of two surface alveoli in isolated, perfused rat lungs. Epithelium labeled with calcein red-orange. Transpulmonary pressure, P_L, as indicated. In bottom images, right alveolus flooded with fluorescein-labeled 5% albumin solution. Air appears black. Sections are 2-µm thick and at 20-µm sub-pleural depth. Flooding right alveolus causes bowing of central "intervening" septum that separates aerated and flooded alveoli (arrows). Scale bars from baseline image are superimposed on all other images. Right alveolus that becomes flooded and left alveolus that remains aerated have areas A_{Edem} and A_{Adj}, respectively. **(B)** Meniscus in flooded alveolus. Image is *y–z* section, constructed from confocal *z*-stack, of an alveolus flooded with fluorescein-labeled 5% albumin solution. Pleural surface is at top of image. Epithelium is unlabeled and, along with air, appears black. Dashed line shows meniscus at mouth of flooded alveolus. **(C)** Schematics of alveolus before (left) and after (right) liquid flooding. Intervening septa separate aerated from flooded alveoli. Radiating septa are directed outward from flooded alveolus and have aerated alveoli to each side. P_{ALV} is alveolar air pressure. P_{LIQ} is flooding liquid pressure. Air–liquid interface in flooded alveolus forms a meniscus. $\Delta P_M = P_{ALV} - P_{LIQ}$ is pressure drop across meniscus. $\Delta P_S = P_{ALV} - P_{LIQ}$ is pressure

(Continued)

FIGURE 1 | Continued
drop across intervening septa. Axial distending force F_A acts at ends of sectioned septa and is greater in radiating septa around flooded alveolus on the right than in normally-stressed septa around aerated alveolus on the left. Ratio of summed F_A over alveolar surface is an effective distending pressure P_D applied to central alveolus. **(D)** Alveolar compliance. Alveolar areas plotted vs. P_L for pairs of adjacent alveoli, one of which becomes flooded as in **(A)**. Slope of lines is a two-dimensional analog of compliance. Statistics: *Area greater at P_L of 15 than 5 cm H_2O ($p < 0.01$), for state before or after one alveolus is flooded. #Area different after than before one alveolus is flooded, at constant P_L ($p < 0.01$). ##Same as "#" but $p < 0.02$. ‡Slope less after than before one alveolus is flooded ($p < 0.01$). **(A,B,D)** Modified, with permission, from Perlman et al. (2011).

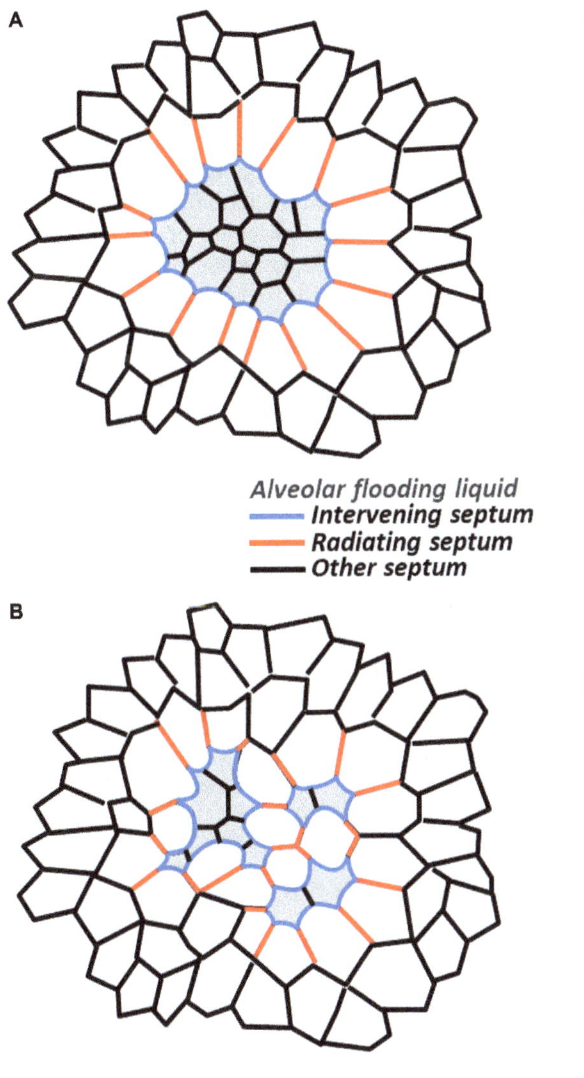

FIGURE 2 | Stress concentrations in injured regions. Schematic representations showing stressed intervening and radiating septa in **(A)** homogeneously and **(B)** heterogeneously flooded regions. While only single layers of radiating septa are shown, computational modeling indicates radiating septa, especially those around a larger injured area, penetrate further into surrounding, aerated parenchyma (see text).

diminished alveolus is subject to a greater P_D than a normal-sized alveolus (Mead et al., 1970; Albert et al., 2019).

At the intermediate scale, a region of homogeneously flooded or collapsed alveoli should have the effect of a giant, individual flooded or collapsed alveolus (**Figure 2A**). In the case of flooding, with menisci present at the mouths of all regional alveoli, or in common ducts, the region as a whole should be diminished below its normal, aerated size. Septa within the region should be shorter than when the regions is aerated and normal-sized and, with equal P_{LIQ} to each side, subject to $\Delta P_S = 0$ cm H_2O and planar. The septa should be subject to reduced stress. Septa composing the perimeter of the flooded region will be intervening septa. If the region as a whole is not too diminished in size, the septa may be sites of stress concentration. (Significant regional diminishment may move the septal endpoints close enough that even bowing does not cause over-distension). And radiating septa splaying outward from the injured region should be sites of stress concentration. Computational modeling indicates that radiating septal stress concentrations are greater and penetrate further into surrounding aerated parenchyma for a multi-alveolar injured region than for a single injured alveolus (Albert et al., 2019). Mead et al.'s (1970) classic model suggests that P_D around a multi-alveolar injured region exceeds the recoil pressure of the lungs. Further, two injured regions in relatively close proximity would be expected to amplify stress concentrations in radiating septa bridging through healthy tissue between the regions. How injured-region size and distance between injured regions affect stress in radiating septa between the regions has yet to be characterized.

For a region with heterogeneous flooding or collapse (**Figure 2B**), stress concentrations within the region should be higher than normal and higher than within a homogeneously flooded region. That is, there will be stressed intervening septa and stressed radiating septa (bridging between two flooded/collapsed alveoli) within a heterogeneously injured region. With the heterogeneously injured region containing injured/diminished and aerated/over-expanded alveoli, the region as a whole should be less diminished in size than if homogenously injured. Thus, intervening septa on the perimeter may well be a site of stress concentration. And radiating septa should be less stressed than those around a homogeneously injured region, though they may still be a site of stress concentration.

At the whole-lung scale, the dependent lung is often a gross region of extensive flooding or collapse (Gattinoni et al., 2001). (Both the flooded dependent lung and aerated non-dependent lung likely comprise, to greater or lesser degrees, sub-regions of homogeneously flooded or collapsed alveoli, heterogeneously flooded or collapsed alveoli, and aerated alveoli). Stress might be expected to be concentrated at the border between the dependent and non-dependent regions. However, CT data show the border region to exhibit an intermediate density between that of the dependent and non-dependent regions (Terragni et al., 2007). Thus, with the caveat that there could be a few layers of stressed, over-distended alveoli or septa in the border region that are not detectable by CT, there is no evidence for stress concentration at the border. There is, however, evidence that diminishment of the flooded dependent lung is marked enough to cause ventilation-induced over-distension injury throughout the non-dependent lung. In a saline lavage-induced high T injury model in rats, high tidal volume, V_T/low positive end-expiratory pressure (PEEP) ventilation caused atelectasis in the dependent lung and greater alveolar injury in the non-dependent than in the dependent lung (Tsuchida et al., 2006). The larger the injured area, it appears, the further acting the effect of interdependence.

Alveolar Compliance and Septal Stress

Consideration of alveolar compliance yields additional insight into the stresses applied to intervening and radiating septa. The injured lung exhibits reduced compliance. Contrary to expectation, however, flooding alone does not alter alveolar compliance. When a single alveolus in a healthy lung is flooded and T remains normal, the alveolus becomes diminished in size but maintains normal compliance (**Figure 1D**) (Perlman et al., 2011). Adjacent aerated alveoli, due to interdependence, become enlarged and, due to the non-linear stress-strain relation of septal tissue (Perlman and Wu, 2014), exhibit reduced compliance.

Lung inflation increases F_A and extends septa. In planar septa, the increase in F_A is balanced by increases in T and tissue stress, σ_T (**Figure 3A**). In intervening septa (**Figure 3B**), the increase in F_A tends to pull apart the septal endpoints and reduce bowing, and the increase in σ_T, which still counters F_A, likewise tends to reduce bowing. However, the inflation-induced increase in T has two opposing effects. Acting along the septum, like σ_T, elevated T tends to reduce bowing. Elevated T also increases ΔP_S, which tends to increase bowing. Thus, lung inflation sometimes increases bowing of intervening septa (**Figure 1A**).

Inflation-induced increase in intervening septal bowing into a flooded alveolus/out of an adjacent aerated alveolus should tend to decrease compliance of the flooded alveolus and increase compliance of the adjacent aerated alveolus. The perimeter of a single flooded alveolus is formed entirely by intervening septa. For a single flooded alveolus to exhibit the same compliance as in its prior aerated state (**Figure 1D**, left) requires that inflation, at the same time as increasing inward bowing of some intervening septa, cause the septal junctions at the alveolar corners to move outward. If inflation moves apart the endpoints of an intervening septum while simultaneously increasing bowing of the septum, then inflation increases stress in the septum. The perimeter of an adjacent aerated alveolus includes one intervening septum and two radiating septa. For an adjacent aerated alveolus to exhibit reduced compliance compared with its state prior to flooding of its neighbor (**Figure 1D**, right) requires that inflation, at the same time as increasing outward bowing of the intervening septum, cause less distension of the radiating septa than prior to flooding of the neighbor. That is, the radiating septa must be stiffer than prior to flooding of the neighbor. Thus, the observation of flooding-induced decrease in compliance in adjacent aerated alveoli supports the prediction from modeling (Mead et al., 1970; Albert et al., 2019) that stress is concentrated in radiating septa.

Dynamic, T-Dependent Stress Concentrations

Oftentimes, there is a threshold opening pressure, P_O, required at the airway entrance to open flooded, collapsed, or injured lung regions, and $P_O \sim T$. For air to enter and cause initial inflation of fluid-filled fetal lungs requires a P_O that is proportional to T (Enhörning and Robertson, 1972). Similarly, for air to enter a fluid-filled region of an injured lung or peel apart apposed septa separated by a thin liquid layer in a collapsed alveolus should require a P_O that is proportional to T (Gaver et al.,

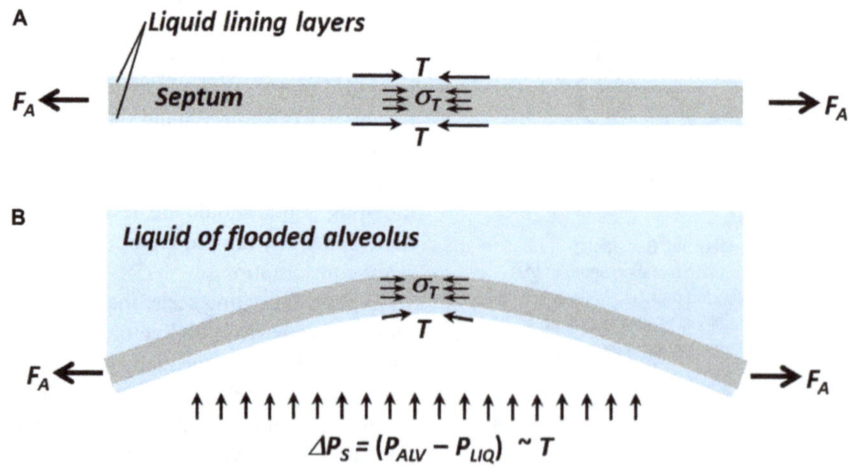

FIGURE 3 | Forces acting on septa. **(A)** Normal planar septum between two aerated alveoli. Distending force F_A applies axial tension. Interfacial surface tension, T, and tissue stress, σ_T, counter F_A. **(B)** Intervening septum separating flooded (top) from aerated (bottom) alveolus. Due to ΔP_S, which is $\sim T$, septum bows into flooded alveolus. Inflation-induced increases in F_A and σ_T tend to reduce bowing. Inflation-induced increase in T acting along septum tends to reduce bowing, but inflation-induced increase in T also increases ΔP_S, which tends to increase bowing. Net result is that inflation sometimes increases bowing (**Figure 1A**).

1990; Rühl et al., 2019). When PEEP < P_O < PIP, intervening and radiating septa around a flooded or collapsed region will be subject to maximal stress, in each ventilation cycle, just before the airway entrance pressure, P_{AW}, exceeds P_O. Thus, maximal stress in the septa surrounding an injured region that cyclically reopens should be proportional to T.

Interestingly, increasing P_{AW} above P_O could be a moving goal post. Once inflation commences, newly opened interfacial area may increase T and thus the P_O required for continued inflation. This scenario is one of negative feedback that may underlie incomplete opening of flooded or injured lung regions, particularly in cases of high T (Enhörning and Robertson, 1972).

Experimental Evidence That Heterogeneous Flooding Causes Injurious Stress Concentrations

To determine whether stress concentrations in regions of heterogeneous flooding are injurious, my group performed experiments in isolated rat lungs.

We developed a local VILI assay in heterogeneously flooded regions of healthy lungs, in which alveolar-capillary barrier permeability was initially normal, and used increase in permeability as an indicator of injurious stress level (**Figure 4A**) (Wu et al., 2014). In isolated perfused rat lungs, we labeled the perfusate with fluorescein. By micropuncture of a surface alveolus, we infused a non-fluorescent solution of 3% albumin in normal saline into a local region of the parenchymal airspace. The infusion resulted in heterogeneous alveolar flooding. In control regions, we omitted the micropuncture and infusion such that all alveoli remained aerated. Following this preparation, we held the lungs at a constant transpulmonary pressure, P_L, of 5 cm H_2O and imaged a flooded or control region at two baseline time points; provided five ventilation breaths with a PEEP of 0–20 cm H_2O (airway pressure adjusted to account for isolated lung with pleural pressure of zero) and a V_T of 6 or 12 ml/kg; and returned the lungs to a constant P_L of 5 cm H_2O for 10 min of post-ventilation imaging. In control regions without alveolar flooding, thus without septal stress concentrations, fluorescein concentration in the alveolar liquid lining layer remained constant at the baseline level, regardless of ventilation settings, over the 10-min post-ventilation period. In flooded regions with stress concentrations, just five breaths with the gentlest ventilation settings caused fluorescein to leak into the alveolar flooding liquid. Further, fluorescein concentration increased continuously over the 10-min post-ventilation period, indicating that transient ventilation caused a sustained increase in barrier permeability. Increasing PEEP or V_T increased the rate of fluorescein entrance into the alveolar liquid.

In a different, global VILI assay, we assessed ventilation-induced increase in T in the presence of heterogeneous flooding throughout the lungs (**Figure 4B**) (Wu et al., 2017). Our protocol was as follows. First, in isolated and perfused but unventilated rat lungs, we raised left atrial pressure to generate hydrostatic edema. We obtained heterogeneous alveolar flooding. Second, we arrested perfusion and determined T at the meniscus of a flooded surface alveolus according to our established method (Kharge et al., 2014). Briefly, following two ventilation cycles between P_L of 5 and 15 cm H_2O, we held the lungs at constant P_L of 15 cm H_2O, determined P_{ALV} with a tracheal transducer, determined P_{LIQ} by servo-nulling pressure measurement, determined three-dimensional interfacial radius of curvature by confocal imaging, and calculated T according to the Laplace relation. We found that hydrostatic flooding did not alter T from normal. [We determined normal T in healthy lungs by applying the same method to the curved interface of the liquid lining layer in the corners of aerated alveoli (Kharge et al., 2014).] Finally, with perfusion still arrested, we gently ventilated the heterogeneously flooded lungs 50 times between P_L of 5 and 10 cm H_2O and then again determined T. The ventilation increased T by 52%; we speculate that, as discussed below, debris from damaged cells caused the increase in T. Thus, again, ventilation exacerbated stress concentrations present due to heterogeneous alveolar flooding and led to lung injury.

We have not, to date, been able to distinguish between injury to intervening vs. radiating septa. However, our studies demonstrate that stress concentration levels are injurious in at least one of the two types of septa.

Spatial Propagation of Injury

Computed tomography analysis, in an acid-induced ARDS animal model and clinical ARDS, showed that ventilation causes injured areas to grow larger over time (Cereda et al., 2017). That over-stressed intervening and radiating septa are located at the perimeters of injured regions suggests that injured areas might grow larger through over-expansion of initially normal alveoli at the borders of injured regions. In this first scenario, high maximum T might be especially problematic. Alternatively, ventilation-induced exacerbation of the condition in an injured region—for example, by transiently high-pressure gradients imposed when $P_{AW} > P_O$ re-expands an injured region (Bilek et al., 2003)—might exacerbate already-elevated barrier permeability and lead to additional extravasation of liquid. The new liquid might extend, and thus generate stress concentrations, beyond the originally-injured area, thus leading to outward expansion of the injured area. In this second scenario, as $P_O \sim T$, high minimum T might be especially problematic. The mechanism of spatial injury propagation remains to be determined.

SURFACE TENSION IN ARDS

Bronchoalveolar lavage fluid (BALF) from ARDS patients exhibits increased adsorption time and elevated minimum surface tension, T_{MIN}, when tested *in vitro* in Langmuir–Wilhelmy troughs and pulsating bubble surfactometers (PBSs) (Hallman et al., 1982; Gregory et al., 1991). These results have overwhelmingly been attributed to the presence of plasma proteins in edema liquid. My group (Kharge et al., 2014) and Holm et al. (1988, 1999) have suggested, as detailed below, that the results are attributable co-adsorption of surfactant and plasma proteins in *in vitro* tests and shown that when an intact surfactant monolayer is present before plasma proteins enter the

A

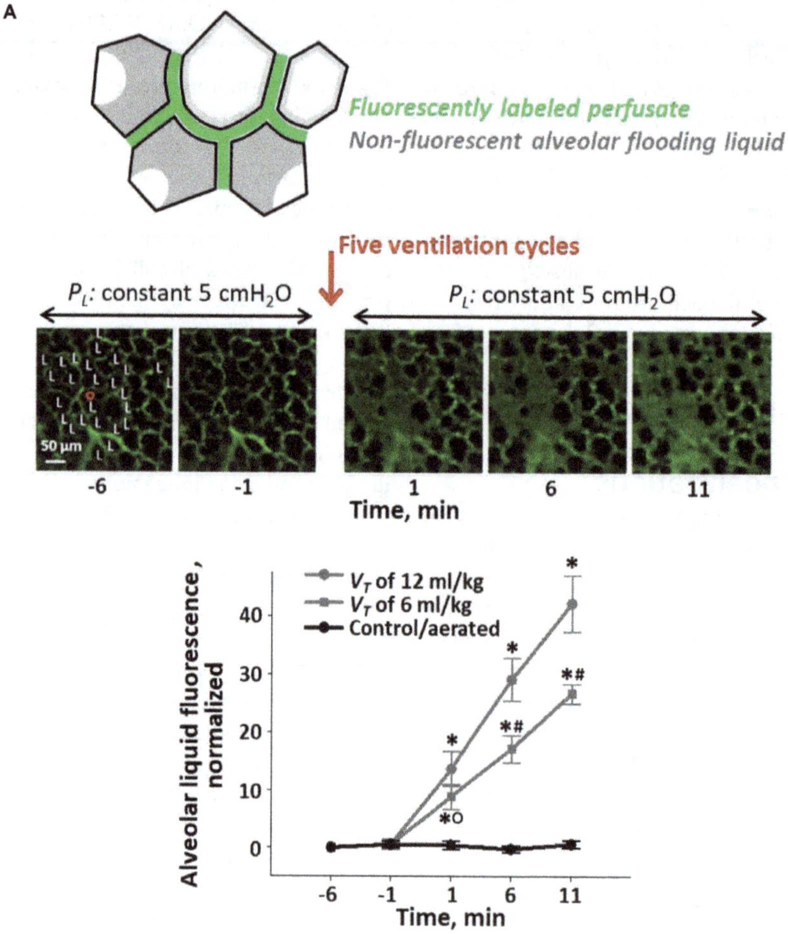

B

Following:	T, mN/m
Lung isolation and perfusion *Data from Kharge et al. (2014)*	11.7 ± 1.1
Hydrostatic edema generation with left atrial pressure of 12 cmH$_2$O and P_L held constant at 5 cmH$_2$O	12.2 ± 1.6
Arrest of perfusion and 50 cycles of mechanical ventilation between P_L of 5 and 10 cmH$_2$O	18.6 ± 1.3*

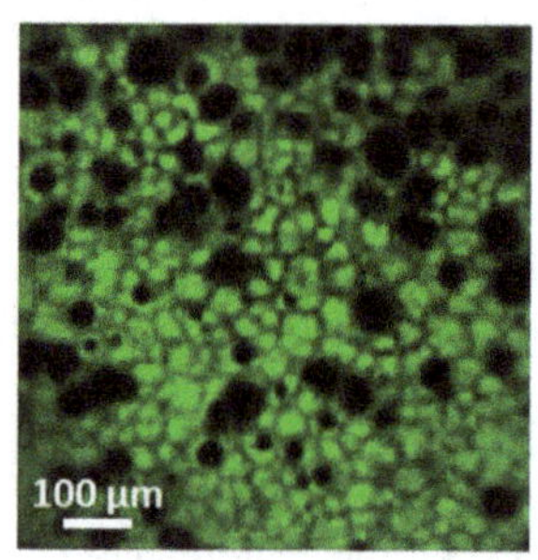

FIGURE 4 | Ventilation-induced lung injury (VILI) assays. **(A)** Local VILI assay of ventilation-induced injury to alveolar–capillary barrier in the presence of heterogeneous alveolar flooding. Top schematic: Isolated lung is perfused with fluorescein-labeled blood/5% albumin mixture. A glass micropipette is used to puncture a surface alveolus and infuse non-fluorescent 3% albumin solution, which causes heterogeneous alveolar flooding in a local region. Menisci are present in flooded alveoli. Middle images: With P_L held at 5 cm H$_2$O, the region is imaged by confocal microscopy over 5-min baseline period. "L" labels alveoli flooded with non-fluorescent liquid. Then, five ventilation cycles are administered with an end-expiratory P_L equivalent to an *in vivo* positive end-expiratory pressure (PEEP) of 10 cm H$_2$O and a tidal volume, V_T, of 12 ml/kg. Following ventilation, P_L is returned to 5 cm H$_2$O, and the region is imaged for 10 additional minutes. Bottom graph: plot of increase above baseline of normalized fluorescence in alveolar liquid vs. time. Gray: experimental, heterogeneously flooded regions in lungs subjected to five ventilation breaths with 10 cm H$_2$O PEEP and V_T as specified (fluorescein intensity quantified in alveolar flooding liquid). Black: control, aerated regions in lungs subjected to five ventilation breaths with 10 cm H$_2$O PEEP and 6 or 12 ml/kg V_T (data for two V_T groups combined; fluorescein intensity quantified in liquid lining layer). Statistics: $^*p < 0.01$ vs. baseline; $\#p < 0.01$ vs. both other groups at the same time point; $^{\circ}p < 0.01$ vs. control group at the same time point. Figure modified, with permission, from Wu et al. (2014). **(B)** Global VILI assay of ventilation-induced increase in T in the presence of heterogeneous alveolar flooding. Table: summary of experimental protocol and T-values, all determined at P_L of 15 cm H$_2$O, at different time points. Statistics: $^*p < 0.05$ vs. T-values at two earlier time points. Image: representative view of alveolar flooding pattern on surface of lungs at final time point after induction of VILI and elevation of T. Alveolar edema liquid labeled by fluorescein administered to the perfusate. Figure modified, with permission, from Wu et al. (2017).

subphase, as occurs in the lungs, plasma proteins do not alter *T*. Other causes of elevated *T* in ARDS have been proposed, and indeed, Günther et al. (1996) showed that ARDS BALF from which proteins were removed still exhibited elevated *T*. However, other purported *T*-raising substances have also generally been tested under co-adsorption conditions. And even if a monolayer is formed first, another consideration is that, in the absence of transformation by rapid compression, *in vitro* monolayers lack the metastability exhibited by surfactant in the lungs (Horie and Hildebrandt, 1971; Smith et al., 2004). The ability of other substances to raise *T* of an intact and metastable monolayer requires testing.

Plasma Components

Proteins are the plasma component in alveolar edema liquid most widely cited as raising *T*. However, plasma proteins have only been shown to raise *T* by competitive adsorption and may not have the opportunity to adsorb in the lungs. With an initially clean interface in a trough with constant interfacial area or a PBS with constant bubble volume, plasma proteins that co-adsorb with surfactant raise *T* (Holm et al., 1988, 1999; Seeger et al., 1993). Proteins that co-adsorb with surfactant in a PBS also raise the T_{MIN} achieved by subsequent bubble pulsation (Seeger et al., 1993; Holm et al., 1999). With an initially-intact interfacial surfactant monolayer in a Langmuir–Wilhelmy trough, plasma proteins injected into the subphase raise T_{MIN} during subsequent 80% cyclic surface area compression (Holm et al., 1999; Warriner et al., 2002). In the Langmuir–Wilhelmy trough, plasma proteins should have the opportunity to co-adsorb after the monolayer is ruptured by compression to 20% of initial area or to adsorb at peak surface area when regions of clean interface are exposed by monolayer expansion into the two-dimensional gaseous phase (Warriner et al., 2002; Wüstneck et al., 2005). However, with an intact surfactant monolayer, plasma proteins lack access to the interface and fail to raise *T*. Holm et al. (1988) showed that albumin injection below a static, intact surfactant monolayer fails to raise *T*. Holm et al. (1999) also generated an intact monolayer in a PBS and then added albumin to the subphase by subphase exchange. Even with subsequent 50% cyclic surface area compression, albumin below the intact monolayer failed to raise T_{MIN}. While 50% is just about the compression that begins to collapse the monolayer (Schürch et al., 1992; Holm et al., 1999), we estimate compression in the lungs to be, at most, ~40% (Kharge et al., 2014). Further, the monolayer in the lungs is always in the liquid-condensed phase (Wüstneck et al., 2005; Kharge et al., 2014; Nguyen and Perlman, 2018) such that even maximal lung inflation should not expose clean interface. Accordingly, in isolated healthy rat lungs held above functional residual capacity (FRC), alveolar injection of 5% albumin solution or blood plasma does not raise *T*. That plasma fails to raise *T* in the lungs indicates that, as discussed previously (Kharge et al., 2014), no plasma protein is likely at physiologic concentration to raise alveolar *T* with an intact surfactant monolayer.

In injured lung regions, it is possible that the surfactant monolayer might collapse, and allow plasma protein adsorption, at the end of expiration. In rat lungs at FRC, P_L is in the range of 3.5–4.5 cm H_2O (Schürch et al., 1976). With albumin present in alveolar flooding liquid, ventilating between P_L of 3 and 30 cm H_2O failed to increase *T*; ventilating between P_L of 1 and 30 cm H_2O caused a transient increase in *T* that was subsequently completely reversed by additional surfactant spreading (Kharge et al., 2014). In injured regions, local volume is certain to be below normal at FRC. Whether that volume is sufficiently low to enable plasma proteins to raise *T*, and whether any increase in *T* would be sustained, remains to be determined.

Another plasma component in alveolar edema liquid suspected of raising *T* is cholesterol. Native surfactant includes 5–10% cholesterol. Additional cholesterol has been mixed with surfactant by organic phase combination or, with cyclodextrin-facilitated solubilization, aqueous phase combination (Gunasekara et al., 2005; Lugones et al., 2018). Cholesterol-induced *T* elevation has been shown, following co-adsoprtion, to depend on concentration, requiring a nominal cholesterol fraction of $\geq$20%, and surfactant composition. However, cholesterol in blood plasma did not raise *T* of an intact surfactant monolayer in the lungs (Kharge et al., 2014).

Debris From Damaged Cells

With elevated barrier permeability and occasional hemorrhagic regions in ARDS, cells including epithelial cells and RBCs are damaged, and their contents should be present in edema liquid (Henzler et al., 2011; Santos et al., 2012). Cellular components including hemoglobin (Hb) from RBCs and phospholipids—particularly unsaturated phospholipids and lysophospholipids—and cholesterol from cell membranes may interfere with surfactant function and raise *T* (Holm and Notter, 1987; Holm et al., 1991, 1999; Hite et al., 2005; van Meer et al., 2008). The ability of Hb and RBC membrane lipids to increase *T* depends on the quantities of these inhibitory factors relative to the quantity of surfactant present (Holm and Notter, 1987; Holm et al., 1991, 1999; Hite et al., 2005). In ARDS edema liquid, my group estimated phospholipid concentration to be 2 mg/ml $\approx$ 2.7 μmol/ml, based on the molecular weight of dipalmitoylphosphatidylcholine (Kharge et al., 2014). At a comparable 2 μmol/ml of lipids in whole lung surfactant, Holm and Notter (1987) found membrane lipids more inhibitory than Hb and >1 μmol/ml membrane lipids necessary to raise T_{MIN}. Holm et al. (1999) also found lysophosphatidylcholine capable of raising *T* of an already-established intact surfactant monolayer. The high cholesterol content of cell membranes might also behave differently than plasma cholesterol and contribute to surfactant dysfunction (Gunasekara et al., 2005; van Meer et al., 2008; Lugones et al., 2018). Thus, cell debris may contribute to the elevated *T* of alveolar edema liquid.

Surfactant Degradation

Surfactant lipids and proteins may be degraded by enzymes or reactive oxygen species (ROS). Inflammatory cells release secretory phospholipase A_2 and certain bacteria, including *Pseudomonas*, release phospholipase C (Holm et al., 1991;

Kitsiouli et al., 2009). Accordingly, in BALF from ARDS patients, elevated phospholipase levels and activity have been observed (Hallman et al., 1982; Seeds et al., 2012). Phospholipases could elevate *T* directly, by reducing the availability of *T*-lowering surfactant phospholipids. Additionally, the products of phospholipase activity, lysophospholipids and fatty acids, raise T_{MIN} in a PBS, perhaps by intercalating into and increasing fluidity of the monolayer (Holm et al., 1991, 1999; Hite et al., 2005). As mentioned, lysophosphatidylcholine, in particular, has been shown to raise *T* of an already-established intact surfactant monolayer (Holm et al., 1999). Thus, phospholipases in alveolar edema liquid may increase *T* in the lungs.

In ARDS, ROS from activated leukocytes and macrophages can attack the surfactant monolayer from below. Oxidation of phospholipids first transforms unsaturated hydrocarbon tails and then causes cleavage, resulting in lysophospholipids and fatty acids (Rodríguez-Capote et al., 2006). Oxidized phospholipids cause only a marginally greater increase in *T* than their unoxidized counterparts and, thus, might not increase *T* much more than any alteration in phospholipid composition due to contamination by lipids of degraded cell membranes. However, ROS-induced generation of lysophospholipids, which increase *T* of an intact surfactant monolayer, has the potential to raise *T*. Oxidation also alters the form and function of surfactant proteins B and C (SP-B and -C) (Rodríguez-Capote et al., 2006). For example, oxidation causes depalmitoylation of SP-C, which is known to inactivate SP-C (Gustafsson et al., 2000). Nonetheless, it is almost entirely oxidation of SP-B that results in elevated *T* (Rodríguez-Capote et al., 2006). The effect of ROS on surfactant proteins has been tested with co-adsorption of reconstituted surfactant components including already-oxidized proteins but not with ROS application below an intact surfactant monolayer.

Surfactant protein alteration might also contribute to the acceleration, in ARDS, of normal surfactant recycling. Surfactant isolated from BALF by centrifugation partitions into surface-active large aggregates and surface-inactive small aggregates. In ARDS, the ratio of large-to-small aggregates decreases (Günther et al., 2002). In addition, conversion of large-to-small aggregates has been shown to be facilitated by serine-active carboxyl esterases (Ruppert et al., 2003). However, whether one of the surfactant proteins might be a substrate of the esterases is not known.

Gastric Liquid Aspiration

Aspiration of acidic gastric contents is a common cause of ARDS. In this situation, low pH gastric contents pass through the airways and mix with airway liquid, *en route* to the alveoli.

Low pH does not appear directly to alter surfactant function. In a PBS, pH as low as 2 did not alter T_{MIN} of the hydrophobic fraction of calf lung surfactant (Haddad et al., 1994). In addition, when we administered pH 1.9 HCl solution by direct micropuncture to surface alveoli of isolated rat lungs, the solution raised alveolar *T* over a period of ~30 min (Nguyen and Perlman, 2018). The time delay in the lungs suggests that low pH might raise *T* indirectly, perhaps by damaging the alveolar epithelium and releasing cell components that subsequently interfere with surfactant function.

Administration of pH 1.9 hydrochloric acid (HCl) solution via the trachea also raised alveolar *T* in isolated rat lungs. Surprisingly, however, this effect was not pH dependent. Tracheal instillation of pH 5.0 normal saline caused the same increase in alveolar *T* (Nguyen and Perlman, 2018). The *T*-raising effect of HCl or saline instillation was not due to surfactant dilution as direct alveolar injection of saline, which should cause greater dilution, did not alter *T* from normal. Further, even tracheal instillation of the surfactant Infasurf raised alveolar *T*. Thus, we suspected the involvement of airway mucins and, indeed, injection into surface alveoli of tracheal lavage liquid raised alveolar *T*. Addition to the tracheal lavage liquid of HCl or calcium, both of which aggregate mucins, reduced or eliminated the effect of tracheal lavage liquid on alveolar *T*. And, following tracheal saline administration, alveolar liquid sampled directly by vacuum suction through a glass micropipette contained mucin 5B. Thus, we demonstrated that tracheal liquid instillation raises alveolar *T* by washing *T*-raising airway mucins to the alveolus.

In gastric aspiration, the effects of pH and mucins should tend to balance one another. If gastric contents mix significantly with airway liquid, then they should be partially buffered but also collect mucins (Kim et al., 2014; Nguyen and Perlman, 2018). The higher pH might not be injurious, but the mucins might elevate *T* (Nguyen and Perlman, 2018). Alternatively, if there is relatively little mixing with airway liquid, there will be relatively little buffering, and pH will remain low. The low pH will tend to aggregate mucins such that the mucins might not contribute to elevated *T* (Hong et al., 2005; Nguyen and Perlman, 2018). The low pH, itself, should lead to elevated *T*, albeit perhaps indirectly via debris from damaged epithelial or other cells. Regardless of the degree of mixing between gastric contents and airway liquid, gastric aspiration is likely to raise alveolar *T*.

MEANS OF REDUCING *T*-DEPENDENT VILI

Surface tension is believed to be elevated in ARDS and is further increased by lung inflation during ventilation. And the static and dynamic stress concentrations described above, which likely contribute to VILI, are proportional to *T*. Thus, lowering *T* should reduce the VILI.

Means of Reducing *T*

Surfactant therapy has been tested for ARDS but, in six randomized controlled clinical trials, failed to reduce mortality (Brower and Fessler, 2011). Certainly, surfactant could lower *T* and yet fail to reduce mortality. However, surfactant therapy only improved oxygenation significantly in one of the six trials and marginally in one other and did not improve compliance in either of the two trials in which compliance was assessed (Weg et al., 1994; Anzueto et al., 1996; Gregory et al., 1997; Spragg et al., 2004, 2011; Kesecioglu et al., 2009), suggesting that it is a challenge for exogenous surfactant to lower alveolar T. Problematic surfactant dosage, administration technique, and formulation have been discussed as possible causes of the failure of surfactant therapy in ARDS (Spragg et al., 2011; Kazemi et al., 2019). My group has identified two new potential causes for the failure of surfactant therapy. First, surfactant delivery appears to be problematic. As detailed above, tracheal instillation of any liquid washes T-raising mucins to the alveolus. Thus, tracheal instillation of surfactant, contrary to expectation, *raises* alveolar T (Nguyen and Perlman, 2018). [Lower mucin production and more airspace liquid to dilute mucins may enable surfactant therapy efficacy in NRDS (Buisine et al., 1999)]. Second, when T is elevated in ARDS, adding more surfactant may fail to reduce T. In isolated rat lungs, we modeled acid-aspiration ARDS by administering pH 1.9 HCl solution to the alveolus by direct micropuncture or indirect tracheal instillation (Nguyen and Perlman, 2018). Both administration methods raised alveolar T. In both cases, however, subsequent alveolar delivery of mucin-free Infasurf by micropuncture failed to reduce T. Whether surfactant, if it could to be delivered mucin-free in a clinical setting, would be effective in other forms of ARDS remains to be determined.

With our T-determination method, we identified a potential alternative means of reducing T in ARDS. We found that that the non-toxic dye sulforhodamine B (SRB) acts in conjunction with albumin present in edema liquid to improve the efficacy of native lung surfactant and lower T 27% below normal in healthy lungs (Kharge et al., 2015). Thus, albumin, generally believed to be detrimental, might beneficially help lower T. Further, SRB, which has a molecular weight of 577 and is water soluble, might be administered intravenously. In this case, SRB would be expected to reach the alveolar liquid, along with albumin, specifically in injured regions where barrier permeability is elevated. Whether SRB will work in the presence of the various factors responsible for elevating T in ARDS remains to be determined.

Effects of Reducing *T*

Reducing T should help reduce VILI via various mechanisms. Direct effects of lowering T are as follows. Lowering T should increase P_{LIQ} in flooded alveoli, thus reduce bowing of and stress concentrations in intervening septa. Lowering T should reduce the diminishment of flooded alveoli and may prevent or reverse alveolar collapse, thus should reduce stress concentrations in radiating septa. And reducing stress concentrations in intervening or radiating septa should reduce VILI. Indeed, with our local VILI assay (**Figure 4A**), we demonstrated that lowering T, including by administration of SRB, reduced ventilation-induced barrier injury (Wu et al., 2014; Kharge et al., 2015).

Lowering T should also indirectly reduce stress concentrations in radiating septa. That is, lowering T should reduce the P_O required for air to enter a flooded region or to peel open the apposed septa of a collapsed region (Enhörning and Robertson, 1972; Gaver et al., 1990). Thus lowering T, by lowering P_O, should reduce the peak cyclic stress applied, just before reopening, to radiating septa around the injured region.

Further, lowering T may reduce VILI by promoting re-aeration of previously flooded or collapsed alveoli. Low T-induced re-aeration of a flooded alveolus is a rapid process in which liquid that has been sequestered in the alveolus redistributes, more equitably, across regional alveoli. In regions of heterogeneous alveolar flooding or collapse (**Figures 2B, 4**), re-aeration should reduce the degree of heterogeneity, thus, the number of intra-regional stress concentrations. For example, in regions of heterogeneous alveolar flooding, considering that bowed intervening septa are likely more stressed than planar septa separating two aerated or two flooded alveoli, we quantified heterogeneity as the percentage of all septa that were intervening septa (Wu et al., 2017). (In this basic analysis, we did not account for the presence of stressed radiating septa within injured regions). We found that heterogeneity peaked when ~50% of alveoli were flooded. Thus with heterogeneous flooding, reducing the number of flooded alveoli should reduce the number of intervening septa in which stress is concentrated and, in turn, VILI. (If >50% of alveoli are initially flooded, reducing the number of flooded alveoli should first exacerbate and then, once alveolar flooding decreases below 50%, relieve VILI). In regions with homogeneous alveolar flooding or collapse, re-aeration is most likely to occur on the periphery of the region (see below). As intervening and radiating septa around the perimeter of a homogeneously injured region are the sites of greatest stress concentration, re-aeration should, by reducing injured region perimeter length, reduce the number of septa in which stress is concentrated and reduce VILI.

Experimental evidence supports the possibility that lowering T may promote rapid re-aeration that could be beneficial in the time period before re-absorption causes the permanent re-aeration of ARDS resolution. Though the mechanism of rapid re-aeration has yet to be fully elucidated, my group has made observations that inform an understanding of the process (Kharge et al., 2015; Wu et al., 2017). (i) Flooded alveoli generally remain flooded and, at normal T, lung inflation does not generally cause re-aeration. However, occasionally, a flooded alveolus will spontaneously re-aerate. (ii) When T is reduced by SRB administration and the lungs are gently ventilated, the frequency of re-aeration increases. The direct effect of lowering T might be amplified by reduced T causing greater tissue stretch and thus contributing to enhanced surfactant secretion. (iii) It is also possible to promote re-aeration by accelerating deflation to increase momentum transfer to the flooding liquid and, essentially, catapult liquid out of alveoli. Accelerated deflation successfully reduces the number of flooded alveoli, and thus flooding heterogeneity, only when T is normal (below-normal T should be even better), and PIP is moderate, such that T at peak inflation is not too high. (iv) When T is elevated ~50% above normal in our model of **Figure 4B**, accelerated deflation still propels liquid out of flooded alveoli, but the high T keeps the liquid aggregated. The liquid transfers *en mass* to a neighboring alveolus that was previously aerated and the number of flooded alveoli remains unchanged. (Consistent with the hydrostatic origin of flooding in this model, the observation

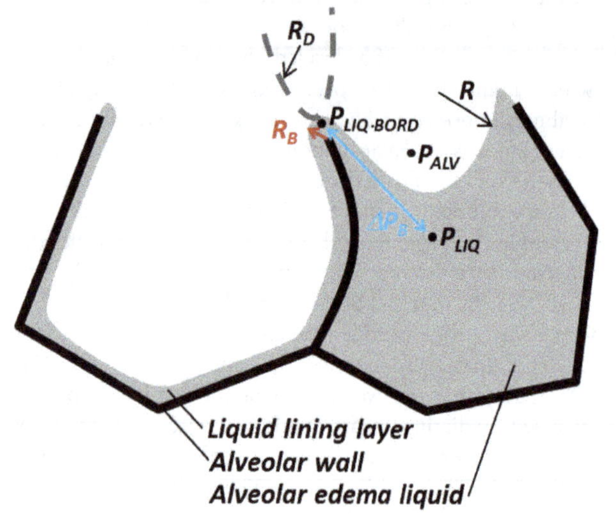

FIGURE 5 | Pressure barrier, ΔP_B, traps liquid in flooded alveoli. According to the Laplace relation, pressure in liquid below meniscus is $P_{LIQ} = P_{ALV} - 2T/R < P_{ALV}$, where R is the meniscus radius. At the border between two adjacent alveoli, shared septum terminates at alveolar duct or sac, and liquid phases of alveoli are presumably continuous. Thus, in the plane of the figure, the interface has a small convex radius R_B at the border of the flooded alveolus. In the plane perpendicular to the figure, the end of the septum and the interface should have larger concave radius R_D of duct or sac, indicated by dashed gray curve. Again, according to the Laplace relation, the liquid phase pressure at the border of the alveolus is $P_{LIQ \cdot BORD} = P_{ALV} + T(1/R_B - 1/R_D) > P_{ALV}$. Thus, pressure barrier $\Delta P_B = P_{LIQ \cdot BORD} - P_{LIQ} = T(1/R_B - 1/R_D + 2/R) > 0$ traps liquid in the flooded alveolus. As $\Delta P_B \sim T$, lowering T lowers ΔP_B and increases the likelihood of liquid escape from the flooded alveolus, i.e., the likelihood of re-aeration. Figure modified, with permission, from Kharge et al. (2015) and Wu et al. (2017).

of liquid transfer between alveoli indicates that alveoli are truly flooded, not collapsed. That is, flooding liquid volume is greater than the aggregated liquid lining layer volume that would be found in the center of a collapsed alveolus). (v) Finally, whether spontaneous or prompted by reduced T or accelerated deflation, we do not observe re-aeration of flooded alveoli surrounded entirely by other flooded alveoli but, rather, always of flooded alveoli that were in contact with one or more aerated alveoli. We interpret that flooded alveoli that are adjacent to at least one aerated alveolus are in a state of T-dependent unstable equilibrium.

The unstable equilibrium of flooded alveoli with aerated neighbors may be attributable to the antagonism across each intervening septum of outward-acting P_D, applied by radiating septa (**Figure 1C**, right), vs. inward-acting ΔP_S (**Figure 3B**). We have not identified the circumstances in which outward P_D sometimes prevails over inward ΔP_S, but note that a greater number of aerated neighbors make this occurrence more likely. Nevertheless, flooded alveoli typically remain flooded. This general stability is assisted by liquid pressure being greater at the border than in the center of flooded alveoli. That is, there is a pressure barrier, ΔP_B, that opposes liquid flow out of flooded alveoli and that is proportional to T (**Figure 5**). By trapping liquid in flooded alveoli, ΔP_B tends to maintain the low P_{LIQ} in flooded alveoli and thus maintain the diminished size of flooded alveoli. However, lowering T reduces ΔP_B and increases the likelihood of re-aeration (Kharge et al., 2015). For this reason, accelerated deflation most effectively clears alveoli when PIP is moderate, such that high elastic recoil for momentum transfer is balanced with low peak T for maintaining a low ΔP_B, and SRB administration increases the frequency of re-aeration during gentle ventilation (Kharge et al., 2015; Wu et al., 2017).

The existence of a pressure barrier is also supported by—and helps to explain—the difference in efficacy between two alternative recruitment maneuvers for initial inflation of immature fetal lungs. In a preterm lamb model, Tingay et al. (2019) showed that a gradual recruitment maneuver increases lung compliance more than an abrupt maneuver. This result might be explained by greater alveolar aeration at moderate P_L values—due to a moderate T and consequently moderate ΔP_B—in the course of the gradual maneuver. Although Tingay et al.'s (2019) direct comparison appears to be unique, other studies suggest that gradual recruitment may also result in greater re-aeration in ARDS. First, ARDS lung volume increased more in response to inflation from P_L of 19 to 28 cm H_2O than from 28 to 40 cm H_2O (Cressoni et al., 2017). Second, in an ARDS recruitment maneuver comprising a 7-s ramp up to a sustained 40 cm H_2O, essentially all of the effected volume increase occurred within the first 10 s after the ramp up period (Arnal et al., 2011). Finally, the response, in ARDS patients, to an abrupt 40 cm H_2O recruitment maneuver was inversely proportional to extravascular lung water index (Smetkin et al., 2012)—suggesting that high pressure may not effectively clear fluid from edematous alveoli, perhaps due to a high ΔP_B. A gradual recruitment maneuver might be more effective than an abrupt maneuver.

Re-aeration, by distributing liquid equitably between alveoli and thereby reducing the prevalence of stress concentrations, should reduce VILI. The balance between entering air (promoted by a high $P_{AW} > P_O$) and escaping liquid (promoted by a low P_L that maintains a low T and low ΔP_B) that causes re-aeration of a flooded alveolus remains to be determined. Such an understanding of the mechanism of flooded alveolar re-aeration might lead to new ventilation and recruitment maneuver protocols for maintaining an open lung.

DISCUSSION AND CONCLUSION

The above analysis stems from observations of T effects on flooded alveolar mechanics and speculates about consequences not yet investigated experimentally. The speculation, however, has limitations. First, the experimental observations were made in alveoli that were generally flooded with proteinaceous model edema liquid but that were otherwise, at least prior to ventilation, normal. The influence of pre-existing injury on flooded alveolar mechanics is not known. For example, whether flooded injured alveoli maintain normal compliance is not known. Second, discussion of T effects in regions of alveolar collapse is speculative. Alveolar collapse in a lung injury model has not, to date, been identified by microscopy on the surface of isolated lungs. Thus, collapse has not been studied, like flooding, with high resolution and tracking across varied inflation pressures. Third, the mechanism of flooded alveolar re-aeration, which should reduce the prevalence of stress concentrations, remains to be elucidated. And the feasibility of permanently re-aerating injured alveoli in ARDS is not known. Nonetheless, evidence suggests that lowering T should reduce alveolar septal stress concentrations and that lowering T in conjunction with application of gradual recruitment maneuvers may improve lung re-aeration. And both interventions should reduce VILI. Treatment with SRB appears a promising avenue of investigation for lowering T and VILI in ARDS.

AUTHOR CONTRIBUTIONS

CP conceived of the subject matter for and wrote this manuscript.

REFERENCES

Albert, R. K., Smith, B., Perlman, C. E., and Schwartz, D. A. (2019). Is progression of pulmonary fibrosis due to ventilation-induced lung injury? *Am. J. Respir. Crit. Care Med.* 200, 140–151. doi: 10.1164/rccm.201903-0497PP

Anzueto, A., Baughman, R. P., Guntupalli, K. K., Weg, J. G., Wiedemann, H. P., Raventós, A. A., et al. (1996). Aerosolized surfactant in adults with sepsis-induced acute respiratory distress syndrome. Exosurf acute respiratory distress syndrome sepsis study group. *N. Engl. J. Med.* 334, 1417–1421. doi: 10.1056/NEJM199605303342201

Arnal, J.-M., Paquet, J., Wysocki, M., Demory, D., Donati, S., Granier, I., et al. (2011). Optimal duration of a sustained inflation recruitment maneuver in ARDS patients. *Intensive Care Med.* 37, 1588–1594. doi: 10.1007/s00134-011-2323-0

Bachofen, H., Schürch, S., Michel, R. P., and Weibel, E. R. (1993). Experimental hydrostatic pulmonary edema in rabbit lungs. Morphology. *Am. Rev. Respir. Dis.* 147, 989–996. doi: 10.1164/ajrccm/147.4.989

Bachofen, H., Schürch, S., Urbinelli, M., and Weibel, E. R. (1987). Relations among alveolar surface tension, surface area, volume, and recoil pressure. *J. Appl. Physiol.* 62, 1878–1887. doi: 10.1152/jappl.1987.62.5.1878

Bilek, A. M., Dee, K. C., and Gaver, D. P. (2003). Mechanisms of surface-tension-induced epithelial cell damage in a model of pulmonary airway reopening. *J. Appl. Physiol.* 94, 770–783. doi: 10.1152/japplphysiol.00764.2002

Brower, R. G., and Fessler, H. E. (2011). Another "negative" trial of surfactant. Time to bury this idea? *Am. J. Respir. Crit. Care Med.* 183, 966–968. doi: 10.1164/rccm.201101-0018ED

Brower, R. G., Matthay, M. A., Morris, A., Schoenfeld, D., Thompson, B. T., Wheeler, A., et al. (2000). Ventilation with lower tidal volumes as compared with traditional tidal volumes for acute lung injury and the acute respiratory distress syndrome. *N. Engl. J. Med.* 342, 1301–1308. doi: 10.1056/NEJM200005043421801

Buisine, M. P., Devisme, L., Copin, M. C., Durand-Réville, M., Gosselin, B., Aubert, J. P., et al. (1999). Developmental mucin gene expression in the human respiratory tract. *Am. J. Respir. Cell Mol. Biol.* 20, 209–218. doi: 10.1165/ajrcmb.20.2.3259

Cereda, M., Xin, Y., Hamedani, H., Bellani, G., Kadlecek, S., Clapp, J., et al. (2017). Tidal changes on CT and progression of ARDS. *Thorax* 72, 981–989. doi: 10.1136/thoraxjnl-2016-209833

Clements, J. A. (1997). Lung surfactant: a personal perspective. *Annu. Rev. Physiol.* 59, 1–21. doi: 10.1146/annurev.physiol.59.1.1

Cressoni, M., Chiumello, D., Algieri, I., Brioni, M., Chiurazzi, C., Colombo, A., et al. (2017). Opening pressures and atelectrauma in acute respiratory distress syndrome. *Intensive Care Med.* 43, 603–611. doi: 10.1007/s00134-017-4754-8

de Prost, N., Feng, Y., Wellman, T., Tucci, M. R., Costa, E. L., Musch, G., et al. (2014). 18F-FDG kinetics parameters depend on the mechanism of injury in early experimental acute respiratory distress syndrome. *J. Nucl. Med.* 55, 1871–1877. doi: 10.2967/jnumed.114.140962

Dreyfuss, D., and Saumon, G. (1998). Ventilator-induced lung injury: lessons from experimental studies. *Am. J. Respir. Crit. Care Med.* 157, 294–323. doi: 10.1164/ajrccm.157.1.9604014

Enhörning, G., and Robertson, B. (1972). Lung expansion in the premature rabbit fetus after tracheal deposition of surfactant. *Pediatrics* 50, 58–66.

Gattinoni, L., Caironi, P., Pelosi, P., and Goodman, L. R. (2001). What has computed tomography taught us about the acute respiratory distress syndrome? *Am. J. Respir. Crit. Care Med.* 164, 1701–1711. doi: 10.1164/ajrccm.164.9.2103121

Gaver, D. P., Samsel, R. W., and Solway, J. (1990). Effects of surface tension and viscosity on airway reopening. *J. Appl. Physiol.* 69, 74–85. doi: 10.1152/jappl.1990.69.1.74

Gil, J., Bachofen, H., Gehr, P., and Weibel, E. R. (1979). Alveolar volume-surface area relation in air- and saline-filled lungs fixed by vascular perfusion. *J. Appl. Physiol. Respir. Environ. Exerc. Physiol.* 47, 990–1001. doi: 10.1152/jappl.1979.47.5.990

Gommers, D., Vilstrup, C., Bos, J. A., Larsson, A., Werner, O., Hannappel, E., et al. (1993). Exogenous surfactant therapy increases static lung compliance, and cannot be assessed by measurements of dynamic compliance alone. *Crit. Care Med.* 21, 567–574. doi: 10.1097/00003246-199304000-00019

Gregory, T. J., Longmore, W. J., Moxley, M. A., Whitsett, J. A., Reed, C. R., Fowler, A. A., et al. (1991). Surfactant chemical composition and biophysical activity in acute respiratory distress syndrome. *J. Clin. Invest.* 88, 1976–1981. doi: 10.1172/JCI115523

Gregory, T. J., Steinberg, K. P., Spragg, R., Gadek, J. E., Hyers, T. M., Longmore, W. J., et al. (1997). Bovine surfactant therapy for patients with acute respiratory distress syndrome. *Am. J. Respir. Crit. Care Med.* 155, 1309–1315. doi: 10.1164/ajrccm.155.4.9105072

Gunasekara, L., Schürch, S., Schoel, W. M., Nag, K., Leonenko, Z., Haufs, M., et al. (2005). Pulmonary surfactant function is abolished by an elevated proportion of cholesterol. *Biochim. Biophys. Acta* 1737, 27–35. doi: 10.1016/j.bbalip.2005.09.002

Günther, A., Schmidt, R., Harodt, J., Schmehl, T., Walmrath, D., Ruppert, C., et al. (2002). Bronchoscopic administration of bovine natural surfactant in ARDS and septic shock: impact on biophysical and biochemical surfactant properties. *Eur. Respir. J.* 19, 797–804. doi: 10.1183/09031936.02.00243302

Günther, A., Siebert, C., Schmidt, R., Ziegler, S., Grimminger, F., Yabut, M., et al. (1996). Surfactant alterations in severe pneumonia, acute respiratory distress syndrome, and cardiogenic lung edema. *Am. J. Respir. Crit. Care Med.* 153, 176–184. doi: 10.1164/ajrccm.153.1.8542113

Gustafsson, M., Palmblad, M., Curstedt, T., Johansson, J., and Schürch, S. (2000). Palmitoylation of a pulmonary surfactant protein C analogue affects the surface associated lipid reservoir and film stability. *Biochim. Biophys. Acta* 1466, 169–178. doi: 10.1016/s0005-2736(00)00198-x

Haagsman, H. P., and van Golde, L. M. (1991). Synthesis and assembly of lung surfactant. *Annu. Rev. Physiol.* 53, 441–464. doi: 10.1146/annurev.ph.53.030191.002301

Haddad, I. Y., Holm, B. A., Hlavaty, L., and Matalon, S. (1994). Dependence of surfactant function on extracellular pH: mechanisms and modifications. *J. Appl. Physiol.* 76, 657–662. doi: 10.1152/jappl.1994.76.2.657

Hallman, M., Spragg, R., Harrell, J. H., Moser, K. M., and Gluck, L. (1982). Evidence of lung surfactant abnormality in respiratory failure. Study of bronchoalveolar lavage phospholipids, surface activity, phospholipase activity, and plasma myoinositol. *J. Clin. Invest.* 70, 673–683. doi: 10.1172/jci110662

Henzler, D., Hochhausen, N., Chankalal, R., Xu, Z., Whynot, S. C., Slutsky, A. S., et al. (2011). Physiologic and biologic characteristics of three experimental models of acute lung injury in rats. *Anesth. Analg.* 112, 1139–1146. doi: 10.1213/ANE.0b013e3182104dac

Hite, R. D., Seeds, M. C., Jacinto, R. B., Grier, B. L., Waite, B. M., and Bass, D. A. (2005). Lysophospholipid and fatty acid inhibition of pulmonary surfactant: non-enzymatic models of phospholipase A2 surfactant hydrolysis. *Biochim. Biophys. Acta* 1720, 14–21. doi: 10.1016/j.bbamem.2005.10.014

Holm, B. A., Enhorning, G., and Notter, R. H. (1988). A biophysical mechanism by which plasma proteins inhibit lung surfactant activity. *Chem. Phys. Lipids* 49, 49–55. doi: 10.1016/0009-3084(88)90063-1

Holm, B. A., Keicher, L., Liu, M. Y., Sokolowski, J., and Enhorning, G. (1991). Inhibition of pulmonary surfactant function by phospholipases. *J. Appl. Physiol.* 71, 317–321. doi: 10.1152/jappl.1991.71.1.317

Holm, B. A., and Notter, R. H. (1987). Effects of hemoglobin and cell membrane lipids on pulmonary surfactant activity. *J. Appl. Physiol.* 63, 1434–1442. doi: 10.1152/jappl.1987.63.4.1434

Holm, B. A., Wang, Z., and Notter, R. H. (1999). Multiple mechanisms of lung surfactant inhibition. *Pediatr. Res.* 46, 85–93. doi: 10.1203/00006450-199907000-00015

Hong, Z., Chasan, B., Bansil, R., Turner, B. S., Bhaskar, K. R., and Afdhal, N. H. (2005). Atomic force microscopy reveals aggregation of gastric mucin at low pH. *Biomacromolecules* 6, 3458–3466. doi: 10.1021/bm0505843

Horie, T., and Hildebrandt, J. (1971). Dynamic compliance, limit cycles, and static equilibria of excised cat lung. *J. Appl. Physiol.* 31, 423–430. doi: 10.1152/jappl.1971.31.3.423

Jobe, A., Ikegami, M., Jacobs, H., Jones, S., and Conaway, D. (1983). Permeability of premature lamb lungs to protein and the effect of surfactant on that permeability. *J. Appl. Physiol. Respir. Environ. Exerc. Physiol.* 55, 169–176. doi: 10.1152/jappl.1983.55.1.169

Kazemi, A., Louis, B., Isabey, D., Nieman, G. F., Gatto, L. A., Satalin, J., et al. (2019). Surfactant delivery in rat lungs: Comparing 3D geometrical simulation model with experimental instillation. *PLoS Comput. Biol.* 15:e1007408. doi: 10.1371/journal.pcbi.1007408

Kesecioglu, J., Beale, R., Stewart, T. E., Findlay, G. P., Rouby, J.-J., Holzapfel, L., et al. (2009). Exogenous natural surfactant for treatment of acute lung injury and the acute respiratory distress syndrome. *Am. J. Respir. Crit. Care Med.* 180, 989–994. doi: 10.1164/rccm.200812-1955OC

Kharge, A. B., Wu, Y., and Perlman, C. E. (2014). Surface tension *in situ* in flooded alveolus unaltered by albumin. *J. Appl. Physiol.* 117, 440–451. doi: 10.1152/japplphysiol.00084.2014

Kharge, A. B., Wu, Y., and Perlman, C. E. (2015). Sulforhodamine B interacts with albumin to lower surface tension and protect against ventilation injury of flooded alveoli. *J. Appl. Physiol.* 118, 355–364. doi: 10.1152/japplphysiol.00818.2014

Kiefmann, M., Tank, S., Tritt, M.-O., Keller, P., Heckel, K., Schulte-Uentrop, L., et al. (2019). Dead space ventilation promotes alveolar hypocapnia reducing surfactant secretion by altering mitochondrial function. *Thorax* 74, 219–228. doi: 10.1136/thoraxjnl-2018-211864

Kim, D., Liao, J., and Hanrahan, J. W. (2014). The buffer capacity of airway epithelial secretions. *Front. Physiol.* 5:188. doi: 10.3389/fphys.2014.00188

Kitsiouli, E., Nakos, G., and Lekka, M. E. (2009). Phospholipase A2 subclasses in acute respiratory distress syndrome. *Biochim. Biophys. Acta* 1792, 941–953. doi: 10.1016/j.bbadis.2009.06.007

Lugones, Y., Blanco, O., López-Rodríguez, E., Echaide, M., Cruz, A., and Pérez-Gil, J. (2018). Inhibition and counterinhibition of Surfacen, a clinical lung surfactant of natural origin. *PLoS ONE* 13:e0204050. doi: 10.1371/journal.pone.0204050

Mead, J., Takishima, T., and Leith, D. (1970). Stress distribution in lungs: a model of pulmonary elasticity. *J. Appl. Physiol.* 28, 596–608. doi: 10.1152/jappl.1970.28.5.596

Nguyen, T. L., and Perlman, C. E. (2018). Tracheal acid or surfactant instillation raises alveolar surface tension. *J. Appl. Physiol.* 125, 1357–1367. doi: 10.1152/japplphysiol.00397.2017

Perlman, C. E., Lederer, D. J., and Bhattacharya, J. (2011). Micromechanics of alveolar edema. *Am. J. Respir. Cell Mol. Biol.* 44, 34–39. doi: 10.1165/rcmb.2009-0005OC

Perlman, C. E., and Wu, Y. (2014). *In situ* determination of alveolar septal strain, stress and effective Young's modulus: an experimental/computational approach. *Am. J. Physiol. Lung Cell Mol. Physiol.* 307, L302–L310. doi: 10.1152/ajplung.00106.2014

Rodríguez-Capote, K., Manzanares, D., Haines, T., and Possmayer, F. (2006). Reactive oxygen species inactivation of surfactant involves structural and functional alterations to surfactant proteins SP-B and SP-C. *Biophys. J.* 90, 2808–2821. doi: 10.1529/biophysj.105.073106

Rühl, N., Lopez-Rodriguez, E., Albert, K., Smith, B. J., Weaver, T. E., Ochs, M., et al. (2019). Surfactant protein B deficiency induced high surface tension: relationship between alveolar micromechanics, alveolar fluid properties and alveolar epithelial cell injury. *Int. J. Mol. Sci.* 20:E4243. doi: 10.3390/ijms20174243

Ruppert, C., Pucker, C., Markart, P., Schmidt, R., Grimminger, F., Seeger, W., et al. (2003). Selective inhibition of large-to-small surfactant aggregate conversion by serine protease inhibitors of the bis-benzamidine type. *Am. J. Respir. Cell Mol. Biol.* 28, 95–102. doi: 10.1165/rcmb.4591

Santos, C. L., Moraes, L., Santos, R. S., Oliveira, M. G., Silva, J. D., Maron-Gutierrez, T., et al. (2012). Effects of different tidal volumes in pulmonary and extrapulmonary lung injury with or without intraabdominal hypertension. *Intensive Care Med.* 38, 499–508. doi: 10.1007/s00134-011-2451-6

Schürch, S., Bachofen, H., Goerke, J., and Green, F. (1992). Surface properties of rat pulmonary surfactant studied with the captive bubble method: adsorption, hysteresis, stability. *Biochim. Biophys. Acta* 1103, 127–136. doi: 10.1016/0005-2736(92)90066-u

Schürch, S., Goerke, J., and Clements, J. A. (1976). Direct determination of surface tension in the lung. *Proc. Natl. Acad. Sci. U.S.A.* 73, 4698–4702. doi: 10.1073/pnas.73.12.4698

Seeds, M. C., Grier, B. L., Suckling, B. N., Safta, A. M., Long, D. L., Waite, B. M., et al. (2012). Secretory phospholipase A2-mediated depletion of phosphatidylglycerol in early acute respiratory distress syndrome. *Am. J. Med. Sci.* 343, 446–451. doi: 10.1097/MAJ.0b013e318239c96c

Seeger, W., Grube, C., Günther, A., and Schmidt, R. (1993). Surfactant inhibition by plasma proteins: differential sensitivity of various surfactant preparations. *Eur. Respir. J.* 6, 971–977.

Smetkin, A. A., Kuzkov, V. V., Suborov, E. V., Bjertnaes, L. J., and Kirov, M. Y. (2012). Increased extravascular lung water reduces the efficacy of alveolar recruitment maneuver in acute respiratory distress syndrome. *Crit. Care. Res. Pract.* 2012:606528. doi: 10.1155/2012/606528

Smith, E. C., Laderas, T. G., Crane, J. M., and Hall, S. B. (2004). Persistence of metastability after expansion of a supercompressed fluid monolayer. *Langmuir* 20, 4945–4953. doi: 10.1021/la036150f

Spragg, R. G., Lewis, J. F., Walmrath, H.-D., Johannigman, J., Bellingan, G., Laterre, P.-F., et al. (2004). Effect of recombinant surfactant protein C-based surfactant on the acute respiratory distress syndrome. *N. Engl. J. Med.* 351, 884–892. doi: 10.1056/NEJMoa033181

Spragg, R. G., Taut, F. J. H., Lewis, J. F., Schenk, P., Ruppert, C., Dean, N., et al. (2011). Recombinant surfactant protein C-based surfactant for patients with severe direct lung injury. *Am. J. Respir. Crit. Care Med.* 183, 1055–1061. doi: 10.1164/rccm.201009-1424OC

Staub, N. C., Nagano, H., and Pearce, M. L. (1967). Pulmonary edema in dogs, especially the sequence of fluid accumulation in lungs. *J. Appl. Physiol.* 22, 227–240. doi: 10.1152/jappl.1967.22.2.227

Terragni, P. P., Rosboch, G., Tealdi, A., Corno, E., Menaldo, E., Davini, O., et al. (2007). Tidal hyperinflation during low tidal volume ventilation in acute respiratory distress syndrome. *Am. J. Respir. Crit. Care Med.* 175, 160–166. doi: 10.1164/rccm.200607-915OC

Tingay, D. G., Pereira-Fantini, P. M., Oakley, R., McCall, K. E., Perkins, E. J., Miedema, M., et al. (2019). Gradual aeration at birth Is more lung protective than a sustained inflation in preterm lambs. *Am. J. Respir. Crit. Care Med.* 200, 608–616. doi: 10.1164/rccm.201807-1397OC

Tsuchida, S., Engelberts, D., Peltekova, V., Hopkins, N., Frndova, H., Babyn, P., et al. (2006). Atelectasis causes alveolar injury in nonatelectatic lung regions. *Am. J. Respir. Crit. Care Med.* 174, 279–289. doi: 10.1164/rccm.200506-1006OC

van Meer, G., Voelker, D. R., and Feigenson, G. W. (2008). Membrane lipids: where they are and how they behave. *Nat. Rev. Mol. Cell Biol.* 9, 112–124. doi: 10.1038/nrm2330

Ware, L. B. (2006). Pathophysiology of acute lung injury and the acute respiratory distress syndrome. *Semin. Respir. Crit. Care Med.* 27, 337–349. doi: 10.1055/s-2006-948288

Warriner, H. E., Ding, J., Waring, A. J., and Zasadzinski, J. A. (2002). A concentration-dependent mechanism by which serum albumin inactivates replacement lung surfactants. *Biophys. J.* 82, 835–842. doi: 10.1016/S0006-3495(02)75445-3

Weg, J. G., Balk, R. A., Tharratt, R. S., Jenkinson, S. G., Shah, J. B., Zaccardelli, D., et al. (1994). Safety and potential efficacy of an aerosolized surfactant in human sepsis-induced adult respiratory distress syndrome. *JAMA* 272, 1433–1438.

Wu, C., Chen, X., Cai, Y., Xia, J., Zhou, X., Xu, S., et al. (2020). Risk factors associated with acute respiratory distress syndrome and death in patients with coronavirus disease 2019 pneumonia in Wuhan, China. *JAMA Intern. Med.* [Epub ahead of print]. doi: 10.1001/jamainternmed.2020.0994

Wu, Y., Kharge, A. B., and Perlman, C. E. (2014). Lung ventilation injures areas with discrete alveolar flooding, in a surface tension-dependent fashion. *J. Appl. Physiol.* 117, 788–796. doi: 10.1152/japplphysiol.00569.2014

Wu, Y., Nguyen, T. L., and Perlman, C. E. (2017). Accelerated deflation promotes homogeneous airspace liquid distribution in the edematous lung. *J. Appl. Physiol.* 122, 739–751. doi: 10.1152/japplphysiol.00526.2016

Wüstneck, R., Perez-Gil, J., Wüstneck, N., Cruz, A., Fainerman, V. B., and Pison, U. (2005). Interfacial properties of pulmonary surfactant layers. *Adv. Colloid Interf. Sci.* 117, 33–58. doi: 10.1016/j.cis.2005.05.001

Yamashita, C., Forbes, A., Tessolini, J. M., Yao, L.-J., Lewis, J. F., and Veldhuizen, R. A. W. (2008). Protective effects of elevated endogenous surfactant pools to injurious mechanical ventilation. *Am. J. Physiol. Lung Cell Mol. Physiol.* 294, L724–L732. doi: 10.1152/ajplung.00389.2007

12

A Physiologically Informed Strategy to Effectively Open, Stabilize and Protect the Acutely Injured Lung

Gary F. Nieman[1], Hassan Al-Khalisy[1,2], Michaela Kollisch-Singule[3], Joshua Satalin[1], Sarah Blair[1], Girish Trikha[1,2], Penny Andrews[4], Maria Madden[4], Louis A. Gatto[1,5] and Nader M. Habashi[4]*

[1] *Department of Surgery, SUNY Upstate Medical University, Syracuse, NY, United States,* [2] *Department of Medicine, SUNY Upstate Medical University, Syracuse, NY, United States,* [3] *Department of Pediatric Surgery, Arkansas Children's Hospital, Little Rock, AR, United States,* [4] *Department of Trauma Critical Care Medicine, R Adams Cowley Shock Trauma Center, University of Maryland School of Medicine, Baltimore, MD, United States,* [5] *Department of Biological Sciences, SUNY Cortland, Cortland, NY, United States*

Correspondence:
Joshua Satalin
SatalinJ@upstate.edu

Acute respiratory distress syndrome (ARDS) causes a heterogeneous lung injury and remains a serious medical problem, with one of the only treatments being supportive care in the form of mechanical ventilation. It is very difficult, however, to mechanically ventilate the heterogeneously damaged lung without causing secondary ventilator-induced lung injury (VILI). The acutely injured lung becomes *time* and *pressure* dependent, meaning that it takes more time and pressure to open the lung, and it recollapses more quickly and at higher pressure. Current protective ventilation strategies, ARDSnet low tidal volume (LVt) and the open lung approach (OLA), have been unsuccessful at further reducing ARDS mortality. We postulate that this is because the LVt strategy is constrained to ventilating a lung with a heterogeneous mix of normal and focalized injured tissue, and the OLA, although designed to fully open and stabilize the lung, is often unsuccessful at doing so. In this review we analyzed the pathophysiology of ARDS that renders the lung susceptible to VILI. We also analyzed the alterations in alveolar and alveolar duct mechanics that occur in the acutely injured lung and discussed how these alterations are a key mechanism driving VILI. Our analysis suggests that the *time* component of each mechanical breath, at both inspiration and expiration, is critical to normalize alveolar mechanics and protect the lung from VILI. Animal studies and a meta-analysis have suggested that the time-controlled adaptive ventilation (TCAV) method, using the airway pressure release ventilation mode, eliminates the constraints of ventilating a lung with heterogeneous injury, since it is highly effective at opening and stabilizing the *time*- and *pressure*-dependent lung. In animal studies it has been shown that by "casting open" the acutely injured lung with TCAV we can (1) reestablish normal expiratory lung volume as assessed by direct observation of subpleural alveoli; (2) return normal parenchymal microanatomical structural support, known as alveolar interdependence and parenchymal tethering, as assessed by morphometric analysis of lung histology; (3) facilitate regeneration of normal surfactant function measured as increases in surfactant proteins A and B; and (4) significantly increase lung compliance, which reduces the pathologic impact of driving pressure and mechanical power at any given tidal volume.

Keywords: ARDS, VILI (ventilator induced lung injury), mechanical ventilalion, APRV, alveolar mechanics

INTRODUCTION

Acute respiratory distress syndrome (ARDS) was initially thought to be a lethal double pneumonia and was identified as a syndrome by Ashbaugh et al. (1967). Unfortunately, in the 50 years since ARDS was identified, only a few treatments have been used, with the mainstay being supportive in the form of mechanical ventilation (Slutsky and Ranieri, 2013). However, mechanical ventilation constrained to the limitations of a heterogeneously injured lung can cause unintended tissue damage, referred to as ventilator-induced lung injury (VILI), which can significantly increase mortality (~40%) as compared to lung protective ventilation (~31%) (Acute Respiratory Distress Syndrome Network, 2000). Initial randomized controlled trials (RCTs) attempting to reduce VILI by lowering tidal volume (Vt) failed to reduce mortality (Stewart et al., 1998; Brower et al., 1999). It was not until the ARDS Network (ARDSnet) conducted the seminal ARMA study, published in 2000, that a reduction in mortality was shown (Acute Respiratory Distress Syndrome Network, 2000). However, most (Phua et al., 2009; Villar et al., 2011; Caser et al., 2014; Bellani et al., 2016; Laffey et al., 2016; Villar et al., 2016; Maca et al., 2017; Raymondos et al., 2017; Rezoagli et al., 2017; Fan et al., 2018; McNicholas et al., 2018; Pham et al., 2019; Shen et al., 2019) but not all (Brun-Buisson et al., 2004; Fan et al., 2005; Putensen et al., 2009; Petrucci and De Feo, 2013; Shen et al., 2019) of the recent statistical- and meta-analyses have shown that ARDS mortality has not been reduced below the 31% "gold standard" of the 2000 ARMA study but rather remains unacceptably high at ~40% (**Figure 1**). Despite these disappointing results, the low-Vt ARDSnet method is still recommended as the standard-of-care protective ventilation strategy for ARDS patients (Fan et al., 2017, 2018; Papazian et al., 2019).

Since outcome data for ARDS patients has not improved for almost 20 years, it is imperative to (1) ascertain the mechanisms of dynamic alveolar and alveolar duct volume change during mechanical ventilation (elastic, viscous, or viscoelastic), (2) characterize ARDS-induced changes in alveolar mechanics (i.e., the dynamic change in alveolar size and shape during mechanical ventilation) (Grune et al., 2019) that drive VILI-induced tissue damage, (3) identify the role of airway pressure and the duration at both inspiration and expiration on alveolar mechanics in the acutely injured lung (Kollisch-Singule et al., 2014a, 2018), and (4) use this knowledge to develop novel ventilation strategies to better reduce VILI and protect the lung. Although pulmonary inflammation (biotrauma) also plays a critical role in ARDS and VILI pathogenesis, the focus of this review will be the mechanical injury to tissue caused during ventilation.

CONSTRAINTS OF VENTILATING THE ACUTELY INJURED LUNG

The current concept is that ARDS causes heterogeneous injury in three general lung compartments that are layered by gravity (**Figure 2**). The first compartment, or the non-dependent area, contains a small number of normal compliant alveoli that remain inflated at end-expiration—functional residual capacity (FRC)—and is referred to as the "baby lung" (Gattinoni and Pesenti, 2005). The second compartment consists of alveoli in the dependent areas that are collapsed and/or edema filled. The third compartment consists of alveoli that remain in the transition zone between healthy and unstable, due to loss of surfactant function, and that open and collapse with every breath.

Consequently, the ARDSnet low-Vt and plateau pressure (Pplat) strategy is constrained to ventilating this heterogeneous lung tissue without causing VILI using a three-tiered approach: (1) *protect* the baby lung by not overdistending the compliant tissue that is open at FRC, (2) *rest* the dependent collapsed and edema-filled tissue by keeping it out of the ventilatory cycle, and (3) *stabilize* the tissue in between by applying positive end-expiratory pressure (PEEP), usually adjusted by oxygenation (**Figure 2**) (Acute Respiratory Distress Syndrome Network, 2000; Del Sorbo et al., 2017).

Problems With Protecting the Baby Lung

Since the baby lung is believed to be a small volume of normal tissue (Gattinoni and Pesenti, 2005), its overdistension has been postulated to be a primary VILI mechanism (Brower et al., 2004). However, in studies in which normal lungs were subjected to excessively high airway pressures (>30 cm H_2O) and strain (2.5 ratio), overdistension-induced VILI did not occur as long as this excessive strain was nearly static. This suggests that overdistension of normal tissue with high volume and pressure is not a primary VILI mechanism unless there is also a large dynamic strain (Seah et al., 2011; Protti et al., 2013b; Jain et al., 2017). It is possible that the baby lung is injured not by overdistension of the normal tissue, but rather by the recruiting and recollapse of unstable tissue in the adjacent collapsed regions (Gattinoni et al., 1995). Thus, lowering Vt and Pplat to reduce overdistension in the open lung tissue, which is surrounded by a large volume of collapsed and unstable tissue of very low compliance, may not reduce VILI. Regional instability and inflammation occur throughout the entire lung, including in tissue that appears to be normal on computed tomography (CT) scan or chest X-ray, and serve as pathologic focal points from which VILI-induced tissue damage expands (Wellman et al., 2014, 2016; Cereda et al., 2016b, 2017). This suggests that to protect the normal lung tissue regional instability must be eliminated.

However, others have shown that overdistension is a major component of VILI pathophysiology in injured lungs (Guldner et al., 2016). Guldner et al. (2016), in a porcine ARDS model, showed that extreme conditions of overdistension resulted in more lung inflammation than did extreme lung collapse, suggesting that static stress and strain are major VILI mechanisms. Although this study clearly showed that volutrauma increased inflammation, histopathology was not measured, and there was no difference in pulmonary edema as measured by lung weight. Thus, it is not clear whether the increase in inflammation caused any lung pathology. In addition, recalculation of the data showed that the average mechanical power in the volutrauma group was 17.12 J/min, more than double that of the atelectrauma group (7.13 J/min) (Tonetti et al., 2017). Others have also

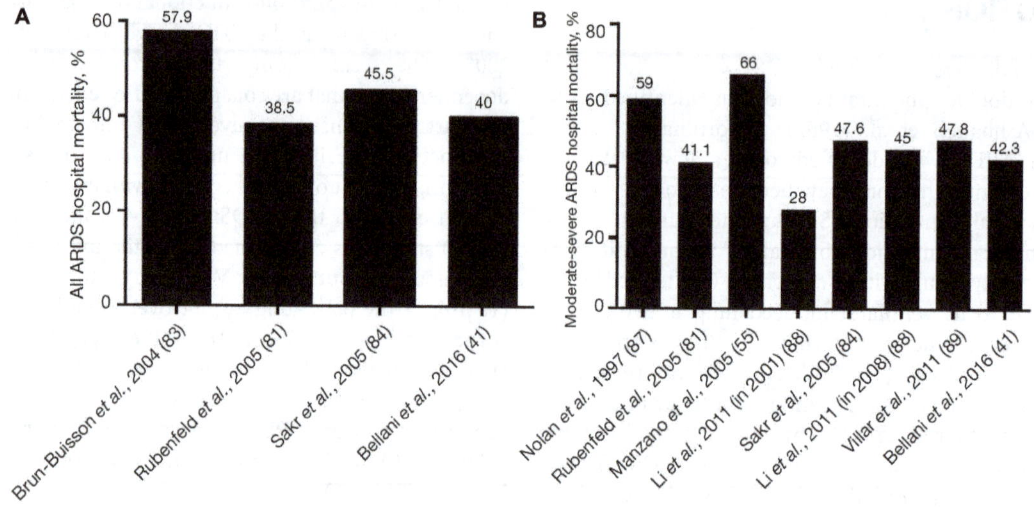

FIGURE 1 | (A) Hospital mortality (%) in the main epidemiological studies for all three American-European Consensus Conference (AECC) classifications of acute respiratory distress syndrome (ARDS – mild, moderate, and severe) and **(B)** mortality (%) for only moderate and severe ARDS. The mean and standard deviation for mortality in all of the studies following the 2000 ARMA study (Acute Respiratory Distress Syndrome Network, 2000) is 45.4 ± 9.5 (Rezoagli et al., 2017). *Permissions obtained from AME Publishing Company, License ID 1017423-1.*

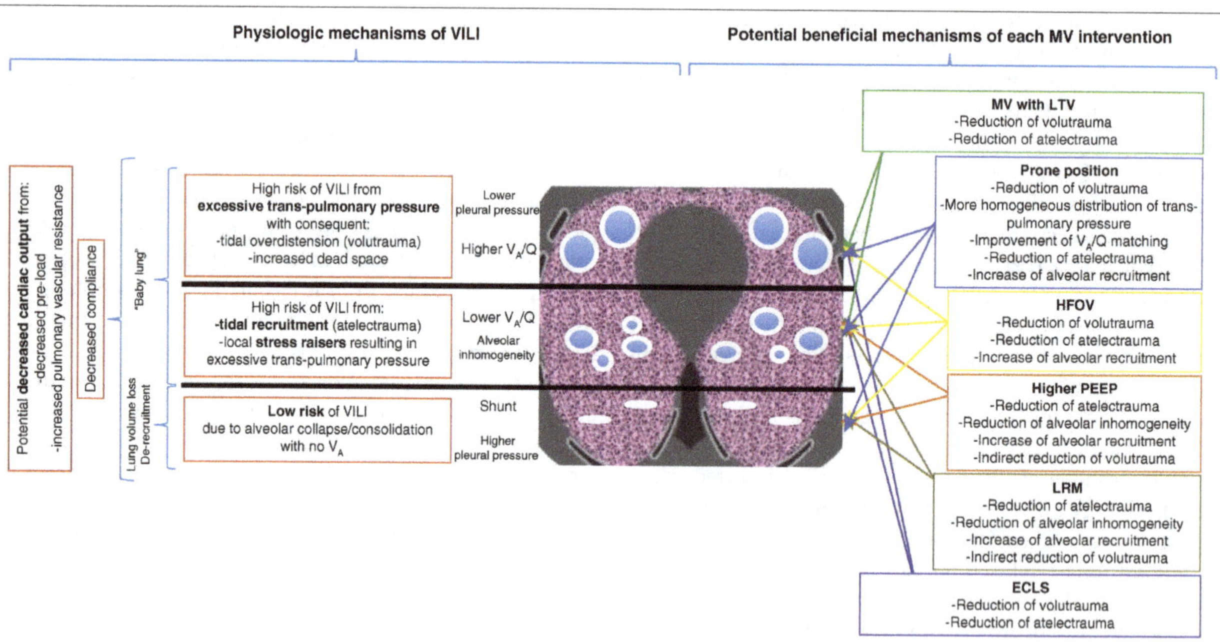

FIGURE 2 | Gravity dependent three-compartment model of acute respiratory distress syndrome (ARDS) pathology: **Left** – Physiological mechanisms of ventilator-induced lung injury (VILI) and **Right** – Potential beneficial mechanisms of various protective ventilation strategies to minimize VILI. Open alveoli are shown as blue circles similar in size (top), unstable alveoli as smaller circles of various sizes (middle), and collapsed alveoli as solid white lines (bottom). The ARDSnet low tidal volume (LVt) method is designed to *protect* compliant open alveoli in the non-dependent lung and *rest* the collapsed tissue in the dependent portion of the lung by keeping it unventilated. Positive end-expiratory pressure (PEEP) is added in an attempt to *stabilize* the alveoli in between (Acute Respiratory Distress Syndrome Network, 2000). High-frequency oscillatory ventilation (HFOV) and lung recruitment maneuvers (LRMs) have been shown ineffective in reducing ARDS mortality (Brower et al., 2004; Meade et al., 2008; Mercat et al., 2008; Ferguson et al., 2013; Young et al., 2013; Cavalcanti et al., 2017; Hodgson et al., 2019). Prone position has been shown effective at reducing mortality (Guerin et al., 2013) by a mechanism of reducing regional alveolar strain and inflammation (Motta-Ribeiro et al., 2018; Xin et al., 2018). VILI, ventilator-induced lung injury; MV, mechanical ventilation; LTV, low tidal volume and inspiratory pressure; PEEP, positive end-expiratory pressure; ECLS, extracorporeal life support; HFOV, high-frequency oscillatory ventilation; LRM, lung recruitment maneuver; Q, perfusion; V_A, alveolar ventilation; V_A/Q, ventilation/perfusion ratio; baby lung, functional residual capacity (FRC) (Del Sorbo et al., 2017). *Permissions to publish obtained from ATS.*

shown that increasing airway pressure in an acutely injured lung will cause a rapid progression of injury in a "rich-get-richer" power-law fashion, supporting the findings in the Guldner study (Hamlington et al., 2018). Combined, these studies suggest that high static stress and strain are associated with volutrauma in acutely injured lung tissue but not in normal lung tissue.

Problems With Resting the Collapsed Lung

When the lung is allowed to collapse below normal FRC, atelectatic, and edema-filled *resting* tissue (1) does not exchange gas; (2) is susceptible to the development of pneumonia (Huynh et al., 2019; Li Bassi et al., 2019); (3) will become fibrotic if not reopened (Burkhardt, 1989; Cabrera-Benitez et al., 2014; Lutz et al., 2015); (4) initiates patient-ventilator dyssynchrony, which is caused by the firing of mechanical stretch, PO_2, PCO_2, and pH receptors (Solomon et al., 2000; Manning and Mahler, 2001; Widdicombe, 2001; Mellott et al., 2009; Burki and Lee, 2010; Yu, 2016; Yoshida et al., 2017) and which is associated with high mortality (Blanch et al., 2015); and (5) creates a stress-focus in the adjacent open alveoli and alveolar ducts, greatly amplifying the forces applied to these parenchymal tissues during tidal ventilation (Mead et al., 1970; Gattinoni et al., 2012; Cressoni et al., 2014; Makiyama et al., 2014; Retamal et al., 2014). It has been shown that letting the lung *rest* in obese bariatric surgery patients is associated with worse oxygenation, longer post-anesthesia care unit stay, and more post-operative pulmonary complications as compared with patients in which the atelectatic *resting* lung was opened and ventilated (Talab et al., 2009). Although, the phrase *resting* the lung sounds protective, the lung is not meant to function in a deflated state, and as listed above, such a state is associated with numerous pathologies. If the lung is to be *rested*, meaning that parenchymal tissue is to be kept from being damaged by mechanical ventilation, the better strategy would be to *rest* it in the natural inflated state (Nieman et al., 2018).

Problems With Stabilizing the Lung

There is no consensus on how best to set PEEP to effectively *stabilize* lung tissue (Coruh and Luks, 2014; Gattinoni et al., 2017; Nieman et al., 2017a; Bergez et al., 2019). The current ARDSnet method for setting PEEP uses a sliding scale of oxygenation (Acute Respiratory Distress Syndrome Network, 2000), but increased oxygenation does not correlate well with an increase in alveolar stability (Andrews et al., 2015), a key VILI mechanism (Wellman et al., 2014, 2016; Cereda et al., 2016b, 2017). Many methods have been used in an attempt to titrate the PEEP to stabilize lung tissue. These methods include using dead space, lung stress and strain, lung compliance, CT, pressure-volume curve inflection points, and electrical impedance tomography, but there is no current bedside technique to determine whether the set PEEP has actually stabilized the lung (Nieman et al., 2017a). The above problems with the ARDSnet *protect, rest,* and *stabilize* method may partially explain the lack of improved outcome in ARDS mortality over the last 20 years (**Figure 1**) (Brun-Buisson et al., 2004; Phua et al., 2009; Villar et al., 2011; Caser et al., 2014; Bellani et al., 2016; Laffey et al., 2016; Villar et al., 2016; Maca et al., 2017; Raymondos et al., 2017; Rezoagli et al., 2017; Fan et al., 2018; McNicholas et al., 2018; Pham et al., 2019). By allowing the lung to remain heterogeneously collapsed, the *protect, rest,* and *stabilize* method is unintendedly preserving the constraints of ventilating the heterogeneously injured lung, which is nearly impossible to do without causing some degree of VILI.

Open Lung Approach (OLA) as a Protective Strategy

The goal of the open lung approach (OLA) is to eliminate the constraints of ventilating a heterogeneously injured lung by normalizing all three pathologic compartments (**Figure 2**). The aim is to reinflate the collapsed tissue using a recruitment maneuver (RM) and to keep it open by using an appropriate level of PEEP. If the entire lung could be recruited and recollapse prevented, the main VILI mechanical mechanisms (dynamic strain and overdistension of alveolar walls in areas of stress-focus) would be eliminated (Nieman et al., 2017b). An RM is an acute event performed by raising the airway pressure (30–40 cm H_2O) and holding it for ~40 s (Fan et al., 2008) or by greatly increasing PEEP (25 cm H_2O) and combining it with 15 cm H_2O of driving pressure above the PEEP (Borges et al., 2006). In the latter strategy, PEEP is increased in 5 cm H_2O increments up to 45 cm H_2O until the lung fully recruits, which was confirmed when $PaO_2 + PaCO_2 > 400$ mmHg (Borges et al., 2006).

Following the RM, PEEP is titrated downward to find the lung recollapse point (usually by a sharp fall in lung compliance), and then PEEP is set 2 cm H_2O above this collapse pressure, following a second RM. However, multiple RCTs testing the OLA in ARDS patients have failed to show significant benefits over standard of care (Brower et al., 2004; Meade et al., 2008; Mercat et al., 2008; Cavalcanti et al., 2017; Hodgson et al., 2019). Reasons for these failures include the following: (1) timing of OLA application [early (Borges et al., 2006) vs. late (Gattinoni et al., 2006)] (2) one-size-fits-all RM strategies, (3) PEEP set inappropriately to keep the recruited lung open, (4) recruiting pressures insufficient to open all of the lung, (5) a patient population of responders (lung recruits) and non-responders (lung does not recruit) (Gattinoni et al., 2006), and (6) application of OLA not as a continuous treatment but rather as a one-time event with a long time period before a second application or with no second application at all (Goligher et al., 2017; Lu et al., 2017; Bhattacharjee et al., 2018; Cui et al., 2019; Hodgson et al., 2019; Kang et al., 2019; van der Zee and Gommers, 2019; Zheng et al., 2019). Most (Bhattacharjee et al., 2018; Cui et al., 2019; Hodgson et al., 2019; Kang et al., 2019; Zheng et al., 2019) but not all (Goligher et al., 2017; Lu et al., 2017) meta-analyses have shown no decrease in ARDS-related mortality associated with the OLA.

To further reduce ARDS mortality and acute lung injury, two pathologic processes must be understood: (1) the pathophysiology of ARDS that predisposes the lung to a secondary VILI and (2) the mechanisms of VILI in the microenvironment (i.e., the terminal airspaces, alveoli, and alveolar ducts). This knowledge informs the design of a

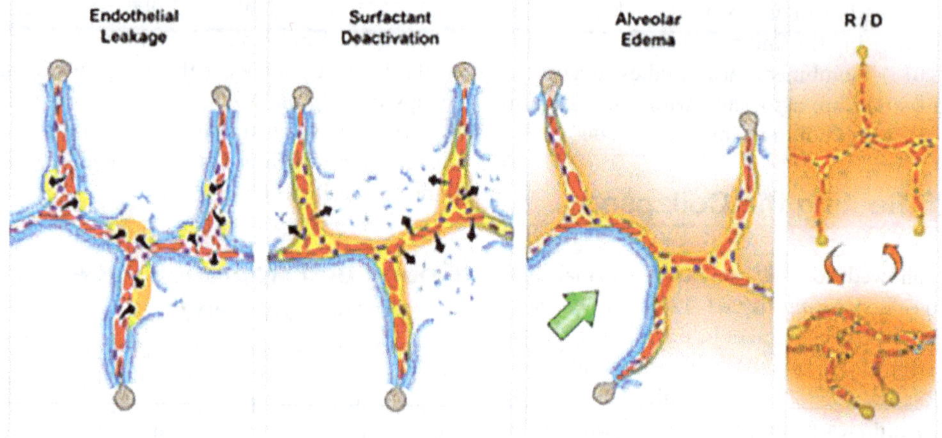

FIGURE 3 | The *pathologic tetrad* of acute respiratory distress syndrome (ARDS). Alveolar walls contain pulmonary capillaries (red circles) and are lined with a liquid hypophase (blue layer inside each alveolus), with an intact pulmonary surfactant layer (small blue ball with tail) layered on the hypophase. The systemic inflammatory response syndrome (SIRS) secondary to sepsis, trauma, burns, pneumonia, and so on increases pulmonary capillary permeability. **Endothelial leakage:** increased microvascular permeability allowing pulmonary edema to move into the alveolus (black arrows and tan edema blebs) (Martin and Brigham, 2012). **Surfactant deactivation:** the continuous layer of pulmonary surfactant molecules is disrupted as the edema blebs expand causing surfactant deactivation (surfactant sluffing off into the alveolar space). Edema usurping surfactant from the alveolar surface, the proteins in the edema fluid deactivating the surfactant (Taeusch et al., 2005), and improper mechanical ventilation (Albert, 2012) causing further surfactant disruption all combine to exacerbate surfactant loss. **Alveolar edema:** increased capillary permeability (Martin and Brigham, 2012) and high alveolar surface tension combine to flood alveoli with edema fluid (tan). **Recruitment/derecruitment (R/D)**: loss of surfactant function results in increased alveolar surface tension causing loss of alveolar stability (i.e., causing alveolar R/D with each breath). Alveoli in the top frame of **R/D** are fully inflated but collapse during expiration in the bottom **R/D** frame. Alveolar R/D, known as atelectrauma, is another key VILI mechanism (Cressoni et al., 2017). **Stress-focus**: edema-filled or collapsed alveoli adjacent to air-filled alveoli create a stress-focus causing the alveolar wall to bend toward the fluid-filled alveolus (green arrow), which can cause stress failure at the alveolar wall (Perlman et al., 2011). Stress-focus is another key mechanism of VILI (Perlman et al., 2011; Chen et al., 2014; Makiyama et al., 2014; Retamal et al., 2014). Thus, the *pathologic tetrad* sets up a vicious cycle of high microvascular permeability → edema → surfactant deactivation → high alveolar surface tension → more edema → alveolar R/D → further increase in microvascular permeability → severe ARDS (Nieman and Bredenberg, 1985).

protective mechanical breath that will allow the lung to heal by eliminating the constraints present when ventilating a heterogeneously injured lung (Nieman et al., 2018).

ARDS PATHOPHYSIOLOGY THAT PREDISPOSES THE LUNG TO VILI

ARDS Is a Pathologic Tetrad

To investigate the relationship between ARDS and VILI, we need to understand the pathology of acute lung injury. Although ARDS is a complex syndrome, it features four well-accepted central components (Thompson et al., 2017) known as the "pathologic tetrad" (**Figure 3**) (Nieman et al., 2018). The components of the tetrad include *increased pulmonary capillary permeability* (**Figure 3**, Endothelial Leakage), which if unchecked will lead to *loss of surfactant function* (**Figure 3**, Surfactant Deactivation) (Lewis et al., 1993). The resultant high alveolar surface tension will exacerbate the permeability-induced increase in *alveolar flooding* with edema fluid (**Figure 3**, Alveolar Edema) (Nieman and Bredenberg, 1985). Surfactant dysfunction will alter alveolar mechanics, resulting in alveolar *recruitment/derecruitment (R/D)* with each breath (**Figure 3**, R/D) (Schiller et al., 2001). Each component of the tetrad has a profound impact on alveolar mechanics. Surfactant deactivation sets the stage for a secondary VILI by promoting heterogeneous lung tissue instability and collapse. In addition, surfactant secretions from type II cells would be inhibited in collapsed areas that are not being stretched during ventilation (Wirtz and Dobbs, 1990; Majumdar et al., 2012). Reduced surfactant secretion would exacerbate and perpetuate the already reduced surfactant function caused by alveolar flooding with edema.

VILI MECHANISMS: HETEROGENEOUS ALVEOLAR INSTABILITY AND COLLAPSE

The hallmark of ARDS is a heterogeneous lung injury encompassing normal, collapsed, edematous, and unstable tissues (**Figure 2**). This pathology alters pulmonary microanatomy and dynamic alveolar inflation physiology, generating three basic VILI mechanisms: *volutrauma* (overdistension of airways), *atelectrauma* (R/D of alveoli), and *biotrauma* (inflammation) (Thompson et al., 2017). From an engineering perspective, volutrauma is caused by excessive static strain and atelectrauma by excessive dynamic strain (Seah et al., 2011; Protti et al., 2013a,b, 2014). In this review we do not discuss biotrauma but rather focus on the unintentional mechanical damage to the pulmonary parenchyma caused during mechanical ventilation.

Mechanical ventilation of the acutely injured lung with altered alveolar opening and collapse time constants can cause tissue

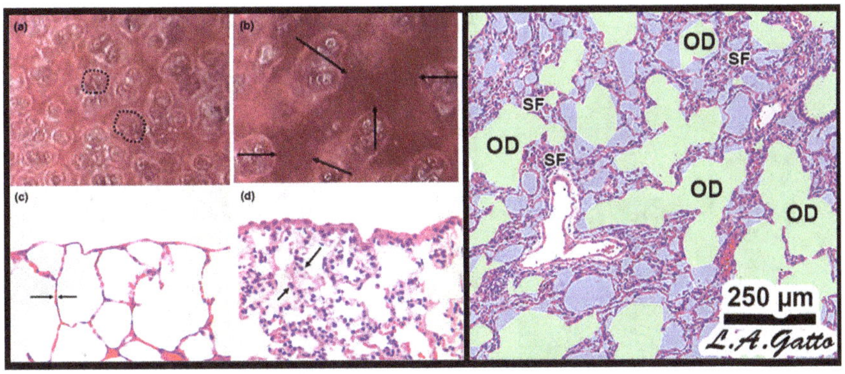

FIGURE 4 | Mechanical mechanisms of ventilator-induced lung injury (VILI) in the microenvironment: Left – *In vivo* subpleural alveoli in an acutely injured rat lung at inspiration **(a)** and expiration **(b)**. Lung histology in the same rat lung injury model fixed at inspiration **(c)** and expiration **(d)** (Pavone et al., 2007). *Alveolar recruitment/derecruitment (R/D)* causing atelectrauma can be seen as fully recruited alveoli filling the microscopic field (white circles, two of which are highlighted with black dotted line) **(a)** that collapse during expiration (red atelectatic areas highlighted by arrows) **(b)**. Histology shows open alveoli at inspiration with a shared alveolar wall highlighted by arrows **(c)** that collapse with expiration by alveolar wall folding, identified by arrows. Right – *Stress-focus (SF)* in areas with collapsed alveoli. SF adjacent to open alveolar ducts, causing alveolar duct *overdistension (OD)*. SF-induced OD causes excessive mechanical stress and strain on alveolar duct walls, resulting in damage to pulmonary parenchymal cells (Ghadiali and Gaver, 2008). Loss of surfactant function results in alveolar instability (**Figure 3**, R/D). Histology at exhalation in a rat Tween-induced surfactant deactivation model with a tidal volume of 6 ml/kg and a PEEP of 5 cm H_2O. Note the heterogeneous collapse of alveoli causing areas of stress-focus (SF). Adjacent to these areas of SF are overdistended (OD) alveolar ducts (Kollisch-Singule et al., 2014b). Summary – R/D causes excessive normal or "peeling" stress as the adhered alveolar walls peel apart during inflation; both R/D and SF cause OD in adjacent open stable tissue. This excessive stress and strain on alveolar walls results in lung parenchymal cell death and is a major VILI mechanism. *Permissions obtained to reuse panels* **(a–d)** (Pavone et al., 2007). *Springer Nature license number 4766000130978.*

stress-failure by the following mechanisms: (1) alveolar R/D-induced excessive stress on the epithelial cells as the alveolar walls in apposition peel apart (Bilek et al., 2003), (2) stress-focusing in areas of open alveoli adjacent to collapsed or edema fill alveoli (Gattinoni et al., 2012; Cressoni et al., 2014; Retamal et al., 2014), and (3) collapsed tissue stretching and overdistending the shared walls of patent alveoli, as alveolar walls are interconnected (**Figure 4**) (Nieman et al., 2017b). Theoretically, if it were possible to minimize or prevent all of the above VILI mechanisms, ARDS associated mortality would be significantly reduced.

In normal pigs ventilated for 54 h, Protti et al. (2013b) examined the impact of high static strain and several levels of dynamic strain. They demonstrated that *high static strain,* using elevated PEEP and minimal Vt, caused little damage, but when PEEP was reduced, producing a *high dynamic strain,* it caused pulmonary edema and death. In subsequent work they showed that high static strain did not merely act as a dam to prevent edema formation by altering the Starling forces (i.e., increasing the pulmonary interstitial pressure) (Effros and Parker, 2009) but rather preserved the integrity of the alveolar-capillary membrane (**Figure 3**, Endothelial Leakage) (Protti et al., 2013a). These findings were supported by Jain et al. (2017) using a porcine heterogeneous lung injury model. They subjected two study groups to high static strain (Pplat = 40 cm H_2O) that was believed to be more than sufficient to cause volutrauma-induced VILI (Acute Respiratory Distress Syndrome Network, 2000; Sahetya et al., 2017). Following heterogeneous lung injury, the animals in the second group were also subjected to high dynamic strain. High static strain did not injure normal open tissue (baby lung), nor did it exacerbate acutely injured tissue. However, combining high static strain with high dynamic strain caused significant damage to both of these tissues (**Figure 5**). Further support for the contention that volutrauma of normal lung tissue is not a primary VILI mechanism comes from the Bates group, who showed that 4 h of mechanical ventilation in mice with high static strain was not associated with lung injury, but when it was combined with high dynamic strain, it caused VILI-induced tissue damage (Seah et al., 2011).

Protti et al. (2014) showed that a large dynamic strain (atelectrauma) is much more harmful to the normal lung than a large static strain (volutrauma), and when combined, the two work additively or synergistically to greatly accelerate tissue damage (Seah et al., 2011; Hamlington et al., 2016; Ruhl et al., 2019). In addition, the heterogeneous injury caused by ARDS establishes many areas of *stress-focus* between the open tissue and collapsed or unstable tissue and have been shown to double the stress and strain calculated for the entire lung (Cressoni et al., 2014). The impact that areas of stress-focus have on the forces generated on alveolar walls during ventilation was first described by Mead et al. (1970) and was more recently analyzed by Makiyama et al. (2014) using computer-simulated alveolar walls. This latter group demonstrated that a Pplat at the upper end of the "safe" level (30 cm H_2O) could result in a local stress-focusing in individual alveolar walls of up to 48 cm H_2O and could concentrate stress in an individual alveolar wall as much as 16-fold (**Figure 6**).

In summary, ARDS results in a heterogeneous loss of surfactant function (**Figure 3**, Surfactant Deactivation) and airway flooding (**Figure 3**, Alveolar Edema) that cause the lung to become *time and pressure dependent,* which means that the lung will collapse in a relatively short time at atmospheric pressure and will require a longer period of time to open

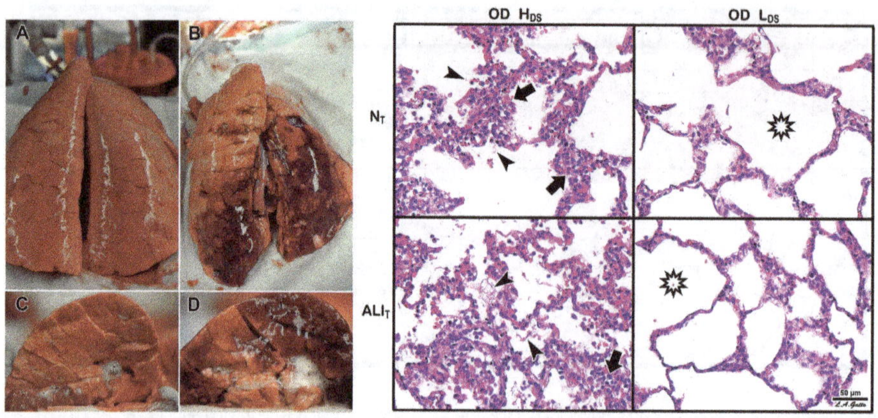

FIGURE 5 | Heterogeneous Tween Injury in pigs ventilated for 6 h. A bronchoscope was used to deliver Tween to the dependent areas of the diaphragmatic or caudal lung lobes. Thus, the upper lobes would be normal homogeneously inflated tissue (i.e., would simulate the baby lung), and the dependent areas of the caudal lobe would model acutely injured tissue that would be either collapsed or unstable during tidal ventilation. Using this injury model we can determine whether a ventilation strategy protects either normal tissue (N_T) or acutely injured lung tissue (ALI_T), protects neither, or protects both. Two groups were studied. Both groups were subjected to a high static strain (Pplat = 40 cm H_2O) hypothesized to be sufficient to cause overdistension (OD)-induced VILI to the baby lung (Acute Respiratory Distress Syndrome Network, 2000). One group was also subject to high dynamic strain (H_{DS}) and the other to low dynamic strain (L_{DS}). The dynamic strain was adjusted using the airway pressure release ventilation (APRV) mode by changing the expiratory duration, which changed tidal volume size. Left – Gross photographs of the whole lung **(A,B)** and cut surface **(C,D)** of the diaphragmatic lung lobe. The L_{DS} group **(A,C)** showed minimal damage in both N_T and ALI_T lung tissue (i.e., no dark red hepatized atelectasis). This was in contrast to the H_{DS} group, in which there was severe injury in both the N_T and ALI_T lung tissues **(B,D)**. Right – In the OD + H_{DS} group (OD + H_{DS}), widespread histopathology typical of ARDS was seen, with inflammatory cell inflation (arrows) and fibrin deposits (arrowheads) in both the N_T and ALI_T lung tissue. In the OD + L_{DS} group, minimal histopathology was seen, and alveoli remained open (stars) in both N_T and ALI_T lung tissue. These data support Protti et al.'s (2013b) work and demonstrate that normal lung tissue is highly resistant to static strain-induced volutrauma. In addition, this study showed that acutely injured lung tissue is also resistant to volutrauma as long as dynamic strain remains low. Both normal and acutely injured lung tissue are highly susceptible to high alveolar R/D-induced VILI when under high inflation pressure (Jain et al., 2017). These data support the rapid progression of lung injury in a power-law fashion when high static and dynamic strain are combined (Hamlington et al., 2018).

even at high inflation pressures (Takahashi et al., 2015). Mechanical ventilation can exacerbate the initial ARDS-induced inflammatory injury (**Figure 3**, Endothelial Leakage, Surfactant Deactivation, and Alveolar Edema) by generating excessive stress and strain on alveolar and alveolar duct walls resulting from a collapsing and reopening of alveoli and heterogeneous areas of stress-focusing in open tissue adjacent to collapsed or edema-filled tissue (**Figure 4**).

It is important to note that parenchymal overdistension following acute lung injury is a regional phenomenon and occurs only in open alveoli and alveolar ducts that are adjacent to the unstable or collapsed tissue (**Figure 7**, PEEP 16, PEEP 5, APRV 10%); it does not occur in homogeneously inflated acutely injured lung tissue (**Figure 7**, APRV 75%) (Nieman et al., 2017b). It has been shown that combining high pressure with alveolar instability greatly exacerbates tissue tearing in a rich-get-richer fashion (i.e., the larger the initial tear in the epithelial membrane the more that this tear will be expanded by increased airway pressure) (**Figure 8**) (Hamlington et al., 2016; Ruhl et al., 2019).

VENTILATING WITHIN THE CONSTRAINTS OF AN ACUTELY INJURED LUNG

The ARDSnet method is a logical physiologically based lung ventilation strategy within the constraints of protecting a heterogeneously injured lung. The better strategy would be to eliminate these constraints by opening and stabilizing the acutely injured lung or, better yet, by applying a protective ventilation strategy early and never letting the lung collapse (Satalin et al., 2018). Gattinoni and Pesenti stressed that in a patient with ARDS the Vt should not be set by body weight (Vt/kg ratio) but rather by the size of the remaining normal open tissue at FRC: the baby lung (Vt/baby lung volume ratio) (Gattinoni and Pesenti, 2005). They hypothesized that the baby lung was the small amount of open tissue at end-expiration (i.e., FRC) surrounded by a large volume of collapsed tissue with very low compliance. Since the specific elastance [E_{spec} = transpulmonary pressure (Ptp)/Vt x baby lung volume, which is the airway pressure at which expiratory lung volume or FRC or baby lung volume doubles in size (i.e., when Vt/baby lung volume = 1)] if the baby lung is postulated to be normal, there would be a greater potential for overdistension in normal lung tissue because of the high compliance at any given level of static strain (Gattinoni and Pesenti, 2005). Both the potential of excessive stress (Ptp) to cause volutrauma and of excessive strain (Vt/end-expiratory lung volume) to cause atelectrauma are linked with the following equation:

$$\text{Ptp (stress)} = E_{spec} \times (\text{Vt/baby lung volume}). \quad (1)$$

(Eq. 1) (Gattinoni and Pesenti, 2005)

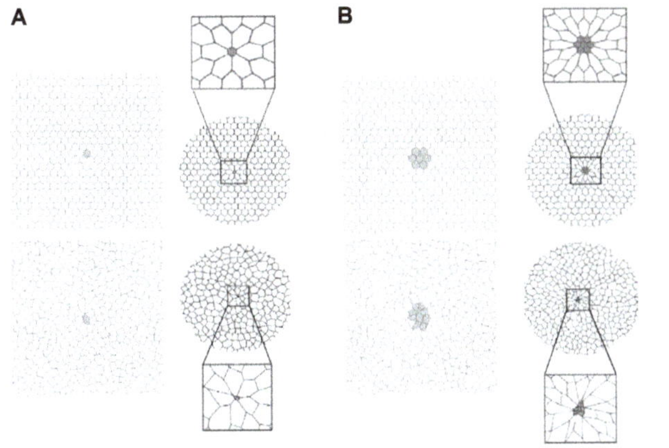

FIGURE 6 | A two-dimensional finite element computational model of interconnected alveolar walls to study the impact of areas of stress-focus (S-F) on stress–strain relationships. Both a hexagonal honeycomb (top) and Voroni honeycombs (bottom) were studied with areas of S-F created by increasing the stiff regions in one **(A)** or nine **(B)** cells. These stiff regions simulate collapsed alveoli adjacent to open alveoli that create an S-F in acute respiratory distress syndrome (ARDS) patients (**Figure 4**) (Cressoni et al., 2014). The entire honeycomb structure was expanded and exposed to strains of 15, 30, 45, and 55% above the resting geometry. Some of the alveolar walls in the Voroni honeycomb were exposed to a S-F ~16 times greater than that applied to uniformly expanded areas. This suggests that ventilation pressures considered safe in ARDS patients (<30 cm H_2O) (Acute Respiratory Distress Syndrome Network, 2000) could be causing local stress concentration on some alveolar walls of approximately 48 cm H_2O, with even higher stress in areas of S-F (Makiyama et al., 2014). *Permissions obtained from Elsevier. License 4699410294890.*

Gattinoni and Pesenti further concluded that the above equation suggests the baby lung must be treated gently, using low Vt, low Ptp, and proning so as not to cause volutrauma. Gently ventilating the lung should be protective, within the constraints of a heterogeneously injured lung (i.e., high E_{spec} and low baby lung volume).

The current strategy of lung protection is designed to minimize normal tissue overdistention (low Vt) and to stabilize (PEEP) injured tissue. Although the current hypothesis is that the primary mechanism of VILI is overdistension of the baby lung (Acute Respiratory Distress Syndrome Network, 2000), recent studies have demonstrated that high Ptp does not result in injury to normal lung tissue (Seah et al., 2011; Protti et al., 2013a,b, 2014; Jain et al., 2017). Since much of the lung remains collapsed and unstable using the ARDSnet method, there are numerous areas of stress-focus, as PEEP adjusted by changes in oxygenation may not be adequate to prevent R/D (Baumgardner et al., 2002; Boehme et al., 2015). Even with low Vt, tissue injury may occur regionally, since overdistension is not global but occurs in the microenvironment. Specifically, alveolar and alveolar duct overdistension occurs in open tissue surrounding a collapsed area of stress-focus or adjacent to areas of alveolar instability (**Figures 4, 6, 7**) (Mead et al., 1970; Cereda et al., 2011, 2013, 2016a; Kollisch-Singule et al., 2014b, 2018; Makiyama et al., 2014; Nieman et al., 2017b; Ruhl et al., 2019). Indeed, it has been shown that atelectasis, not high Vt, causes overdistension

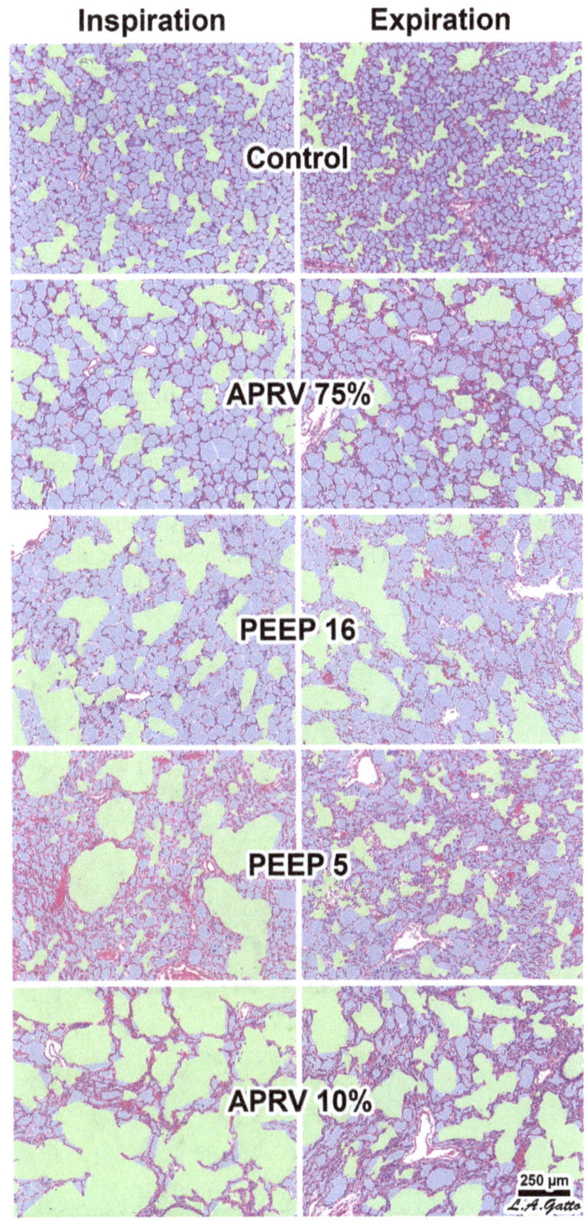

FIGURE 7 | Rat lungs fixed at inspiration and expiration in normal lungs (**Control**) and in a Tween lavage ARDS model with four ventilation strategies: (1) the TCAV method setting airway pressure release ventilation (APRV) with the expiratory flow termination (E_{FT}) at 75% of expiratory flow peak (E_{FP}) (E_{FT}/E_{FP} = 75%) (**APRV 75%**) (Habashi, 2005; Jain et al., 2016); (2) E_{FT}/E_{FP} = 10% (**APRV 10%**), which significantly increased expiratory time; (3) controlled mandatory ventilation (CMV) with low tidal volume (6 mL/kg) with 5 cm H_2O positive end-expiratory pressure (**PEEP 5**); or (4) CMV with low tidal volume (6 mL/kg) with 16 cm H_2O PEEP (**PEEP 16**). **APRV 10%** (not the TCAV method) significantly increased expiratory duration, allowing sufficient time for alveoli to collapse. The conducting airways are depicted in green; alveoli in lilac; and remaining interstitium, blood vessels, and lymphatics in magenta. The size of each microanatomical area was quantified using computer image analysis. In the **Control** group all alveoli were inflated surrounding normally distended alveolar ducts. Following Tween-induced ARDS, alveolar ducts in all ventilation groups were increased in size. In the CMV groups alveolar ducts were overdistended at both inspiration and

(Continued)

FIGURE 7 | Continued
expiration in **PEEP16.** In the **PEEP5** group alveolar ducts were relatively normal size at expiration but greatly overdistended at inspiration with areas of alveolar collapse (i.e., high dynamic strain) at both inspiration and expiration. **APRV 10%** resulted in highly overdistended alveolar ducts at both inspiration and expiration with large areas of collapsed alveoli. **APRV 75%** (i.e., the TCAV method) resulted in the smallest increase in alveolar duct size, with uniformly open, homogeneously ventilated alveoli that were closest to those seen in the **Control** group (Kollisch-Singule et al., 2014b). *Permissions obtained from Elsevier. License 4732510649425.*

in the adjacent patent alveoli and that alveolar size actually decreases with increased airway pressure (i.e., PEEP) if lung tissue is recruited by a mechanism of gas redistribution (Cereda et al., 2011, 2013, 2016a). It has also been shown that gas redistribution in the microenvironment is not only *pressure* dependent but also *time* dependent (i.e., the longer the pressure is applied, the better the gas redistribution) (**Figure 7**) (Kollisch-Singule et al., 2014b).

Animal studies have shown that the OLA can protect the lung from VILI even if ΔP is not reduced (Tojo et al., 2018). Recruiting the lung with PEEP has been shown to reduce tissue damage secondary to spontaneous breathing (SB) by two mechanisms: (1) the intensity of the SB is reduced via neuromechanical uncoupling, and (2) the reduced amount of atelectatic tissue decreases the volume of stress-focus areas (Morais et al., 2018). Other studies using animal models have also shown the physiologic and pathologic benefit of opening the acutely injured lung (Faridy et al., 1966; Webb and Tierney, 1974; Dreyfuss et al., 1988; Muscedere et al., 1994; Nakazawa et al., 2007; Nieman et al., 2015; Magalhaes et al., 2018). Additionally, animal studies have shown that to successfully implement the OLA, the RM and subsequent PEEP level must be applied properly, or the approach may actually increase lung damage. Farias et al. (2005) showed that an RM increased lung pathology if PEEP was not set sufficiently high to prevent recollapse of the newly opened tissue, a finding that is supported by direct *in vivo* observation of subpleural alveoli (Halter et al., 2003). In light of

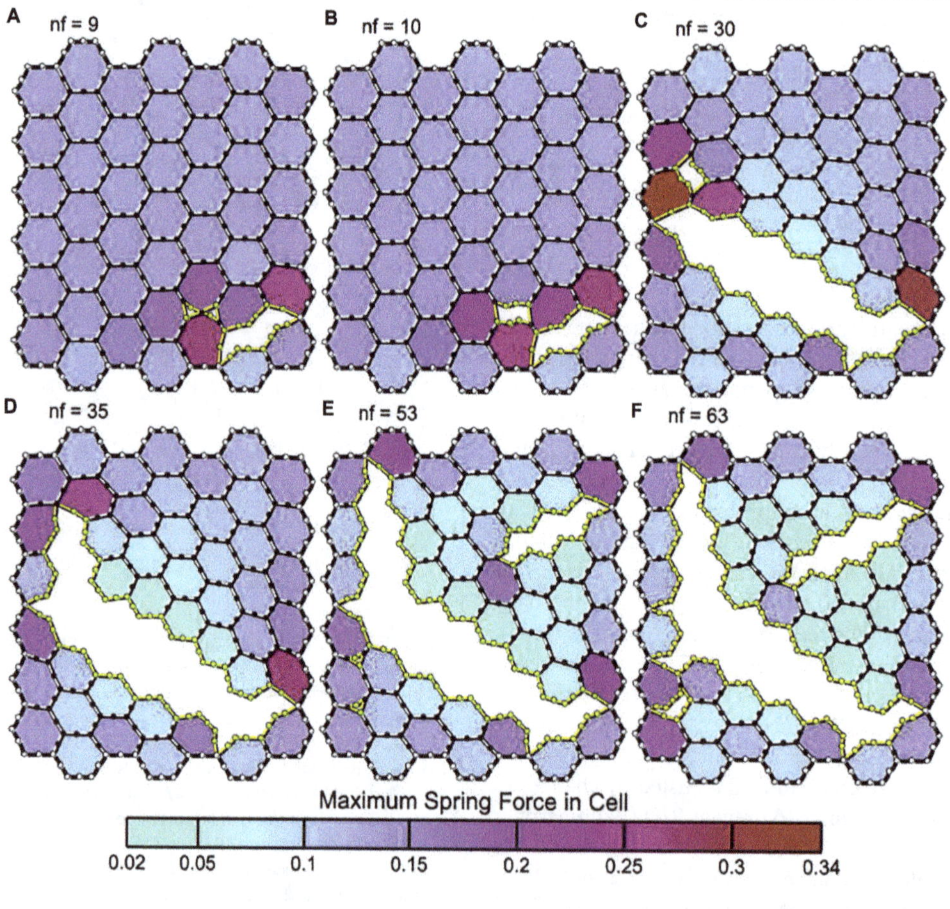

FIGURE 8 | Panels **(A–F)** depict leak progression caused by an applied stretch force. A single node fails (nf) at each time point with nf indicating the number of nodes that have failed in each panel. Computational model of an epithelial monolayer to simulate leak progression due to overdistension. Leak progression in a 45-cell (hexagon) network caused by applied stretch (i.e., Vt). After the force required to initiate the leak was reached, the leak area increased at a constant rate as the force increased further (Hamlington et al., 2016). Atelectrauma caused the initial tears, after which volutrauma expanded those tears. The tears progressed in a rich-get-richer mechanism in which the likelihood of a tear getting larger increased with the size of the initial tear. This mechanism explains why atelectrauma appears to be essential to the initiation of VILI in a normal lung, and why atelectrauma and volutrauma act synergistically once VILI is underway (Hamlington et al., 2018). *Permissions obtained from Springer Nature. License 4699410825602.*

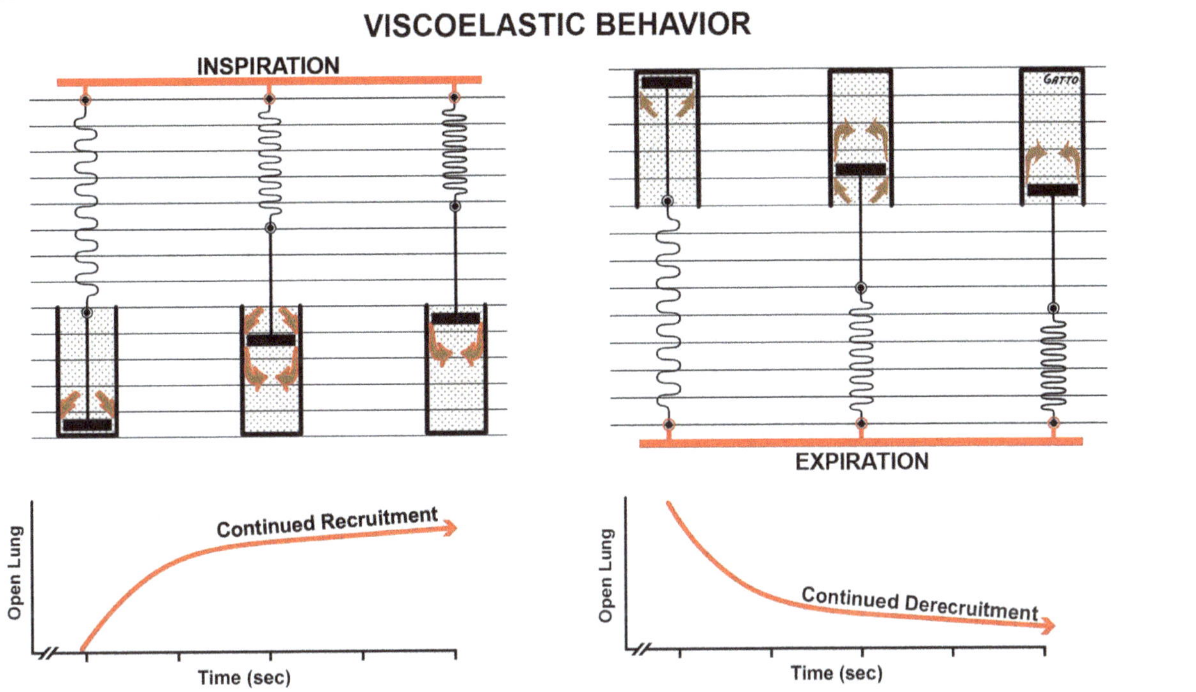

FIGURE 9 | Viscoelastic behavior of alveolar recruitment and derecruitment described using a spring and dashpot model. During inspiration the spring is rapidly stretched, whereas the dash in the pot moves more slowly as fluid squeezes around it (brown arrows), in response to the applied force (i.e., tidal volume – red bar). The effect of this viscoelastic behavior is continual alveolar recruitment as long as inspiration is held (open lung/time curve). Viscoelastic behavior during expiration shows a rapid collapse of the spring and a much slower collapse of the dash in the pot. This is shown in the open lung/time curve as continuous alveolar collapse or derecruitment over time. Viscoelastic alveolar opening and collapse suggests that the longer inspiration is held, the more alveoli are recruited, and the shorter the expiratory time, the fewer the alveoli that collapse.

this evidence, discarding the OLA does not seem logical, since it is unclear whether the RCTs testing the OLA actually opened and stabilized the lung. A better strategy might be to identify ventilation strategies that are most likely to accomplish the goals of the OLA (Sahetya and Brower, 2017).

A PHYSIOLOGICALLY INFORMED STRATEGY TO EFFECTIVELY OPEN AND STABILIZE THE LUNG

Surfactant deactivation and edema flooding with acute lung injury cause alveolar collapse; the result is very "sticky" and does not reopen easily (**Figure 3**) (Crotti et al., 2001; Gattinoni et al., 2003). This tissue has a very long opening time constant, and thus it will take an extended period of time at any given pressure to recruit these surfactant deficient and edematous tissues. Once the collapsed alveoli are recruited, the opposite problem develops; the newly opened alveoli have a very brief collapse time constant (Neumann et al., 1998a,b, 2000). Thus, alveoli collapse quickly ($\leq$0.5 s) once a critical collapse airway pressure is reached (i.e., collapse is *time* and *pressure* dependent) (Kollisch-Singule et al., 2014a,b).

To effectively implement the OLA, the entire mechanical breath pattern (MBP), including all airway volumes, flows, pressure, rates, and the times during which they apply during inspiration and expiration, must be analyzed (Kollisch-Singule et al., 2014a). The current OLA ventilation strategies do not consider the pathophysiological changes that occur in alveolar opening and collapse time constants. Attempting to recruit large volumes of collapsed lung with a single RM over a very brief period of time is often not physiologically possible depending on the degree of surfactant damage and edema. A more effective strategy may be a ventilation method that "nudges" the lung open over an extended period of time (6–24 h) using a high mean airway pressure held for most of each breath. Likewise, the very fast alveolar collapse time constants are not considered when setting PEEP with expiratory durations in the 2- to 3-s range. A more effective strategy may be to use a ventilator method with a very brief ($\leq$0.5 s) expiratory time while maintaining a level of time-controlled PEEP (TC-PEEP). Greatly limiting the expiratory duration ($\leq$0.5 s) keeps the lung from emptying completely, maintaining a TC-PEEP that is related to expiratory duration and the collapse time constant of the lung. Thus, for any given collapse time constant, the shorter the expiratory time, the higher the TC-PEEP and vice versa. In addition, since alveolar collapse is viscoelastic in nature (**Figure 9**), the very short expiratory duration would work synergistically with TC-PEEP to prevent alveolar collapse – alveoli simply would not have sufficient time to derecruit (Nieman et al., 2019). Analysis of the change in alveolar opening and collapse time constants with acute lung injury suggests that the time component of the

MB_P (Kollisch-Singule et al., 2014a) can be used to improve the ability to recruit and stabilize acutely injured lung tissue, which is necessary to successfully implement the OLA.

In addition to the time component of MB_P, the dynamic physiology of alveolar R/D must also be understood to design a mechanical breath for the OLA. Alveoli and alveolar ducts inflate and deflate as a viscoelastic system (Denny and Schroter, 2000; Escolar and Escolar, 2004; Farias et al., 2005; Carvalho and Zin, 2011; Suki and Bates, 2011; Nieman et al., 2017b). The model most used to analyze viscoelastic behavior is the spring and dashpot (**Figure 9**). The most important thing to know about a viscoelastic system, in relation to lung opening and collapse, is that there is a time lag from when the force (inspiratory pressure) is applied until alveoli begins to open and a lag between when force is removed (expiratory pressure) and when alveoli begin to collapse. Thus, the longer the inspiratory time, the more lung tissue that will be recruited, and the shorter the expiratory time, the less lung tissue that will be allowed to recollapse (**Figure 9**). A collapsed airway inflates after the opening threshold pressure is reached, and the pressure then propagates down the airway, inflating more airways and alveoli. This process progresses in an avalanche manner with power-law distributions of both the size of and intervals between avalanches (Suki et al., 1994; Alencar et al., 2002). It has been postulated that as the lung opens, the increase in parenchymal tethering of airways (Broche et al., 2017) and alveolar interdependence improves lung function as a power-law function (Nieman et al., 2019). These new perspectives inform the quest for novel protective ventilation strategies. Indeed, our work in translational animal models and a meta-analysis of data on surgical intensive care unit (SICU) patients has shown that our time-controlled adaptive ventilation (TCAV) method, using airway pressure release ventilation (APRV) mode, is highly effective at keeping the lung open and stable, significantly reducing morbidity in translational animal models and reducing the ARDS incidence and mortality rates of SICU patients at high risk of developing ARDS (Roy et al., 2012; Andrews et al., 2013; Emr et al., 2013; Roy S.K. et al., 2013; Kollisch-Singule et al., 2014a,b, 2015a,b, 2017; Nieman et al., Nieman et al., 2015, 2017a,b, 2018; Smith et al., 2015; Jain et al., 2016, 2017; Satalin et al., 2018; Silva et al., 2018; Mahajan et al., 2019).

Others have shown the importance of ventilation time on lung mechanics. Saddy et al. (2013) calculated a pressure-time product (PTP)/breath as the integral of the change in esophageal pressure over time. They found that, when using biphasic positive airway pressure, PTP significantly increased when the rate of time-cycled control breaths was at 50 breaths/min as compared to when it was 100 or 75 breaths/min. The energetics of ventilation also contain components of ventilator time. Power is defined as work per unit time and is thus equal to pressure x (volume/time) (Marini, 2018). Most of the energy applied to the lung during inflation is accounted for in elastic storage and airway resistance. It is postulated that the damage due to power is caused by the energy that is dissipated and unrecovered during exhalation. In addition, it is not just the power but also the changes in the microenvironment that result in tissue damage. Regional alveolar instability can develop during ARDS and can greatly amplify energy dissipation locally. Regional instability acts as a stress-focus, and once a microstrain threshold is reached, the unrecovered energy will cause a rapid progression of lung tissue injury in a power-law fashion (Hamlington et al., 2018).

ELIMINATING CONSTRAINTS OF VENTILATING THE ACUTELY INJURED LUNG

It was recently shown in ARDS patients that low Vt and Pplat do not correlate well with reduced patient mortality, whereas low ΔP correlated strongly with improved survival (Amato et al., 2015). The critical lesson is that it is not the settings dialed into the ventilator (i.e., Vt, Pplat, and so on) that are key to improved survival, but rather the impact of these settings on lung physiology measured as a change in ΔP (Kollisch-Singule et al., 2014a,b, 2015b).

Using the ARDSnet method, the Vt was set at 6 cc/kg, the Pplat was set at < 30 cm H_2O, and PEEP was set on a sliding oxygenation scale; the mechanism of improved mortality was assumed to be due to these parameters. The Amato study clearly demonstrated that the mechanism of increased survival was not these desired setting values, because none correlated with outcome (Amato et al., 2015). Lower ΔP, on the other hand, strongly correlated with reduced mortality. Respiratory system compliance (C_{RS}) was used to calculate driving pressure ($\Delta P = Vt/C_{RS}$), which was shown to decrease in patients who survived, reflecting a desirable change in lung physiology caused by recruitment.

The ARDSnet method assumes that the constraints of ventilating a heterogeneously collapsed lung are unavoidable, in which case the Ptp is high due to the high E_{spec} value and low baby lung (FRC) volume. However, if the entire lung could be fully recruited, these constraints would be eliminated, E_{spec} reduced, and FRC increased, resulting in a significant reduction in the applied stress (i.e., Ptp) for any given Vt. Rahaman used a stress equation similar to Eq. 1 to analyze the mathematics of VILI (Rahaman, 2017). He concluded that stress increases for any given Vt and PEEP with an increase in respiratory rate (RR). This conclusion assumes that the clinician is constrained in ventilating a heterogeneously collapsed lung such that neither FRC (i.e., the size of the baby lung) nor E_{spec} can be changed. When these conditions are true, the conclusion that Vt, PEEP, and RR must be kept low to reduce stress is correct. Conversely, our perspective is the better strategy is to treat the lung by reinflating the collapsed tissue, increase FRC (eliminating the baby lung), and decreasing E_{spec}. This combination will reduce lung stress (Ptp) during ventilation even at higher Vt, PEEP, and RR (Eq. 1).

Of course the strategy of "casting" the broken lung open until it heals would be clinically effective only with a ventilation strategy that could perform such a feat (Nieman et al., 2018). Unfortunately, the current OLA strategies have not been shown effective at opening and stabilizing the lung (Bhattacharjee et al., 2018; Cui et al., 2019; Hodgson et al., 2019; Kang et al., 2019; Zheng et al., 2019), and the recent ART trial showed an increase in

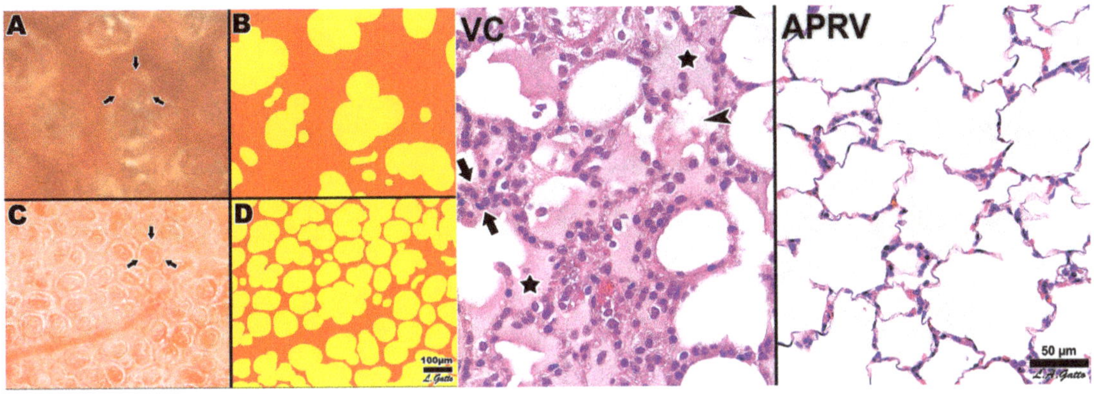

FIGURE 10 | Left – Subpleural alveoli seen using *in vivo* microscopy in a rat hemorrhagic shock-induced ARDS model ventilated with volume cycled ventilation (*VC*; **A,B**) or airway pressure release ventilation (*APRV*) using the time controlled adaptive ventilation (TCAV) method (*APRV*; **C,D**). Individual alveoli are shown by arrows. Inflated alveoli were color coded yellow, and alveolar number, size, and surface area were measured by computer image analysis in each group. TCAV significantly improved alveolar patency and stability as compared with the VC group. Right – The *APRV* group delivered using the TCAV method stabilized alveoli that was associated with a significant reduction in lung histopathology as evidenced by open alveoli and reduced intra-alveolar edema (purple areas) as compared with the collapsed and edema-filled alveoli (stars), fibrinous deposits in the air compartment (arrowheads), and white cell infiltration (between arrows) in the *VC* group (Roy S.K. et al., 2013). *Permissions obtained from Wolters Kluwer Health, Inc. License 4699411295724.*

mortality using the OLA (Brower et al., 2004; Meade et al., 2008; Mercat et al., 2008; Cavalcanti et al., 2017).

THE TCAV METHOD TO OPEN AND STABILIZE THE ACUTELY INJURED LUNG

Our TCAV method using the APRV mode has been discussed in detail elsewhere (Habashi, 2005; Jain et al., 2016; Nieman et al., 2018, 2019; Kollisch-Singule et al., 2019). Briefly, TCAV consists of an extended (4–5 s) open valve continuous positive airway pressure (CPAP) phase with a very short ($\leq$0.5 s) release phase. The inspiratory:expiratory ratio is ~10:1. The open valve allows the patient to spontaneously breath (inspiration or expiration) with little resistance. Tidal volume (Vt) is not set but rather is a product of the CPAP level and lung compliance. A heterogeneously collapsed lung will have a very low Vt because the compliance will be low, but as the lung gradually recruits over time, the compliance will increase and so will the Vt. Since the Vt is set based on lung compliance, a high Vt will never be delivered to a non-compliant collapsed lung using the TCAV method. Thus, the Vt size is personalized and adaptive as the patient's lung gets better or worse, directed by changes in lung compliance. The extended CPAP time will gradually nudge viscoelastic alveoli open over several hours until the lung is fully inflated. The newly recruited alveoli will be prevented from recollapse through the use of a very short expiratory duration (release phase). Expiratory time is very short ($\leq$0.5 s), and thus the lung is reinflated (CPAP phase) before it has time to completely empty, maintaining a TC-PEEP. The very short expiratory time is not sufficient for viscoelastic alveoli to collapse and when combined with the TC-PEEP is highly effective at preventing alveolar derecruitment.

Our group has investigated the physiological impact of the TCAV method in both mechanistic and efficacy animal studies (Roy et al., 2012; Emr et al., 2013; Roy S.K. et al., 2013; Roy S. et al., 2013; Kollisch-Singule et al., 2014a,b, 2015a,b, 2017; Smith et al., 2015; Silva et al., 2018) and in a meta-analysis of data on SICU patients (Andrews et al., 2013). In addition, the TCAV method is the primary ventilator strategy used at the R Adam Cowley Shock Trauma Center in Baltimore, with well over 1,000,000 h of ventilator time. Below, we discuss the results from our animal data and our clinical statistical analysis as evidence for the TCAV method's mechanisms and efficacy.

In rat VILI and hemorrhagic shock models, it was shown that ventilation for 6 h using the TCAV method was superior to volume-controlled ventilation (VCV; Vt 10 ml/kg, PEEP 0.5 cm H_2O) at preventing the development of ARDS and that lung protection was associated with stabilization of alveoli (**Figure 10**) (Emr et al., 2013; Roy S.K. et al., 2013). The TCAV method was also shown to be lung protective in a preterm piglet model of infant respiratory distress syndrome (Kollisch-Singule et al., 2017). These data were supported by mechanistic studies showing the ability of the TCAV method to normalize alveolar and alveolar duct microanatomy (Kollisch-Singule et al., 2014b) (**Figure 7**) and to reduce dynamic alveolar strain (Kollisch-Singule et al., 2014a, 2015b; Smith et al., 2015). We developed a 48-hr clinically applicable, high-fidelity, porcine peritoneal sepsis (PS) plus gut ischemia/reperfusion (I/R), multiple organ dysfunction syndrome (MODS) and ARDS model. In three studies using this clinically applicable model, we demonstrated that the TCAV method was superior to VC or the ARDSnet method at blocking progressive acute lung injury and preventing ARDS development (**Figure 11**) (Roy et al., 2012; Roy S. et al., 2013; Kollisch-Singule et al., 2015a). In addition, we have shown that surfactant proteins A and B are both better preserved with the TCAV as compared with the ARDSnet method, suggesting that there is sufficient lung volume change with TCAV to preserve stretch-induced surfactant release (Roy et al., 2012; Emr et al., 2013; Roy S.K. et al., 2013; Roy S. et al., 2013; Kollisch-Singule et al., 2015a). Lastly, in a

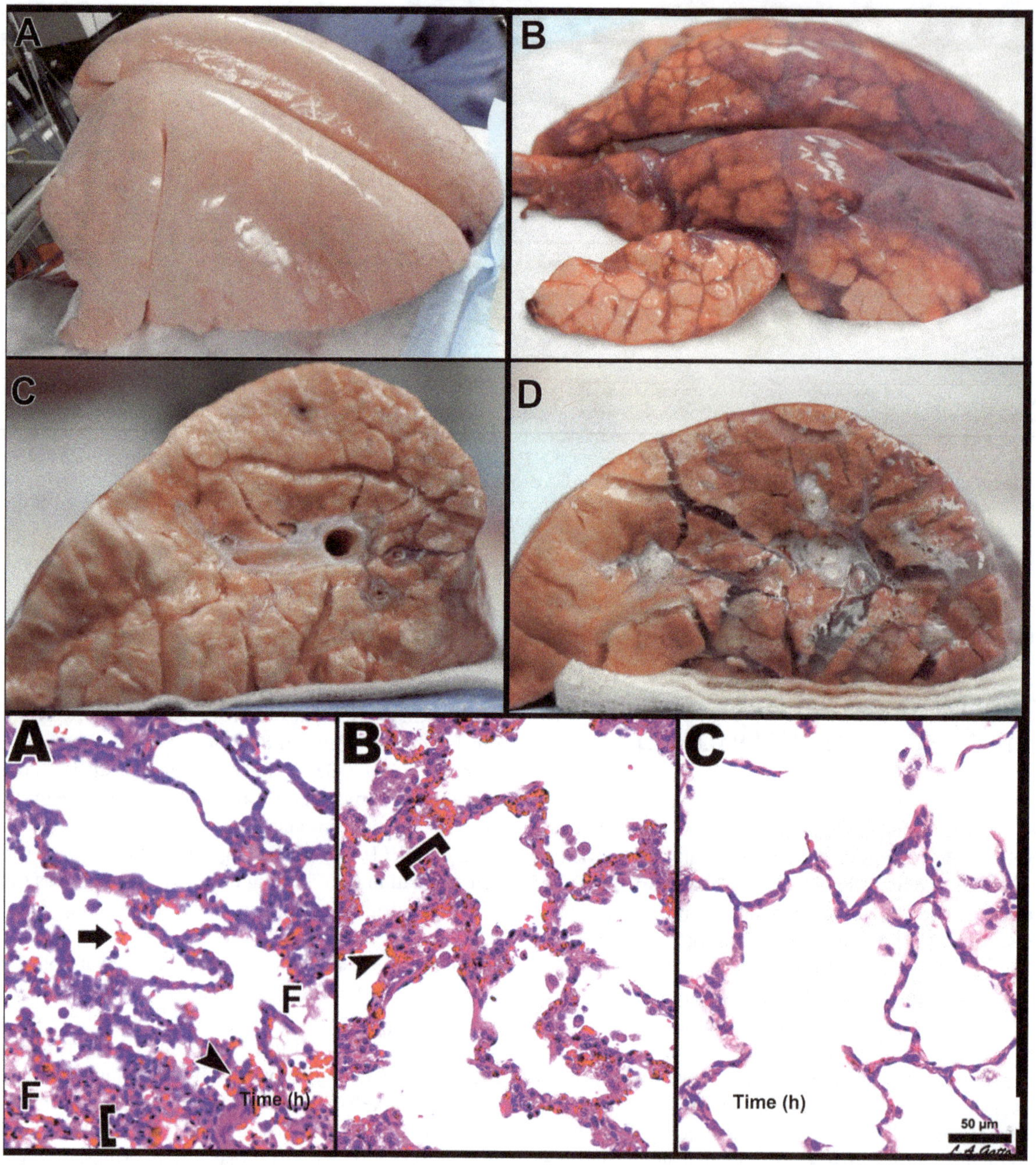

FIGURE 11 | Three groups of pigs were ventilated for 48 h with a clinically applicable, high-fidelity porcine peritoneal sepsis (PS) and gut ischemia/reperfusion (I/R) acute respiratory distress syndrome (ARDS) model: (1) *Control* group without PS + I/R injury ventilated with a tidal volume (Vt) of 10 cc/kg and a positive end-expiratory pressure (PEEP) of 5 cm H_2O. (2) *ARDSnet* group using a low-Vt ventilation method, applied following PS + I/R injury at the time point at which the animal reached the oxygen saturation limit listed in the ARDSnet protocol, with PEEP and FiO_2 adjusted by oxygenation (Acute Respiratory Distress Syndrome Network, 2000). (3) Time-controlled adaptive ventilation (*TCAV*) method using the airway pressure release ventilation (APRV) mode applied immediately after PS + I/R injury (Habashi, 2005; Jain et al., 2016). **Upper** – Gross lung photographs after 48 h of ventilation following PS + I/R injury at necropsy (*Control* not shown). In the *TCAV* group **(A,B)**, lungs inflated fully to near total lung capacity at 25 cm H_2O without any gross atelectasis. The cut surface of the diaphragmatic lobe also showed no interstitial or airway edema and no atelectasis. Lungs in the *ARDSnet* group **(C,D)** also inflated to 25 cm H_2O showed low lung volume with heterogeneous collapse and atelectasis and were wet and "boggy." The cut surface showed both interstitial and airway edema. **Lower** – Photomicrographs of representative lung sections of specimens from the *Control* **(A)**, *ARDSnet* **(B)**, and *TCAV* **(C)** groups each at 40× magnification. F, fibrinous deposit in the air compartment; arrow, blood in alveolus; arrowhead, congested alveolar capillary; bracket, thickened alveolar wall. **(A)** *Control*: animals received 48 h of mechanical ventilation without PS + I/R injury. Specimen shows typical early acute lung injury pathology including fibrinous deposits, blood in alveolus, congested capillaries, and thickened alveolar walls. **(B)** *ARDSnet*: animals received PS + I/R injury, and LVt ventilation was applied after the onset of acute lung injury (i.e., PaO_2/FiO_2 ratio <300). Specimen shows typical advanced acute lung injury pathology including fibrinous deposits, blood in alveolus, congested capillaries, leukocyte infiltration, and thickened alveolar walls. **(C)** *TCAV*: specimen shows normal pulmonary architecture, alveoli are well-expanded and thin walled, and there are no exudates (Roy S. et al., 2013). *Permissions obtained from Wolters Kluwer Health, Inc. License 4699411460832.*

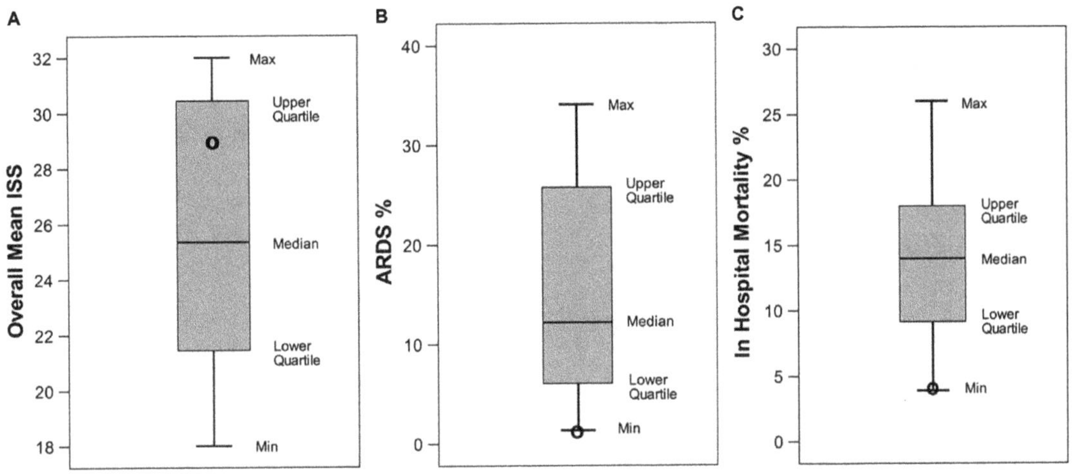

FIGURE 12 | A systematic review of data from trauma patients who were ventilated with either conventional mechanical ventilation (CMV) or the time-controlled adaptive ventilation (TCAV) method using the airway pressure release ventilation (APRV) mode. Boxplots are mean and standard error for **(A)** Injury Severity Score (ISS), **(B)** percentage of patients who developed ARDS (ARDS%), and **(C)** in-hospital mortality (%) from 16 published papers using standard of care CMV. Black circles indicate the results in each category using the TCAV method at the *R Adam Cowley Shock Trauma Center* in Maryland. Although patients in the TCAV group were in the high-ISS range, they had the lowest levels of both ARDS incidence (ARDS%) and in-hospital mortality (%) as compared with patients ventilated using CMV (Andrews et al., 2013). *Permissions obtained from Wolters Kluwer Health, Inc. License 4699420119915.*

statistical analysis of data from SICU patients, the TCAV method was associated with a significant reduction in ARDS incidence and mortality as compared to standard of care ventilation in 15 SICUs (**Figure 12**) (Andrews et al., 2013).

It is important to remember that if the acutely injured lung can be fully recruited, it will remain *time* and *pressure* dependent (i.e., will collapse quickly at atmospheric pressure) for a period of hours to days (Takahashi et al., 2015). Once the acutely injured lung is opened, the ventilator pressure/time support necessary to keep it open cannot be reduced until the lung "heals." Gradually pulmonary edema will be reabsorbed and surfactant function restored (Vazquez de Anda et al., 2000). As more and more lung tissue is recruited, reestablishing alveolar interdependence (**Figure 6**) (Mead et al., 1970; Makiyama et al., 2014) and parenchymal tethering (Perun and Gaver, 1995), the lung will once again become stable at atmospheric airway pressure, and the weaning process can begin (Mead et al., 1970; Perun and Gaver, 1995; Makiyama et al., 2014).

Recent RCTs have shown mixed results in ARDS patients using APRV (but not utilizing the TCAV method). Zhou et al. (2017) randomized patients with a PaO_2/FiO_2 (P/F) ratio < 200 to either ARDSnet LVt or APRV with TCAV-like settings. The APRV group demonstrated significant decreases in length of ICU stay, tracheostomy requirement, ventilator days, and mortality. The APRV group also had significant reductions in the need for prone positioning, sedation, and neuromuscular blockade.

Lalgudi Ganesan et al. (2018) conducted an RCT in children with ARDS, who were randomized to receive either standard LVt strategy or APRV. The APRV group was shown not to be lung protective, and the trial was terminated early. We postulate the failure was due to fundamental misconceptions as to the MB_P necessary to protect the lung. A key objective in our TCAV method is to gradually nudge the lung open. In the Ganesan study, the CPAP pressure was reduced to generate a low Vt, and thus the CPAP level was likely not above the lung critical opening pressure, meaning the lung was not inflated. In the TCAV method, Vt is not set (see TCAV description above), so an increase in release volume (analogous to Vt) during the release phase and an increase in C_{RS} are positive signs and indictive of lung recruitment (Roy et al., 2012; Roy S. et al., 2013; Kollisch-Singule et al., 2015a). If the ventilation strategy used does not actually open the lung, the VILI mechanisms associated with heterogeneous ventilation will not be prevented (**Figure 4**). We postulate that this is also the reason for the failed RCTs using an RM and titrated PEEP (Brower et al., 2004; Meade et al., 2008; Mercat et al., 2008; Cavalcanti et al., 2017).

Hirshberg et al. (2018) conducted an RCT in adults, and similarly to the Ganesan study, targeted a Vt at ~6 mL/kg. The study was stopped early, in part because the Vt often exceeded 12 mL/kg, even though there were no significant differences between groups in pneumothorax, sedation, vasoactive medications, P/F ratio, or outcome (Hirshberg et al., 2018). As stated above, when the TCAV method is used, an increase in Vt is indicative of lung recruitment and is a positive effect. Thus, one of the critical protective mechanisms of the TCAV method, the ability to fully open the lung, was not incorporated into the APRV setting in either the Hirshberg or Ganesan study. The conclusion from these clinical studies should not be that "APRV is not lung protective" but rather that the Zhou (Zhou et al., 2017) and TCAV methods (Andrews et al., 2013) are superior to the Ganesan (Lalgudi Ganesan et al., 2018) and Hirshberg (Hirshberg et al., 2018) methods for lung protection. Two recent statistical reviews and meta-analyses of RCTs have shown the APRV mode is associated with a mortality benefit, improved oxygenation, and a greater number of ventilator-free days when compared with conventional ventilation strategies,

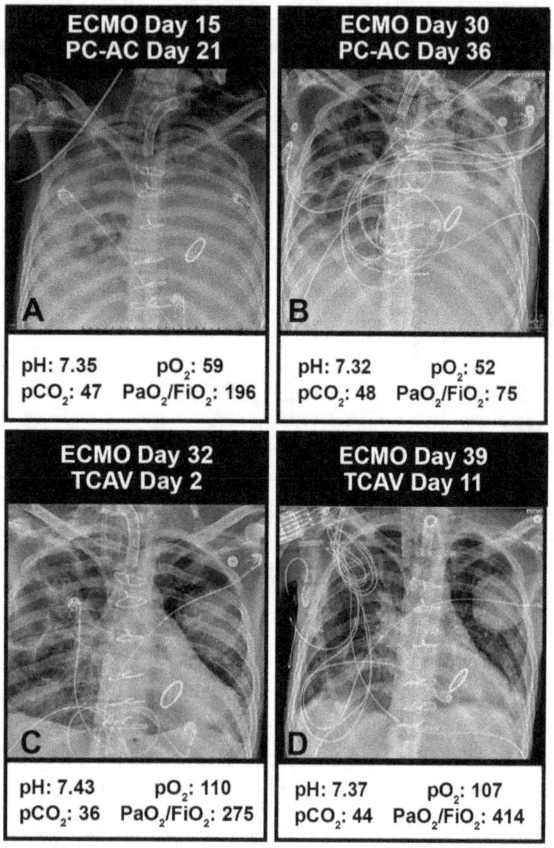

FIGURE 13 | Chest X-rays (CXRs) and blood gases in a patient with respiratory failure on extracorporeal membrane oxygenation (ECMO). **(A)** CXR and blood gases (arterial pH, PCO_2, and PO_2 with the calculated PaO_2/FiO_2 ratio) at 15 days on ECMO and protective ARDSnet pressure-control assist-control ventilation (PC-AC). Bilateral infiltrates can be seen throughout the lung with a PaO_2/FiO_2 ratio of 196. **(B)** After 30 days on ECMO and PC-AC, the patient showed some clearing in the upper right quadrant but a worsening PaO_2/FiO_2 ratio of 75. **(C)** Two days after conversion to the TCAV method, the patient showed marked improvement in CXR and PaO_2/FiO_2 ratio (275). **(D)** After 11 days on the TCAV method, the patient showed a cleared CXR and normalized PaO_2/FiO_2 ratio (414). The patient came off of ECMO and was extubated. *Written informed consent obtained for the use of these images.*

without any negative hemodynamic impact or higher risk of barotrauma (Carsetti et al., 2019; Lim and Litton, 2019).

An example of the TCAV method's effectiveness when applied to a patient on extracorporeal membrane oxygenation (ECMO) with respiratory failure is seen in **Figure 13**. A 35-year-old man with a history of systemic lupus erythematous, with catastrophic antiphospholipid syndrome, underwent a coronary artery bypass graft with mitral valve repair and was placed on protective pressure-control assist-control ventilation (PC-AC) with protective settings using the ARDSnet method. Chest X-rays (CXRs) on PC-AC for 21 days, 15 of those days on ECMO, showed widespread infiltrates (**Figure 13A**). Another 15 days on ECMO (30 days on ECMO total) and PC-AC showed minimal change in CXRs and worsening lung function assessed by P/F ratio (A: 196, B: 75) (**Figure 13B**). Conversion to the TCAV method for 2 days resulted in a marked improvement in CXRs and P/F ratio (275) (**Figure 13C**). After 11 days on TCAV, the patient had a clear CXR and normal P/F ratio (414) (**Figure 13D**). **Figure 13D** was 6 h prior to decannulation and liberation from ECMO. After 39 days on PC-AC with worsening lung function, it took only 2 days on the TCAV method to reopen and stabilize the patient's lung, and after 11 days the patient was disconnected from ECMO, extubated, and removed from mechanical ventilation.

CONCLUSION

Current protective ventilation strategies have not significantly reduced ARDS-related mortality in the 20 years since the ARMA study, possibly because strategies are constrained to ventilating the heterogeneously collapsed and unstable lung. In addition, current protective ventilation strategies have not considered all of the physiological parameters necessary to protect the acutely injured lung. Alveoli and alveolar ducts open and collapse as a viscoelastic system such that there is a time lag between when the airway pressure is applied and alveoli open, and between when the airway pressure is removed and alveoli collapse. Loss of pulmonary surfactant function, a key ARDS pathology, amplifies these viscoelastic properties, rendering the lung *time* and *pressure* dependent, such that it takes an extended time at the higher pressure for lung tissue to open and a very brief time, even with an elevated airway pressure, for the lung to recollapse.

This knowledge suggests that to eliminate VILI the ventilation strategy must open and stabilize the lung. Current ventilation strategies attempting this OLA have not reduced mortality in clinical trials. Since alveolar volume change is viscoelastic in nature, the *time* at both inspiration and expiration would be critical to accomplishing the OLA goals. We have developed a time-controlled adaptive ventilation TCAV method using the APRV mode and have shown that it is highly effective at opening and stabilizing the lung, which significantly reduces VILI-induced lung damage in animal ARDS models. We have also shown that preemptive application of the TCAV method in trauma patients significantly reduces ARDS incidence and mortality. Recent RCTs using the APRV mode but not adjusted with the TCAV method have shown mixed results, suggesting that properly adjusted APRV is critical to clinical success.

AUTHOR CONTRIBUTIONS

GN drafted the manuscript. HA-K, MK-S, JS, SB, GT, PA, MM, LG, and NH critically revised the manuscript. All authors read and approved the final manuscript.

REFERENCES

Albert, R. K. (2012). The role of ventilation-induced surfactant dysfunction and atelectasis in causing acute respiratory distress syndrome. *Am. J. Respir. Crit. Care Med.* 185, 702–708.

Alencar, A. M., Arold, S. P., Buldyrev, S. V., Majumdar, A., Stamenovic, D., Stanley, H. E., et al. (2002). Dynamic instabilities in the inflating lung. *Nature* 417, 809–811. doi: 10.1038/417809b

Amato, M. B., Meade, M. O., Slutsky, A. S., Brochard, L., Costa, E. L., Schoenfeld, D. A., et al. (2015). Driving pressure and survival in the acute respiratory distress syndrome. *N. Engl. J. Med.* 372, 747–755. doi: 10.1056/NEJMsa1410639

Andrews, P. L., Sadowitz, B., Kollisch-Singule, M., Satalin, J., Roy, S., Snyder, K., et al. (2015). Alveolar instability (atelectrauma) is not identified by arterial oxygenation predisposing the development of an occult ventilator-induced lung injury. *Intensive Care Med. Exp.* 3:16. doi: 10.1186/s40635-015-0054-1

Andrews, P. L., Shiber, J. R., Jaruga-Killeen, E., Roy, S., Sadowitz, B., O'Toole, R. V., et al. (2013). Early application of airway pressure release ventilation may reduce mortality in high-risk trauma patients: a systematic review of observational trauma ARDS literature. *J. Trauma Acute Care Surg.* 75, 635–641.

Acute Respiratory Distress Syndrome Network (2000). Ventilation with lower tidal volumes as compared with traditional tidal volumes for acute lung injury and the acute respiratory distress syndrome. The acute respiratory distress syndrome network. *N. Engl. J. Med.* 342, 1301–1308. doi: 10.1056/nejm200005043421801

Ashbaugh, D. G., Bigelow, D. B., Petty, T. L., and Levine, B. E. (1967). Acute respiratory distress in adults. *Lancet* 2, 319–323.

Baumgardner, J. E., Markstaller, K., Pfeiffer, B., Doebrich, M., and Otto, C. M. (2002). Effects of respiratory rate, plateau pressure, and positive end-expiratory pressure on PaO2 oscillations after saline lavage. *Am. J. Respir. Crit. Care Med.* 166(12 Pt 1), 1556–1562. doi: 10.1164/rccm.200207-717oc

Bellani, G., Laffey, J. G., Pham, T., Fan, E., Brochard, L., Esteban, A., et al. (2016). Epidemiology, patterns of care, and mortality for patients with acute respiratory distress syndrome in intensive care units in 50 countries. *J. Am. Med. Assoc.* 315, 788–800.

Bergez, M., Fritsch, N., Tran-Van, D., Saghi, T., Bounkim, T., Gentile, A., et al. (2019). PEEP titration in moderate to severe ARDS: plateau versus transpulmonary pressure. *Ann. Intensive Care.* 9:81. doi: 10.1186/s13613-019-0554-3

Bhattacharjee, S., Soni, K. D., and Maitra, S. (2018). Recruitment maneuver does not provide any mortality benefit over lung protective strategy ventilation in adult patients with acute respiratory distress syndrome: a meta-analysis and systematic review of the randomized controlled trials. *J. Intensive Care* 6:35.

Bilek, A. M., Dee, K. C., and Gaver, D. P. (2003). Mechanisms of surface-tension-induced epithelial cell damage in a model of pulmonary airway reopening. *J. Appl. Physiol.* 94, 770–783. doi: 10.1152/japplphysiol.00764.2002

Blanch, L., Villagra, A., Sales, B., Montanya, J., Lucangelo, U., Lujan, M., et al. (2015). Asynchronies during mechanical ventilation are associated with mortality. *Intensive Care Med.* 41, 633–641. doi: 10.1007/s00134-015-3692-6

Boehme, S., Bentley, A. H., Hartmann, E. K., Chang, S., Erdoes, G., Prinzing, A., et al. (2015). Influence of inspiration to expiration ratio on cyclic recruitment and derecruitment of atelectasis in a saline lavage model of acute respiratory distress syndrome. *Crit. Care Med.* 43, e65–e74. doi: 10.1097/CCM.0000000000000788

Borges, J. B., Okamoto, V. N., Matos, G. F., Caramez, M. P., Arantes, P. R., Barros, F., et al. (2006). Reversibility of lung collapse and hypoxemia in early acute respiratory distress syndrome. *Am. J. Respir. Crit. Care Med.* 174, 268–278. doi: 10.1164/rccm.200506-976oc

Broche, L., Perchiazzi, G., Porra, L., Tannoia, A., Pellegrini, M., Derosa, S., et al. (2017). Dynamic mechanical interactions between neighboring airspaces determine cyclic opening and closure in injured lung. *Crit. Care Med.* 45, 687–694. doi: 10.1097/CCM.0000000000002234

Brower, R. G., Lanken, P. N., MacIntyre, N., Matthay, M. A., Morris, A., Ancukiewicz, M., et al. (2004). Higher versus lower positive end-expiratory pressures in patients with the acute respiratory distress syndrome. *N. Engl. J. Med.* 351, 327–336. doi: 10.1056/nejmoa032193

Brower, R. G., Shanholtz, C. B., Fessler, H. E., Shade, D. M., White, P. Jr., Wiener, C. M., et al. (1999). Prospective, randomized, controlled clinical trial comparing traditional versus reduced tidal volume ventilation in acute respiratory distress syndrome patients. *Crit. Care Med.* 27, 1492–1498. doi: 10.1097/00003246-199908000-00015

Brun-Buisson, C., Minelli, C., Bertolini, G., Brazzi, L., Pimentel, J., Lewandowski, K., et al. (2004). Epidemiology and outcome of acute lung injury in European intensive care units. Results from the ALIVE study. *Intensive Care Med.* 30, 51–61. doi: 10.1007/s00134-003-2022-6

Burkhardt, A. (1989). Alveolitis and collapse in the pathogenesis of pulmonary fibrosis. *Am. Rev. Respir. Dis.* 140, 513–524. doi: 10.1164/ajrccm/140.2.513

Burki, N. K., and Lee, L. Y. (2010). Mechanisms of dyspnea. *Chest* 138, 1196–1201. doi: 10.1378/chest.10-0534

Cabrera-Benitez, N. E., Laffey, J. G., Parotto, M., Spieth, P. M., Villar, J., Zhang, H., et al. (2014). Mechanical ventilation-associated lung fibrosis in acute respiratory distress syndrome: a significant contributor to poor outcome. *Anesthesiology* 121, 189–198. doi: 10.1097/ALN.0000000000000264

Carsetti, A., Damiani, E., Domizi, R., Scorcella, C., Pantanetti, S., Falcetta, S., et al. (2019). Airway pressure release ventilation during acute hypoxemic respiratory failure: a systematic review and meta-analysis of randomized controlled trials. *Ann. Intensive Care* 9:44. doi: 10.1186/s13613-019-0518-7

Carvalho, A. R., and Zin, W. A. (2011). Respiratory system dynamical mechanical properties: modeling in time and frequency domain. *Biophys. Rev.* 3:71. doi: 10.1007/s12551-011-0048-5

Caser, E. B., Zandonade, E., Pereira, E., Gama, A. M., and Barbas, C. S. (2014). Impact of distinct definitions of acute lung injury on its incidence and outcomes in Brazilian ICUs: prospective evaluation of 7,133 patients*. *Crit. Care Med.* 42, 574–582. doi: 10.1097/01.ccm.0000435676.68435.56

Cavalcanti, A. B., Suzumura, E. A., Laranjeira, L. N., Paisani, D. M., Damiani, L. P., Guimaraes, H. P., et al. (2017). Effect of lung recruitment and titrated positive end-expiratory pressure (PEEP) vs low PEEP on mortality in patients with acute respiratory distress syndrome: a randomized clinical trial. *JAMA* 318, 1335–1345. doi: 10.1001/jama.2017.14171

Cereda, M., Emami, K., Kadlecek, S., Xin, Y., Mongkolwisetwara, P., Profka, H., et al. (2011). Quantitative imaging of alveolar recruitment with hyperpolarized gas MRI during mechanical ventilation. *J. Appl. Physiol.* 110, 499–511. doi: 10.1152/japplphysiol.00841.2010

Cereda, M., Emami, K., Xin, Y., Kadlecek, S., Kuzma, N. N., Mongkolwisetwara, P., et al. (2013). Imaging the interaction of atelectasis and overdistension in surfactant-depleted lungs. *Crit. Care Med.* 41, 527–535. doi: 10.1097/CCM.0b013e31826ab1f2

Cereda, M., Xin, Y., Hamedani, H., Bellani, G., Kadlecek, S., Clapp, J., et al. (2017). Tidal changes on CT and progression of ARDS. *Thorax* 72, 981–989. doi: 10.1136/thoraxjnl-2016-209833

Cereda, M., Xin, Y., Hamedani, H., Clapp, J., Kadlecek, S., Meeder, N., et al. (2016a). Mild loss of lung aeration augments stretch in healthy lung regions. *J. Appl. Physiol.* 120, 444–454. doi: 10.1152/japplphysiol.00734.2015

Cereda, M., Xin, Y., Meeder, N., Zeng, J., Jiang, Y., Hamedani, H., et al. (2016b). Visualizing the propagation of acute lung injury. *Anesthesiology* 124, 121–131. doi: 10.1097/ALN.0000000000000916

Chen, Z. L., Chen, Y. Z., and Hu, Z. Y. (2014). A micromechanical model for estimating alveolar wall strain in mechanically ventilated edematous lungs. *J. Appl. Physiol.* 117, 586–592. doi: 10.1152/japplphysiol.00072.2014

Coruh, B., and Luks, A. M. (2014). Positive end-expiratory pressure. When more may not be better. *Ann. Am. Thorac. Soc.* 11, 1327–1331. doi: 10.1513/annalsats.201404-151cc

Cressoni, M., Cadringher, P., Chiurazzi, C., Amini, M., Gallazzi, E., Marino, A., et al. (2014). Lung inhomogeneity in patients with acute respiratory distress syndrome. *Am. J. Respir. Crit. Care Med.* 189, 149–158. doi: 10.1164/rccm.201308-1567OC

Cressoni, M., Chiumello, D., Algieri, I., Brioni, M., Chiurazzi, C., Colombo, A., et al. (2017). Opening pressures and atelectrauma in acute respiratory distress syndrome. *Intensive Care Med.* 43, 603–611. doi: 10.1007/s00134-017-4754-8

Crotti, S., Mascheroni, D., Caironi, P., Pelosi, P., Ronzoni, G., Mondino, M., et al. (2001). Recruitment and derecruitment during acute respiratory failure: a clinical study. *Am. J. Respir. Crit. Care Med.* 164, 131–140. doi: 10.1164/ajrccm.164.1.2007011

Cui, Y., Cao, R., Wang, Y., and Li, G. (2019). Lung recruitment maneuvers for ARDS patients: a systematic review and meta-analysis. *Respiration* 1–13. doi: 10.1159/000501045 [Epub ahead of print].

de Anda, G. F., Gommers, D., Verbrugge, S. J., De Jaegere, A., and Lachmann, B. (2000). Mechanical ventilation with high positive end-expiratory pressure and small driving pressure amplitude is as effective as high-frequency oscillatory ventilation to preserve the function of exogenous surfactant in lung-lavaged rats. *Crit. Care Med.* 28, 2921–2925. doi: 10.1097/00003246-200008000-00039

Del Sorbo, L., Goligher, E. C., McAuley, D. F., Rubenfeld, G. D., Brochard, L. J., Gattinoni, L., et al. (2017). Mechanical ventilation in adults with acute respiratory distress syndrome. Summary of the experimental evidence for the clinical practice guideline. *Ann. Am. Thorac. Soc.* 14(Suppl. 4), S261–S270.

Denny, E., and Schroter, R. C. (2000). Viscoelastic behavior of a lung alveolar duct model. *J. Biomech. Eng.* 122, 143–151. doi: 10.1115/1.429644

Dreyfuss, D., Soler, P., Basset, G., and Saumon, G. (1988). High inflation pressure pulmonary edema. Respective effects of high airway pressure, high tidal volume, and positive end-expiratory pressure. *Am. Rev. Respir. Dis.* 137, 1159–1164. doi: 10.1164/ajrccm/137.5.1159

Effros, R. M., and Parker, J. C. (2009). Pulmonary vascular heterogeneity and the starling hypothesis. *Microvas. Res.* 78, 71–77. doi: 10.1016/j.mvr.2009.03.004

Emr, B., Gatto, L., Roy, S., Satalin, J., Ghosh, A., Snyder, K., et al. (2013). Airway pressure release ventilation prevents ventilator-induced lung injury in normal lungs. *JAMA Surg.* 148, 1005–1012. doi: 10.1001/jamasurg.2013.3746

Escolar, J. D., and Escolar, A. (2004). Lung hysteresis: a morphological view. *Histol. Histopathol.* 19, 159–166. doi: 10.14670/HH-19.159

Fan, E., Brodie, D., and Slutsky, A. S. (2018). Acute respiratory distress syndrome: advances in diagnosis and treatment. *JAMA* 319, 698–710.

Fan, E., Del Sorbo, L., Goligher, E. C., Hodgson, C. L., Munshi, L., Walkey, A. J., et al. (2017). An official American Thoracic society/European society of intensive care medicine/society of critical care medicine clinical Practice Guideline: mechanical ventilation in adult patients with acute respiratory distress syndrome. *Am. J. Respir. Crit. Care Med.* 195, 1253–1263. doi: 10.1164/rccm.201703-0548ST

Fan, E., Needham, D. M., and Stewart, T. E. (2005). Ventilatory management of acute lung injury and acute respiratory distress syndrome. *JAMA* 294, 2889–2896.

Fan, E., Wilcox, M. E., Brower, R. G., Stewart, T. E., Mehta, S., Lapinsky, S. E., et al. (2008). Recruitment maneuvers for acute lung injury: a systematic review. *Am. J. Respir. Crit. Care Med.* 178, 1156–1163. doi: 10.1164/rccm.200802-335OC

Farias, L. L., Faffe, D. S., Xisto, D. G., Santana, M. C., Lassance, R., Prota, L. F., et al. (2005). Positive end-expiratory pressure prevents lung mechanical stress caused by recruitment/derecruitment. *J. Appl. Physiol.* 98, 53–61. doi: 10.1152/japplphysiol.00118.2004

Faridy, E. E., Permutt, S., and Riley, R. L. (1966). Effect of ventilation on surface forces in excised dogs' lungs. *J. Appl. Physiol.* 21, 1453–1462. doi: 10.1152/jappl.1966.21.5.1453

Ferguson, N. D., Cook, D. J., Guyatt, G. H., Mehta, S., Hand, L., Austin, P., et al. (2013). High-frequency oscillation in early acute respiratory distress syndrome. *N. Engl. J. Med.* 368, 795–805. doi: 10.1056/NEJMoa1215554

Gattinoni, L., Caironi, P., Cressoni, M., Chiumello, D., Ranieri, V. M., Quintel, M., et al. (2006). Lung recruitment in patients with the acute respiratory distress syndrome. *N. Engl. J. Med.* 354, 1775–1786.

Gattinoni, L., Carlesso, E., and Caironi, P. (2012). Stress and strain within the lung. *Curr. Opin. Crit. Care* 18, 42–47. doi: 10.1097/mcc.0b013e32834f17d9

Gattinoni, L., Collino, F., Maiolo, G., Rapetti, F., Romitti, F., Tonetti, T., et al. (2017). Positive end-expiratory pressure: how to set it at the individual level. *Ann. Transl. Med.* 5:288. doi: 10.21037/atm.2017.06.64

Gattinoni, L., Pelosi, P., Crotti, S., and Valenza, F. (1995). Effects of positive end-expiratory pressure on regional distribution of tidal volume and recruitment in adult respiratory distress syndrome. *Am. J. Respir. Crit. Care Med.* 151, 1807–1814. doi: 10.1164/ajrccm.151.6.7767524

Gattinoni, L., and Pesenti, A. (2005). The concept of "baby lung". *Intensive Care Med.* 31, 776–784. doi: 10.1007/s00134-005-2627-z

Gattinoni, L., Vagginelli, F., Carlesso, E., Taccone, P., Conte, V., Chiumello, D., et al. (2003). Decrease in PaCO2 with prone position is predictive of improved outcome in acute respiratory distress syndrome. *Crit. Care Med.* 31, 2727–2733. doi: 10.1097/01.ccm.0000098032.34052.f9

Ghadiali, S. N., and Gaver, D. P. (2008). Biomechanics of liquid-epithelium interactions in pulmonary airways. *Respir. Physiol. Neurobiol.* 163, 232–243. doi: 10.1016/j.resp.2008.04.008

Goligher, E. C., Hodgson, C. L., Adhikari, N. K. J., Meade, M. O., Wunsch, H., Uleryk, E., et al. (2017). Lung recruitment maneuvers for adult patients with acute respiratory distress syndrome. a systematic review and meta-analysis. *Ann. Am. Thorac. Soc.* 14(Suppl. 4), S304–S311.

Grune, J., Tabuchi, A., and Kuebler, W. M. (2019). Alveolar dynamics during mechanical ventilation in the healthy and injured lung. *Intensive Care Med. Exp.* 7(Suppl. 1):34. doi: 10.1186/s40635-019-0226-5

Guerin, C., Reignier, J., and Richard, J. C. (2013). Prone positioning in the acute respiratory distress syndrome. *N. Engl. J. Med.* 369, 980–981.

Guldner, A., Braune, A., Ball, L., Silva, P. L., Samary, C., Insorsi, A., et al. (2016). Comparative effects of volutrauma and atelectrauma on lung inflammation in experimental acute respiratory distress syndrome. *Crit. Care Med.* 44, e854–e865. doi: 10.1097/CCM.0000000000001721

Habashi, N. M. (2005). Other approaches to open-lung ventilation: airway pressure release ventilation. *Crit. Care Med.* 33(Suppl. 3), S228–S240.

Halter, J. M., Steinberg, J. M., Schiller, H. J., DaSilva, M., Gatto, L. A., Landas, S., et al. (2003). Positive end-expiratory pressure after a recruitment maneuver prevents both alveolar collapse and recruitment/derecruitment. *Am. J. Respir. Crit. Care Med.* 167, 1620–1626. doi: 10.1164/rccm.200205-435oc

Hamlington, K. L., Bates, J. H. T., Roy, G. S., Julianelle, A. J., Charlebois, C., Suki, B., et al. (2018). Alveolar leak develops by a rich-get-richer process in ventilator-induced lung injury. *PLoS One* 13:e0193934. doi: 10.1371/journal.pone.0193934

Hamlington, K. L., Ma, B., Smith, B. J., and Bates, J. H. (2016). Modeling the progression of epithelial leak caused by overdistension. *Cell. Mol. Bioeng.* 9, 151–161. doi: 10.1007/s12195-015-0426-3

Hirshberg, E. L., Lanspa, M. J., Peterson, J., Carpenter, L., Wilson, E. L., Brown, S. M., et al. (2018). Randomized feasibility trial of a low tidal volume-airway pressure release ventilation protocol compared with traditional airway pressure release ventilation and volume control ventilation protocols. *Crit. Care Med.* 46, 1943–1952. doi: 10.1097/CCM.0000000000003437

Hodgson, C. L., Cooper, D. J., Arabi, Y., King, V., Bersten, A., Bihari, S., et al. (2019). Maximal Recruitment open lung ventilation in acute respiratory distress syndrome (PHARLAP): a phase II, multicenter, randomized, controlled trial. *Am. J. Respir. Crit. Care Med.* 200, 1363–1372. doi: 10.1164/rccm.201901-0109OC

Huynh, T. T., Liesching, T. N., Cereda, M., Lei, Y., Frazer, M. J., Nahouraii, M. R., et al. (2019). Efficacy of oscillation and lung expansion in reducing postoperative pulmonary complication. *J. Am. Coll. Surg.* 229, 458.e–466.e. doi: 10.1016/j.jamcollsurg.2019.06.004

Jain, S. V., Kollisch-Singule, M., Sadowitz, B., Dombert, L., Satalin, J., Andrews, P., et al. (2016). The 30-year evolution of airway pressure release ventilation (APRV). *Intensive Care Med. Exp.* 4:11. doi: 10.1186/s40635-016-0085-2

Jain, S. V., Kollisch-Singule, M., Satalin, J., Searles, Q., Dombert, L., Abdel-Razek, O., et al. (2017). The role of high airway pressure and dynamic strain on ventilator-induced lung injury in a heterogeneous acute lung injury model. *Intensive Care Med. Exp.* 5:25. doi: 10.1186/s40635-017-0138-1

Kang, H., Yang, H., and Tong, Z. (2019). Recruitment manoeuvres for adults with acute respiratory distress syndrome receiving mechanical ventilation: a systematic review and meta-analysis. *J. Crit. Care* 50, 1–10. doi: 10.1016/j.jcrc.2018.10.033

Kollisch-Singule, M., Andrews, P., Satalin, J., Gatto, L. A., Nieman, G. F., and Habashi, N. M. (2019). The time-controlled adaptive ventilation protocol: mechanistic approach to reducing ventilator-induced lung injury. *Eur. Respir. Rev.* 28:180126. doi: 10.1183/16000617.0126-2018

Kollisch-Singule, M., Emr, B., Jain, S. V., Andrews, P., Satalin, J., Liu, J., et al. (2015a). The effects of airway pressure release ventilation on respiratory mechanics in extrapulmonary lung injury. *Intensive Care Med. Exp.* 3:35.

Kollisch-Singule, M., Emr, B., Smith, B., Roy, S., Jain, S., Satalin, J., et al. (2014a). Mechanical breath profile of airway pressure release ventilation: the effect on alveolar recruitment and microstrain in acute lung injury. *JAMA Surg.* 149, 1138–1145. doi: 10.1001/jamasurg.2014.1829

Kollisch-Singule, M., Emr, B., Smith, B., Ruiz, C., Roy, S., Meng, Q., et al. (2014b). Airway pressure release ventilation reduces conducting airway micro-strain in lung injury. *J. Am. Coll. Surg.* 219, 968–976. doi: 10.1016/j.jamcollsurg.2014.09.011

Kollisch-Singule, M., Jain, S., Andrews, P., Smith, B. J., Hamlington-Smith, K. L., Roy, S., et al. (2015b). Effect of airway pressure release ventilation on dynamic alveolar heterogeneity. *JAMA Surg.* 151, 64–72. doi: 10.1001/jamasurg.2015.2683

Kollisch-Singule, M., Jain, S. V., Satalin, J., Andrews, P., Searles, Q., Liu, Z., et al. (2017). Limiting ventilator-associated lung injury in a preterm porcine neonatal model. *J. Pediatr. Surg.* 52, 50–55. doi: 10.1016/j.jpedsurg.2016.10.020

Kollisch-Singule, M. C., Jain, S. V., Andrews, P. L., Satalin, J., Gatto, L. A., Villar, J., et al. (2018). Last word on viewpoint: looking beyond macrovenitlatory parameters and rethinking ventilator-induced lung injury. *J. Appl. Physiol.* 124, 1220–1221. doi: 10.1152/japplphysiol.00049.2018

Laffey, J. G., Bellani, G., Pham, T., Fan, E., Madotto, F., Bajwa, E. K., et al. (2016). Potentially modifiable factors contributing to outcome from acute respiratory distress syndrome: the LUNG SAFE study. *Intensive Care Med.* 42, 1865–1876. doi: 10.1007/s00134-016-4571-5

Lalgudi Ganesan, S., Jayashree, M., Singhi, S. C., and Bansal, A. (2018). Airway pressure release ventilation in pediatric acute respiratory distress syndrome: a randomized controlled trial. *Am. J. Respir. Crit. Care Med.* 198, 1199–1207. doi: 10.1164/rccm.201705-0989oc

Lewis, J. F., Ikegami, M., Jobe, A. H., and Absolom, D. (1993). Physiologic responses and distribution of aerosolized surfactant (Survanta) in a nonuniform pattern of lung injury. *Am. Rev. Respir. Dis.* 147(6 Pt 1), 1364–1370. doi: 10.1164/ajrccm/147.6_pt_1.1364

Li Bassi, G., Marti, J. D., Comaru, T., Aguilera-Xiol, E., Rigol, M., Ntoumenopoulos, G., et al. (2019). Short-term appraisal of the effects and safety of manual versus ventilator hyperinflation in an animal model of severe pneumonia. *Respir. Care* 64, 760–770. doi: 10.4187/respcare.06487

Lim, J., and Litton, E. (2019). Airway pressure release ventilation in adult patients with acute hypoxemic respiratory failure: a systematic review and meta-analysis. *Crit. Care Med.* 47, 1794–1799. doi: 10.1097/ccm.0000000000003972

Lu, J., Wang, X., Chen, M., Cheng, L., Chen, Q., Jiang, H., et al. (2017). An open lung strategy in the management of acute respiratory distress syndrome: a systematic review and meta-analysis. *Shock* 48, 43–53. doi: 10.1097/shk.0000000000000822

Lutz, D., Gazdhar, A., Lopez-Rodriguez, E., Ruppert, C., Mahavadi, P., Gunther, A., et al. (2015). Alveolar derecruitment and collapse induration as crucial mechanisms in lung injury and fibrosis. *Am. J. Respir. Cell Mol. Biol.* 52, 232–243. doi: 10.1165/rcmb.2014-0078OC

Maca, J., Jor, O., Holub, M., Sklienka, P., Bursa, F., Burda, M., et al. (2017). Past and present ARDS mortality rates: a systematic review. *Respir. Care* 62, 113–122. doi: 10.4187/respcare.04716

Magalhaes, P. A. F., Padilha, G. A., Moraes, L., Santos, C. L., Maia, L. A., Braga, C. L., et al. (2018). Effects of pressure support ventilation on ventilator-induced lung injury in mild acute respiratory distress syndrome depend on level of positive end-expiratory pressure: a randomised animal study. *Eur. J. Anaesthesiol.* 35, 298–306. doi: 10.1097/EJA.0000000000000763

Mahajan, M., DiStefano, D., Satalin, J., Andrews, P., Al-Khalisy, H., Baker, S., et al. (2019). Time-controlled adaptive ventilation (TCAV) accelerates simulated mucus clearance via increased expiratory flow rate. *Intensive Care Med. Exp.* 7:27. doi: 10.1186/s40635-019-0250-5

Majumdar, A., Arold, S. P., Bartolak-Suki, E., Parameswaran, H., and Suki, B. (2012). Jamming dynamics of stretch-induced surfactant release by alveolar type II cells. *J. Appl. Physiol.* 112, 824–831. doi: 10.1152/japplphysiol.00975.2010

Makiyama, A. M., Gibson, L. J., Harris, R. S., and Venegas, J. G. (2014). Stress concentration around an atelectatic region: a finite element model. *Respir. Physiol. Neurobiol.* 201, 101–110. doi: 10.1016/j.resp.2014.06.017

Manning, H. L., and Mahler, D. A. (2001). Pathophysiology of dyspnea. *Monaldi Arch. Chest Dis.* 56, 325–330.

Marini, J. J. (2018). Dissipation of energy during the respiratory cycle: conditional importance of ergotrauma to structural lung damage. *Curr. Opin. Crit. Care* 24, 16–22. doi: 10.1097/MCC.0000000000000470

Martin, G. S., and Brigham, K. L. (2012). Fluid flux and clearance in acute lung injury. *Compr. Physiol.* 2, 2471–2480. doi: 10.1002/cphy.c100050

McNicholas, B. A., Rooney, G. M., and Laffey, J. G. (2018). Lessons to learn from epidemiologic studies in ARDS. *Curr. Opin. Crit. Care* 24, 41–48. doi: 10.1097/MCC.0000000000000473

Mead, J., Takishima, T., and Leith, D. (1970). Stress distribution in lungs: a model of pulmonary elasticity. *J. Appl. Physiol.* 28, 596–608. doi: 10.1152/jappl.1970.28.5.596

Meade, M. O., Cook, D. J., Guyatt, G. H., Slutsky, A. S., Arabi, Y. M., Cooper, D. J., et al. (2008). Ventilation strategy using low tidal volumes, recruitment maneuvers, and high positive end-expiratory pressure for acute lung injury and acute respiratory distress syndrome: a randomized controlled trial. *JAMA* 299, 637–645.

Mellott, K. G., Grap, M. J., Munro, C. L., Sessler, C. N., and Wetzel, P. A. (2009). Patient-ventilator dyssynchrony: clinical significance and implications for practice. *Crit. Care Nurse* 29, 41–55 quiz 1 p following 55.

Mercat, A., Richard, J. C., Vielle, B., Jaber, S., Osman, D., Diehl, J. L., et al. (2008). Positive end-expiratory pressure setting in adults with acute lung injury and acute respiratory distress syndrome: a randomized controlled trial. *JAMA* 299, 646–655.

Morais, C. C. A., Koyama, Y., Yoshida, T., Plens, G. M., Gomes, S., Lima, C. A. S., et al. (2018). High positive end-expiratory pressure renders spontaneous effort noninjurious. *Am. J. Respir. Crit. Care Med.* 197, 1285–1296. doi: 10.1164/rccm.201706-1244OC

Motta-Ribeiro, G. C., Hashimoto, S., Winkler, T., Baron, R. M., Grogg, K., Paula, L., et al. (2018). Deterioration of regional lung strain and inflammation during early lung injury. *Am. J. Respir. Crit. Care Med.* 198, 891–902. doi: 10.1164/rccm.201710-2038OC

Muscedere, J. G., Mullen, J. B., Gan, K., and Slutsky, A. S. (1994). Tidal ventilation at low airway pressures can augment lung injury. *Am. J. Respir. Crit. Care Med.* 149, 1327–1334. doi: 10.1164/ajrccm.149.5.8173774

Nakazawa, K., Yokoyama, K., Yamakawa, N., and Makita, K. (2007). Effect of positive end-expiratory pressure on inflammatory response in oleic acid-induced lung injury and whole-lung lavage-induced lung injury. *J. Anesth.* 21, 47–54. doi: 10.1007/s00540-006-0465-y

Neumann, P., Berglund, J. E., Andersson, L. G., Maripu, E., Magnusson, A., and Hedenstierna, G. (2000). Effects of inverse ratio ventilation and positive end-expiratory pressure in oleic acid-induced lung injury. *Am. J. Respir. Crit. Care Med.* 161, 1537–1545. doi: 10.1164/ajrccm.161.5.9906060

Neumann, P., Berglund, J. E., Fernandez Mondejar, E., Magnusson, A., and Hedenstierna, G. (1998a). Dynamics of lung collapse and recruitment during prolonged breathing in porcine lung injury. *J. Appl. Physiol.* 85, 1533–1543. doi: 10.1152/jappl.1998.85.4.1533

Neumann, P., Berglund, J. E., Mondejar, E. F., Magnusson, A., and Hedenstierna, G. (1998b). Effect of different pressure levels on the dynamics of lung collapse and recruitment in oleic-acid-induced lung injury. *Am. J. Respir. Crit. Care Med.* 158(5 Pt 1), 1636–1643. doi: 10.1164/ajrccm.158.5.9711095

Nieman, G., Gatto, L., Andrews, P., Satalin, J., Camporota, L., Daxon, B., et al. (2019). Prevention and treatment of acute lung injury with time controlled adaptive ventilation. *Ann. Intensive Care* 10:3.

Nieman, G. F., Andrews, P., Satalin, J., Wilcox, K., Kollisch-Singule, M., Madden, M., et al. (2018). Acute lung injury: how to stabilize a broken lung. *Critical Care* 22:136. doi: 10.1186/s13054-018-2051-8

Nieman, G. F., and Bredenberg, C. E. (1985). High surface tension pulmonary edema induced by detergent aerosol. *J. Appl. Physiol.* 58, 129–136. doi: 10.1152/jappl.1985.58.1.129

Nieman, G. F., Gatto, L. A., and Habashi, N. M. (2015). Impact of mechanical ventilation on the pathophysiology of progressive acute lung injury. *J. Appl. Physiol.* 119, 1245–1261. doi: 10.1152/japplphysiol.00659.2015

Nieman, G. F., Satalin, J., Andrews, P., Aiash, H., Habashi, N. M., and Gatto, L. A. (2017a). Personalizing mechanical ventilation according to physiologic parameters to stabilize alveoli and minimize ventilator induced lung injury (VILI). *Intensive Care Med. Exp.* 5:8. doi: 10.1186/s40635-017-0121-x

Nieman, G. F., Satalin, J., Kollisch-Singule, M., Andrews, P., Aiash, H., Habashi, N. M., et al. (2017b). Physiology in medicine: understanding dynamic alveolar physiology to minimize ventilator-induced lung injury. *J. Appl. Physiol.* 122, 1516–1522. doi: 10.1152/japplphysiol.00123.2017

Papazian, L., Aubron, C., Brochard, L., Chiche, J. D., Combes, A., Dreyfuss, D., et al. (2019). Formal guidelines: management of acute respiratory distress syndrome. *Ann. Intensive Care* 9:69. doi: 10.1186/s13613-019-0540-9

Pavone, L. A., Albert, S., Carney, D., Gatto, L. A., Halter, J. M., and Nieman, G. F. (2007). Injurious mechanical ventilation in the normal lung causes a progressive pathologic change in dynamic alveolar mechanics. *Critical Care* 11:R64.

Perlman, C. E., Lederer, D. J., and Bhattacharya, J. (2011). Micromechanics of alveolar edema. *Am. J. Respir. Cell Mol. Biol.* 44, 34–39. doi: 10.1165/rcmb.2009-0005OC

Perun, M. L., and Gaver, D. P. (1995). Interaction between airway lining fluid forces and parenchymal tethering during pulmonary airway reopening. *J. Appl. Physiol.* 79, 1717–1728. doi: 10.1152/jappl.1995.79.5.1717

Petrucci, N., and De Feo, C. (2013). Lung protective ventilation strategy for the acute respiratory distress syndrome. *Cochrane Database Syst. Rev.* 2013:CD003844.

Pham, T., Serpa Neto, A., Pelosi, P., Laffey, J. G., De Haro, C., Lorente, J. A., et al. (2019). Outcomes of patients presenting with mild acute respiratory distress syndrome: insights from the LUNG SAFE study. *Anesthesiology* 130, 263–283. doi: 10.1097/ALN.0000000000002508

Phua, J., Badia, J. R., Adhikari, N. K., Friedrich, J. O., Fowler, R. A., Singh, J. M., et al. (2009). Has mortality from acute respiratory distress syndrome decreased over time: a systematic review. *Am. J. Respir. Crit. Care Med.* 179, 220–227. doi: 10.1164/rccm.200805-722OC

Protti, A., Andreis, D. T., Iapichino, G. E., Monti, M., Comini, B., Milesi, M., et al. (2013a). High positive end-expiratory pressure: only a dam against oedema formation? *Crit. Care* 17:R131. doi: 10.1186/cc12810

Protti, A., Andreis, D. T., Monti, M., Santini, A., Sparacino, C. C., Langer, T., et al. (2013b). Lung stress and strain during mechanical ventilation: any difference between statics and dynamics? *Crit. Care Med.* 41, 1046–1055. doi: 10.1097/CCM.0b013e31827417a6

Protti, A., Votta, E., and Gattinoni, L. (2014). Which is the most important strain in the pathogenesis of ventilator-induced lung injury: dynamic or static? *Curr. Opin. Crit. Care* 20, 33–38. doi: 10.1097/MCC.0000000000000047

Putensen, C., Theuerkauf, N., Zinserling, J., Wrigge, H., and Pelosi, P. (2009). Meta-analysis: ventilation strategies and outcomes of the acute respiratory distress syndrome and acute lung injury. *Ann. Intern. Med.* 151, 566–576.

Rahaman, U. (2017). Mathematics of ventilator-induced lung injury. *Indian J. Crit. Care Med.* 21, 521–524.

Raymondos, K., Dirks, T., Quintel, M., Molitoris, U., Ahrens, J., Dieck, T., et al. (2017). Outcome of acute respiratory distress syndrome in university and non-university hospitals in Germany. *Crit. Care* 21:122. doi: 10.1186/s13054-017-1687-0

Retamal, J., Bergamini, B. C., Carvalho, A. R., Bozza, F. A., Borzone, G., Borges, J. B., et al. (2014). Non-lobar atelectasis generates inflammation and structural alveolar injury in the surrounding healthy tissue during mechanical ventilation. *Critical Care* 18:505. doi: 10.1186/s13054-014-0505-1

Rezoagli, E., Fumagalli, R., and Bellani, G. (2017). Definition and epidemiology of acute respiratory distress syndrome. *Ann Transl Med.* 5:282. doi: 10.21037/atm.2017.06.62

Roy, S., Habashi, N., Sadowitz, B., Andrews, P., Ge, L., Wang, G., et al. (2013). Early airway pressure release ventilation prevents Ards-a novel preventive approach to lung injury. *Shock* 39, 28–38. doi: 10.1097/SHK.0b013e31827b47bb

Roy, S., Sadowitz, B., Andrews, P., Gatto, L. A., Marx, W., Ge, L., et al. (2012). Early stabilizing alveolar ventilation prevents acute respiratory distress syndrome: a novel timing-based ventilatory intervention to avert lung injury. *J. Trauma Acute Care Surg.* 73, 391–400. doi: 10.1097/ta.0b013e31825c7a82

Roy, S. K., Emr, B., Sadowitz, B., Gatto, L. A., Ghosh, A., Satalin, J. M., et al. (2013). Preemptive application of airway pressure release ventilation prevents development of acute respiratory distress syndrome in a rat traumatic hemorrhagic shock model. *Shock* 40, 210–216. doi: 10.1097/SHK.0b013e31829efb06

Ruhl, N., Lopez-Rodriguez, E., Albert, K., Smith, B. J., Weaver, T. E., Ochs, M., et al. (2019). Surfactant protein B deficiency induced high surface tension: relationship between alveolar micromechanics, alveolar fluid properties and alveolar epithelial cell injury. *Int. J. Mol. Sci.* 20:4243. doi: 10.3390/ijms20174243

Saddy, F., Moraes, L., Santos, C. L., Oliveira, G. P., Cruz, F. F., Morales, M. M., et al. (2013). Biphasic positive airway pressure minimizes biological impact on lung tissue in mild acute lung injury independent of etiology. *Crit. Care* 17:R228. doi: 10.1186/cc13051

Sahetya, S. K., and Brower, R. G. (2017). Lung recruitment and titrated PEEP in moderate to severe ARDS: is the door closing on the open lung? *JAMA* 318, 1327–1329.

Sahetya, S. K., Mancebo, J., and Brower, R. G. (2017). Fifty years of research in ARDS. Vt selection in acute respiratory distress syndrome. *Am. J. Respir. Crit. Care Med.* 196, 1519–1525. doi: 10.1164/rccm.201708-1629CI

Satalin, J., Habashi, N. M., and Nieman, G. F. (2018). Never give the lung the opportunity to collapse. *Trends Anaesth. Crit. Care* 22, 10–16. doi: 10.1016/j.tacc.2018.05.007

Schiller, H. J., McCann, U. G., Carney, D. E., Gatto, L. A., Steinberg, J. M., and Nieman, G. F. (2001). Altered alveolar mechanics in the acutely injured lung. *Crit. Care Med.* 29, 1049–1055. doi: 10.1097/00003246-200105000-00036

Seah, A. S., Grant, K. A., Aliyeva, M., Allen, G. B., and Bates, J. H. T. (2011). Quantifying the roles of tidal volume and PEEP in the pathogenesis of ventilator-induced lung injury. *Ann. Biomed. Eng.* 39, 1505–1516. doi: 10.1007/s10439-010-0237-6

Shen, Y., Cai, G., Gong, S., Dong, L., Yan, J., and Cai, W. (2019). Interaction between low tidal volume ventilation strategy and severity of acute respiratory distress syndrome: a retrospective cohort study. *Critical Care* 23:254. doi: 10.1186/s13054-019-2530-6

Silva, P. L., Cruz, F. F., Samary, C. D. S., Moraes, L., de Magalhaes, R. F., Fernandes, M. V. S., et al. (2018). Biological response to time-controlled adaptive ventilation depends on acute respiratory distress syndrome etiology. *Critical Care Med.* 46, e609–e617. doi: 10.1097/CCM.0000000000003078

Slutsky, A. S., and Ranieri, V. M. (2013). Ventilator-induced lung injury. *N. Engl. J. Med.* 369, 2126–2136.

Smith, B. J., Lundblad, L. K., Kollisch-Singule, M., Satalin, J., Nieman, G., Habashi, N., et al. (2015). Predicting the response of the injured lung to the mechanical breath profile. *J. Appl. Physiol.* 118, 932–940. doi: 10.1152/japplphysiol.00902.2014

Solomon, I. C., Edelman, N. H., and Neubauer, J. A. (2000). Pre-Botzinger complex functions as a central hypoxia chemosensor for respiration in vivo. *J. Neurophysiol.* 83, 2854–2868. doi: 10.1152/jn.2000.83.5.2854

Stewart, T. E., Meade, M. O., Cook, D. J., Granton, J. T., Hodder, R. V., Lapinsky, S. E., et al. (1998). Evaluation of a ventilation strategy to prevent barotrauma in patients at high risk for acute respiratory distress syndrome. Pressure- and volume-limited ventilation strategy group. *N. Engl. J. Med.* 338, 355–361. doi: 10.1056/nejm199802053380603

Suki, B., Barabasi, A. L., Hantos, Z., Petak, F., and Stanley, H. E. (1994). Avalanches and power-law behaviour in lung inflation. *Nature* 368, 615–618. doi: 10.1038/368615a0

Suki, B., and Bates, J. H. (2011). Emergent behavior in lung structure and function. *J. Appl. Physiol.* 110, 1109–1110. doi: 10.1152/japplphysiol.00179.2011

Taeusch, H. W., Bernardino de la Serna, J., Perez-Gil, J., Alonso, C., and Zasadzinski, J. A. (2005). Inactivation of pulmonary surfactant due to serum-inhibited adsorption and reversal by hydrophilic polymers: experimental. *Biophys. J.* 89, 1769–1779. doi: 10.1529/biophysj.105.062620

Takahashi, A., Bartolak-Suki, E., Majumdar, A., and Suki, B. (2015). Changes in respiratory elastance after deep inspirations reflect surface film functionality in mice with acute lung injury. *J. Appl. Physiol.* 119, 258–265. doi: 10.1152/japplphysiol.00476.2014

Talab, H. F., Zabani, I. A., Abdelrahman, H. S., Bukhari, W. L., Mamoun, I., Ashour, M. A., et al. (2009). Intraoperative ventilatory strategies for prevention of pulmonary atelectasis in obese patients undergoing laparoscopic bariatric surgery. *Anesth. Analg.* 109, 1511–1516. doi: 10.1213/ANE.0b013e3181ba7945

Thompson, B. T., Chambers, R. C., and Liu, K. D. (2017). Acute respiratory distress syndrome. *N. Engl. J. Med.* 377, 1904–1905.

Tojo, K., Yoshida, T., Yazawa, T., and Goto, T. (2018). Driving-pressure-independent protective effects of open lung approach against experimental acute respiratory distress syndrome. *Crit. Care* 22:228. doi: 10.1186/s13054-018-2154-2

Tonetti, T., Cressoni, M., Collino, F., Maiolo, G., Rapetti, F., Quintel, M., et al. (2017). Volutrauma, atelectrauma, and mechanical power. *Crit. Care Med.* 45, e327–e328. doi: 10.1097/ccm.0000000000002193

van der Zee, P., and Gommers, D. (2019). Recruitment maneuvers and higher PEEP, the so-called open lung concept, in patients with ARDS. *Crit. Care* 23:73. doi: 10.1186/s13054-019-2365-1

Villar, J., Blanco, J., Anon, J. M., Santos-Bouza, A., Blanch, L., Ambros, A., et al. (2011). The ALIEN study: incidence and outcome of acute respiratory distress syndrome in the era of lung protective ventilation. *Intensive Care Med.* 37, 1932–1941. doi: 10.1007/s00134-011-2380-4

Villar, J., Blanco, J., and Kacmarek, R. M. (2016). Current incidence and outcome of the acute respiratory distress syndrome. *Curr. Opin. Crit. Care.* 22, 1–6. doi: 10.1097/MCC.0000000000000266

Webb, H. H., and Tierney, D. F. (1974). Experimental pulmonary edema due to intermittent positive pressure ventilation with high inflation pressures. Protection by positive end-expiratory pressure. *Am. Rev. Respir. Dis.* 110, 556–565.

Wellman, T. J., de Prost, N., Tucci, M., Winkler, T., Baron, R. M., Filipczak, P., et al. (2016). Lung metabolic activation as an early biomarker of acute respiratory distress syndrome and local gene expression heterogeneity. *Anesthesiology* 125, 992–1004. doi: 10.1097/aln.0000000000001334

Wellman, T. J., Winkler, T., Costa, E. L., Musch, G., Harris, R. S., Zheng, H., et al. (2014). Effect of local tidal lung strain on inflammation in normal and lipopolysaccharide-exposed sheep. *Crit. Care Med.* 42, e491–e500. doi: 10.1097/CCM.0000000000000346

Widdicombe, J. (2001). Airway receptors. *Respir. Physiol.* 125, 3–15.

Wirtz, H. R., and Dobbs, L. G. (1990). Calcium mobilization and exocytosis after one mechanical stretch of lung epithelial cells. *Science* 250, 1266–1269. doi: 10.1126/science.2173861

Xin, Y., Cereda, M., Hamedani, H., Pourfathi, M., Siddiqui, S., Meeder, N., et al. (2018). Unstable inflation causing injury. Insight from prone position and paired computed tomography scans. *Am. J. Respir. Crit. Care Med.* 198, 197–207. doi: 10.1164/rccm.201708-1728OC

Yoshida, T., Fujino, Y., Amato, M. B., and Kavanagh, B. P. (2017). nisms, and management. *Am. J. Respir. Crit. Care Med.* 195, 985–992. doi: 10.1164/rccm.201604-0748CP

Young, D., Lamb, S. E., Shah, S., MacKenzie, I., Tunnicliffe, W., Lall, R., et al. (2013). High-frequency oscillation for acute respiratory distress syndrome. *N. Engl. J. Med.* 368, 806–813. doi: 10.1056/NEJMoa1215716

Yu, J. (2016). Deflation-activated receptors, not classical inflation-activated receptors, mediate the Hering-Breuer deflation reflex. *J. Appl. Physiol.* 121, 1041–1046. doi: 10.1152/japplphysiol.00903.2015

Zheng, X., Jiang, Y., Jia, H., Ma, W., Han, Y., and Li, W. (2019). Effect of lung recruitment and titrated positive end-expiratory pressure (PEEP) versus low PEEP on patients with moderate-severe acute respiratory distress syndrome: a systematic review and meta-analysis of randomized controlled trials. *Ther. Adv. Respir. Dis.* 13:1753466619858228. doi: 10.1177/1753466619858228

Zhou, Y., Jin, X., Lv, Y., Wang, P., Yang, Y., Liang, G., et al. (2017). Early application of airway pressure release ventilation may reduce the duration of mechanical ventilation in acute respiratory distress syndrome. *Intensive Care Med.* 43, 1648–1659. doi: 10.1007/s00134-017-4912-z

13

Surfactant-Mediated Airway and Acinar Interactions in a Multi-Scale Model of a Healthy Lung

*Haoran Ma [1], Hideki Fujioka [2], David Halpern [3] and Donald P. Gaver III [1]**

[1] Department of Biomedical Engineering, Tulane University, New Orleans, LA, United States, [2] Center for Computational Science, Tulane University, New Orleans, LA, United States, [3] Department of Mathematics, University of Alabama, Tuscaloosa, AL, United States

We present a computational multi-scale model of an adult human lung that combines dynamic surfactant physicochemical interactions and parenchymal tethering between ~16 generations of airways and subtended acini. This model simulates the healthy lung by modeling nonlinear stress distributions from airway/alveolar interdependency. In concert with multi-component surfactant transport processes, this serves to stabilize highly compliant interacting structures. This computational model, with ~10 k degrees of freedom, demonstrates physiological processes in the normal lung such as multi-layer surfactant transport and pressure–volume hysteresis behavior. Furthermore, this model predicts non-equilibrium stress distributions due to compliance mismatches between airway and alveolar structures. This computational model provides a baseline for the exploration of multi-scale interactions of pathological conditions that can further our understanding of disease processes and guide the development of protective ventilation strategies for the treatment of acute respiratory distress syndrome (ARDS).

Keywords: biofluid mechanics, surfactant, multi-scale modeling, fluid–structure interactions, high-performance computing, acute respiratory distress syndrome

***Correspondence:**
Donald P. Gaver III
dpg@tulane.edu

INTRODUCTION

The lung is an extraordinary example of a physiological organ whose stability and function depends critically upon multiscale geometric interactions and processes that interlink tissue and biofluid mechanics. Airflow during inspiration and expiration changes the lung volume, causing the geometric change of highly compliant pulmonary tissues. During this volume change, tissue-level interactions like parenchymal tethering and molecular level interactions like surfactant re-distribution take place simultaneously in order to stabilize the lung. The lung's large surface area to volume ratio suggests the great importance of surfactant-mediated surface tension to lung stability. Meanwhile, the mechanical interdependency of lung units provides parenchymal tethering support for compliant airways that is instrumental to stabilizing the lung by maintaining adequate airflow to foam-like acinar structures that, in turn, support compliant airways. The large liquid-covered surface of the pulmonary tissue requires surfactant transport to dynamically modulate the surface tension during volume cycling in order to prevent fluid–structure instabilities, as it reduces the work of breathing (West, 1977, 2012; Notter, 2000). In this paper, we describe the development of a multi-scale model of a healthy lung from which future studies of pathophysiological systems can be explored.

The computational investigations of lung mechanics have been conducted on different scales. For example, at the organ level, our model is based upon an algorithm developed by Tawhai et al. who presented a computational method for generating the conducting airway network (Tawhai et al., 2000). At the tissue level, Lambert et al. (1982) and Fujioka et al. (2013) have developed computational models to describe the non-linear properties of the acinus and conductive airways, respectively. Micro-mechanical models of parenchyma support are based upon the recent work by Ryans et al. (2019), that is based on the foundational work of Wilson (1972), Lai-Fook et al. (1977, 1978), and Anafi and Wilson (2001). Surfactant transport properties are based on multilayer transport processes described by Krueger and Gaver (2000), which models surfactant behavior originally described by Clements (1957), Horn and Davis (1975), Smith and Stamenovic (1986), and Schurch (1995).

While these and many other studies have provided useful information and analysis about pulmonary mechanics on separate scales, the interactions between all of these interlinking processes have not been modeled directly. Ryans et al. demonstrated a reduced-dimension modeling approach for investigating the recruitment/de-recruitment of the airways without full fluid–structure interactions or surfactant transport processes (Ryans et al., 2016). Wall et al. (2010) developed a 3-D lung model with CT-based geometries up to a maximum of approximately seven generations, including not only airway wall deformability but also the influence of surrounding lung tissue. Filoche et al. (2015) presented a mathematical model of surfactant replacement therapy in a 3-D lung structure to investigate whether the instilled surfactant mixture actually reaches the adult alveoli/acinus in therapeutic amounts. Interlinking the multiscale processes is likely to introduce forcing and response characteristics that are not investigated in isolated models of isolated scales. For example, the multilayer surfactant behavior has heretofore been modeled in an oscillating bubble system with a pre-defined bubble radius. In contrast, in the pulmonary system the radius of airways and acini are driven by an oscillating pleural pressure on the surface of the lung. This, in turn, induces a heterogeneous distribution of mechanical stresses within the lung that dynamically modifies the lung sub-structure. In this process, the geometry of the airways and alveoli are modified, which induces surfactant transport that modulates the surface tension of the lining fluid on the internal structures of the airways and alveoli and, once again, modulates the tethering pressure and geometry of the system (Perun and Gaver, 1995). These feedback processes, when fully modeled, may elucidate pulmonary behavior that cannot understood from the reductionist approach and may exhibit emergent behavior (Suki and Bates, 1985).

In this study, our goal is to build a computational model of an adult human lung that combines dynamic multi-scale interactions between ~16 generations of airways and subtended acini generated by a space filling algorithm, including airflow, multilayer surfactant transport and airway/alveolar interdependency. We explore this system under an oscillating pleural pressure that is applied to simulate the breathing of a healthy lung. Our goal is to develop this model as a useful tool to understand the multi-scale lung mechanics and a critical baseline for the future study of the pathological conditions.

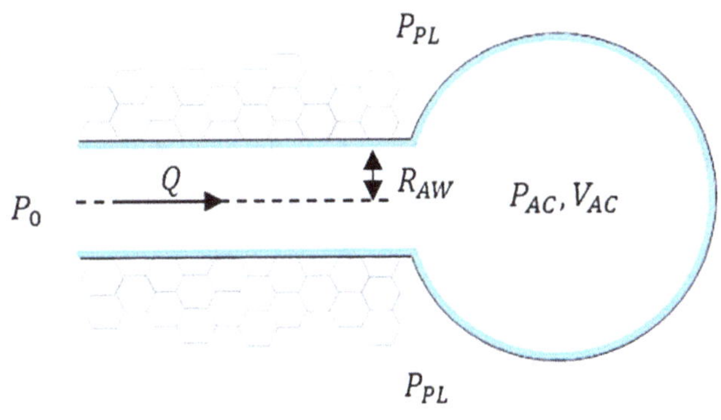

FIGURE 1 | Schematic of a "simple" lung unit with one terminal airway attached to an acinus.

MATERIALS AND METHODS

Conceptual Formulation

Framework

We have developed a rational engineering design approach for elucidating the surfactant physicochemical interactions and the mechanical interdependency within a healthy lung. It is assumed that under healthy conditions, the pleural pressure (P_{PL}) is always negative and varies with time during the normal breathing cycle. The framework of this simulation approach is based upon three components:

I. Tissue Components represent the series and parallel segments of airways and acini. The 3-D structure of airways and acini is determined using an anatomically based space-filling algorithm (Tawhai et al., 2000) in order to introduce inter-connections between airways and acini via parenchymal tethering, which is heterogeneously distributed.
II. Air Components represent the volume of the air spaces, with temporal changes based upon the flow rate within each segment. Segmental flow rates are determined by regional pressure differences and the status of each of the compliant airways and acini as determined from the Tissue Component.
III. Liquid Components represent the lining fluid and surfactant in the airways and acini, which dynamically modulate the surface tension. This, in turn, influences the Tissue Component stresses and thus affects flow rate.

Interactions Among Components

To illustrate the concept of interactions among the three components, consider the presence of a terminal airway surrounded by parenchyma and connected to an acinus at one end as seen in **Figure 1**, where P_{PL} is the pleural pressure, P_{AC} is internal acinar pressure, R_{AW} is the radius of airway, Q is the airflow toward the acinus. The pressure at the open end of the airway is considered a constant P_0 to simplify this situation.

I. Tissue Components

These are defined by airways and acini, shown in simplified form in **Figure 1**. The components are defined by

a. Airways: The dynamic radius of the airway is defined by the tube law (Lambert et al., 1982) as a function of the airway transmural pressure ($P_{TM,AW}$), described conceptually as:

$$P_{TM,AW} = P_{int,AW} - P_{ext,AW}, \tag{1}$$

where $P_{int,AW}$ represents the internal pressure from the internal air pressure and the Laplace pressure drop from surface tension, and thus is modulated by Air and Liquid Components. $P_{ext,AW}$ represents the external stresses from the time-dependent pleural pressure (P_{PL}) and is modulated by the parenchymal tethering using a shear modulus (G_{eff}) representation of the acinar support as described in Ryans et al. (2019).

b. Acinus: Similarly, from Fujioka et al. (2013), the volume of acinus is a function of acinar transmural pressure

$$P_{TM,AC} = P_{int,AC} - P_{ext,AC}, \tag{2}$$

where $P_{int,AC}$ represents the internal pressure from the acinus air pressure and the Laplace pressure drop from surface tension within alveoli that create the acinus, and $P_{ext,AC} = P_{PL}$.

In addition to structural coupling that exists through $P_{int,AW}$ and tethering forces between the acini and the exterior of airways, internal coupling exists through internal pressures because $P_{int,AC}$ is a function of the acinus volume. This sets P_{AC} as the end-condition of the Air Component system, which is necessary for determining the flow rates in the system, as described below.

II. Air Components

These are driven by airflow to and from airways and the subtending downstream acinus in the following manner:

a. Airflow (Q): Determined by the pressure difference at the two ends of the airway (P_{AW}), and the conductance (C) of the airway, $Q = CP_{AW}$.
b. Air Conductance (C): We simplify conductance as a function of the pressure-dependent airway radius, viscosity and length, following a Poiseuille relationship.
c. Conservation of volume dictates that the flow determines the change of volume of the downstream acinus (V_{AC}).

As can be seen from the above descriptions, the Air Components create an internal coupling to the Tissue components through $P_{int,AW}$ and $P_{int,AC}$.

III. Liquid Components

These determine the distribution of fluid in the airways and alveoli. Two fundamental aspects are imposed:

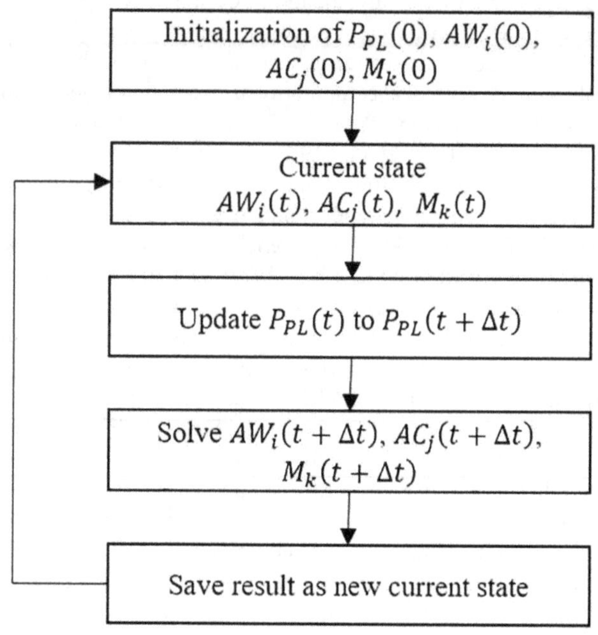

FIGURE 2 | Schematic flow chart of the of system evolution for the simulation model.

a. Conservation of mass: The volume of liquid is conserved within each airway and acinus. So, as an airway or acinus changes shape, the liquid film thickness changes accordingly.
b. Surfactant physicochemical interactions: Conservation of mass of surfactant is enforced. As the airway and alveolar surface areas change, this triggers multilayer surfactant transport (Krueger and Gaver, 2000). Through a surface tension equation of state, a dynamic surface tension exists and leads to a realistic full-lung pressure–volume loop.

As can be seen from these interactions, the liquid components directly influence $P_{int,AW}$ and $P_{int,AC}$ in Tissue Components.

System Evolution

The key to the modeling approach is the evolution of the system as each component interacts with each other. To evolve the system, the time-dependent pleural pressure P_{PL} (t) is prescribed and the rest of the system is updated with an adaptive time increment t from the current state. The new state after the time increment is solved by the method described in the Modeling Implementation section and the breathing cycle is tracked.

Modeling Implementation

Modeling Overview

To investigate surfactant-surface tension interactions and the mechanical interdependency within a healthy lung, the algorithm shown in **Figure 2** was used to simulate the whole lung respiration. Initially the time-dependent pleural pressure P_{PL} (t) is prescribed at the beginning of each time step. This provides the driving pressure for ventilation, as exists for normal respiration. We define the fundamental solution vectors for the airways, acini

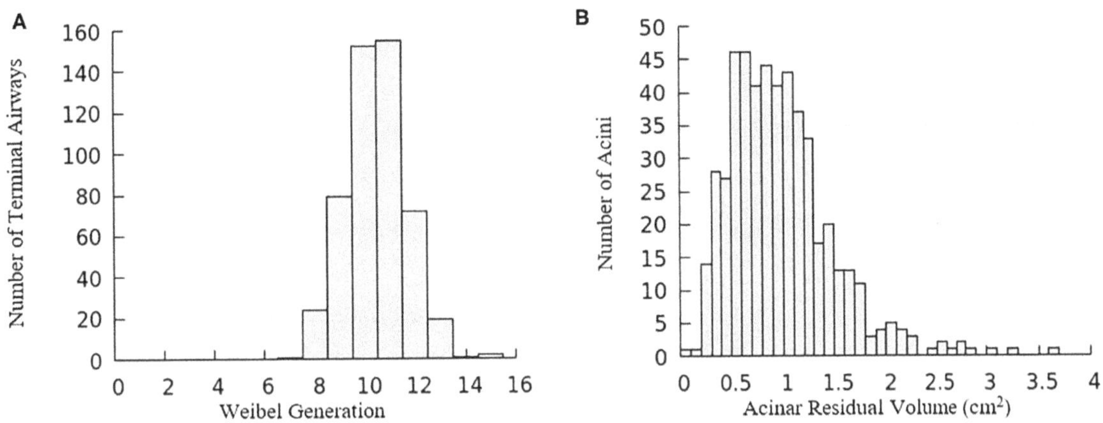

FIGURE 3 | Distribution relationships for the computational model of a half-lung. **(A)** The Weibel generation of the terminal airways connecting to acinar regions, **(B)** the residual volume of the acini connecting to the terminal airways.

and surfactant as $AW_i(t) = [P(t), R(t)]_i$, $AC_j(t) = [P(t), V(t)]_j$, and $M_k(t) = [M_p(t), M_s(t), M_b(t)]_k$, respectively, where P is airway/acinus pressure, R is airway radius, V is volume of acinus, M is a vector consists of the surfactant masses in each region of the multilayer structure, including M_p for the primary layer, M_s for the secondary layer, M_b for the bulk liquid. Each airway or acinus is represented by two solution vectors, one of which is $AC_i(t)$ or $AW_j(t)$ containing tissue component properties, and the other is $M_k(t)$ containing liquid component properties. $AC_i(t)$, $AW_j(t)$ and $M_k(t)$ are solved simultaneously based on the mechanical relationship described in Network Flow Dynamics using a differential-algebraic equation systems solver.

Tissue Components

I. Airway Morphology

The domain of one half of the lung is generated using an anatomically based space-filling algorithm from Tawhai et al. (2000). It consists of a network of airways that has up to an equivalent Horsfield 15th generation (bottom-up with terminal airway defined as generation 1) that terminate into acinar regions with mechanical properties described in the "Acinus Component" section (Fujioka et al., 2013). The equivalent Weibel generation (top-down from trachea as generation 0) of terminal airways and the residual volume of their attached acini are shown in **Figure 3**. We note that structural differences exist among airways and acini, which will appear as important contributors to the heterogeneity in surface tension and parenchymal tethering described in the "Results and Discussion" section.

Airways and acini are positioned in a 3-D space in order to build inter-connections between the airways and acini (Tawhai et al., 2000). The morphology of the pulmonary airways was based on Lambert et al. by providing the airway maximum radius ($R_{AW,max}$) and normalized cross-sectional area α at $P_{TM,AW} = 0$, i.e., $\alpha_0 = \frac{A_0}{A_{max}}$ (Lambert et al., 1982).

II. Compliant Airway Components

We used the airway morphological data to construct a tube law that describes the radius of a compliant airway as a function of the airway transmural pressure. For a healthy lung, we assume

TABLE 1 | Generation-based constants used for the tube law used in Equation (3).

Generation (*n*)	*A*	*b*
1	0.0354	0.8486
2	0.0841	0.3504
3	0.0947	0.1004
4	0.0969	−0.0889
5	0.1115	−0.2347
6–15	0.1219	−0.3506

that the acinus is the most compliant region of the system, so that the parenchyma tethers the embedded airway open during inspiration, as described in the "Parenchymal Tethering" section, below. To do so, we defined a tube-law that follows a sigmoidal form that matches the airway-based morphological parameters. The general form of the tube-law is defined as

$$\frac{R_{AW}}{R_{AW,max}} = \sqrt{0.5 \times \left[1 + \mathrm{erf}\left(aP_{TM,AW} + b\right)\right]}, \qquad (3)$$

where $P_{TM,AW}$ is the transmural pressure defined in Equation (1), $R_{AW,max}$ is the maximum radius of this airway. The parameters a and b are generation-based constants shown in **Table 1**. The tube law behavior through the Weibel 6th generation as well as experimental data for the first 3 generations are shown in **Figure 4** (Lambert et al., 1982).

The internal airway pressure $P_{int,AW}$ is subject to the airway pressure determined by the average of the upstream and downstream pressure as well as the Laplace pressure drop from the liquid lining of the airway. The Laplace pressure drop and airway pressure can be expressed respectively as

$$P_{int,AW} = P_{AW} - \frac{\gamma}{R_{in,AW}}, \text{ and} \qquad (4)$$

$$P_{AW} = \frac{P_{DN} + P_{UP}}{2}, \qquad (5)$$

where P_{AW} is the airway pressure, γ is the surface tension of the liquid lining, $R_{in,AW}$ is the radius from the center line

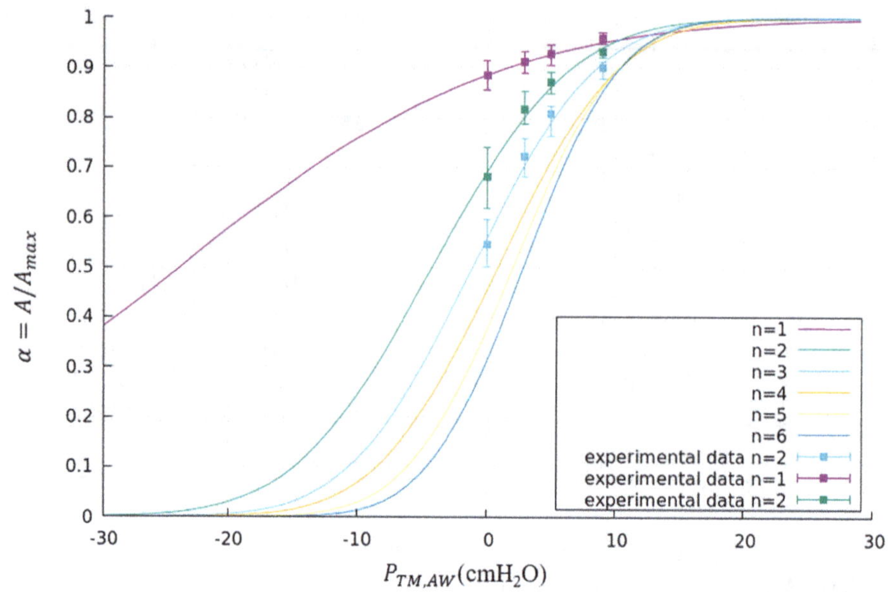

FIGURE 4 | Tube law through the Weibel 6th generation. Airways smaller than the 6th generation are assumed to have the same tube law as the 6th generation. Experimental data is shown for the first 3 generations.

of the airway to the interior surface of the liquid lining, P_{DN} is the downstream pressure, P_{UP} is the upstream pressure. For the airway shape calculation, we assumed the pressure is uniform within an airway and determined the average pressure by Equation (5).

The external airway pressure $P_{ext,AW}$ is subject to the pleural pressure and the parenchymal tethering from surrounding acini. We modeled tidal breathing by forcing the pleural pressure to be prescribed by a sinusoidally varying waveform with a 1:2 inspiration–expiration ratio that varies between -5 cmH_20 and -8.2 cmH_20 with a period of 5 s (Swan et al., 2012). The parenchymal tethering pressure is determined based on the work from Ryans et al. detailed in Parenchymal Tethering (Ryans et al., 2019). The peri airway pressure can be expressed as

$$P_{ext,AW} = P_{PL} + 2G_{eff}\left(\frac{\Delta R}{R}\right), \quad (6)$$

where P_{PL} is the pleural pressure, G_{eff} is the effective parenchyma shear modulus, $\frac{\Delta R}{R}$ is the fractional radius change from the "hole" radius of parenchyma as described below in Equation (12). From Equations (4) to (6), Equation (1) can be rewritten as

$$P_{TM,AW}(t) = P_{AW} - 2G_{eff}\left(\frac{\Delta R}{R}\right) - P_{PL}(t) - \frac{\gamma}{R_{in,AW(t)}}, \quad (7)$$

where the transmural pressure varies with time due to the change in pleural pressure and radius change of compliant airways.

To determine the length of airways, it is assumed that the length change of airways is proportional to the size change of their surrounding parenchyma. The parenchyma model is described in Parenchymal Tethering.

III. Acinus Component

The morphological information of the representative acinar regions connected to the terminal airways of the lung is based on the octahedral models depicted in Fujioka et al. (2013). We represent the behavior of a block of alveoli (~1,200 alveoli representing ~1.7 × 10^{-3} cc of tissue) by a pressure-volume relationship derived from simulation results of this block. We follow the form suggested by Venegas et al. (1985) that successfully models whole-lung mechanics. As such, the pressure-volume relationship of this model is governed by

$$\frac{V_{AC}}{V_{RV}} = a + \frac{b}{1+\exp\left[-(P_{TM,AC}-c)/d\right]}, \quad (8)$$

where V_{AC} is the acinar volume, V_{RV} is the acinar volume at residual volume (RV), $P_{TM,AC}$ is the acinar transmural pressure defined in Equation (2), a–d are constants that describe the mechanical characteristics of the parenchyma. Since we add the dynamic surface tension to the Laplace pressure drop in our form of $P_{TM,AC}$ in Equation (11), this structural component is based upon parameters describing the tissue behavior only (zero surface tension model) with a = 1.03, b = 4.95, c = 5.04, d = 1.02.

The external and internal acinar pressure are

$$P_{ext,AC} = P_{PL}, \text{ and} \quad (9)$$

$$P_{int,AC} = P_{AC} - \frac{2\gamma}{R_{\overline{ALV}}}, \quad (10)$$

where P_{AC} is the acinar pressure, P_{PL} is pleural pressure, γ is the surface tension of the liquid lining and $R_{\overline{ALV}}$ represents the mean radius of the interior surface of the alveolar lining fluid inside the acinus. At this stage, alveoli are assumed to be spherical. From Equations (9) and **(10)**, Equation (2) can be rewritten as

$$P_{TM,AC} = P_{AC} - \frac{2\gamma}{R_{\overline{ALV}}} - P_{PL}, \quad (11)$$

IV. Parenchymal Tethering

We utilized the parenchyma model from Ryans et al. (2019) to describe the tethering pressure. In that model, a cylindrical "hole" is surrounded by an annular region of parenchyma. An airway is laminated inside this parenchymal hole. Without the laminated airway, the equilibrium hole radius is defined as R_H so that when the strain in the annular parenchyma is uniform, this yields $P_{ext,AW} = P_{PL}$. For non-uniform strain, following Lai-Fook et al. (1978), we define the effective parenchyma shear modulus G_{eff} by

$$\frac{\Delta R}{R} = \frac{R_{AW}-R_H}{R_H} = \frac{P_{ext,AW}-P_{PL}}{2G_{eff}}, \quad (12)$$

where R_{AW} is the airway radius, $P_{ext,AW}$ is the peri-airway pressure, P_{PL} is the pleural pressure. From analyses performed by Ryans et al. (2019), we assume the equilibrium hole radius is proportional to the cubic root of the weighted average of acinus volume within a distance of $5R_{AW,0}$ from the airway axis, where $R_{AW,0}$ is R_{AW} at zero transmural pressure. This behavior is consistent with the finite-element model by Ma et al. (2013). We also assumed the equilibrium hole radius $R_{H,FRC}$ is equal to $R_{AW,FRC}$ when the surrounding acinus volume is at the Functional Residual Capacity, V_{FRC}. Since the exact value of FRC is unknown before the simulation, $R_{H,FRC}$ and $R_{AW,FRC}$ are estimated from the isolated airway and acini model. We note that the equilibrium hole radius setpoint at FRC is an assumption that should be experimentally validated and is related to positive strain-deviation of terminal airways, as described in section Parenchymal Tethering and Strain Deviation.

From computational simulations as described from Ryans et al., the effective parenchyma shear modulus G_{eff} is empirically determined as a function of mean transpulmonary pressure (Ryans et al., 2019). The transpulmonary pressure and effective parenchyma shear modulus can be expressed as

$$\overline{P_{TP}} = \overline{P_{ALV}} - P_{PL}, \ and \quad (13)$$

$$G_{eff} = Ae^{b\overline{P_{TP}}^3}, \quad (14)$$

where $\overline{P_{TP}}$ is average transpulmonary pressure, $\overline{P_{ALV}}$ is the weighted average of surrounding acinar pressures within a distance of $5R_{AW,0}$ from the airway axis, $A = 4.75$ cmH$_2$O, $B = 5.17 \times 10^{-4}$ cmH$_2$O^{-3}.

Air Component

I. Air Conductance

We assume that all air flows are laminar and fully developed. Airflow throughout the lung model is described using a Poiseuille relationship at each airway. From Poiseuille's law, the conductance of a compliant airway is prescribed as a function of its radius and length:

$$C_{AW} = \frac{\pi R_{in,AW}{}^4}{8\mu L}, \quad (15)$$

where C_{AW} is the conductance of airway, $R_{in,AW}$ is the radius from the center line of the airway to the interior surface of the liquid lining, μ is the viscosity of air, L is the length of the airway. We acknowledge that this is inaccurate when Reynolds numbers are high, as in the central airways (trachea and mainstem bronchi) and first generations of the model of the lung. We also neglect the loss of pressure at bifurcations.

II. Network Flow Dynamics

In our model, the axial component of the pressure gradient inside each airway is assumed to be a constant. We also assume that all air flows through airways are fully developed and without turbulence. The flow rates at the airway level are determined by

$$Q_{AW,i} = C_{AW,i}\left(P_{UP,i} - P_{DN,i}\right), \quad (16)$$

where $Q_{AW,i}$ is the flow rate of the airway, $C_{AW,i}$ is the conductance of the airway, $P_{UP,i}$ and $P_{DN,i}$ are the upstream and downstream pressure of the airway, respectively.

At the terminal end of the system (acinus), the flow changes the acinus volume as

$$Q_{AW,i} = C_{AW,i}\left(P_{UP,i} - P_{AC,i}\right) = \frac{dV_{AC,i}}{dt}, \quad (17)$$

where $P_{AC,i}$ is the acinus pressure, $V_{AC,i}$ is the acinus volume.

We assume that there is no pressure loss at the bifurcations. Conservation of flow rate at each bifurcation is satisfied by an equation of the form

$$Q_{AW,P} + Q_{AW,D1} + Q_{AW,D2} = 0, \quad (18)$$

where P stands for the parent airway, and D stands for the daughter airways.

Equations (16)–(18) are applied to each acinus, airway and bifurcation to build the differential-algebraic equation system. We note that we neglect the loss of pressure at the airway bifurcation (Filoche et al., 2015).

Liquid Components

I. Conservation of Liquid Phase

We assume the amount of liquid is conserved within each airway/alveolus. Thus the liquid film thickness has to varies with time due to changes in radius of airway/alveolus. A parameter which characterizes this change is defined as

$$\varepsilon = \frac{R_{out}-R_{in}}{R_{out}}, \quad (19)$$

where R_{out} is the airway/alveolus radius, R_{in} is the radius from the center(line) to the liquid lining that determines the Laplace pressure drop. The change in the volume of the airways and alveolus therefore modulates the film thickness, which feeds back to the stress balance Equations (7) and (11). We note that the change of airway caliber as well as length is accounted for in the conservation of mass calculation for determining the dynamic film thickness.

II. Surfactant Physicochemical Interactions

The mechanism of surfactant transport was based on the multilayer surfactant behavior analysis done by Krueger and Gaver (2000). Soluble surfactant in the liquid lining of airways/acini exists in the bulk fluid and two surface layers: primary and secondary layers. The primary layer is in direct contact with the air-liquid interface, while the secondary layer is created by collapse of the primary layer and resides between the primary layer and the bulk fluid. Adsorption/desorption can only happen between the bulk liquid and the primary layer. Only the surfactant in the primary layer can reduce the surface tension. The surface tension of water $\gamma_0 = 72\frac{dyne}{cm}$. From Krueger and Gaver (2000), the equilibrium surface tension $\gamma_\infty = 22\frac{dyne}{cm}$ at the equilibrium surfactant concentration $\Gamma_\infty = 3\times10^{-4}\frac{mg}{cm^2}$. The minimum surface tension $\gamma_{min} = 4\frac{dyne}{cm}$ occurs at the maximum surfactant concentration $\Gamma_{max} = 3.3\times10^{-4}\frac{mg}{cm^2}$. We assumed the relationship between the primary layer surfactant concentration and surface tension is linear from $(0, \gamma_0)$ to $(\Gamma_\infty, \gamma_\infty)$ and from $(\Gamma_\infty, \gamma_\infty)$ to $(\Gamma_{max}, \gamma_{min})$ with a slope of m and m', respectively. The surface tension equation of state can be expressed as

$$\gamma = \begin{cases} m\Gamma_1 + \gamma_0, & if\ \Gamma_1 < \Gamma_\infty \\ m'(\Gamma_1 - \Gamma_{max}) + \gamma_{min} & if\ \Gamma_1 \geq \Gamma_\infty \end{cases}, \tag{20}$$

where $m = -1.7 \times 10^5\ dyne \cdot \frac{cm}{mg}$, $m' = -5.3 \times 10^5\ dyne \cdot \frac{cm}{mg}$. **Figure 5** demonstrates an example hysteresis behavior of alveolar unit as determined from Equations (21) to (25) below.

In **Figure 5**, $\Gamma_{max} = 4.2 \times 10^{-4}\ mg/cm^2$ is the maximum surfactant concentration, $\gamma_{min} = 2\ dyne/cm$ is the surface tension when $\Gamma_1 = \Gamma_{max}$, $\Gamma_\infty = 3 \times 10^{-4}\ mg/cm^2$ is the surfactant concentration at equilibrium state, $\gamma_\infty = 22\ dyne/cm$ is the surface tension when $\Gamma_1 = \Gamma_\infty$.

As described by **Figure 5**, the alveolar unit starts contracting from the maximum volume point (top right corner). During the contraction, the surface tension decreases as the monolayer surfactant concentration increases with simultaneous adsorption/desorption occurring between the surface and bulk phases. When the monolayer surfactant concentration exceeds Γ_∞, the adsorption from the bulk stops. At this time, the monolayer cannot sustain further compression without collapsing to create a multi-layer with surfactant molecules exuded from the primary to the secondary layer as the alveolar unit continues contracting. Desorption between the primary layer and bulk fluid continues as Γ_1 exceeds Γ_∞ and simultaneously the primary layer (Γ_1) collapses to transport mass to the secondary layer (Γ_2). At the bottom right corner, the primary layer concentration reaches Γ_{max}. The speed of collapse increases by an order of magnitude when $\Gamma_1 > \Gamma_{max}$. Therefore $\Gamma_1 \sim \Gamma_{max}$ as the contraction continues, highly enriching the secondary layer. At the bottom left corner, the alveolar unit starts to expand. The surface tension increases during this expansion due to the decreasing concentration of the primary layer. When the concentration of the primary layer begins to fall below Γ_∞, respreading starts from the secondary layer to the primary layer, and surfactant molecules are once again adsorbed from the bulk. This hysteresis loop is a key characteristic relating surfactant physicochemical behavior to the stabilizing properties associated with dynamic surface tension in the healthy lung (Notter, 2000).

The governing equations of the surfactant transport are

$$\begin{aligned} \frac{dM_1}{dt} &= (-j_c + j_r + j_a - j_d)\,A \\ \frac{dM_2}{dt} &= (j_c - j_r)\,A, \\ \frac{dM_b}{dt} &= (-j_a + j_d)\,A \end{aligned} \tag{21}$$

where M_1 is the surfactant mass in the primary layer, M_2 is the surfactant mass in the secondary layer, M_b is the surfactant mass in the bulk liquid, A is the surface area of the air–liquid interface, j terms represent the transport between bulk and surface layers. Terms for collapse and respreading are defined as

$$j_c = \begin{cases} C_{collapse}\frac{\Gamma_1^2}{\Gamma_1^2+\Gamma_{max}^2} max\left(\frac{\Gamma_1-\Gamma_\infty}{\Gamma_\infty}, 0\right), & if\ \Gamma_\infty < \Gamma_1 < \Gamma_{max} \\ \exp\left[1000^*\left(\frac{\Gamma_1}{\Gamma_{max}} - 1\right)\right] \cdot C_{collapse}\frac{\Gamma_1^2}{\Gamma_1^2+\Gamma_{max}^2} max\left(\frac{\Gamma_1-\Gamma_\infty}{\Gamma_\infty}, 0\right), & if\ \Gamma_1 > \Gamma_{max} \end{cases}, \ and \tag{22}$$

$$j_r = C_{respread}\frac{\Gamma_1^2}{\Gamma_1^2+\Gamma_{mls}^2} max\left(\frac{\Gamma_\infty-\Gamma_1}{\Gamma_\infty}, 0\right)\frac{\Gamma_2}{\Gamma_\infty}, \tag{23}$$

where Γ_1 is the primary layer surfactant concentration, Γ_2 is the secondary layer concentration, $C_{collapse} = 2 \times 10^{-4}\ (\frac{mg}{s\cdot cm^2})$, $C_{respread} = 5\times10^{-2}\ (\frac{mg}{s\cdot cm^2})$, $\Gamma_{mls} = 2.34\ mg/cm^2$ is the multilayer respreading concentration (corresponds to $\gamma_{mls} = 33\ dyne/cm$), $max\left(\frac{\Gamma_1-\Gamma_\infty}{\Gamma_\infty}, 0\right)/max(\frac{\Gamma_\infty-\Gamma_1}{\Gamma_\infty}, 0)$ serve as a switch to turn on the collapse/respreading when Γ_1 is above/below Γ_∞, and describes the relationship between concentration and speed of transport together with the sigmoidal function $\frac{\Gamma_1^2}{\Gamma_1^2+\Gamma_{max}^2}$ and $\frac{\Gamma_2^2}{\Gamma_2^2+\Gamma_{mls}^2}$. The collapse term increases exponentially when Γ_1 is greater than Γ_{max} based on the experimental evidence (Clements, 1957; Horn and Davis, 1975; Schurch, 1995; Krueger and Gaver, 2000). Note that we have modified the collapse and respreading terms from that originally introduced by Krueger and Gaver (2000) in order to stabilize the computations. In the present model we assume that collapse can be initiated (albeit slowly) as soon as the primary layer concentration exceeds Γ_∞, and this collapse rate increases substantially as Γ_1 increases to Γ_{max}. Likewise, respreading initiates when the primary layer concentration falls below Γ_∞, and the respreading rate increases substantially near Γ_{mls}.

Terms for adsorption and desorption are defined as

$$j_a = \begin{cases} K_a c_{bulk} (\Gamma_\infty - \Gamma_1)\left(1 - \frac{\Gamma_2}{2\Gamma_\infty}\right), \; when \; \Gamma_1 < \Gamma_\infty \\ 0, \; otherwise \end{cases}, \; and \tag{24}$$

$$j_d = K_d \Gamma_1 \left(1 - \frac{\Gamma_2}{2\Gamma_\infty}\right), \tag{25}$$

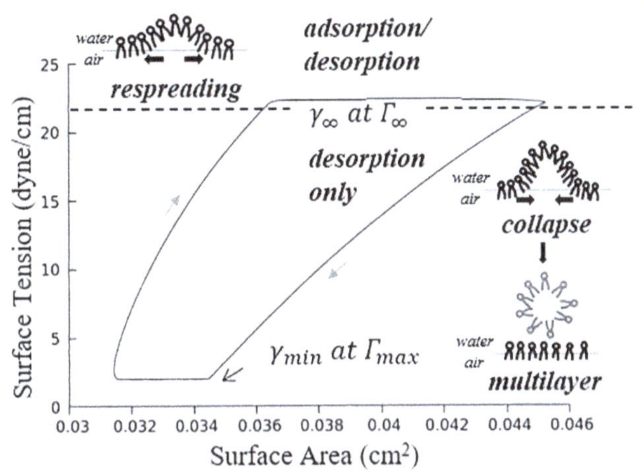

FIGURE 5 | Example hysteresis loop of an alveolus. Γ_1 is inversely proportional to the interfacial area. The primary layer begins to collapse when $\Gamma_1 \geq \Gamma_\infty$, forming a secondary layer between the bulk and primary layer. When $\Gamma_1 < \Gamma_\infty$, the secondary layer dynamically respreads, which stabilizes the surface tension.

where c_{bulk} is the bulk concentration, $K_a = 1.7(\frac{cm^3}{mg \cdot s})$, $K_d = 1.7 \times 10^{-2}(\frac{1}{s})$, $\left(1 - \frac{\Gamma_2}{2\Gamma_\infty}\right) A$ is the effective surface area.

Computational Methods

High-performance computing simulations were conducted on Tulane's Cypress supercomputer. The code was constructed in C++ and utilized MPI library. The differential-algebraic equation systems solver used in the code was SUNDIALS IDAS solver with adaptive time stepping (Hindmarsh et al., 2005). The simulation utilizes 8 Intel Xeon E5-2680 v2 CPUs and 128 GB of RAM. Total CPU time for one simulation (180 s of breathing) is ~5 h.

RESULTS AND DISCUSSION

Overview

In this study, pleural pressure forcing was assumed to be periodic with $-5 \leq P_{PL} \leq -8.2$ cmH_2O and a frequency of 12 min^{-1} to simulate tidal breathing (Swan et al., 2012). The inhalation–exhalation time ratio is assumed to be to be 1:2. As an initial condition, the dimensionless liquid film thickness ε, and the total amount of surfactant, $M_{total} = M_1 + M_2 + M_b$ were prescribed at each airway as well as each acinus when the lung is at its residual volume (RV). In this study, we assumed the minimum alveolar radius equals 100 μm, and the alveolar liquid film thickness equals 0.1 μm at residual lung volume (Bastacky et al., 1985), so $\varepsilon = 1 \times 10^{-3}$ at RV in the acinus components. For airway components, the initial ε is assumed to be 0.02 (Cassidy et al., 1985). We initially apply a uniform bulk surfactant concentration $c_{aiway} = 6\frac{mg}{ml}$ for airway components, and $c_{alveolus} = 35\ \frac{mg}{ml}$ for acinar components. During initialization, the equilibrium

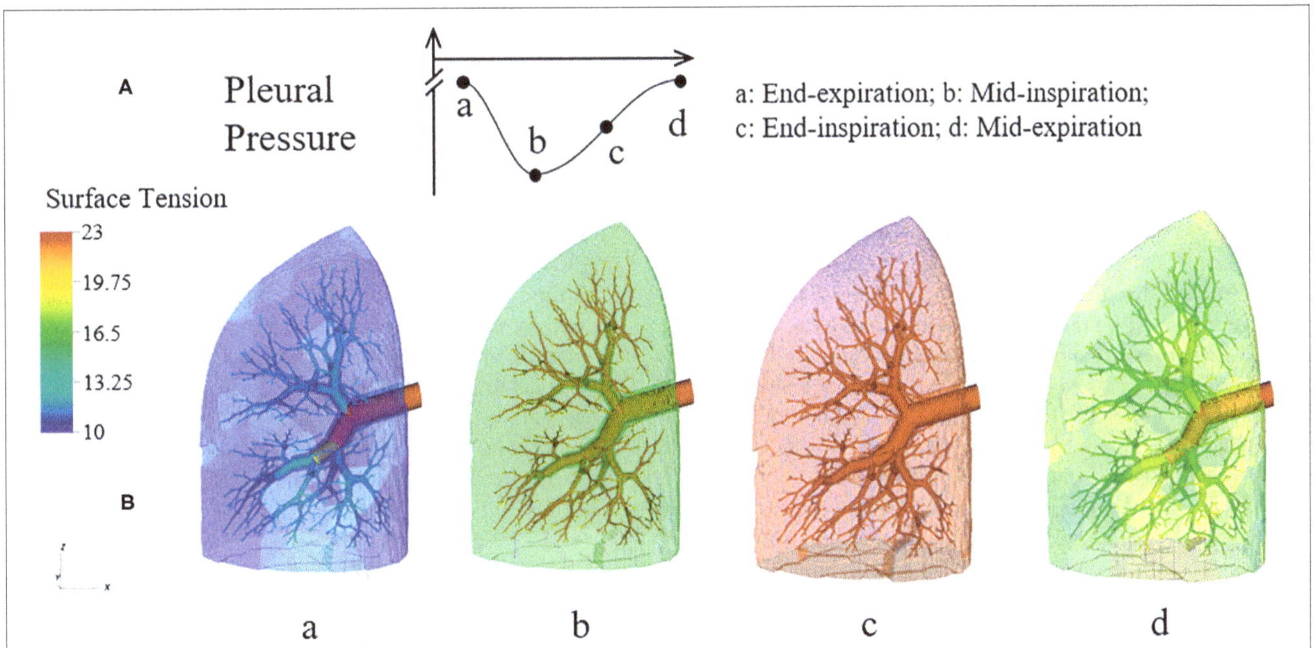

FIGURE 6 | Dynamic surface tension of the lung. **(A)** Specific time points during breathing cycle. **(B)** 3-D figure of the half-lung at four time points. The color scale in the legend denotes the surface tension. Statistical variation is documented in **Figure 8**.

surface concentrations are determined according to the defined bulk concentration and the physicochemical description above. True surfactant concentration values in the healthy lung are not known, but $c_{alveolus}$ equals the concentration of the exogenous surfactant Infasurf (ONY, Inc; Amherst, NY).

During the simulation, states of each component are recorded to track the evolution of the system. For visualization, a 3-D figure of the half-lung was generated. This figure reflects the space distribution of each airway and acinus as well as their real-time states. Our simulation was performed for several breathing cycles until stationary states were achieved.

Figure 6 demonstrates the changes of surface tension in the lung (consisting of airways and acini) at four different time points (a–d) during a breathing cycle. Starting with end-exhalation (a), the surface tension in acini and small airways is as small as 8 dynes/cm, which is far below the equilibrium surface tension (22 dynes/cm) and can be achieved only due to the dynamic transport of surfactant. This low surface tension occurs because the air-liquid interface in each component contracts, increasing the primary layer interfacial surfactant concentration, and decreasing the surface tension (as surfactant also loads the secondary layer). As the lung volume increases during inspiration (b), the surface tension increases, implying a decrease of primary layer surfactant concentration. At the end of inspiration (c), the surface tension attains close to a maximum value in both acini and airways. During expiration (d), the volume of the lung decreases and thus the inner surface area of acini and airways are decreased, reducing the surface tension.

We note that at points a and c, the lung volumes and surface tensions are not respectively the minimum and maximum due to the airway network resistance and the Laplace pressure drop explained in the Pressure–Volume Curve section. Likewise, the lung volumes as well as the surface tensions at points b and d are not identical, even though these represent identical P_{PL} values. The differentials in lung volume and surface tension are related to the phase-lag that occurs in the system, described below.

Pressure–Volume Behavior

The pressure-volume behavior described here reflects both lungs, that is twice the size of our computational domain. Our lung model has a full lung residual volume (RV) of 1.0 L. Assuming homogeneous acinar behavior, following Equation (8) the total lung capacity (TLC) is 6.0 L. The dynamic properties of the lung are determined by pressure cycling and **Figure 7** presents the pressure-volume (PV) relationship for the entire lung. Under the given pleural pressure range investigated for normal breathing, the tidal volume (TV) equals 0.82 L, with a functional residual capacity (FRC) of ~2.30 L. From these simulations of normal breathing, the maximum flow rate at the trachea is ~0.92 L/s. The average compliance of the lung during tidal breathing is ~0.25 L/cmH_2O, while the accepted normal value is 0.2 L/cmH_2O in human lungs (Harris, 2005). TV and compliance of our model is higher than the normal values because the simulated airway resistance is unrealistically low due to the assumptions of laminar, fully developed flow in "Modeling Implementation" as described in "Limitations". The total airway resistance excluding upper airways ranges from 0.6 to 0.9 cmH_2O/L/s with lung volume

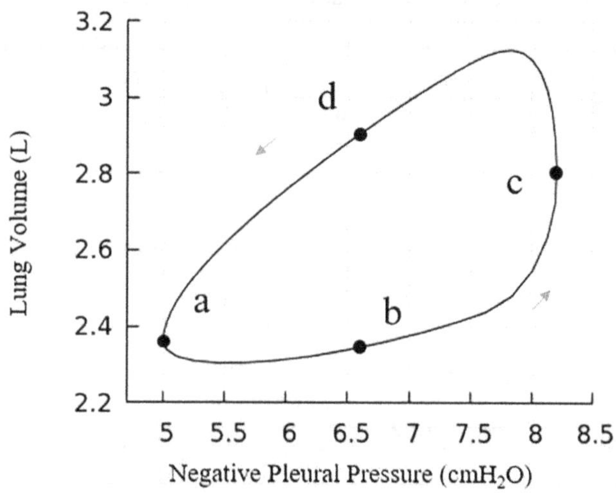

FIGURE 7 | Pressure vs. volume curve of the entire lung. The points (a), (b), (c), and (d) relate to **Figure 6**. Note, this figure demonstrates a portion of the total PV curve for volumes between end-inspiration and end-expiration for normal tidal volume breathing (~0.82 L).

oscillating between 2.30 L (38% of TLC) and 3.12 L (52% of TLC), which is less than the predicted flow resistance at low equivalent lung volumes predicted by Pedley et al. (1970).

Our model presents a typical PV hysteresis behavior, i.e., the compliance of the lung ($\Delta volume/pressure$) is different between the inspiration and expiration phase. The PV phase lag that is demonstrated in **Figure 6** is evident from points a–d in **Figure 7**.

Figure 8 further elucidates the acinar contributions to PV hysteresis behavior—here we present the behavior in terms of local forcing ($\Delta P_{AC} = P_{AC} - P_{PL}$, represented by the blue curve), and global forcing (P_{PL}, represented by the red curve). The global forcing demonstrates a rounded behavior similar to the full lung in **Figure 7**. However, the behavior of a specific acinus is best understood from the local forcing, ΔP_{AC}.

This analysis demonstrates that the hysteretic behavior is reflected by two factors:

a. The flow resistance of airways. As seen in **Figure 8A**, the hysteresis area of the $\Delta P_{AC}V$ curve is much smaller than $P_{PL}V$, which results from the network airflow resistance. The time lag between the global and local pressure changes caused by the airway network resistance can be observed in **Figure 8B**, and causes the lung volume to lag the changes in P_{PL}, as demonstrated by **Figure 6**.
b. The Laplace pressure drop. The hysteresis area of the local PV curve (ΔP_{AC}, represented by the blue curve) results from the behavior of surfactant transport as shown in **Figure 5**, as described in the next section.

Surfactant Transport

In order to understand the PV relationships in **Figure 8**, it is necessary to explore the dynamic surface tension behavior at the alveolar and airway levels (**Figure 9**). As seen in **Figure 9A**, the surface tension hysteresis behavior of acinus components

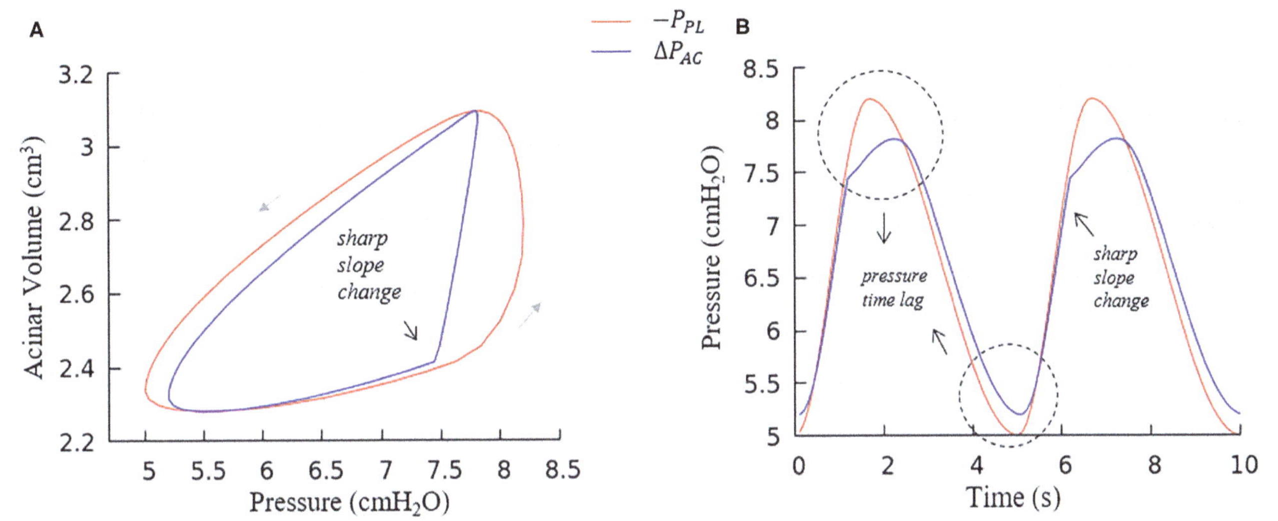

FIGURE 8 | Average acinar global forcing vs. local forcing. **(A)** PV relationship, **(B)** pressure vs. time, global ($-P_{PL}$, red), local ($\Delta P_{AC} = P_{AC} - P_{PL}$, blue). Airway resistance leads to the hysteresis area difference between global and local forcing shown in **(A)** and the pressure time lag shown in **(B)**, contributes to the global PV hysteresis behavior.

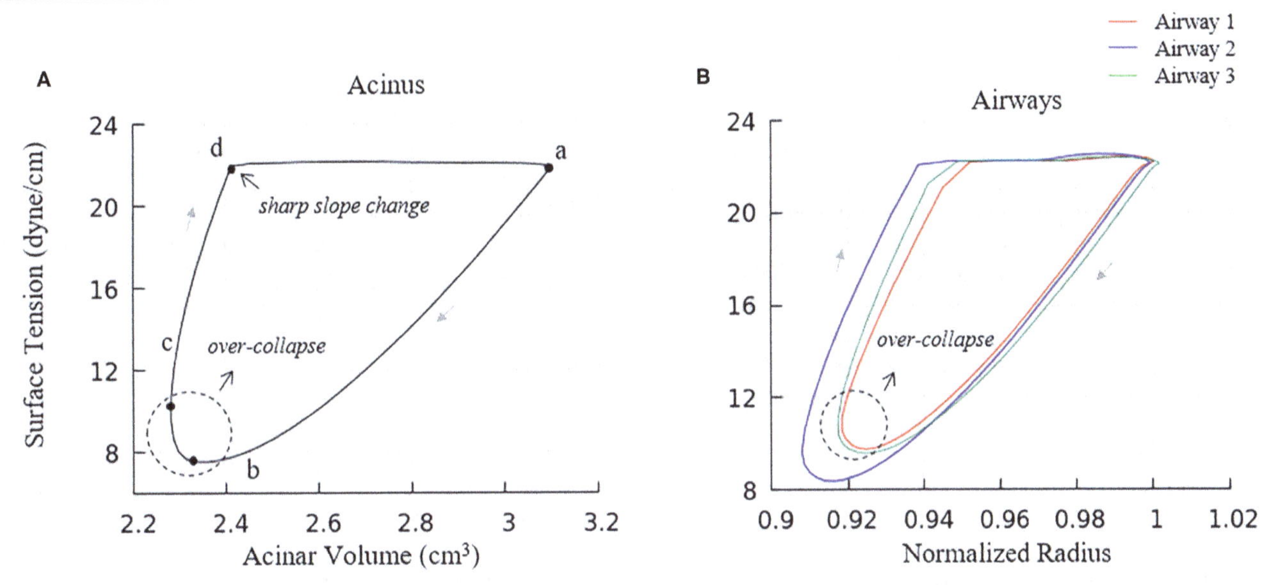

FIGURE 9 | Surface tension behavior of model elements. **(A)** Average surface-tension vs. volume of acinar units. Statistical variation of these element is provided in **Figure 10A**. **(B)** Representative surface-tension *vs.* normalized surface area of airways demonstrating variations in behavior. The acinar and airway surface tension hysteresis behavior is similar to the isolated model in **Figure 5** and contributes to the PV hysteresis behavior of the entire lung. Surface tension variation of airways corresponds to observations in **Figure 6**.

is similar to the isolated interface model (**Figure 5**) except that a minimum surface tension plateau does not exist at the lowest acinar volumes. This deviation occurs because the surfactant concentration of the acinus model does not approach Γ_{max} under the breathing conditions imposed by this simulation. In this model, "collapse" refers to the transport of surfactant from the primary to secondary layers. This transport occurs if $\Gamma_1 > \Gamma_\infty$, and occurs at a greater rate as Γ_1 increases, to a point where saturation will occur if $\Gamma_1 \geq \Gamma_\infty$. In our full-lung model, the rate of interfacial contraction is not large enough to hyper-concentrate the alveolar primary layer to a level that leads to secondary layer saturation. Nevertheless, a significant secondary layer does exist in acinus components.

We note that there is a sharp slope change in the local PV curve in **Figure 8A**. This abrupt change in compliance is due to

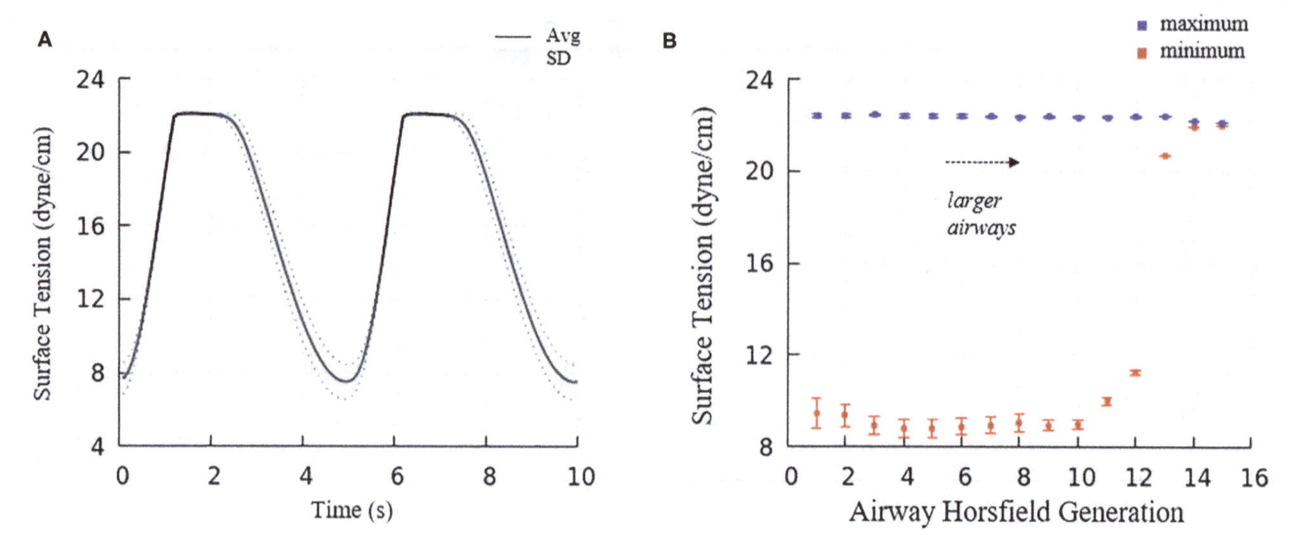

FIGURE 10 | (A) Average acinar surface tension with standard deviation. Secondary layer respreading stabilizes surface tension near γ_∞. Low surface tension demonstrates surfactant collapse behavior. **(B)** The average maximum and minimum surface tension of each airway generation together with standard deviation by Horsfield generation. The minimum surface tension decreases with more compliant (smaller) airways. The secondary layer respreading stabilizes the maximum surface tension near γ_∞.

the secondary layer respreading, which reduces surface tension and work of breathing. This sharp slope change corresponds to the slope change at point d in **Figure 9A**.

Airways (**Figure 9B**) in our model have surface tension hysteresis behaviors similar to acini. Airways exhibit hysteresis areas that varies due to geometrical as well as tethering pressure difference. This corresponds to observations in **Figure 6**.

We also note that the surface tension increases slightly prior to alveolar and airway expansion (dotted circles), which is likewise observed in the acinar PV relationship (**Figure 8A**). We attribute this behavior to surfactant over-collapse. In our model, the direction of transport between the primary and secondary layer is only determined by the value of Γ_1. During most of the phase a–b–c–d in **Figure 9A**, the primary layer concentration exceeds Γ_∞, so surfactant transport from the primary to secondary layer occurs. However, as described above, this rate of transport is not large enough to saturate the secondary layer. Nevertheless, the secondary layer is able to respread to the primary layer during the phase d-a in **Figure 9A**. In phase a– and c–d, the surface concentration is dominated by the surface area change, i.e., the surface concentration increases/decreases as the surface area decreases/increases. However, due to the sinusoidal pleural pressure, the change rate of the surface area in phase c-d decreases dramatically, while the collapse term in Equation (22) does not have any abrupt changes. Here, the surface concentration becomes transport-dominated, i.e., the surface concentration decreases as surfactant being exuded from the primary layer.

Figure 6 demonstrated the surface tension in our model and shows spatial variation. This variation is due to physiologically based heterogeneity that is inherent in our model. For example, there are geometrical differences that exist from generation to generation based upon the space-filling algorithm used to construct the airway tree (Tawhai et al., 2000). Acini are likewise non-uniform because they fill different-sized regions of the lung depending upon the location of the terminal airways. The local surface tension depends upon the lining fluid/surfactant that is distributed within the alveolar components of the acini. While this is assumed to be a uniform concentration, the local strain-field is nonuniform. The physicochemical interactions from variable strain result in transport behavior that leads to non-uniform heterogeneous surface tensions in this dynamic model. **Figure 10A** demonstrates the average and standard deviations of the acinar surface tension. This figure demonstrates an upper limit of surface tension near γ_∞ with an insignificant variation. This occurs as the secondary layer respreads, and is indicated by point d in **Figure 9A**. In contrast, at low surface tension the variation is much greater.

The acinar minimum surface tension is found to be corelated to its residual volume, as shown in **Figure 11A**. We subdivide the data into two groups: (1) symmetrical acini that are created at the ends of two equivalent daughter terminal airways, and (2) an asymmetrical acinus that develops from a single terminal airway, with the other daughter airway non-terminal (see figure inset). We investigate the linear regressions using the form $\gamma_{min} = aV_{RV} + b$. On average, symmetrically produced acini have higher the surface tensions than asymmetric acini. We also explored the influence of central airway-to-acinus path length on the surface tension (**Figure 11B**) and found no correlation between these values.

For airways, the surface tension heterogeneity also exists. **Figure 10B** shows the relationship between airway generation (Horsfield) and maximum/minimum airway surface tension. The points represent the average value of all the airways in

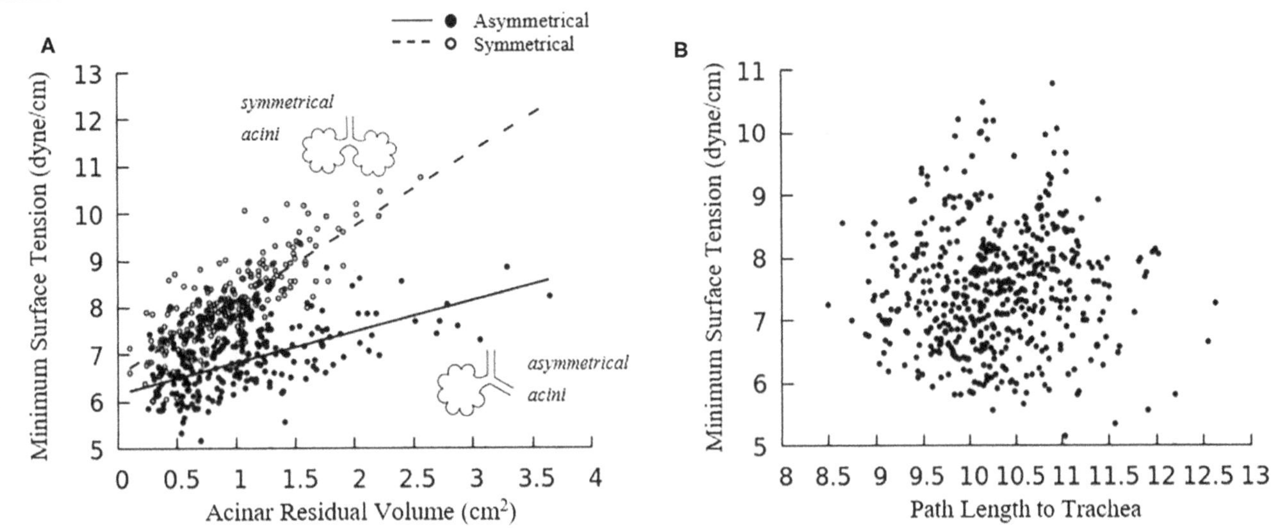

FIGURE 11 | (A) Acinar residual volume plotted against the minimum surface tension. Regressions of (1) symmetrical (a = 1.58 and b = 6.56, reduced chi-square=0.22) and (2) asymmetrical acini (a = 0.66 and b = 6.16, reduced chi-square = 0.28) show that the surface tension is lower in asymmetrical acini. **(B)** Minimum surface tension plotted against the flow path length to the trachea. No correlation exists.

that generation in one breathing cycle, and the bars represent the standard deviation. Similar to acini, the variation of the maximum surface tension is insignificant due to the surfactant transport mechanism, while a much greater variation of the minimum exists in each generation. The difference among generations can be found to correlate with the tube law defined by Equation (3) and **Table 1**.

To investigate the impact of a sigh to enhance surfactant surface-layer sorption, we introduced a sigh-like maneuver by temporarily tripling the magnitude of pleural pressure (from 3.2 to 9.6 cmH_2O), and doubling the time period (from 5 to 10 s per breath). During this cycle, the maximum lung volume increased to 5.96 L. As shown in **Figure 12**, this high increment of lung volume temporarily depletes the secondary layer and reduces the surfactant concentration of the primary layer, and allows for greater sorption from the bulk to the interface. Upon exhalation, the primary layer is highly concentrated and significantly reduces the surface tension to very low values (<5 dynes/cm). Simultaneously, transfer to the secondary layer occurs, and this leads to a lower surface tension on the following inspiration compared to that observed during the stationary state of tidal breathing.

Parenchymal Tethering and Strain Deviation

As the red curve in **Figure 13A** shown, airways in our model has a hysteresis pressure-radius behavior similar to the acini. As discussed in the previous sections, this hysteresis behavior is a result from the flow resistance of the airway network and the surfactant behavior (same mechanics as in acini), and more importantly, the pressure-related tethering force. To describe the tethering effect of the parenchyma, we rewrite Equation (12) and define $\Delta Strain$ as

$$\Delta Strain = \frac{R_H - R_{AW}}{R_H}, \tag{26}$$

where R_H is the hole radius of the parenchyma, R_{AW} is the airway radius. If $\Delta Strain$ is negative, it means $R_H < R_{AW}$, and the tethering force is compressing the airway. Likewise, if $\Delta Strain$ is positive, $R_H > R_{AW}$, and the tethering force is pulling the airway open. In **Figure 14**, the strain deviation at four different time point of the breathing cycle are shown.

It can be observed in **Figure 14** that $\Delta Strain$ is positive almost all the time, which indicates that airways are pulled outward by parenchyma. To elucidate this stabilizing force, we investigate the parenchyma effect $\left[2G_{eff}\left(\frac{\Delta R}{R}\right)\right]$ and airways' own properties $\left[P_{AW} - P_{PL}(t)\frac{\gamma}{R_{in,AW(t)}}\right]$ in Equation (7) separately. We simulate the system without tethering, i.e., forcing $2G_{eff}\left(\frac{\Delta R}{R}\right) = 0$ in Equation (7).

Figure 13A demonstrates the terminal airway radius with and without tethering ($R_{AW,\frac{w}{p}}$, and $R_{AW,\frac{w}{o}P}$, respectively) compared to the size of the hole radius, R_H. This figure shows that R_H is greater than the size of the terminal airways. This induces an outward tethering stress that increases the airway radius, so $R_{AW,\frac{w}{p}} > R_{AW,\frac{w}{o}P}$. This stent-like behavior depends upon the set-point for the equilibrium hole-radius (set at V_{FRC}) as described in "Parenchymal Tethering." This assumption leads to physiologically reasonable positive strain-deviations during normal breathing for nearly all generations of airways, indicating that the parenchymal tethering supports the airway structure in this healthy lung model. We found that reducing the set-point of the equilibrium hole-radius to volumes below V_{FRC} results in negative-strain deviation

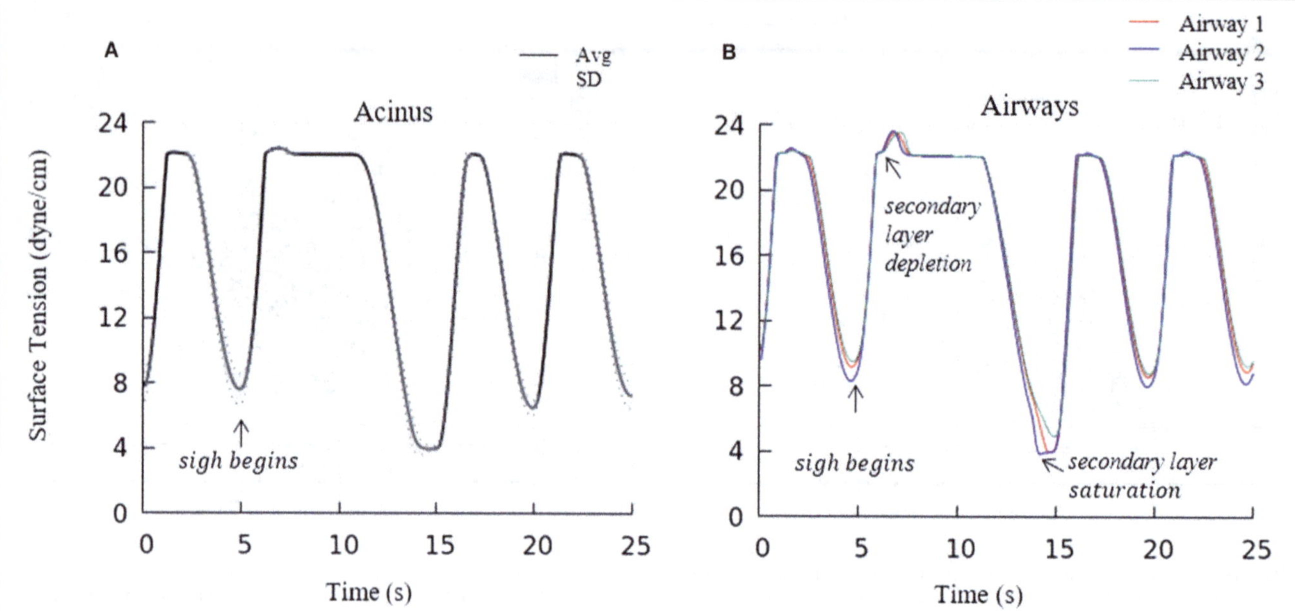

FIGURE 12 | Acinar **(A)** and representative airways, **(B)** surface tension after a deep sigh. The secondary layer respreading stabilizes the surface tension around γ_∞. In airways, secondary layer depletion can be seen where the surface tension rises rapidly again after being stabilized around γ_∞ for a short period. Compared to the stationary tidal breathing state, the additional surfactant in the primary layer by respreading from the secondary layer and adsorption from the bulk during sigh leads to a lower surface tension at end-expiration. The representative airways are the same as those shown in **Figure 9**.

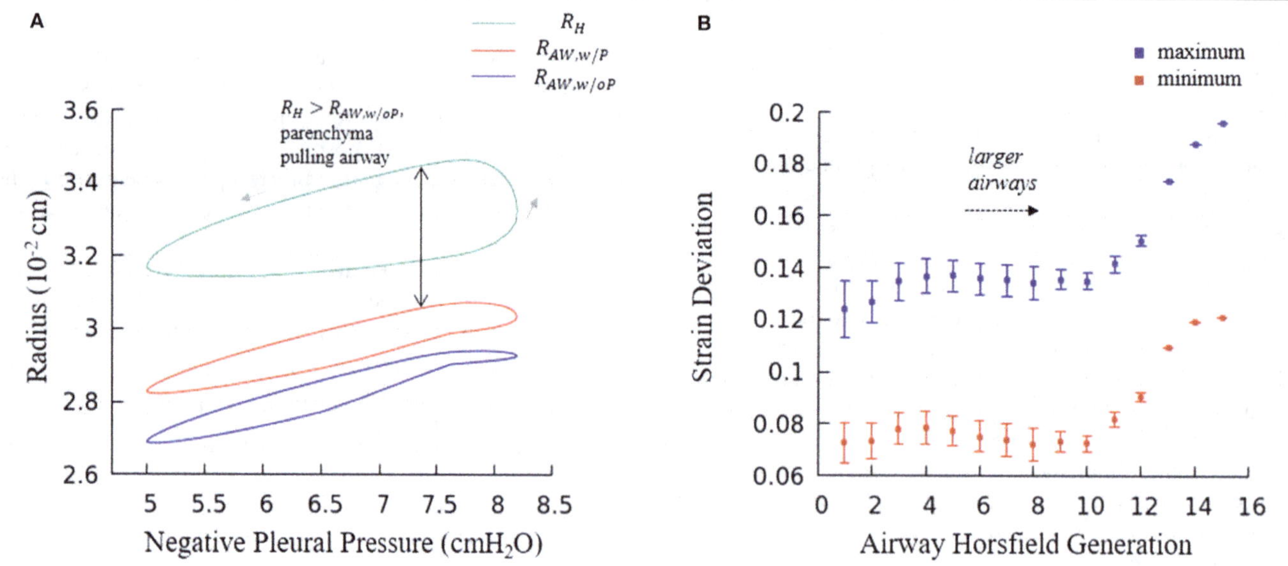

FIGURE 13 | (A) Predictions of terminal airway radius with and without parenchymal tethering. Parenchymal hole radius R_H (green), airway radius with parenchymal tethering, $R_{AW,\frac{w}{P}}$ (red), and predicted airway radius without parenchymal tethering, $R_{AW,\frac{w}{o}P}$ (blue). This figure demonstrates the important feature that in this healthy lung model, $R_H > R_{AW,\frac{w}{o}P}$. This implies that parenchyma provides an outwardly directed mechanical stress that stabilizes compliant airways. **(B)** The average maximum and minimum strain deviation of each Horsfield airway generation. Bars represent the standard deviation.

during portions of the ventilation cycle for mid-generation and terminal airways (data not shown). This behavior could be destabilizing because it would reduce the caliber of compliant airways and lead to an enhanced proclivity for airway obstruction. This parenchymal support behavior is consistent with earlier simulations conducted by Ryans et al. (2019). The tethering force is important to stabilize the open airway and maintain air flow, though surfactant deficiency can still lead to airway closure or meniscus obstruction in the unhealthy lung (Notter, 2000; West, 2012).

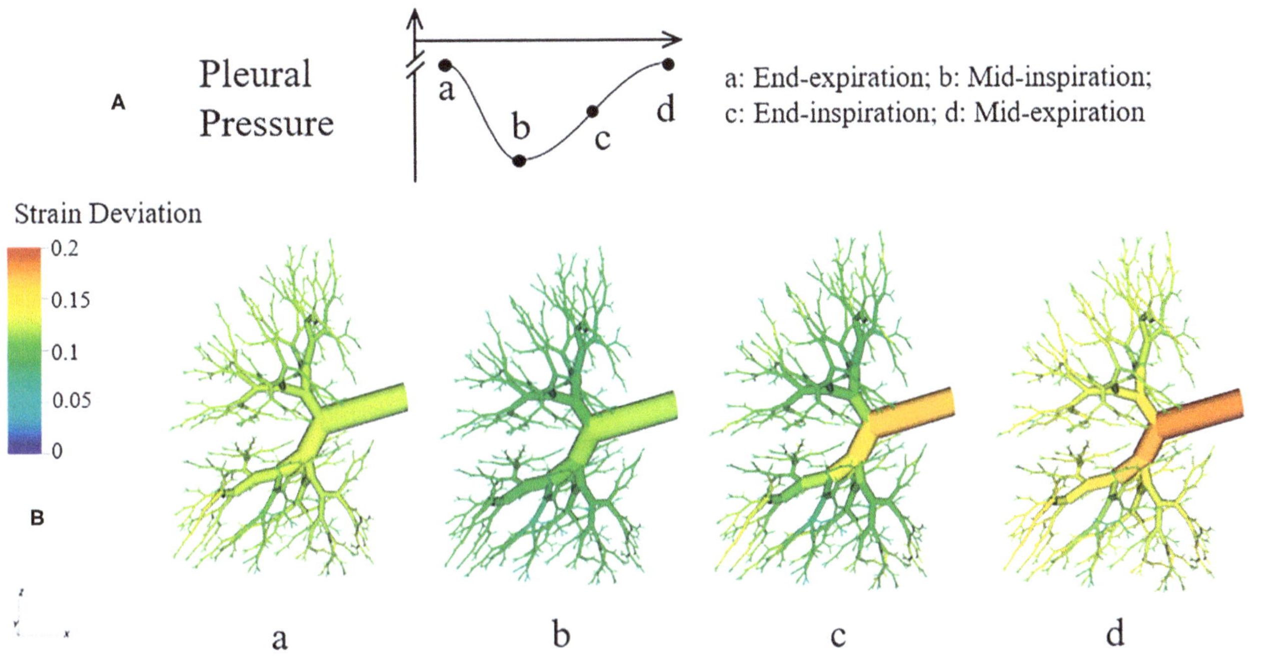

FIGURE 14 | Dynamic strain deviation in the lung model. **(A)** Specific time points during breathing cycle, **(B)** 3-D figure of the airway network at four time points, with color representing the strain deviation from the equilibrium parenchymal state.

Figure 13B demonstrates the relationship between airway generation (Horsfield) and strain deviation Equation (26). The points represent the average value of all airways in that generation in one breathing cycle, and the bars represent the standard deviation. Small strain deviations exist in the most compliant airways, and this deviation is due to time-dependence in the acinar response related to Equation (17), since the compliance of the airways is approximately equal to the acini. In contrast, for larger airways, significantly positive strain deviation exists due to several factors: (1) a compliance differences between the acinus and airway, (2) the pressure differences associated with large path-lengths between the large airways and surrounding acinus, and (3) the time-dependence in the acinar response.

Limitations

While this model provides a useful tool for simulating the multi-scale interactions of the lung, there are significant limitations due to the assumed idealized conditions. For example, we neglect gravitational effects and assume a uniform pleural pressure distribution. As such, this model cannot yet simulate ventilation dependency that is linked to orientation. This model also neglects smooth muscle biomechanics that may be neuromodulated. Furthermore, we neglect important pressure losses due to turbulence and entrance-flow effects (Filoche et al., 2015). Our simulations of normal breathing induce a maximum flow rate of ~0.92 L/s in the trachea. The Reynolds number is large ($Re > 2,000$) in airways of generations $n \leq 3$ and the Womersley parameter indicates unsteady flow in generations $n \leq 4$. Furthermore, we have assumed fully developed flow, which does not occur near bifurcations. Thus, we can expect that these regions will have greater pressure-drops than those predicted by this model. We also assume that each airway and acinus is initialized with the same dimensionless film thickness ε and a uniform surfactant concentration, and we do not allow for inter-airway or airway-to-acinar transport. Since this is a model of a healthy lung, we do not incorporate interfacial instabilities that can create plugs or regions of atelectasis. Despite these limitations, this multi-scale model a significant step in the development of a multi-scale model of the entire lung, and is capable of reproducing physiologically realistic behavior.

It should be noted that there are a large number of parameters in our system. Some of these are simple physical constants such as viscosity, equilibrium surface tension, adsorption/desorption rates, etc. that can be determined independently. Other parameters include physiological model constants related to the tube law, the set-point for tethering between parenchyma and airways, airway parent-daughter branch angles, etc. Some of these are better known than others, and could be patient specific. These might be considered "tunable" in the sense that they can be subject to revision when more information is available. With present technology, we cannot hope to create patient-specific geometric models of all branching airways and alveoli, lining fluid distributions and regionally dependent surfactant physico-chemical behavior. Despite the inability to define this type of specific information, when fully developed for healthy and pathological states, we will seek to determine the sensitivity of physiological behavior to key measurable parameters. This could provide insight into pathophysiological behavior and system interdependency that is not available from simpler systems. With this understanding, the step toward patient-specific analyses will become clearer.

CONCLUSIONS

We have developed and investigated a computational 3-D lung model that simulates multi-scale pulmonary interactions under healthy conditions. This model includes the airflow between airways and acini, surfactant transport in the liquid lining, and parenchymal tethering between the acini that surrounds airways. As shown above, these simulations demonstrate physiologically realistic macroscale PV relationships and predict microscale strain distributions that deviate from the uniform strain state (Ma et al., 2013). This deviation occurs due to ventilation-induced airflow pressures and non-equilibrium Laplace pressures resulting from surfactant physicochemical interactions (West, 1977, 2012; Krueger and Gaver, 2000; Notter, 2000). In the future, this model will provide a baseline for the study of pathological conditions; for example, airway closure and liquid plug movement that may be important contributors to the etiology of ARDS and ventilator-induced lung injury. Simulations of pathophysiological conditions may foster the development of improved methods of ventilation (Kollisch-Singule et al., 2014; Gaver et al., 2020).

AUTHOR CONTRIBUTIONS

HM, HF, and DG conceived, designed research, analyzed data, interpreted results of experiments, prepared figures, and drafted manuscript. HM and HF performed experiments. HM, HF, DH, and DG edited, revised manuscript, and approved final version of manuscript. All authors contributed to the article and approved the submitted version.

REFERENCES

Anafi, R. C., and Wilson, T. A. (2001). Airway stability and heterogeneity in the constricted lung. *J. Appl. Physiol.* 91, 1185–1192. doi: 10.1152/jappl.2001.91.3.1185

Bastacky, J., Lee, C. Y., Goerke, J., Koushafar, H., Yager, D., Kenaga, L., et al. (1985). Alveolar lining layer is thin and continuous: low-temperature scanning electron microscopy of rat lung. *J. Appl. Physiol.* 79, 1615–1628. doi: 10.1152/jappl.1995.79.5.1615

Cassidy, K. J., Halpern, D., Ressler, B. G., and Grotberg, J. B. (1985). Surfactant effects in model airway closure experiments. *J. Appl. Physiol.* 87, 415–427. doi: 10.1152/jappl.1999.87.1.415

Clements, J. A. (1957). Surface tension of lung extracts. *Proc. Soc. Exp. Biol. Med.* 95, 170–172. doi: 10.3181/00379727-95-23156

Filoche, M., Tai, C. F., and Grotberg, J. B. (2015). Three-dimensional model of surfactant replacement therapy. *Proc. Nat. Acad. Sci. U.S.A.* 112, 9287–9292. doi: 10.1073/pnas.1504025112

Fujioka, H., Halpern, D., and Gaver, D.P. 3rd. (2013). A model of surfactant-induced surface tension effects on the parenchymal tethering of pulmonary airways. *J. Biomech.* 46, 319–328. doi: 10.1016/j.jbiomech.2012.11.031

Gaver D. P. III, Nieman, G. F., Gatto, L. A., Cereda, M., Habashi, N. M., and Bates, J. H. (2020). The POOR Get POORer: a hypothesis for the pathogenesis of ventilator-induced lung injury. *Am. J. Respir. Crit. Care Med.* doi: 10.1164/rccm.202002-0453CP. [Epub ahead of print].

Harris, R.S. (2005). Pressure–volume curves of the respiratory system. *Respir. Care* 50, 78–98.

Hindmarsh, A. C., Brown, P. N., Grant, K. E., Lee, S. L., Serban, R., Shumaker, D.E., et al. (2005). SUNDIALS: suite of nonlinear and differential/algebraic equation solvers. *ACM Trans. Math. Softw.* 31, 363–396. doi: 10.1145/1089014.1089020

Horn, L.W., and Davis, S. H. (1975). Apparent surface tension hysteresis of a dynamical system. *J. Colloid Interface Sci.* 51, 459–476. doi: 10.1016/0021-9797(75)90143-5

Kollisch-Singule, M., Emr, B., Smith, B., Roy, S., Jain, S., Satalin, J., et al. (2014). Mechanical breath profile of airway pressure release ventilation: the effect on alveolar recruitment and microstrain in acute lung injury. *JAMA Surg.* 149, 1138–1145. doi: 10.1001/jamasurg.2014.1829

Krueger, M. A., and Gaver, D. P. (2000). A theoretical model of pulmonary surfactant multilayer collapse under oscillating area conditions. *J. Colloid Interface Sci.* 229, 353–364. doi: 10.1006/jcis.2000.7029

Lai-Fook, S. J., Hyatt, R. E., and Rodarte, J. R. (1978). Effect of parenchymal shear modulus and lung volume on bronchial pressure-diameter behavior. *J. Appl. Physiol. Respir. Environ. Exerc. Physiol.* 44, 859–68. doi: 10.1152/jappl.1978.44.6.859

Lai-Fook, S. J., Hyatt, R. E., Rodarte, J. R., and Wilson, T. A. (1977). Behavior of artificially produced holes in lung parenchyma. *J. Appl. Physiol. Respir. Environ. Exerc. Physiol.* 43, 648–655. doi: 10.1152/jappl.1977.43.4.648

Lambert, R. K., Wilson, T. A., Hyatt, R. E., and Rodarte, J. R. (1982). A computational model for expiratory flow. *J. Appl. Physiol.* 52, 44–56. doi: 10.1152/jappl.1982.52.1.44

Ma, B., Breen, B., and Bates, J. H. (2013). Influence of parenchymal heterogeneity on airway-parenchymal interdependence. *Respir. Physiol. Neurobiol.* 188, 94–101. doi: 10.1016/j.resp.2013.06.005

Notter, R. H. (2000). *Lung Surfactants: Basic Science and Clinical Applications. Lung Biology in Health and Disease.* New York, NY: Marcel Dekker, 444p. doi: 10.1201/9781482270426

Pedley, T., Schroter, R., and Sudlow, M. (1970). The prediction of pressure drop and variation of resistance within the human bronchial airways. *Respir. Physiol.* 9, 387–405. doi: 10.1016/0034-5687(70)90094-0

Perun, M. L., and Gaver, D. P. (1995). Interaction between airway lining fluid forces and parenchymal tethering during pulmonary airway reopening. *J. Appl. Physiol.* 79, 1717–1728. doi: 10.1152/jappl.1995.79.5.1717

Ryans, J., Fujioka, H., Halpern, D. and Gaver, D. P. (2016). Reduced-dimension modeling approach for simulating recruitment/de-recruitment dynamics in the lung. *Ann. Biomed. Eng.* 44, 3619–3631. doi: 10.1007/s10439-016-1672-9

Ryans, J. M., Fujioka, H., and, Gaver D. P. 3rd. (2019). Microscale to mesoscale analysis of parenchymal tethering: the effect of heterogeneous alveolar pressures on the pulmonary mechanics of compliant airways. *J. Appl. Physiol.* 126, 1204–1213. doi: 10.1152/japplphysiol.00178.2018

Schurch, S. (1995). Surface tension—area relations. *Pediatr. Pulmonol.* 20, 324–326. doi: 10.1002/ppul.1950200513

Smith, J. C., and Stamenovic, D. (1986). Surface forces in lungs. 1. Alveolar surface tension-lung volume relationships. *J. Appl. Physiol.* 60, 1341–1350. doi: 10.1152/jappl.1986.60.4.1341

Suki, B., and Bates, J. H. (1985). Lung tissue mechanics as an emergent phenomenon. *J. Appl. Physiol.* 110, 1111–1118. doi: 10.1152/japplphysiol.01244.2010

Swan, A. J., Clark, A. R., and Tawhai, M. H. (2012). A computational model of the topographic distribution of ventilation in healthy human lungs. *J. Theor. Biol.* 300, 222–231. doi: 10.1016/j.jtbi.2012.01.042

Tawhai, M. H., Pullan, A. J., and Hunter, P. J. (2000). Generation of an anatomically based three-dimensional model of the conducting airways. *Ann. Biomed. Eng.* 8, 793–802. doi: 10.1114/1.1289457

Venegas, J. G., Harris, R. S., and Simon, B. A. (1985). A comprehensive equation for the pulmonary pressure-volume curve. *J. Appl. Physiol.* 84, 389–395. doi: 10.1152/jappl.1998.84.1.389

Wall, W. A., Wiechert, L., Comerford, A., and Rausch, S. (2010). Towards a comprehensive computational model for the respiratory system. *Int. J. Numer. Methods Biomed. Eng.* 26, 807–827. doi: 10.1002/cnm.1378

West, J. B. (1977). *Bioengineering Aspects of the lung. Lung Biology in Health and Disease.* New York, NY: Marcel Dekker, 583p.

West, J. B. (2012). *Respiratory Physiology: The Essentials. 9th Edn.* Philadelphia, PA: Wolters Kluwer Health/Lippincott Williams and Wilkins, 200p.

Wilson, T. A. (1972). A continuum analysis of a two-dimensional mechanical model of the lung parenchyma. *J. Appl. Physiol.* 33, 472–478. doi: 10.1152/jappl.1972.33.4.472

14

Lung Mechanics Over the Century: From Bench to Bedside and Back to Bench

Paolo Jose Cesare Biselli[1], Fernanda Degobbi Tenorio Quirino Dos Santos Lopes[2], Renato Fraga Righetti[2,3], Henrique Takachi Moriya[4], Iolanda Fátima Lopes Calvo Tibério[2] and Milton Arruda Martins[2]*

[1]*Intensive Care Unit, University Hospital, University of Sao Paulo, Sao Paulo, Brazil,* [2]*Laboratory of Experimental Therapeutics, Department of Clinical Medicine, School of Medicine, University of Sao Paulo, Sao Paulo, Brazil,* [3]*Hospital Sírio-Libanês, Serviço de Reabilitação, São Paulo, Brazil,* [4]*Biomedical Engineering Laboratory, Escola Politecnica, University of Sao Paulo, Sao Paulo, Brazil*

Correspondence:
Paolo Jose Cesare Biselli
p_biselli@hotmail.com

Lung physiology research advanced significantly over the last 100 years. Respiratory mechanics applied to animal models of lung disease extended the knowledge of the workings of respiratory system. In human research, a better understanding of respiratory mechanics has contributed to development of mechanical ventilators. In this review, we explore the use of respiratory mechanics in basic science to investigate asthma and chronic obstructive pulmonary disease (COPD). We also discuss the use of lung mechanics in clinical care and its role on the development of modern mechanical ventilators. Additionally, we analyse some bench-developed technologies that are not in widespread use in the present but can become part of the clinical arsenal in the future. Finally, we explore some of the difficult questions that intensive care doctors still face when managing respiratory failure. Bringing back these questions to bench can help to solve them. Interaction between basic and translational science and human subject investigation can be very rewarding, as in the conceptualization of "Lung Protective Ventilation" principles. We expect this interaction to expand further generating new treatments and managing strategies for patients with respiratory disease.

Keywords: lung mechanics modelling, equation of motion, constant-phase model, respiratory diseases, animal models—rodent, critical care, mechanical ventilalion, lung physiology

INTRODUCTION

Respiratory mechanics has been extensively studied during the last century (RAHN et al., 1946; Otis, 1977; Collett et al., 1985; Bates, 2005) with resultant improvement in our understanding of the function of the respiratory system in health and disease states (MEAD et al., 1955; Reinert and Trendelenburg, 1972; Dodd et al., 1988; Mador, 1991). Newfound knowledge of respiratory mechanics has also been applied to different animal models of respiratory disease (Wanner and Abraham, 1982; Wanner et al., 1990; Irvin and Bates, 2003).

Over the years, accumulated knowledge in respiratory mechanics has been incorporated into mechanical ventilators and respiratory functional assessment of patients (Younes, 1992; Sinderby et al., 1999; Jonkman et al., 2020). Respiratory mechanics became not only a tool for investigating lung disorders. It was also used in developing treatments for failing respiratory system and in designing strategies to prevent lung injury (Henderson et al., 2017).

A Single Frequency

Equation of Motion

$$Paw = Flow.R + Vol.E + P0$$

Functional Parameters

R: Respiratory System Resistance ($cmH_2O.s/mL$)
E: Respiratory System Elastance (cmH_2O/mL)

B Multiple Frequencies

Constant-Phase Model

$$\alpha = \frac{2}{\pi}.tan^{-1}.\left(\frac{Htis}{Gtis}\right)$$

$$Z(f) = \frac{P(f)}{Flow(f)} = Raw + i.2.\pi.f.Iaw + \frac{(Gtis - i.Htis)}{(2.\pi.f)^{\alpha}}$$

Functional Parameters

Raw: Airway Resistance ($cmH_2O.s/mL$)
Gtis: Tissue Resistance (cmH_2Os (1-alfa) /mL)
Htis: Tissue Elastance (cmH_2Os (1-alfa) /mL)

FIGURE 1 | Mathematical models used to obtain functional parameters. **(A)**. The equation of Motion: Paw (cmH_2O) is airway pressure, measured at airway opening, Flow (mL/s) is airway flow, R is Respiratory System Resistance ($cmH_2O.s/mL$), Vol (mL) is the Volume of air that has entered the lungs since the beginning of inspiration, E (cmH_2O/mL) is Respiratory System Elastance and P0 (cmH_2O) is the airway pressure at the beginning of inspiration. **(B)**. The Constant Phase Model (Z(f), $cmH_2O.s/mL$) is calculated as the pressure response (P(f), cmH_2O) divided by ventilator generated flow (Flow(f), mL/s) at each frequency (f). Raw represents Newtonian resistance ($cmH_2O.s/mL$); i is imaginary number; Iaw is airway inertance ($cmH_2O.s^2/mL$), Gtis is tissue viscance (cm $H_2O.s^{(1-\alpha)}/mL$); Htis is tissue elastance (cm $H_2O.s^{(1-\alpha)}/mL$).

In this review, we describe some of the mathematical approaches used in respiratory mechanics in animal models and in patients and their application in the development of mechanical ventilation. Finally, we will discuss how respiratory mechanics is still important for both research and clinical care and how it can provide insightful information moving respiratory science forward.

RESPIRATORY MECHANICS IN ANIMAL MODELS

Animal models have been extensively used to elucidate different physiological mechanisms leading to respiratory disease development, such as asthma and chronic obstructive pulmonary disease (COPD).

Generally, the assessment of respiratory mechanics in animal models is based on the acquisition of pressure and volume/flow data. From these data, mathematical models whose parameters have physiological significance are applied (Bates, 2005).

The most used model for evaluating respiratory mechanics is known as the "equation of motion." It is a linear one-compartment model that assumes the respiratory system is excited at a single frequency, usually very close to the respiratory rate (**Figure 1**) (Bates, 2005). The parameters of this model are respiratory system resistance, representing the amount of pressure required to generate flows; and respiratory system elastance, which is the amount of pressure required to maintain volume changes in the respiratory system.

The equation of motion does not contemplate viscoelastic phenomenon. Viscoelasticity is the property to accommodate stress following changes in volume (stress relaxation) (Faffe and Zin, 2009). It can be observed in pressure-time graph once inspiratory flow is abruptly stopped. The slow pressure decrease after inspiratory pause reveals stress relaxation (**Figure 2A**). It results from parenchymal fiber conformational adaptation (Faffe and Zin, 2009), changes in surface tension in water-air interfaces or redistribution of air within lung regions (Bates, 2009). Measurements in viscoelasticity add complexity to equation of motion model.

The respiratory system has a high frequency dependence. This led to the use of excitations with more than one frequency in order to calculate the respiratory impedance that basically characterizes the biomechanical behaviour of the respiratory system in the frequencies contained in the excitation (**Figure 1**) (Hantos et al., 1992).

For a better physiological understanding of respiratory impedance, models are used whose parameters are correlated with dissipative (airway resistance and tissue viscosity) and conservative (elastance or tissue compliance) components. The most used model for understanding respiratory impedance in small rodents is the constant-phase model (Bates and Irvin, 2003). This model provides more detailed information on lung mechanics comparing to equation of motion. It describes proximal and distal airways with different parameters, which can be useful to evaluate obstructive diseases.

Respiratory Mechanics in Animal Models of Lung Disease

Respiratory mechanics have been studied in several animal models of respiratory diseases. In experimental emphysema, researchers observed a decrease in tissue elastance and viscosity (see section "Respiratory mechanics in animal

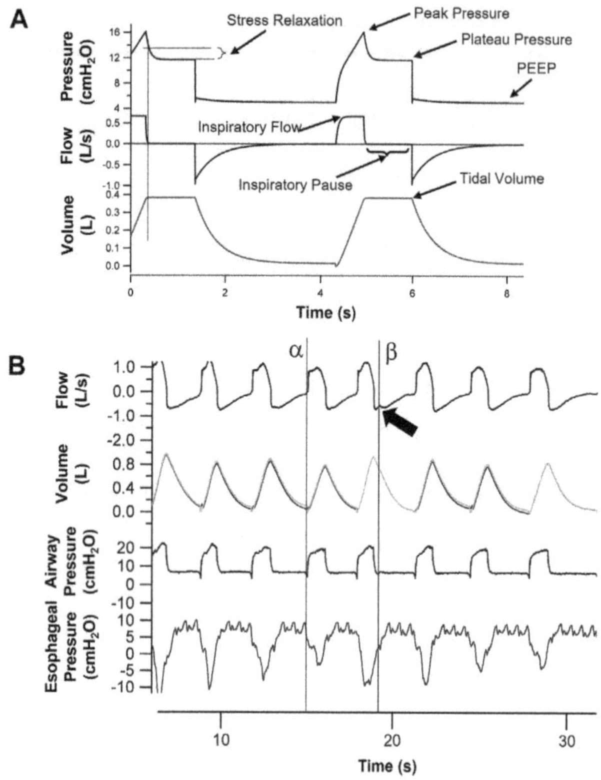

$$Airway\ Pressure = Po + Resistance * Flow + \frac{Tidal\ Volme}{Compliance}$$

$$Static\ Compliance = \frac{Tidal\ Volme}{Plateau\ Pressure - PEEP}$$

$$Resistance = \frac{Peak\ Pressure - Plateau\ Pressure}{Inspiratory\ Flow}$$

$$Airway\ Pressure + Pmus = Po + Resistance * Flow + \frac{Tidal\ Volme}{Compliance}$$

FIGURE 2 | Respiratory mechanics in paralyzed and spontaneously breathing patients. **(A)**. This is a representation of Flow, Volume and Pressure signals over time for a patient under sedation and neuromuscular blockage. Since there is no respiratory muscle activity, equation of motion (see **Figure 1A**) can be applied. Compliance (inverse of Elastance, displayed in **Figure 1**) and Resistance can be found using minimum square method or by the inspiratory pause special case displayed in **(A)**. Applying an inspiratory pause will simplify the equation allowing measurement of Static Compliance and Resistance. It also allows observation of viscoelastic properties of the respiratory system, with the slow decrease in pressure (Stress Relaxation) once flow is abruptly stopped. **(B)**. In non-sedated patients, respiratory muscles interact with the ventilator. In this example, we show Pressure, Flow, Volume and Esophageal Pressure signal over time in a patient ventilated in Pressure Support Mode. Muscle activity can be measured with an esophageal catheter. In this scenario, equation of motion needs to be adapted to include pressure generated by respiratory muscles (Pmus). The model becomes less stable but esophageal pressure reveals several features of patient ventilator interaction. The observed changes in tidal volumes over several breaths is caused by a change in patient's effort detected by esophageal pressure. Additionally, we can observe the inspiratory effort triggering mechanical ventilator (line α) and the prolongation of patient's inspiratory effort into ventilator expiration (line β), distorting expiratory flow curve (arrow).

models") related to alveolar destruction and loss of viscoelastic properties (Bates, 2009; Ito et al., 2019a, 2019b). On the other hand, repairing lung tissue with different components of extracellular matrix also alters lung function. Changes in collagen fibers types I and III and elastin in lung parenchyma leads to loss of lung elasticity (Fietzek and Kuehn, 1976; Shifren et al., 2007; Suki and Bates, 2008; Koenders, 2009).

Airway resistance increase is usually detected in experimental models of asthma where structural changes in airways are the major histological finding (Bates, 2009). Edema in peribronchovascular areas also increases viscoelastic properties. Airway hyperresponsiveness can be detected with a dose-response curve to methacholine or the antigen itself (Wang et al., 1986). Both constant phase model and equation of motion can be used to describe respiratory function in these animals (Bates, 2009) (see **Figure 1** and section "Respiratory mechanics in animal models" above).

Camargo et al. (2020) showed in an experimental model of asthma in mice sensitized with ovalbumin that there was an increased response of airway resistance when compared to the control group. In addition, Possa et al. (2012); Righetti et al. (2014) and Pigati et al. (2015), in an experimental model of asthma showed that the worsening in mechanical parameters had a positive correlation with markers of eosinophilic inflammation, Th2 profile cytokines, oxidative stress (iNOS and 8- iso-PGF2alpha), and extracellular matrix remodelling.

Oscillatory mechanics and the constant phase model (see **Figure 1** and section "Respiratory mechanics in animal models" above) can be applied not only to whole lung, but also to lung tissue *in vitro*. Using this technique, it is possible to calculate resistance and elastance of lung tissue strips (Leite-Júnior et al., 2003). For oscillatory mechanics, subpleural parenchyma strips of the lower lobes are cut and the resting length (Lr) and wet weight (W0) of each strip are measured (Aristoteles et al., 2013; Righetti et al., 2014). Lung tissue strips are composed of 86–90% alveoli, 5–8% blood vessels and 0.4–5% airways (Ludwig and Dallaire, 1994; Aristoteles et al., 2013). The tissue lungs are infused with Krebs solution (in mM: NaCl, 118;

KCl, 4.5; $NaHCO_3$, 25.5; $CaCl_2$, 2.5; $MgSO_4$, 1.2; KH_2PO_4, 1.2; glucose 10) and metal clips are glued to either end of the tissue strips with cyanoacrylate. Steel wires are attached to the clips; one side is connected to a force transducer and the other side is connected to a servo-controlled lever arm. The lever arm is capable of peak-to-peak length excursions. It is connected to a function generator, which controlled the frequency, amplitude, and waveform of the device oscillation (Ebihara et al., 2000; Pigati et al., 2015). The resting tension (T) is set by the movement of a screw thumb wheel system, which effected slow vertical displacements of the force transducer. Length and force signals are converted from analog to digital with an analog-to-digital converter and recorded by a compatible computer. The resistance (R) and elastance (E) of the lung tissue strip are estimate by the recursive least-squares algorithm to the equation of motion (Ludwig and Dallaire, 1994; Aristoteles et al., 2013; Righetti et al., 2014; Pigati et al., 2015).

$$T = E\Delta 1 + R\left(\Delta 1/_{\Delta t}\right) + K$$

Where T is tension, l is length, Δl/Δt is the length change per unit of time, and K is a constant reflecting resting tension. The unstressed cross-sectional area (*A*0) of the strip was obtained from the formula:

$$A0\ (\mathrm{cm}^2) = \mathrm{W0}/(\mathrm{p\ x\ Lr})$$

In this sense, Nakashima et al. (Nakashima et al., 2008) evaluated the active process of lung immune unresponsiveness with oral ingestion of ovalbumin (oral tolerance) in guinea pigs sensitized with ovalbumin and Starling (Starling et al., 2009) evaluated the use of nitric oxide synthetase inhibitor in an experimental model of asthma. In both studies oscillatory mechanics identified the improvement in lung tissue resistance and elastance parameters as a result of treatment. Furthermore, changes in lung resistance and elastance also correlate with changes in inflammation, oxidative stress, and remodelling in the lung parenchyma (Righetti et al., 2014; Pigati et al., 2015). Pigati et al. 2015 showed similar changes in resistance and elastance of the respiratory system and lung tissue strip. Moreover, tissue strip oscillatory mechanics can also include dose-response curves after challenges with antigen or methacholine. (Lanças et al., 2006). In recent decades, several studies used this technique for measuring lung tissue resistance and elastance *in vitro* (Xisto et al., 2005; Santos et al., 2008; Starling et al., 2009; Aristoteles et al., 2013; Righetti et al., 2014; Pigati et al., 2015) and these studies helped to support the importance of alterations in the lung parenchyma of asthmatic patients (Tulić and Hamid, 2003; Mauad et al., 2004; Martin, 2008).

Lung mechanics produces a simple description of the function of the lungs and can be used to detect diseases and to analyse the effects of potential treatments. The new methodologies (lung strip mechanics and oscillatory mechanics) described above allowed a more complex and accurate description of lung function (Bates and Irvin, 2003; Leite-Júnior et al., 2003; Lanças et al., 2006). In the decades to come, lung mechanics will continue to play a fundamental role in respiratory research and clinical care.

LUNG PHYSIOLOGY IN HUMAN SUBJECTS: MECHANICAL VENTILATION AND LUNG ASSESSMENT

Lung Physiology and Evolution of Mechanical Ventilators

Besides allowing mechanistic investigation on several lung diseases, respiratory physiology largely contributed to evolution of mechanical ventilation. In the past century, mechanical ventilation evolved from bulky and cumbersome negative pressure chambers (iron lungs) to modern positive pressure ventilators (Kacmarek, 2011). Over decades, many features and ventilatory modes were added to ventilators. This process was greatly assisted by knowledge gained in basic lung physiology.

Incorporation of positive end expiratory pressure (PEEP) to mechanical ventilators became widespread after the description of Acute Respiratory Distress Syndrome (ARDS) in 1967 (Ashbaugh et al., 1967) and observations of hypoxemia improvement with the use of PEEP (Ashbaugh et al., 1969). Measurements of lung compliance using equation of motion and responses to PEEP were important for defining the new syndrome. Although compliance is not part of current ARDS definition (Ranieri et al., 2012), it has been used in initial characterizations of the syndrome (Ashbaugh et al., 1967; Murray et al., 1988). Later, investigations on the role of PEEP and tidal volume in ARDS contributed to understanding Ventilation Induced Lung Injury (VILI) (Parker et al., 1990a; Corbridge et al., 1990; Dreyfuss and Saumon, 1993); and were the basis for developing Lung Protective Ventilation (Amato et al., 1998; The Acute Respiratory Distress Syndrome Network, 2000).

Some ventilatory modes added in time to ventilators were largely based on lung physiology. In Proportional Assist Ventilation (PAV), lung compliance and resistance are used to determine the amount of airway pressure delivered by the ventilator (Younes, 1992). In Neurally-Adjusted Ventilatory Assist (NAVA), electrical impulses generated by depolarization of diaphragm fibers are captured and control the level of ventilatory support (Sinderby et al., 1999). In Automatic Tube Compensation (ATC), mechanical ventilators provide additional pressure proportional to flow and endotracheal tube resistance (Guttmann et al., 1993; L'Her, 2012).

Respiratory Mechanics Applied to Clinical Care

Assessment of lung mechanics is used in daily clinical care. In patients receiving invasive mechanical ventilation, the equation of motion is used to describe lung mechanics and to assist in the characterization of respiratory failure (Pham et al., 2017). Physicians can measure increases in resistance (**Figure 2**) in respiratory failure in patients with obstructive disease. Changes

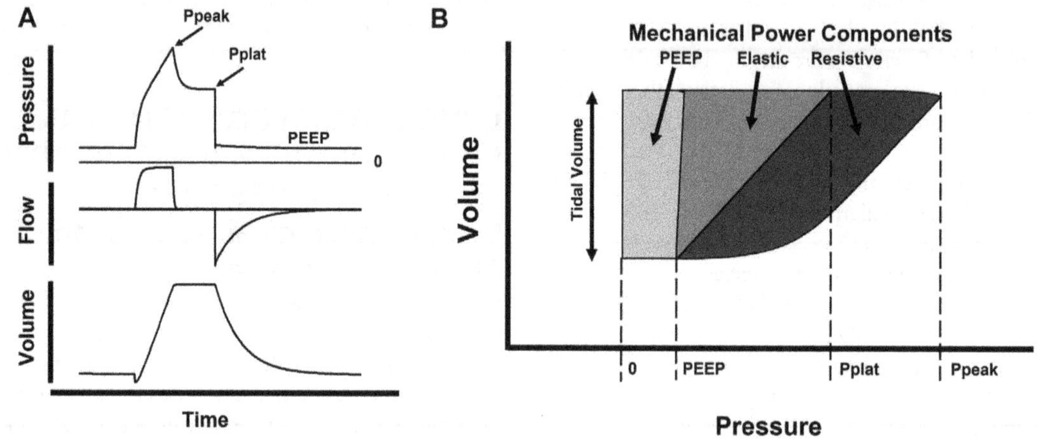

FIGURE 3 | Schematic representation of Mechanical Power. In panel **(A)** we display a single breath of a patient ventilated with Volume Assist Control. Graphs show changes in Pressure, Flow and Volume over time and highlight points of interest: PEEP, peak pressure (Ppeak) and plateau pressure (Pplat, at end of inspiratory pause). In figure **(B)**, we display a Volume-Pressure loop with the same points of interest observed in panel **(A)**. Dark gray area represents Resistive Mechanical Power, change in pressure to overcome resistive respiratory forces integrated over change in volume (tidal volume); middle gray area represents Elastic mechanical power, change in pressure to overcome elastic respiratory forces integrated over change in volume; light gray area represents PEEP mechanical power, a static component of pressure representing baseline tension on the respiratory system also integrated over change in tidal volume. (Adapted from Silva et al., 2019).

in resistance over the course of treatment can indicate worsening or improvement of disease status and guide ventilatory support.

In ARDS, measurements of lung compliance (**Figure 2**) inform the clinician about disease severity (Morales-Quinteros et al., 2019; Panwar et al., 2020; Boscolo et al., 2021). In COVID pandemic, lung compliance was employed to describe specific phenotypes: patients with hypoxemia but little amount of lung collapse and high compliance versus very low compliant lungs with large amount of lung collapse (Gattinoni et al., 2020b). The authors suggested different phenotypes could benefit from different ventilatory strategies (Gattinoni et al., 2020a). This approach was disputed by other researchers, who demonstrated respiratory compliance in COVID patients were similar to values previously reported in ARDS (Tobin, 2020; Ziehr et al., 2020; Sjoding et al., 2021) and treatment should not be changed. Early findings during a pandemic should be carefully evaluated before changing current practice (Meyer et al., 2021). Despite the controversy, use of physiological parameters to further classify ARDS patients highlights the heterogeneity of the disease (Khan et al., 2021). In the future, we might be able to learn what parameters could determine changes in treatment strategies.

Over decades, different physiological approaches have been proposed to properly set PEEP levels in ARDS patients. Obtaining lung pressure-volume curve and selecting PEEP levels according to best compliance was initially used by Amato (Amato et al., 1998). This is rather laborious and measuring lung compliance at different PEEP levels after lung recruitment could be a suitable simplification of this method. Calculating dead space and shunt fraction was also used for PEEP selection (Ferluga et al., 2018; Karbing et al., 2020; Tusman et al., 2020). Recently, measuring potential recruitment has also been proposed (Chen et al., 2020). And Talmor et al. (2008) proposed setting PEEP levels to maintain a positive transpulmonary pressure, measured using an esophageal catheter. They have shown improvements in oxygenation but failed to demonstrate decrease in mortality with this technique (Beitler et al., 2019). Unfortunately, an ideal method for PEEP selection has not been found. Some authors have used a FiO_2-based table to guide PEEP setting. This method can be suitable in the busy ICU environment but did not reduce ARDS mortality (Brower et al., 2004). Additionally, setting PEEP based on FiO_2 level ignores that patients might respond very differently. Physiological approaches could still be useful in addressing this problem.

More recently, Gattinoni proposed the use of Mechanical power, a new measurement of stress applied to lungs based on energy delivered during mechanical ventilation (Gattinoni et al., 2016). Mechanical power was based on equation of motion and incorporated concepts of mechanical work displayed on Campbell's diagram (Cabello and Mancebo, 2006). Each component of the equation of motion was multiplied by the change in volume and Respiratory rate (**Figure 3**) to evaluate the individual contribution to lung injury (Silva et al., 2019). The usefulness of this new analysis is still under investigation. Some authors believe it does not add substantial new information to mechanical ventilation management (Costa et al., 2021). On the other hand, mechanical power can be associated to biomarkers of lung deterioration (Rocco et al., 2020). At a minimum, it underscored the importance of respiratory rate as a source of stress to lungs during ventilation.

The assessment of respiratory mechanics in spontaneously breathing patients has always been a challenge. Respiratory effort should be accounted for when applying equation of motion (Grinnan and Truwit, 2005). Esophageal catheters can be used to measure patients' effort (Baydur et al., 1982), allowing the use of equation of motion even in non-paralyzed patients (**Figure 2**). On the other hand, new lung mechanics techniques evolving from experimental physiology can be used in spontaneously ventilated patients. Notably, forced oscillation technique, or oscillometry, has contributed to a better understanding of lung function in clinical routine and in research, particularly in patients with obstructive disease (Peterson-Carmichael et al., 2016; Hantos, 2021; Lundblad and Robichaud, 2021).

Lung Protective Ventilation. Tidal Volume Challenge

Initial basic research on the effects of PEEP and tidal volume in ARDS (Parker et al., 1990b; Carlton et al., 1990; Corbridge et al., 1990; Dreyfuss and Saumon, 1993) later translated in trials investigating mechanical ventilation management strategies (Amato et al., 1998; The Acute Respiratory Distress Syndrome Network, 2000). Current guidelines for ARDS management suggest limiting tidal volume to 6 ml/kg and plateau pressure to 30 cm H_2O (Griffiths et al., 2019; Papazian et al., 2019). This strategy was named lung protective ventilation. It revealed that mechanical ventilation can be harmful to lungs and defined new targets for the health team. It also introduced the challenging idea that aiming normal blood gas values during mechanical ventilation could lead to worse outcomes. Higher pCO_2 levels (permissive hypercapnia) generated by reduction tidal volume were initially regarded as benign. Later, some authors recognized hypercapnia was associated to impaired immunologic response and vascular tonus dysfunction. Hypercapnia increases pulmonary resistance and can contribute to acute cor pulmonale (Repessé and Vieillard-Baron, 2017; Barnes et al., 2018). Nevertheless, the best current evidence still recommends limiting tidal volume for ARDS patients despite CO_2 elevation. Patients with hypercapnia in this setting could be managed with additional rescue strategies (Repessé and Vieillard-Baron, 2017).

Lung protective ventilation concepts were further explored in a later reanalysis of the initial ARDS trials (Amato et al., 2015). The authors used a multilevel mediation analysis to conclude that driving pressure (plateau pressure—PEEP) was the variable most significantly associated to mortality. Although ARDS guidelines advised against the use of targets of driving pressure (Papazian et al., 2019), this measurement integrates the concepts of disease severity (lung compliance) and ventilator management (tidal volume). Further prospective trials are required but driving pressure could become an essential parameter to monitor in the future.

The success of managing mechanical ventilation during ARDS led several authors to suggest the use of lung protective ventilation in all patients receiving mechanical ventilation. Indeed, initial observational studies suggested better outcomes or decreased inflammatory cytokine production when limiting tidal volume in non-ARDS patients (Determann et al., 2010; Neto et al., 2012; Fuller et al., 2013). The initial observations were not confirmed in a properly conducted clinical trial (Simonis et al., 2018). As surprising this might look, one must remember that patients with ARDS have lungs very different from normal and from other patients on mechanical ventilation. Limiting tidal volume can be useful in some scenarios, as operating rooms, but can be very challenging in ICU. Some individuals would require deep sedation and muscle paralysis to limit tidal volume regardless of the ventilatory mode selected, adding significant morbidity to patient care. Patients waking from sedation after uneventful surgery that develop large tidal volume on spontaneous breathing should probably be extubated and not deeply sedated. COPD patients could benefit from lowering tidal volume and minute ventilation, but probably would handle very poorly high respiratory rates that might be required if tidal volumes are greatly reduced (Marini, 2011).

Even in ARDS patients, duration of strict protective ventilation can bring challenges to caring team. Although essential in the beginning of care, limiting tidal volumes can be difficult in some patients once sedation and muscle paralysis are withdrawn. Maintaining long periods of sedation and paralysis can lead to muscle weakening and prolong time on mechanical ventilation (Kress et al., 2000; Girard et al., 2008; Reade and Finfer, 2014). On the other hand, patients with high ventilatory drive will produce large tidal volumes regardless of ventilatory mode selected (Yoshida et al., 2013; Papazian et al., 2019).

The importance of ventilatory drive and its contribution to lung injury is still under investigation. It has been recognized that patients can generate significant amount of inspiratory pressure during respiratory failure, both before and after being intubated. Large inspiratory pressure swings will translate into large transpulmonary pressure irrespective of the settings on non-invasive ventilation device (before intubation) or mechanical ventilator (after intubation) (Brochard et al., 2017). Even when volume assist control mode is selected, patients with large swings generate intrathoracic pressure reduction that can produce lung edema, increases in left ventricle afterload and double triggering in ventilator, which doubles or triples tidal volumes (Pohlman et al., 2008; Pinsky, 2018; Sottile et al., 2020). The contribution or spontaneous breathing patterns to lung injury has been named P-SILI (Patient Self Inflicted Lung Injury). Although some authors have advised against using those new concepts to manage ventilator at this stage due to lack of experimental and clinical data (Tobin et al., 2020), this will be an important topic to explore. The relative importance of spontaneous effort in producing lung injury will need to be balanced against the deleterious effects of extending sedation and muscle paralysis.

Guidelines for properly managing those patients are still missing. We will need further cooperation between basic and clinical science to understand the limits of lung protective ventilation. We need to understand when this strategy is absolutely required warranting muscle paralysis; and when we can be more flexible on these rules. We also need to understand what other lung disorders require limiting tidal volume.

Respiratory Mechanics in Obstructive Lung Diseases

Patients with respiratory failure secondary to obstructive lung disease can require mechanical ventilation. Ventilatory strategies for these patients are designed to avoid air trapping and intrinsic PEEP (PEEPi) generation (Reddy and Guntupalli, 2007). PEEPi is produced when expiratory time is insufficient to allow complete tidal volume exhalation, usually when both airway resistance and respiratory rate increase. Air is trapped inside the lungs, increasing intrathoracic pressure, decreasing venous return and increasing patients' effort to trigger the ventilator and generate inspiratory flows (Pepe and Marini, 1982; Marini, 2011). Mechanical ventilator settings should allow enough expiratory time to minimize the impact of PEEPi. Although limiting tidal volume can be beneficial, low minute ventilation and high expiratory time should be main targets (Reddy and Guntupalli, 2007).

In obstructive patients, equation of motion can be used to measure lung resistance and monitor the response to treatments: bronchodilators, antibiotics and management of airway secretion. PEEPi can be measured with expiratory pause, informing bedside decisions on setting ventilator parameters.

However, there are limitations for the use of lung mechanics in those patients. Equation of motion is usually applied only to inspiratory phase, where airway pressure variation is significant. Measurement of airway resistance during expiration is often neglected despite its importance in generating PEEPi. Some patients in respiratory failure reach a condition of expiratory flow limitation, where airways collapse at the mid-end expiration (Bates, 2009). In this scenario, expiratory flow becomes independent of pressure gradient and expiratory airway resistance cannot be defined using equation of motion.

Additionally, patients on mechanical ventilators are often awake and have spontaneous breathing. In this setting, if pressure generated by respiratory muscles is not measured (**Figure 2B**), lung mechanics cannot be properly assessed. PEEPi measurement requires long expiratory pause which is usually not possible in patients with spontaneous breathing (Grinnan and Truwit, 2005). And since PEEPi is highly dependent on respiratory rate, values of PEEPi obtained during neuromuscular block are hardly valid when patients resume respiratory effort.

In the future, widespread use of esophageal pressure catheters can allow monitoring of respiratory effort and assessment of lung mechanics in patients with spontaneous breathing (Grinnan and Truwit, 2005). PEEPi can also be measured using esophageal pressure monitoring (Marini, 2011). Methods for measuring expiratory resistance and detecting expiratory flow limitation can become easier. Finally, oscillatory mechanics at the bedside can provide information on dissipative forces of the respiratory system even in patients with spontaneous breathing (see section Oscillometry). It could then allow the analysis of lung resistance in patients with obstructive lung disease without the requirement of deep sedation.

LUNG PHYSIOLOGY STILL NOT AT BEDSIDE PRIMETIME

For different reasons, several physiological approaches developed in the lab did not reach bedside yet and will be discussed in the paragraphs below. Some of these techniques are laborious or provide data clinicians are not ready to use. Some techniques, on the other hand, did become commercially available but are still seldom employed.

Multiple inert gas elimination technique (MIGET) was designed for determining ventilation/perfusion distribution throughout the lungs using several gases with different solubility on blood. MIGET advanced knowledge of respiratory physiology in different species and elucidated mechanisms of hypoxia in different disorders (Wagner, 2008). The technique is very laborious and requires not only injection of several gases but also a pulmonary catheter for measuring cardiac output and gas detector. It provides useful clinical information and could be used to select PEEP levels or describe functional lung behaviour during treatment. Its complexity, however, prevented widespread clinical application.

Electrical Impedance Tomography (EIT) evolved from very simple and inaccurate devices to monitor respiratory rate into complex continuous monitors of lung ventilation. Recent advances in the technique also included perfusion and V/Q distribution measurement using electrocardiography-gated impedance signals or following hypertonic saline infusion (Costa et al., 2009; Nguyen et al., 2012). There should be some caution in interpreting perfusion measured by impedance technique. Impedance signals should not be able to detect perfusion defects in small capillaries if pulmonary blood flow to major arteries remains unchanged (Deibele et al., 2008). Therefore, some authors believe perfusion EIT will be more useful as a non-invasive tool for diagnosing pulmonary embolism rather than small V/Q mismatch (Maciejewski et al., 2021). However, the technology is still evolving and methods for diagnosing small perfusion defects could arise.

Although not used in many ICUs, EIT became commercially available and can provide useful information on ventilation during patient care. It can be used to improve PEEP titration since it displays both overdistention and lung collapse. It also provides a visual and numerical analysis of ventilation homogeneity, can detect pneumothorax in real time and displays patterns of ventilation during spontaneous efforts (Coppadoro et al., 2020; Maciejewski et al., 2021). In the present, there is not enough supporting evidence for the use of EIT, but it can become an important monitoring device in the future.

Measuring resting lung volumes has always been difficult in clinical and research settings. Nitrogen-washout measurements have been proposed by some authors. The technique uses changes in FiO_2 concentrations and nitrogen dilution to estimate lung volumes (Olegård et al., 2005; Dellamonica et al., 2011). The process, however, is time-consuming and cannot be applied continuously in a busy ICU. Nevertheless, measuring resting lung volumes can be used to properly set tidal volumes. Guidelines for ARDS management suggest limiting tidal volumes to 6 ml/kg of ideal body weight, which is calculated based on patient height to correct for different lung sizes (Papazian et al., 2019). However, ARDS patients have different lung volumes not only because of different body constitution but also because of extension of the disease (Chiumello et al., 2008; Mattingley et al., 2011). Scaling tidal volume to actual size of lungs could allow settings targeted not only to each patient, but also to each phase of the disease (Chiumello et al., 2008; Macintyre, 2016; Umbrello et al., 2017; Pelosi et al., 2021).

Patients effort monitoring has been possible to measure for decades using esophageal catheters (Baydur et al., 1982). Although commercially available and proposed by many different research groups, the technique is seldom employed (Akoumianaki et al., 2014). Misplacement of the catheter, patients' discomfort and lack of clear clinical benefit could explain the low enthusiasm for the approach. On the other hand, as we manage patients with less sedation and greater levels of interaction with ventilators, measuring effort can become important. If future research relates respiratory effort to lung injury, spontaneous breathing should be carefully handled.

Oscillometry

Oscillometry or forced oscillation technique consists of applying flow or pressure oscillations at the entrance of the airways and monitoring the response obtained with the oscillations in order to calculate the impedance of the respiratory system. Impedance is the mechanical load of the respiratory system to ventilation.

Initially, the forced oscillation technique was used in apnea situations so that voluntary respiratory efforts did not mask the actual physiological condition of the respiratory system. However, with signal processing techniques, it became possible to use oscillometry in spontaneously ventilating patients by superimposing a high-frequency pressure waveform on the tidal breathing pattern (Peterson-Carmichael et al., 2016) and still calculate the impedance of the respiratory system with the effects of breathing minimized.

The constant-phase model (see section 'Respiratory mechanics in animal models' and **Figure 1**) applied in small rodents is not suitable for patients because of the low frequency broadband excitation needed (Lundblad and Robichaud, 2021). So, the analysis of the human respiratory impedance is based mostly on the frequency response behaviour of impedance, a complex mathematical function with real and imaginary components. This analysis strongly helps the understanding of respiratory physiology, as the real component is related to dissipative energy (resistance) and the imaginary component is related to conservative energy (elastance) of the respiratory system (Lundblad and Robichaud, 2021).

According to Hantos (Hantos, 2021), manoeuvres using oscillometry involving large but slow changes in lung volume allows for fine mapping of respiratory mechanics exceeding the tidal range and a novel intra-breath modality is capable of tracking the dynamic changes in respiratory system.

Technical standards for respiratory oscillometry have been published (King et al., 2020) and commercial devices are becoming popular.

BACK TO BENCH

Basic science and lung physiology helped to develop and advance mechanical ventilation at bedside and they still can be very important for the challenges ahead.

Lung protective ventilation does not answer all questions in respiratory failure. It was crafted long ago, when mechanical ventilation care was substantially different. Awake patients interacting with ventilators bring additional challenges. How far should we go to limit tidal volume? Should we continue to keep low levels of sedation in patients with high respiratory drive? Should we tolerate higher tidal volumes once the initial inflammatory phase of ARDS is over and oxygenation starts to improve? And how should we handle patients without ARDS with high respiratory drive and tidal volumes?

Measuring effort, lung volumes, lung inhomogeneities, pattern of ventilation and V/Q distribution or mechanical power can provide some of these answers. At the same time, ventilators used for small animals incorporated some of the technologies developed at the bedside, as pressure support ventilation. P-SILI and the effects of respiratory effort can be further investigated in animal models.

The advent of ECMO (extracorporeal membrane oxygenation) has brough additional complexity to the field. Once limited to operating rooms, ECMO use in ICU became more popular after influenza (H1N1 in 2009) and COVID (2020) pandemics (Combes et al., 2018; Barbaro et al., 2020). Although very expensive and invasive, ECMO can provide all the respiratory support required by some patients. Ventilators can then be adjusted to provide very minimum ventilation. The optimal setting and how long a patient should be maintained in ECMO are still under investigation (Tonna et al., 2021).

CONCLUSION

The study of lung mechanics has substantially contributed to development of knowledge of respiratory diseases. It was also a cornerstone in the creation and evolution of mechanical ventilation. The combination of basic, translational and applied sciences has proved very useful in respiratory physiology leading not only to better understanding physiopathology but also to designing supportive treatment. In the years to come, we expect this partnership to continue as we face new challenges in managing patients with respiratory failure.

AUTHOR CONTRIBUTIONS

PB, FD, IT, and MM contributed to conception and design of the study. HM and RR wrote sections of the manuscript. All authors contributed to manuscript revision, read, and approved the submitted version.

REFERENCES

Akoumianaki, E., Maggiore, S. M., Valenza, F., Bellani, G., Jubran, A., and Loring, S. H. (2014). The Application of Esophageal Pressure Measurement in Patients with Respiratory Failure. *Am. J. Respir. Crit. Care Med.* 189, 520–531. doi:10.1164/rccm.201312-2193CI

Amato, M. B., Barbas, C. S., Medeiros, D. M., Magaldi, R. B., Schettino, G. P., Lorenzi-Filho, G., et al. (1998). Effect of a Protective-Ventilation Strategy on Mortality in the Acute Respiratory Distress Syndrome. *N. Engl. J. Med.* 338, 347–354. doi:10.1056/NEJM199802053380602

Amato, M. B. P., Meade, M. O., Slutsky, A. S., Brochard, L., Costa, E. L. v., Schoenfeld, D. A., et al. (2015). Driving Pressure and Survival in the Acute Respiratory Distress Syndrome. *N. Engl. J. Med.* 372, 747–755. doi:10.1056/NEJMsa1410639

Aristoteles, L. R. C. R. B., Righetti, R. F., Pinheiro, N. M., Franco, R. B., Starling, C. M., da Silva, J. C. P., et al. (2013). Modulation of the Oscillatory Mechanics of Lung Tissue and the Oxidative Stress Response Induced by Arginase Inhibition in a Chronic Allergic Inflammation Model. *BMC Pulm. Med.* 13, 52. doi:10.1186/1471-2466-13-52

Ashbaugh, D. G., Petty, T. L., Bigelow, D. B., and Harris, T. M. (1969). Continuous Positive-Pressure Breathing (CPPB) in Adult Respiratory Distress Syndrome. *J. Thorac. Cardiovasc Surg.* 57, 31–41. doi:10.1016/s0022-5223(19)42760-8

Ashbaugh, D. G., Boyd Bigelow, D., Petty, T. L., and Levine, B. E. (1967). Acute Respiratory Distress in Adults. *Lancet* 290. doi:10.1016/S0140-6736(67)90168-7

Barbaro, R. P., MacLaren, G., Boonstra, P. S., Iwashyna, T. J., Slutsky, A. S., Fan, E., et al. (2020). Extracorporeal Membrane Oxygenation Support in COVID-19: an International Cohort Study of the Extracorporeal Life Support Organization Registry. *Lancet* 396, 1071–1078. doi:10.1016/S0140-6736(20)32008-0

Barnes, T., Zochios, V., and Parhar, K. (2018). Re-examining Permissive Hypercapnia in ARDS: A Narrative Review. *Chest* 154. doi:10.1016/j.chest.2017.11.010

Bates, J. H. T., and Irvin, C. G. (2003). Measuring Lung Function in Mice: The Phenotyping Uncertainty Principle. *J. Appl. Physiology* 94, 1297–1306. doi:10.1152/japplphysiol.00706.2002

Bates, J. H. T. (2009). *Lung Mechanics: An Inverse Modeling Approach.* Cambridge University Press. doi:10.1017/CBO9780511627156

Bates, J. (2005). "Measuring Techniques in Respiratory Mechanics," in *Physiologic Basis of Respiratory Disease.* Editors Q. Hamid, J. Shannon, and J. Martin, 623–637.

Baydur, A., Behrakis, P. K., Zin, W. A., Jaeger, M. J., and Milic-Emili, J. (1982). Simple Method for Assessing the Validity of the Esophageal Balloon Technique. *Am. Rev. Respir. Dis.*, 126788–791. doi:10.1164/arrd.1982.126.5.788

Beitler, J. R., Sarge, T., Banner-Goodspeed, V. M., Gong, M. N., Cook, D., Novack, V., et al. (2019). Effect of Titrating Positive End-Expiratory Pressure (PEEP) with an Esophageal Pressure-Guided Strategy vs an Empirical High PEEP-F Io 2 Strategy on Death and Days Free from Mechanical Ventilation Among Patients with Acute Respiratory Distress Syndrome: A Randomized Clinical Trial. *JAMA - J. Am. Med. Assoc.* 321 (9), 846–857. doi:10.1001/jama.2019.0555

Boscolo, A., Sella, N., Lorenzoni, G., Pettenuzzo, T., Pasin, L., Pretto, C., et al. (2021). Static Compliance and Driving Pressure Are Associated with ICU Mortality in Intubated COVID-19 ARDS. *Crit. Care* 25, 263. doi:10.1186/s13054-021-03667-6

Brochard, L., Slutsky, A., and Pesenti, A. (2017). Mechanical Ventilation to Minimize Progression of Lung Injury in Acute Respiratory Failure. *Am. J. Respir. Crit. Care Med.* 195, 438–442. doi:10.1164/rccm.201605-1081CP

Brower, R. G., Hopkins Uni-versity, J., Lanken, P. N., MacIntyre, N., Matthay, M. A., Morris, A., et al. (2004). Higher versus Lower Positive End-Expiratory Pressures in Patients with the Acute Respiratory Distress Syndrome the Members of the Writing Committee. *N. Engl. J. Med.* 351 (4), 327–336. Available at: www.ardsnet.org. doi:10.1056/NEJMoa032193

Cabello, B., and Mancebo, J. (2006). Work of Breathing. *Intensive Care Med.* 32, 1311–1314. doi:10.1007/s00134-006-0278-3

Camargo, L. do N., Santos, T. M. dos, Andrade, F. C. P. de, Fukuzaki, S., dos Santos Lopes, F. D. T. Q., de Arruda Martins, M., et al. (2020). Bronchial Vascular Remodeling Is Attenuated by Anti-IL-17 in Asthmatic Responses Exacerbated by LPS. *Front. Pharmacol.* 11. doi:10.3389/fphar.2020.01269

Carlton, D. P., Cummings, J. J., Scheerer, R. G., Poulain, F. R., and Bland, R. D. (1990). Lung Overexpansion Increases Pulmonary Microvascular Protein Permeability in Young Lambs. *J. Appl. Physiology* 69, 577–583. doi:10.1152/jappl.1990.69.2.577

Chen, L., del Sorbo, L., Grieco, D. L., Junhasavasdikul, D., Rittayamai, N., Soliman, I., et al. (2020). Potential for Lung Recruitment Estimated by the Recruitment-To-Inflation Ratio in Acute Respiratory Distress Syndrome a Clinical Trial. *Am. J. Respir. Crit. Care Med.* 201, 178–187. doi:10.1164/rccm.201902-0334OC

Chiumello, D., Carlesso, E., Cadringher, P., Caironi, P., Valenza, F., Polli, F., et al. (2008). Lung Stress and Strain during Mechanical Ventilation for Acute Respiratory Distress Syndrome. *Am. J. Respir. Crit. Care Med.* 178, 346–355. doi:10.1164/rccm.200710-1589OC

Collett, P. W., Perry, C., and Engel, L. A. (1985). Pressure-time Product, Flow, and Oxygen Cost of Resistive Breathing in Humans. *J. Appl. Physiology* 58, 1263–1272. doi:10.1152/jappl.1985.58.4.1263

Combes, A., Hajage, D., Capellier, G., Demoule, A., Lavoué, S., Guervilly, C., et al. (2018). Extracorporeal Membrane Oxygenation for Severe Acute Respiratory Distress Syndrome. *N. Engl. J. Med.* 378. doi:10.1056/nejmoa1800385

Coppadoro, A., Grassi, A., Giovannoni, C., Rabboni, F., Eronia, N., Bronco, A., et al. (2020). Occurrence of Pendelluft under Pressure Support Ventilation in Patients Who Failed a Spontaneous Breathing Trial: an Observational Study. *Ann. Intensive Care* 10. doi:10.1186/s13613-020-00654-y

Corbridge, T. C., Wood, L. D. H., Crawford, G. P., Chudoba, M. J., Yanos, J., and Sznajder, J. I. (1990). Adverse Effects of Large Tidal Volume and Low PEEP in Canine Acid Aspiration. *Am. Rev. Respir. Dis.* 142. doi:10.1164/ajrccm/142.2.311

Costa, E. L. V., Lima, P. G., and Amato, M. B. R. (2009). Electrical Impedance Tomography. *Curr. Opin. Crit. Care* 15. doi:10.1097/MCC.0b013e3283220e8c

Costa, E. L. V., Slutsky, A. S., Brochard, L. J., Brower, R., Serpa-Neto, A., Cavalcanti, A. B., et al. (2021). Ventilatory Variables and Mechanical Power in Patients with Acute Respiratory Distress Syndrome. *Am. J. Respir. Crit. Care Med.* 204, 303–311. doi:10.1164/rccm.202009-3467OC

Deibele, J. M., Luepschen, H., and Leonhardt, S. (2008). Dynamic Separation of Pulmonary and Cardiac Changes in Electrical Impedance Tomography. *Physiol. Meas.* 29. doi:10.1088/0967-3334/29/6/S01

Dellamonica, J., Lerolle, N., Sargentini, C., Beduneau, G., di Marco, F., Mercat, A., et al. (2011). Accuracy and Precision of End-Expiratory Lung-Volume Measurements by Automated Nitrogen Washout/washin Technique in Patients with Acute Respiratory Distress Syndrome. *Crit. Care* 15. doi:10.1186/cc10587

Determann, R. M., Royakkers, A., Wolthuis, E. K., Vlaar, A. P., Choi, G., Paulus, F., et al. (2010). Ventilation with Lower Tidal Volumes as Compared with Conventional Tidal Volumes for Patients without Acute Lung Injury: A Preventive Randomized Controlled Trial. *Crit. Care* 14. doi:10.1186/cc8230

Dodd, D. S., Yarom, J., Loring, S. H., and Engel, L. A. (1988). O2 Cost of Inspiratory and Expiratory Resistive Breathing in Humans. *J. Appl. Physiology* 65. doi:10.1152/jappl.1988.65.6.2518

Dreyfuss, D., and Saumon, G. (1993). Role of Tidal Volume, FRC, and End-Inspiratory Volume in the Development of Pulmonary Edema Following Mechanical Ventilation. *Am. Rev. Respir. Dis.* 148. doi:10.1164/ajrccm/148.5.1194

Ebihara, T., Venkatesan, N., Tanaka, R., and Ludwig, M. S. (2000). Changes in Extracellular Matrix and Tissue Viscoelasticity in Bleomycin-Induced Lung Fibrosis: Temporal Aspects. *Am. J. Respir. Crit. Care Med.* 162. doi:10.1164/ajrccm.162.4.9912011

Faffe, D. S., and Zin, W. A. (2009). Lung Parenchymal Mechanics in Health and Disease. *Physiol. Rev.* 89. doi:10.1152/physrev.00019.2007

Ferluga, M., Lucangelo, U., and Blanch, L. (2018). Dead Space in Acute Respiratory Distress Syndrome. *Ann. Transl. Med.* 6. doi:10.21037/atm.2018.09.46

Fietzek, P. P., and Kuehn, K. (1976). The Primary Structure of Collagen. *Int. Rev. Connect. Tissue Res.* 7. doi:10.1016/b978-0-12-363707-9.50007-1

Fuller, B. M., Mohr, N. M., Drewry, A. M., and Carpenter, C. R. (2013). Lower Tidal Volume at Initiation of Mechanical Ventilation May Reduce Progression to Acute Respiratory Distress Syndrome: A Systematic Review. *Crit. Care* 17. doi:10.1186/cc11936

Gattinoni, L., Chiumello, D., Caironi, P., Busana, M., Romitti, F., Brazzi, L., et al. (2020a). COVID-19 Pneumonia: Different Respiratory Treatments for

Different Phenotypes? *Intensive Care Med.* 46. doi:10.1007/s00134-020-06033-2

Gattinoni, L., Coppola, S., Cressoni, M., Busana, M., Rossi, S., and Chiumello, D. (2020b). COVID-19 Does Not Lead to a "Typical" Acute Respiratory Distress Syndrome. *Am. J. Respir. Crit. Care Med.* 201, 1299–1300. doi:10.1164/rccm.202003-0817LE

Gattinoni, L., Tonetti, T., Cressoni, M., Cadringher, P., Herrmann, P., Moerer, O., et al. (2016). Ventilator-related Causes of Lung Injury: the Mechanical Power. *Intensive Care Med.* 42, 1567–1575. doi:10.1007/s00134-016-4505-2

Girard, T. D., Kress, J. P., Fuchs, B. D., Thomason, J. W., Schweickert, W. D., Pun, B. T., et al. (2008). Efficacy and Safety of a Paired Sedation and Ventilator Weaning Protocol for Mechanically Ventilated Patients in Intensive Care (Awakening and Breathing Controlled Trial): a Randomised Controlled Trial. *Lancet* 371, 126–134. doi:10.1016/S0140-6736(08)60105-1

Griffiths, M. J. D., McAuley, D. F., Perkins, G. D., Barrett, N., Blackwood, B., Boyle, A., et al. (2019). Guidelines on the Management of Acute Respiratory Distress Syndrome. *BMJ Open Respir. Res.* 6, e000420. doi:10.1136/bmjresp-2019-000420

Grinnan, D. C., and Truwit, J. D. (2005). Clinical Review: Respiratory Mechanics in Spontaneous and Assisted Ventilation. *Crit. Care* 9, 472–484. doi:10.1186/cc3516

Guttmann, J., Eberhard, L., Fabry, B., Bertschmann, W., and Wolff, G. (1993). Continuous Calculation of Intratracheal Pressure in Tracheally Intubated Patients. *Anesthesiology* 79. doi:10.1097/00000542-199309000-00014

Hantos, Z., Daroczy, B., Suki, B., Nagy, S., and Fredberg, J. J. (1992). Input Impedance and Peripheral Inhomogeneity of Dog Lungs. *J. Appl. Physiology* 72. doi:10.1152/jappl.1992.72.1.168

Hantos, Z. (2021). Intra-breath Oscillometry for Assessing Respiratory Outcomes. *Curr. Opin. Physiology* 22. doi:10.1016/j.cophys.2021.05.004

Henderson, W. R., Chen, L., Amato, M. B. P., and Brochard, L. J. (2017). Fifty Years of Research in ARDS: Respiratory Mechanics in Acute Respiratory Distress Syndrome. *Am. J. Respir. Crit. Care Med.* 196, 822–833. doi:10.1164/rccm.201612-2495CI

Irvin, C. G., and Bates, J. H. T. (2003). Measuring the Lung Function in the Mouse: The Challenge of Size. *Respir. Res.* 4. doi:10.1186/rr199

Ito, J. T., de Brito Cervilha, D. A., Lourenço, J. D., Gonçalves, N. G., Volpini, R. A., Caldini, E. G., et al. (2019a). Th17/Treg Imbalance in COPD Progression: A Temporal Analysis Using a CS-Induced Model. *PLoS ONE* 14. doi:10.1371/journal.pone.0209351

Ito, J. T., Lourenço, J. D., Righetti, R. F., Tibério, I. F. L. C., Prado, C. M., and Lopes, F. D. T. Q. S. (2019b). Extracellular Matrix Component Remodeling in Respiratory Diseases: What Has Been Found in Clinical and Experimental Studies? *Cells* 8, 342. doi:10.3390/cells8040342

Jonkman, A. H., Rauseo, M., Carteaux, G., Telias, I., Sklar, M. C., Heunks, L., et al. (2020). Proportional Modes of Ventilation: Technology to Assist Physiology. *Intensive Care Med.* 46. doi:10.1007/s00134-020-06206-z

Kacmarek, R. M. (2011). The Mechanical Ventilator: Past, Present, and Future. *Respir. Care* 56, 1170–1180. doi:10.4187/respcare.01420

Karbing, D. S., Panigada, M., Bottino, N., Spinelli, E., Protti, A., Rees, S. E., et al. (2020). Changes in Shunt, Ventilation/perfusion Mismatch, and Lung Aeration with PEEP in Patients with ARDS: A Prospective Single-Arm Interventional Study. *Crit. Care* 24. doi:10.1186/s13054-020-2834-6

Khan, Y. A., Fan, E., and Ferguson, N. D. (2021). Precision Medicine and Heterogeneity of Treatment Effect in Therapies for ARDS. *Chest* 160. doi:10.1016/j.chest.2021.07.009

King, G. G., Bates, J., Berger, K. I., Calverley, P., de Melo, P. L., Dellacà, R. L., et al. (2020). Technical Standards for Respiratory Oscillometry. *Eur. Respir. J.* 55. doi:10.1183/13993003.00753-2019

Koenders, C. M. A. (2009). Wave Propagation through Elastic Granular and Granular Auxetic Materials. *Phys. Status Solidi (B) Basic Res.* 246. doi:10.1002/pssb.200982039

Kress, J. P., Pohlman, A. S., O'Connor, M. F., and Hall, J. B. (2000). Daily Interruption of Sedative Infusions in Critically Ill Patients Undergoing Mechanical Ventilation. *N. Engl. J. Med.* 342, 1471–1477. doi:10.1056/NEJM200005183422002

Lanças, T., Kasahara, D. I., Prado, C. M., Tibério, I. F. L. C., Martins, M. A., and Dolhnikoff, M. (2006). Comparison of Early and Late Responses to Antigen of Sensitized guinea Pig Parenchymal Lung Strips. *J. Appl. Physiology* 100. doi:10.1152/japplphysiol.00828.2005

Leite-Júnior, J. H., Rocco, P. R. M., Faffe, D. S., Romero, P. v., and Zin, W. A. (2003). On the Preparation of Lung Strip for Tissue Mechanics Measurement. *Respir. Physiology Neurobiol.* 134. doi:10.1016/S1569-9048(02)00217-3

L'Her, E. (2012). Automatic Tube Compensation: Is it Worthwhile? *Respir. Care* 57. doi:10.4187/respcare.01865

Ludwig, M. S., and Dallaire, M. J. (1994). Structural Composition of Lung Parenchymal Strip and Mechanical Behavior during Sinusoidal Oscillation. *J. Appl. Physiology* 77. doi:10.1152/jappl.1994.77.4.2029

Lundblad, L. K. A., and Robichaud, A. (2021). Oscillometry of the Respiratory System. A Translational Opportunity Not to be missed. *Am. J. Physiology - Lung Cell. Mol. Physiology* 320. doi:10.1152/AJPLUNG.00222.2020

Maciejewski, D., Putowski, Z., Czok, M., and Krzych, Ł. J. (2021). Electrical impedance tomography as a tool for monitoring mechanical ventilation. An introduction to the technique. *Adv. Med. Sci.* 66. doi:10.1016/j.advms.2021.07.010

Macintyre, N. R. (2016). Lung protective ventilator strategies: Beyond scaling tidal volumes to ideal lung size. *Crit. Care Med.* 44. doi:10.1097/CCM.0000000000001454

Mador, M. J. (1991). Respiratory muscle fatigue and breathing pattern. *Chest* 100. doi:10.1378/chest.100.5.1430

Marini, J. J. (2011). Dynamic hyperinflation and auto-positive end-expiratory pressure lessons learned over 30 years. *Am. J. Respir. Crit. Care Med.* 184, 756–762. doi:10.1164/rccm.201102-0226PP

Martin, R. J. (2008). Exploring the distal lung: New direction in asthma. *Israel Med. Assoc. J.* 10 (12), 846–849.

Mattingley, J. S., Holets, S. R., Oeckler, R. A., Stroetz, R. W., Buck, C. F., and Hubmayr, R. D. (2011). Sizing the lung of mechanically ventilated patients. *Crit. Care* 15, R60. doi:10.1186/cc10034

Mauad, T., Silva, L. F. F., Santos, M. A., Grinberg, L., Bernardi, F. D. C., Martins, M. A., et al. (2004). Abnormal alveolar attachments with decreased elastic fiber content in distal lung in fatal asthma. *Am. J. Respir. Crit. Care Med.* 170. doi:10.1164/rccm.200403-305OC

Mead, J., Lindgren, I., and Gaensler, E. A. (1955). The mechanical properties of the lungs in emphysema. *J. Clin. Investig.* 34. doi:10.1172/jci103150

Meyer, N. J., Gattinoni, L., and Calfee, C. S. (2021). Acute respiratory distress syndrome. *Lancet* 398, 622–637. doi:10.1016/S0140-6736(21)00439-6

Morales-Quinteros, L., Schultz, M. J., Bringué, J., Calfee, C. S., Camprubí, M., Cremer, O. L., et al. (2019). Estimated dead space fraction and the ventilatory ratio are associated with mortality in early ARDS. *Ann. Intensive Care* 9, 128. doi:10.1186/s13613-019-0601-0

Murray, J. F., Matthay, M. A., Luce, J. M., and Flick, M. R. (1988). An expanded definition of the adult respiratory distress syndrome. *Am. Rev. Respir. Dis.* 138, 720–723. doi:10.1164/ajrccm/138.3.720

Nakashima, A. S., Prado, C. M., Lanças, T., Ruiz, V. C., Kasahara, D. I., Leick-Maldonado, E. A., et al. (2008). Oral tolerance attenuates changes in *In Vitro* lung tissue mechanics and extracellular matrix remodeling induced by chronic allergic inflammation in guinea pigs. *J. Appl. Physiology* 104, 1778–1785. doi:10.1152/japplphysiol.00830.2007

Neto, A. S., Cardoso, S. O., Manetta, J. A., Pereira, V. G. M., Espósito, D. C., Pasqualucci, M. D. O. P., et al. (2012). Association between use of lung-protective ventilation with lower tidal volumes and clinical outcomes among patients without acute respiratory distress syndrome: A meta-analysis. *JAMA - J. Am. Med. Assoc.* 308. doi:10.1001/jama.2012.13730

Nguyen, D. T., Jin, C., Thiagalingam, A., and McEwan, A. L. (2012). A review on electrical impedance tomography for pulmonary perfusion imaging. *Physiol. Meas.* 33. doi:10.1088/0967-3334/33/5/695

Olegård, C., Söndergaard, S., Houltz, E., Lundin, S., and Stenqvist, O. (2005). Estimation of functional residual capacity at the bedside using standard monitoring equipment: A modified nitrogen washout/washin technique requiring a small change of the inspired oxygen fraction. *Anesth. Analgesia* 101. doi:10.1213/01.ANE.0000165823.90368.55

Otis, A. B. (1977). Pressure-flow relationships and power output of breathing. *Respir. Physiol.* 30. doi:10.1016/0034-5687(77)90017-2

Panwar, R., Madotto, F., Laffey, J. G., and van Haren, F. M. P. (2020). Compliance phenotypes in early acute respiratory distress syndrome before the COVID-19 pandemic. *Am. J. Respir. Crit. Care Med.* 202. doi:10.1164/rccm.202005-2046OC

Papazian, L., Aubron, C., Brochard, L., Chiche, J. D., Combes, A., Dreyfuss, D., et al. (2019). Formal guidelines: management of acute respiratory distress syndrome. *Ann. Intensive Care* 9. doi:10.1186/s13613-019-0540-9

Parker, J. C., Hernandez, L. A., Longenecker, G. L., Peevy, K., and Johnson, W. (1990a). Lung edema caused by high peak inspiratory pressures in dogs. Role of increased microvascular filtration pressure and permeability. *Am. Rev. Respir. Dis.* 142. doi:10.1164/ajrccm/142.2.321

Parker, J. C., Hernandez, L. A., Longenecker, G. L., Peevy, K., and Johnson, W. (1990b). Lung edema caused by high peak inspiratory pressures in dogs. Role of increased microvascular filtration pressure and permeability. *Am. Rev. Respir. Dis.* 142. doi:10.1164/ajrccm/142.2.321

Pelosi, P., Ball, L., Barbas, C. S. V., Bellomo, R., Burns, K. E. A., Einav, S., et al. (2021). Personalized mechanical ventilation in acute respiratory distress syndrome. *Crit. Care* 25. doi:10.1186/s13054-021-03686-3

Pepe, P. E., and Marini, J. J. (1982). Occult positive end-expiratory pressure in mechanically ventilated patients with airflow obstruction: the auto-PEEP effect. *Am. Rev. Respir. Dis.* 126, 166–170. doi:10.1164/arrd.1982.126.1.166

Peterson-Carmichael, S., Seddon, P. C., Cheifetz, I. M., Frerichs, I., Hall, G. L., Hammer, J., et al. (2016). An official American thoracic society/european respiratory society workshop report: Evaluation of respiratory mechanics and function in the pediatric and neonatal intensive care units. *Ann. Am. Thorac. Soc.* 13, S1–S11. doi:10.1513/AnnalsATS.201511-730ST

Pham, T., Brochard, L. J., and Slutsky, A. S. (2017). Mechanical Ventilation: State of the Art. *Mayo Clin. Proc.* 92, 1382–1400. doi:10.1016/j.mayocp.2017.05.004

Pigati, P. A., Righetti, R. F., Possa, S. S., Romanholo, B. S., Rodrigues, A. P. D., dos Santos, A. S. A., et al. (2015). Y-27632 is associated with corticosteroid-potentiated control of pulmonary remodeling and inflammation in guinea pigs with chronic allergic inflammation. *BMC Pulm. Med.* 15. doi:10.1186/s12890-015-0073-4

Pinsky, M. R. (2018). Cardiopulmonary interactions: Physiologic basis and clinical applications. *Ann. Am. Thorac. Soc.* doi:10.1513/AnnalsATS.201704-339FR

Pohlman, M. C., McCallister, K. E., Schweickert, W. D., Pohlman, A. S., Nigos, C. P., Krishnan, J. A., et al. (2008). Excessive tidal volume from breath stacking during lung-protective ventilation for acute lung injury. *Crit. Care Med.* 36. doi:10.1097/CCM.0b013e31818b308b

Possa, S. S., Charafeddine, H. T., Righetti, R. F., da Silva, P. A., Almeida-Reis, R., Saraiva-Romanholo, B. M., et al. (2012). Rho-kinase inhibition attenuates airway responsiveness, inflammation, matrix remodeling, and oxidative stress activation induced by chronic inflammation. *Am. J. Physiology - Lung Cell. Mol. Physiology* 303. doi:10.1152/ajplung.00034.2012

Rahn, H., Otis, A., and Fenn, W. O. (1946). The pressure-volume diagram of the thorax and lung. *Fed. Proc.* 5. doi:10.1152/ajplegacy.1946.146.2.161

Ranieri, V. M., Rubenfeld, G. D., Thompson, B. T., Ferguson, N. D., Caldwell, E., Fan, E., et al. (2012). Acute respiratory distress syndrome: The Berlin definition. *JAMA - J. Am. Med. Assoc.* 307. doi:10.1001/jama.2012.5669

Reade, M. C., and Finfer, S. (2014). Sedation and Delirium in the Intensive Care Unit. *N. Engl. J. Med.* 370, 444–454. doi:10.1056/nejmra1208705

Reddy, R. M., and Guntupalli, K. K. (2007). Review of ventilatory techniques to optimize mechanical ventilation in acute exacerbation of chronic obstructive pulmonary disease. *Int. J. COPD* 2.

Reinert, M., and Trendelenburg, F. (1972). Correlation between parameters of breathing mechanics, respiratory gases and blood gases in patients with chronic bronchial obstruction. *Respiration* 29. doi:10.1159/000192889

Repessé, X., and Vieillard-Baron, A. (2017). Hypercapnia during acute respiratory distress syndrome: The tree that hides the forest. *J. Thorac. Dis.* 9. doi:10.21037/jtd.2017.05.69

Righetti, R. F., Pigati, P. A. da S., Possa, S. S., Habrum, F. C., Xisto, D. G., Antunes, M. A., et al. (2014). Effects of Rho-kinase inhibition in lung tissue with chronic inflammation. *Respir. Physiology Neurobiol.* 192. doi:10.1016/j.resp.2013.12.012

Rocco, P. R. M., Silva, P. L., Samary, C. S., Hayat Syed, M. K., and Marini, J. J. (2020). Elastic power but Not driving power is the key promoter of ventilator-induced lung injury in experimental acute respiratory distress syndrome. *Crit. Care* 24. doi:10.1186/s13054-020-03011-4

Santos, F. B., Garcia, C. S. N. B., Xisto, D. G., Negri, E. M., Capelozzi, V. L., Faffe, D. S., et al. (2008). Effects of amiodarone on lung tissue mechanics and parenchyma remodeling. *Respir. Physiology Neurobiol.* 162. doi:10.1016/j.resp.2008.05.004

Shifren, A., Woods, J. C., Rosenbluth, D. B., Officer, S., Cooper, J. D., and Pierce, R. A. (2007). Upregulation of elastin expression in constrictive bronchiolitis obliterans. *Int. J. COPD* 2.

Silva, P. L., Ball, L., Rocco, P. R. M., and Pelosi, P. (2019). Power to mechanical power to minimize ventilator-induced lung injury? *Intensive Care Med. Exp.* 7. doi:10.1186/s40635-019-0243-4

Simonis, F. D., Serpa Neto, A., Binnekade, J. M., Braber, A., Bruin, K. C. M., Determann, R. M., et al. (2018). Effect of a Low vs Intermediate Tidal Volume Strategy on Ventilator-Free Days in Intensive Care Unit Patients Without ARDS: A Randomized Clinical Trial. *JAMA - J. Am. Med. Assoc.* 320, 1872–1880. doi:10.1001/jama.2018.14280

Sinderby, C., Navalesi, P., Beck, J., Skrobik, Y., Comtois, N., Friberg, S., et al. (1999). Neural control of mechanical ventilation in respiratory failure. *Nat. Med.* 5. doi:10.1038/71012

Sjoding, M. W., Admon, A. J., Saha, A. K., Kay, S. G., Brown, C. A., Co, I., et al. (2021). Comparing Clinical Features and Outcomes in Mechanically Ventilated Patients with COVID-19 and the Acute Respiratory Distress Syndrome. *Ann. Am. Thorac. Soc.* 18 (11), 1876–1885. doi:10.1513/annalsats.202008-1076oc

Sottile, P. D., Albers, D., Smith, B. J., and Moss, M. M. (2020). Ventilator dyssynchrony-Detection, pathophysiology, and clinical relevance: A Narrative review. *Ann. Thorac. Med.* 15, 190–198. doi:10.4103/atm.ATM_63_20

Starling, C. M., Prado, C. M., Leick-Maldonado, E. A., Lanças, T., Reis, F. G., Aristóteles, L. R. C. B. R., et al. (2009). Inducible nitric oxide synthase inhibition attenuates lung tissue responsiveness and remodeling in a model of chronic pulmonary inflammation in guinea pigs. *Respir. Physiology Neurobiol.* 165. doi:10.1016/j.resp.2008.11.011

Suki, B., and Bates, J. H. T. (2008). Extracellular matrix mechanics in lung parenchymal diseases. *Respir. Physiology Neurobiol.* 163. doi:10.1016/j.resp.2008.03.015

Talmor, D., Sarge, T., Malhotra, A., O'Donnell, C. R., Ritz, R., Lisbon, A., et al. (2008). Mechanical Ventilation Guided by Esophageal Pressure in Acute Lung Injury. *N. Engl. J. Med.* 359, 2095–2104. doi:10.1056/nejmoa0708638

The Acute Respiratory Distress Syndrome Network (2000). Ventilation with lower tidal volumes as compared with traditional tidal volumes for acute lung injury and the acute respiratory distress syndrome. The Acute Respiratory Distress Syndrome Network. *N. Engl. J. Med.* 342, 1301–1308. doi:10.1056/NEJM200005043421801

Tobin, M. J. (2020). Does Making a Diagnosis of ARDS in Patients With Coronavirus Disease 2019 Matter? *Chest* 158, 2275–2277. doi:10.1016/j.chest.2020.07.028

Tobin, M. J., Laghi, F., and Jubran, A. (2020). Caution about early intubation and mechanical ventilation in COVID-19. *Ann. Intensive Care* 10, 78. doi:10.1186/s13613-020-00692-6

Tonna, J. E., Abrams, D., Brodie, D., Greenwood, J. C., Rubio Mateo-Sidron, J. A., Usman, A., et al. (2021). Management of Adult Patients Supported with Venovenous Extracorporeal Membrane Oxygenation (VV ECMO): Guideline from the Extracorporeal Life Support Organization (ELSO). *ASAIO J.* doi:10.1097/MAT.0000000000001432

Tulić, M. K., and Hamid, Q. (2003). Contribution of the distal lung to the pathologic and physiologic changes in asthma: Potential therapeutic target - Roger S. Mitchell Lecture. *Chest* 123 348S–355S. doi:10.1378/chest.123.3_suppl.348S

Tusman, G., Gogniat, E., Madorno, M., Otero, P., Dianti, J., Ceballos, I. F., et al. (2020). Effect of PEEP on dead space in an experimental model of ARDS. *Respir. Care* 65, 11–20. doi:10.4187/respcare.06843

Umbrello, M., Marino, A., and Chiumello, D. (2017). Tidal volume in acute respiratory distress syndrome: How best to select it. *Ann. Transl. Med.* 5, 287. doi:10.21037/atm.2017.06.51

Wagner, P. D. (2008). The multiple inert gas elimination technique (MIGET). *Intensive Care Med.* 34. doi:10.1007/s00134-008-1108-6

Wang, C. G., Dimaria, G., Bates, J. H. T., Guttmann, R. D., and Martin, J. G. (1986). Methacholine-induced airway reactivity of inbred rats. *J. Appl. Physiology* 61. doi:10.1152/jappl.1986.61.6.2180

Wanner, A., Abraham, W. M., Douglas, J. S., Drazen, J. M., Richerson, H. B., and Ram, J. S. (1990). Models of airway hyperresponsiveness. in American Review of Respiratory Disease. doi:10.1164/ajrccm/141.1.253

Wanner, A., and Abraham, W. M. (1982). Experimental models of asthma. *Lung* 160, 231–243. doi:10.1007/BF02719297

Xisto, D. G., Farias, L. L., Ferreira, H. C., Picanço, M. R., Amitrano, D., Lapa E Silva, J. R., et al. (2005). Lung parenchyma remodeling in a murine model of chronic allergic inflammation. *Am. J. Respir. Crit. Care Med.* 171. doi:10.1164/rccm.200408-997OC

Yoshida, T., Torsani, V., Gomes, S., Santis, R. R. D., Beraldo, M. A., Costa, E. L. V., et al. (2013). Spontaneous effort causes occult pendelluft during mechanical ventilation. *Am. J. Respir. Crit. Care Med.* 188. doi:10.1164/rccm.201303-0539OC

Younes, M. (1992). Proportional assist ventilation, a new approach to ventilatory support: Theory. *Am. Rev. Respir. Dis.* 145. doi:10.1164/ajrccm/145.1.114

Ziehr, D. R., Alladina, J., Petri, C. R., Maley, J. H., Moskowitz, A., Medoff, B. D., et al. (2020). Respiratory pathophysiology of mechanically ventilated patients with COVID-19: A cohort study. *Am. J. Respir. Crit. Care Med.* 201. doi:10.1164/rccm.202004-1163LE

15

FGF Signaling in Lung Development and Disease: Human Versus Mouse

*Soula Danopoulos, Jessica Shiosaki and Denise Al Alam**

Saban Research Institute, Children's Hospital Los Angeles, Los Angeles, CA, United States

Correspondence:
Denise Al Alam
dalalam@chla.usc.edu

Fibroblast growth factor 10 (FGF10) plays an important role in mouse lung development, injury, and repair. It is considered the main morphogen driving lung branching morphogenesis in rodents. While many studies have found FGF10 SNPs associated with COPD and branch variants in COPD smokers, there is no evidence of a causative role for FGF10 or these SNPs in human lung development and pediatric lung diseases. We and others have shown divergent roles for FGF10 in mouse lung development and early human lung development. Herein, we only review the existing literature on FGF signaling in human lung development and pediatric human lung diseases, comparing what is known in mouse lung to that in human lung.

Keywords: FGF10, human lung, development, disease, FGF signaling

INTRODUCTION

The mammalian lung is derived from invagination of the foregut endoderm that ultimately forms the primitive lung buds. These buds undergo a series of branching, proliferation, and differentiation to eventually become a fully functioning air exchange organ. Stages of lung development are thought to be comparable among mammalian species, primarily between humans and rodents, thus making rodents a very widely used model to study lung development and disease. The knowledge gained from rodent studies has been crucial in advancing our understanding of basic biological processes in the lung. However, in light of the low success rate in clinical trials [14% reported in 2018 (Wong et al., 2018)], the necessity to better understand human lung biology has become increasingly important.

Although there are numerous similarities between the mouse and human lung, many differences have also been noted at the structural, cellular, and molecular levels. Grossly, the structure, size, and scale of the lung are notably different between the two species. Although they are both five lobed units, the mouse lung comprises a single large left lobe and four right lobes (cranial lobe, middle lobe, caudal lobe, and accessory lobe), whereas the human lung has two left lobes (superior lobe of left lung and inferior lobe of left lung) and three right lobes (superior lobe of right lung, middle lobe of right lung, and inferior lobe of right lung). Embedded in these lobes is the highly structured, arborized, epithelial tree. Starting from the trachea as generation 0 and moving down to the bronchioles, the human lung contains a total of 17–21 branch generations, whereas in mouse, there are only 13–17 branch generations (Irvin and Bates, 2003). This also reflects differences in total lung capacity, alveolar numbers and volume. The total lung capacity is 6×10^3 ml in adult humans compared to 1 ml in adult mouse (Irvin and Bates, 2003). The volume of one alveolus is 4.2×10^6 μm³ in humans compared to 2.2×10^4 μm³ in mouse (Wansleeben et al., 2013), and the estimated average number of alveoli is 4.8×10^8 in humans compared to 2.31×10^6 in mouse (Ochs et al., 2004; Knust et al., 2009). In addition to the very apparent differences in size and structure, there have also been multiple cellular and molecular differences that have been described during development and adulthood. For instance, cartilaginous rings are restricted to the trachea and main bronchi in mouse, whereas in humans, these extend into the bronchioles (**Figure 1**). Similarly, submucosal glands are only present in the upper part of the mouse trachea, whereas in humans, they extend further down into the respiratory bronchioles. Differences in epithelial structure and cell type distribution are further detailed in **Figure 1**. These changes in cellular composition result in different molecular interactions and expression patterns.

For years, it was well-established that the progenitor cell population of the proximal epithelium in the developing mouse lung is Sox2+, whereas that of the distal epithelium is solely Sox9+. We and others have demonstrated that during the pseudoglandular stage of human lung development, the distal epithelial cells express a double positive SOX2/SOX9 progenitor cell population that is no longer present during the canalicular stage of development, suggesting its importance to human lung branching morphogenesis (**Figure 2**) (Nikolic et al., 2017; Miller et al., 2018; Danopoulos et al., 2018a). This difference of progenitor cell populations is accompanied by a change in smooth muscle cell expression. In mouse, ACTA2+ cells are primarily localized in the proximal region of the epithelium, surrounding the Sox2+ cells, whereas in humans, we showed that the ACTA2+ cells extend to the most distal region of the developing lung, surrounding the SOX2+ cells of the proximal epithelium, as well as being located between the clefts of branch points, yet not extending into the region of the SOX2/SOX9 population (**Figure 2**) (Danopoulos et al., 2018a). Nikolic et al. performed transcriptomic analyses of these SOX2/SOX9 positive cells as well as SOX2 stalk cells and compared them to available transcriptomic data from mouse lung epithelial tips. The authors showed that the transcriptomic profile of these SOX2/SOX9 epithelial tips shares similarities with mouse epithelial tips, but more importantly, they showed that some genes were unique to mouse and others were unique to humans, claiming about 348 total unique genes in human lung tips (Nikolic et al., 2017). These analyses were performed only in epithelial lung tip cells, excluding the many other cell types in the lung. Similar comparison and observations were also made by Miller et al. (2018). Many of these molecular and cellular differences between mouse and human lung development are of great significance and may pertain to lung branching morphogenesis such as the SOX2/SOX9 double positive population shown to be required for proper lung branching (Danopoulos et al., 2018a).

Recent advances in human lung development and the *in vitro* models used for these studies have been recently reviewed by Nikolic et al. (2018). Other reviews by Prince and Yuan et al. have also extensively reviewed the role of FGF10 in lung development, homeostasis, and disease, across the life span and in animal models (Prince, 2018; Yuan et al., 2018). In the present concise review, we mainly focus on FGF signaling during human lung development and congenital/pediatric human lung diseases.

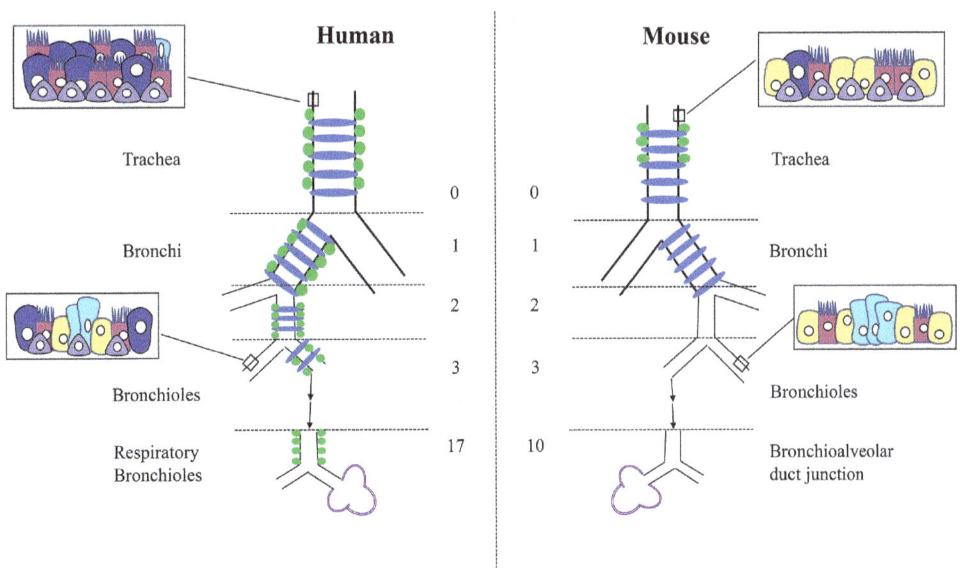

FIGURE 1 | Differences in structure and cellular composition between human and mouse lungs. Cartilage rings (blue) extend into the bronchioles in human lungs but are present only in the trachea and bronchi in mouse. Submucosal glands (green) are limited to the trachea in mouse but are present into the smaller respiratory bronchioles in humans. In mouse, only the trachea and main stem bronchi are lined with pseudostratified epithelium, whereas in humans, all the conducting airways from the trachea to the bronchioles are lined with pseudostratified epithelium. Basal cells (purple) are found deeper into the bronchioles only in humans. The human lung consists of more goblet cells (dark blue) in the proximal epithelium, with Club cells (yellow) mostly restricted to the smaller airways. Conversely, the mouse lung contains more Club cells (yellow) through the trachea and bronchi, with less goblet cells throughout. Neuroendocrine cells (light blue) are present within the bronchioles in clusters in the mouse and isolated or in much smaller clusters throughout the entire epithelial tree in human. Club cells = yellow, Ciliated cells = pink, Basal cells = purple, Goblet cells = dark blue, Neuroendocrine cells = light blue.

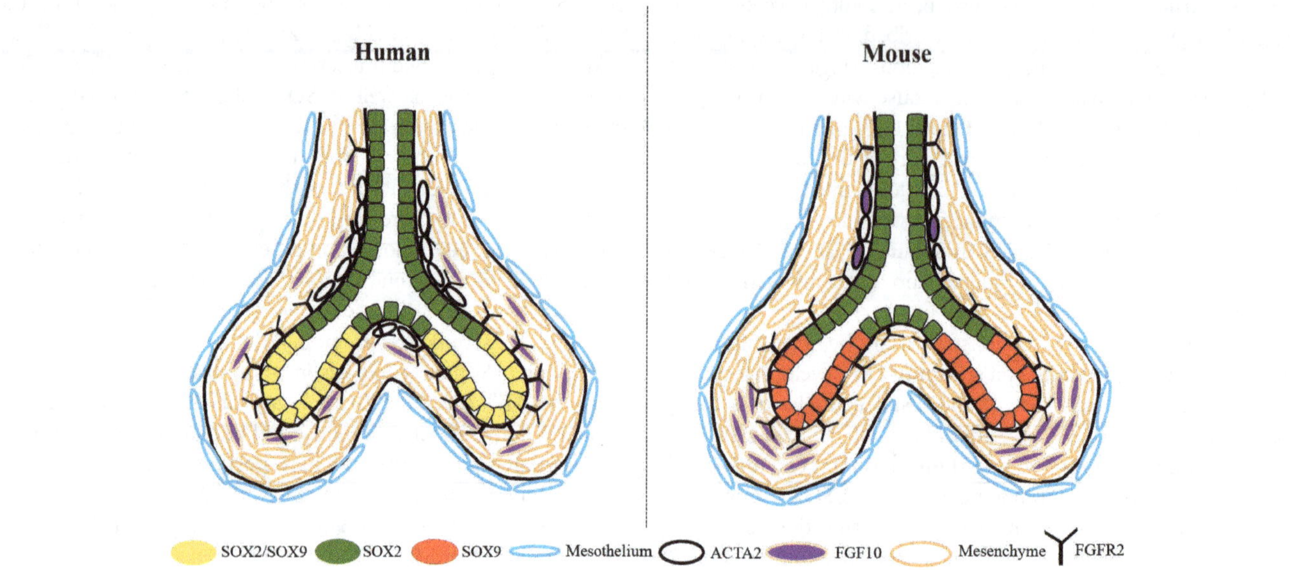

FIGURE 2 | Schematic depiction of the differential expression of SOX2, SOX9, ACTA2, and FGF10 between the developing human and mouse lung during the pseudoglandular stage. SOX2/SOX9 double positive progenitor cells are present in the distal epithelial tips of the human lung, whereas only SOX9+ cells are present in the distal tips of the mouse. ACTA2+ smooth muscle cells are found in both human and mouse surrounding the proximal airway, but extend more distally into the human lung and are closely associated with SOX2+ cells only, they are also in human at the bifurcation of the branch tips. In mouse lung, *Fgf10* is highly expressed in the mesenchyme adjacent to the epithelial tips and in the smooth muscle cells surrounding the airways; whereas in humans *FGF10+* cells are found dispersed throughout the mesenchyme with little expression in the smooth muscle cells.

FGF FAMILY

Fibroblast growth factors are a family of growth factors described in many multicellular species such as xenopus, drosophila, zebrafish, rodents, and humans and are known to be involved in a wide range of biological processes, including organogenesis, homeostasis, repair, and metabolism. There are 22 known FGFs in both human and mouse that have been divided into seven different subfamilies (FGF1, FGF4, FGF7, FGF8, FGF9, FGF11, and FGF15/19), which are categorized according to similarities in biochemical function, sequence, and evolutionary relationships (Ornitz and Itoh, 2015). The FGF1, FGF4, FGF7, FGF8, and FGF9 subfamilies are known as the canonical FGFs, suggesting that they function in a paracrine/autocrine manner, binding to one of the FGFRs (FGFR1-FGFR4, with FGFR1-FGFR3 having a IIIb or IIIc splice variant), with heparin or heparan sulfate as a cofactor (Ornitz and Itoh, 2015). This in turn activates phosphorylation of a specific tyrosine residue on the FGFR, resulting in the initiation of downstream intracellular signaling pathway: RAS-MAPK, PI3K-AKT, PLCγ, or STAT. FGF10 is a canonical FGF and belongs to the FGF7 family (Furdui et al., 2006; Ornitz and Itoh, 2015). The FGF11 subfamily, consisting of FGF11, FGF12, FGF13, and FGF14, is categorized as the intracellular/intracrine FGFs, which as a result do not bind to any of the FGFRs (Olsen et al., 2003). The members of this subfamily are associated with voltage-gated sodium channels and the regulation of neuron activity. The FGFs associated in the final subfamily (FGF15/19, FGF21, and FGF23), the FGF15/19, are also known as the endocrine FGFs. This is where human and mouse differ in terms of FGF expression. In humans, there is no Fgf15, whereas in rodents (mice and rats), there is no expression of FGF19. Therefore, it is believed that Fgf15 and FGF19 are orthologous genes (Wright et al., 2004). The endocrine FGFs do bind to FGFRs; however, in order to increase the affinity to the receptor, it is necessary to have the presence of an additional single pass transmembrane protein known as Klotho (alpha or beta) to act as a cofactor and ensure binding efficiency (Hu et al., 2013). With the presence of 22 different ligands and 4 receptors, not including the different isoforms, it is quite evident that FGF signaling is very complex.

FGFS AND FGFRS MUTATIONS ARE ASSOCIATED WITH HUMAN LUNG DISEASES

Although there is a clear association between *Fgf10* mutations and lung malformation in mouse, such is not evident in humans. The two most familiar conditions associated with human *FGF10* mutations are autosomal dominant aplasia of lacrimal and salivary glands (ALSG) (Entesarian et al., 2005; Seymen et al., 2017) and lacrimo-auriculo-dento-digital syndrome (LADD) (Milunsky et al., 2006; Rohmann et al., 2006), with both conditions lacking a primary lung complication. LADD patients also harbor mutations in the *FGFR2* and *FGFR3* genes (Rohmann et al., 2006), suggesting that additional FGFs may be contributing factors to the syndrome. Although one study demonstrated that ALSG patients displayed lower lung function (reduced FEV1) and irreversible airway obstruction consistent with chronic obstructive pulmonary disease (COPD) (Klar et al., 2011), 6 of the 12 patients studied had asthma and another four had other allergies. Therefore, it is unclear whether lung function changes were a direct cause of *FGF10* mutations or other unrelated factors. Furthermore, none of these patients were diagnosed with lung malformation (Klar et al., 2011). Another study suggested that single nucleotide polymorphisms (SNPs) in the *FGF10* gene may be associated with COPD (Ren et al., 2013). Interestingly, it has also been shown that *FGF10* SNPs are associated with airway branch variants, where the right medial basal segmental airway was absent in smoker COPD patients but remained unaffected in nonsmoker COPD patients (Smith et al., 2018). In addition, significant associations between lung function and SNPs in the FGF10 gene have been found (Jackson et al., 2018). However, combined, these studies still do not establish a direct causative role for *FGF10* mutations/SNPs in human congenital lung malformations, specifically in branching defects. Importantly, the effect of these SNPs on *FGF10* gene expression is unclear. A recent study by Karolak et al. demonstrated the presence of rare FGF10 and TBX4 mutations in lethal pulmonary acinar dyslasia and alveolar dysplasia (Karolak et al., 2019). They showed that FGF10 mutations or SNPs are mostly associated with alveolar dysplasia occurring past the pseudoglandular stage of development. However, the study suggested that these mutations alone are not sufficient to cause these severe lung phenotypes but rather support complex compound inheritance of additional noncoding variants or a genetic modifiers other places in the genome (Karolak et al., 2019). Finally, one cannot exclude that homozygous mutations in FGF10 might cause yet undocumented lethality in early fetal life.

Alternatively, FGF receptors have been associated with lung or airway anomalies. Activating mutations of FGFR2 cause Crouzon, Apert, and Pfeiffer syndromes (Robertson et al., 1998). While these syndromes are primarily characterized by craniofacial and skeletal defects, defects in tracheal cartilaginous ring formation resulting in mortality due to respiratory distress have also been reported (Devine et al., 1984; Cinalli et al., 1995; Gonzales et al., 2005). In these patients, the only lung associated deficiency witnessed is a cartilaginous sleeve that surrounds the trachea with no visible cartilage rings. In contrast, homozygous FGFR2 loss of function mutation (p.R255Q) results in ectrodactyly and pulmonary acinar dysplasia, a rare congenital lung malformation characterized by in utero arrest of lung development at the pseudoglandular stage (Barnett et al., 2016). This suggests that *FGFR2* signaling plays a key role in the progression of lung development from the pseudoglandular stage onwards. However, it is unclear which *FGFR2* ligands are responsible for this effect.

Moreover, SNPs in the *FGFR4* gene were shown to be associated with bronchopulmonary dysplasia (BPD) and respiratory distress syndrome (RDS), whereas SNPs in the *FGFR2* gene had no association with neither BPD nor RDS (Rezvani et al., 2013). SNPs in *FGF3* and *FGF7* but not *FGF2*, *FGF4*, or *FGF18* showed associations with RDS only but not BPD (Rezvani et al., 2013). These findings suggest *FGFR4, FGF3, and FGF7* play an important role in human distal lung growth.

FGF10 IN HUMAN LUNG DEVELOPMENT

Several FGF ligands and receptors have been shown to play important roles in organogenesis of multiple organ systems including the lung. In particular, *Fgf10* has been shown to be the main morphogen driving lung branching morphogenesis in mouse. Absence of *Fgf10* or its receptor *Fgfr2b* results in complete lung agenesis in mouse (Sekine et al., 1999; De Moerlooze et al., 2000). Until recently, the temporal and spatial expression of *FGF10* and its receptors in the developing human lung were unknown. We showed that *FGF10* is expressed throughout human lung development from 10 weeks of gestation up to 21 weeks of gestation (Al Alam et al., 2015; Danopoulos et al., 2018b). Unlike mouse where *Fgf10* expression increases during the pseudoglandular stage, in humans, *FGF10* expression was stable in the pseudoglandular stage and increased significantly in the canalicular stage (Al Alam et al., 2015; Danopoulos et al., 2018b). Fluorescent *in situ* hybridization allowed us to assess the spatial distribution of *FGF10* in the developing human lung and we showed that *FGF10* is expressed throughout the lung parenchyma with some expression in the airway and vascular smooth muscle cells (Danopoulos et al., 2018b). This expression was different than what has been described in mouse where *Fgf10* is abundantly expressed in the distal mesenchyme adjacent to epithelial buds (Bellusci et al., 1997). FGF10 receptors, *FGFR1* and *FGFR2*, are expressed in both epithelium and mesenchyme of the human developing lung between 11–18 weeks of gestation (Danopoulos et al., 2018b) with a stronger expression of *FGFR2* in the distal epithelium as compared to proximal epithelium, comparable to what is observed in mouse. The importance of FGF10 localization for directed branching has been reported in several mouse studies (Bellusci et al., 1997; Hirashima et al., 2009; Makarenkova et al., 2009) though others suggest that this localization is not important for the branching process (Volckaert et al., 2013).

The role of FGF10 in human lung development was unexplored until recently, and it remains incompletely understood. A report by Graeff et al. in 1999 showed that FGF7 and FGF10 both induced liquid secretion and enlargement in distal tips in human fetal lung explants cultured *in vitro* (Graeff et al., 1999). In mouse lung explants in vitro, FGF10 induces branch formation and allows the maintenance of the proximal-distal patterning characterized by SOX2 expression proximally and SOX9 expression distally (Volckaert et al., 2013). We performed more in depth analyses of the effect of FGF10, but also FGF7 and FGF9 on human lung explants cultured in vitro. We demonstrated, similar to the previous work, that FGF10 induces distal bud cysting and inhibits branching in human lung explants in vitro (Danopoulos et al., 2018b). Moreover, FGF10 does not modulate proliferation of either the epithelium or the mesenchyme following 48 hours culture in vitro (Danopoulos et al., 2018b); though an increase in p-ERK was seen, demonstrating that FGF10 successfully binds to its receptor(s) and induces downstream signaling activation in our culture conditions. Other groups have used in vitro organoid cultures from 12 weeks post conception human fetal lung distal epithelial tips to assess the role of growth factors on growth, branching, and self-renewal (Nikolic et al., 2017; Miller et al., 2018). Miller et al. initially showed that these organoids grow and expand up to 6 weeks in presence of FGF7, CHIR99021 (GSK3 inhibitor), retinoic acid (RA), and FGF10. However, removal of FGF10 alone from the media did not affect the growth or expression of the distal tip markers SOX2 and SOX9, suggesting that FGF10 is dispensable for the maintenance and growth of these human bud tips. Similar results were obtained on organoids derived from human pluripotent stem cells (hPSCs) (Miller et al., 2018). Nikolic et al. grew 5–9 weeks postconception human fetal lung tips with a combination of 7 factors (EGF, FGF7, FGF10, NOGGIN, RSPO1, CHIR99021, and the TGFβ inhibitor SB431542) (Nikolic et al., 2017). They showed that removal of FGF10 from the culture media at day 13 (during the branching period) did not affect the initial establishment of the organoid. Following passaging of the organoids, withdrawal of FGF10 only at day 6 of culture (when organoids are spherical) for 3 days did not alter organoid morphology or RNA expression of *SOX2* and *SOX9*, whereas a decrease in SOX2/SOX9 double positive cells was seen by IF. Taken together, these studies suggest that FGF10 is not required for the initial establishment of SOX2/SOX9 double positive progenitors and for human lung branching, while FGF signaling is important in this process. However, both of these studies used a GSK3 inhibitor CHIR99021 that could possibly compensate for the removal of FGF10, as FGF10 is a major activator of ß-catenin signaling. Interestingly, a more recent study showed that treatment of foregut spheroids with 1% serum and high concentrations of FGF10 was sufficient to the generation of lung organoids containing airway like structures, mesenchymal cells, and cells expressing alveolar epithelial cells type I and type II markers (Miller et al., 2019). But, FGF10 alone was not sufficient to give rise to the bud tip progenitor population co-expressing SOX2 and SOX9. Together, this suggests an important role for FGF10 signaling in later stages of human lung development, more specifically the establishment of the distal fate past the pseudoglandular into canalicular stage and alveolar formation, as well as during the differentiation of airway epithelial cells. Furthermore, it is still unclear whether another FGF ligand or a combination of ligands plays the role in human lung branching that FGF10 plays in mouse lung branching.

FGF10 IN PEDIATRIC HUMAN LUNG DISEASES

Whereas FGF10 mutations alone may not be sufficient to cause severe human lung malformations or congenital lung disease, alterations in *FGF10* expression have been described in bronchopulmonary dysplasia (BPD). The number of mesenchymal cells staining positive for FGF10 was decreased in the lung of BPD patients as compared to controls (Benjamin et al., 2007). In contrast, two independent GWAS studies found no association between BPD and FGF10 SNPs and no change in *FGF10* gene expression between BPD and controls (Bhattacharya et al., 2012; Li et al., 2015; Hamvas et al., 2018). Additionally, in congenital cystic adenomatoid malformation (CCAM), *FGF10, FGF7*, and *FGFR2* gene levels are unchanged in the lung mesenchyme (Cass et al., 1998; Jancelewicz et al., 2008), whereas epithelial *FGF9* expression is increased 4-fold in the CCAM samples compared to controls (Jancelewicz et al., 2008 Furthermore, there is no evidence of altered *FGF10* expression or signaling in human congenital small lung or lung hypoplasia, although its expression is different in mouse and rat experimental models of hypoplasia (Teramoto et al., 2003; Wang et al., 2018 However, a decrease in *FGF18* expression has been described in hypoplastic lungs from patients with congenital diaphragmatic hernia (Boucherat et al., 2007). In cystic fibrosis, fluid secretion and transport defects play an important role in the pathogenesis of the disease. While there is no clear evidence in human data sets of a role for FGF10 and/or FGF10 signaling in cystic fibrosis, studies in pig models showed that FGF10 treatment induced fluid secretion in non-CF fetal lung explants but was unable to do so in CF fetal lung explants (Meyerholz et al., 2018), suggesting that FGF10 signaling may play an important role in the pathogenesis of the disease.

CONCLUSION

The role of FGF10 signaling in human lung development and disease remains poorly understood. Despite the limitations associated with the use and manipulation of human tissues, studies in human development and disease are necessary to better understand the role of FGF10 and other pathways that have been shown to be important in mouse, e.g., FGF, Wnt, and Hippo pathways. The disappointingly high failure rate of clinical trials has made studying human tissues critical, along with the necessity to accelerate the development of therapies for pediatric lung diseases. FGF10, under the drug name Repifermin, failed to prove efficacy in clinical trials for wound healing, mucositis, and ulcerative colitis (Freytes et al., 2004 though it had highly protective and therapeutic effects in animal models. Understanding the role of FGF signaling in human lung development and disease will help tailor its possible therapeutic effects and targets, if any, to the appropriate site of action and patient population.

AUTHOR CONTRIBUTIONS

SD, JS and DA reviewed the literature, wrote the review, edited and approved the final version.

REFERENCES

Al Alam, D., El Agha, E., Sakurai, R., Kheirollahi, V., Moiseenko, A., Danopoulos, S., et al. (2015). Evidence for the involvement of fibroblast growth factor 10 in lipofibroblast formation during embryonic lung development. *Development* 142, 4139–4150. doi: 10.1242/dev.109173

Barnett, C. P., Nataren, N. J., Klingler-Hoffmann, M., Schwarz, Q., Chong, C. E., Lee, Y. K., et al. (2016). Ectrodactyly and lethal pulmonary acinar dysplasia associated with homozygous FGFR2 mutations identified by exome sequencing. *Hum. Mutat.* 37, 955–963. doi: 10.1002/humu.23032

Bellusci, S., Grindley, J., Emoto, H., Itoh, N., and Hogan, B. L. (1997). Fibroblast growth factor 10 (FGF10) and branching morphogenesis in the embryonic mouse lung. *Development* 124, 4867–4878.

Benjamin, J. T., Smith, R. J., Halloran, B. A., Day, T. J., Kelly, D. R., and Prince, L. S. (2007). FGF-10 is decreased in bronchopulmonary dysplasia and suppressed by Toll-like receptor activation. *Am. J. Phys. Lung Cell. Mol. Phys.* 292, L550–L558. doi: 10.1152/ajplung.00329.2006

Bhattacharya, S., Go, D., Krenitsky, D. L., Huyck, H. L., Solleti, S. K., Lunger, V. A., et al. (2012). Genome-wide transcriptional profiling reveals connective tissue mast cell accumulation in bronchopulmonary dysplasia. *Am. J. Respir. Crit. Care Med.* 186, 349–358. doi: 10.1164/rccm.201203-0406OC

Boucherat, O., Benachi, A., Barlier-Mur, A. M., Franco-Montoya, M. L., Martinovic, J., Thebaud, B., et al. (2007). Decreased lung fibroblast growth factor 18 and elastin in human congenital diaphragmatic hernia and animal models. *Am. J. Respir. Crit. Care Med.* 175, 1066–1077. doi: 10.1164/rccm.200601-050OC

Cass, D. L., Quinn, T. M., Yang, E. Y., Liechty, K. W., Crombleholme, T. M., Flake, A. W., et al. (1998). Increased cell proliferation and decreased apoptosis characterize congenital cystic adenomatoid malformation of the lung. *J. Pediatr. Surg.* 33, 1043–1046. discussion 1047. doi: 10.1016/S0022-3468(98)90528-0

Cinalli, G., Renier, D., Sebag, G., Sainte-Rose, C., Arnaud, E., and Pierre-Kahn, A. (1995). Chronic tonsillar herniation in Crouzon's and Apert's syndromes: the role of premature synostosis of the lambdoid suture. *J. Neurosurg.* 83, 575–582. doi: 10.3171/jns.1995.83.4.0575

Danopoulos, S., Alonso, I., Thornton, M. E., Grubbs, B. H., Bellusci, S., Warburton, D., et al. (2018a). Human lung branching morphogenesis is orchestrated by the spatiotemporal distribution of ACTA2, SOX2, and SOX9. *Am. J. Phys. Lung Cell. Mol. Phys.* 314, L144–L149. doi: 10.1152/ajplung.00379.2017

Danopoulos, S., Thornton, M. E., Grubbs, B. H., Frey, M. R., Warburton, D., Bellusci, S., et al. (2018b). Discordant roles for FGF ligands in lung branching morphogenesis between human and mouse. *J. Pathol.* 247, 254–265. doi: 10.1002/path.5188

De Moerlooze, L., Spencer-Dene, B., Revest, J. M., Hajihosseini, M., Rosewell, I., and Dickson, C. (2000). An important role for the IIIb isoform of fibroblast growth factor receptor 2 (FGFR2) in mesenchymal-epithelial signalling during mouse organogenesis. *Development* 127, 483–492.

Devine, P., Bhan, I., Feingold, M., Leonidas, J. C., and Wolpert, S. M. (1984). Completely cartilaginous trachea in a child with Crouzon syndrome. *Am. J. Dis. Child.* 138, 40–43. doi: 10.1001/archpedi.1984.02140390032010

Entesarian, M., Matsson, H., Klar, J., Bergendal, B., Olson, L., Arakaki, R., et al. (2005). Mutations in the gene encoding fibroblast growth factor 10 are associated with aplasia of lacrimal and salivary glands. *Nat. Genet.* 37, 125–127. doi: 10.1038/ng1507

Freytes, C. O., Ratanatharathorn, V., Taylor, C., Abboud, C., Chesser, N., Restrepo, A., et al. (2004). Phase I/II randomized trial evaluating the safety and clinical effects of repifermin administered to reduce mucositis in patients undergoing autologous hematopoietic stem cell transplantation. *Clin. Cancer Res.* 10, 8318–8324. doi: 10.1158/1078-0432.CCR-04-1118

Furdui, C. M., Lew, E. D., Schlessinger, J., and Anderson, K. S. (2006). Autophosphorylation of FGFR1 kinase is mediated by a sequential and precisely ordered reaction. *Mol. Cell* 21, 711–717. doi: 10.1016/j.molcel.2006.01.022

Gonzales, M., Heuertz, S., Martinovic, J., Delahaye, S., Bazin, A., Loget, P., et al. (2005). Vertebral anomalies and cartilaginous tracheal sleeve in three patients with Pfeiffer syndrome carrying the S351C FGFR2 mutation. *Clin. Genet.* 68, 179–181. doi: 10.1111/j.1399-0004.2005.00477.x

Graeff, R. W., Wang, G., and McCray, P. B. Jr. (1999). KGF and FGF-10 stimulate liquid secretion in human fetal lung. *Pediatr. Res.* 46, 523–529. doi: 10.1203/00006450-199911000-00006

Hamvas, A., Feng, R., Bi, Y., Wang, F., Bhattacharya, S., Mereness, J., et al. (2018). Exome sequencing identifies gene variants and networks associated with extreme respiratory outcomes following preterm birth. *BMC Genet.* 19:94. doi: 10.1186/s12863-018-0679-7

Hirashima, T., Iwasa, Y., and Morishita, Y. (2009). Mechanisms for split localization of Fgf10 expression in early lung development. *Dev. Dyn.* 238, 2813–2822. doi: 10.1002/dvdy.22108

Hu, M. C., Shiizaki, K., Kuro-o, M., and Moe, O. W. (2013). Fibroblast growth factor 23 and Klotho: physiology and pathophysiology of an endocrine network of mineral metabolism. *Annu. Rev. Physiol.* 75, 503–533. doi: 10.1146/annurev-physiol-030212-183727

Irvin, C. G., and Bates, J. H. (2003). Measuring the lung function in the mouse: the challenge of size. *Respir. Res.* 4:4. doi: 10.1186/rr199

Jackson, V. E., Latourelle, J. C., Wain, L. V., Smith, A. V., Grove, M. L., Bartz, T. M., et al. (2018). Meta-analysis of exome array data identifies six novel genetic loci for lung function. *Wellcome Open Res.* 3:4. doi: 10.12688/wellcomeopenres.12583.3

Jancelewicz, T., Nobuhara, K., and Hawgood, S. (2008). Laser microdissection allows detection of abnormal gene expression in cystic adenomatoid malformation of the lung. *J. Pediatr. Surg.* 43, 1044–1051. doi: 10.1016/j.jpedsurg.2008.02.027

Karolak, J. A., Vincent, M., Deutsch, G., Gambin, T., Cogne, B., Pichon, O., et al. (2019). Complex compound inheritance of lethal lung developmental disorders due to disruption of the TBX-FGF pathway. *Am. J. Hum. Genet.* 104, 213–228. doi: 10.1016/j.ajhg.2018.12.010

Klar, J., Blomstrand, P., Brunmark, C., Badhai, J., Hakansson, H. F., Brange, C. S., et al. (2011). Fibroblast growth factor 10 haploinsufficiency causes chronic obstructive pulmonary disease. *J. Med. Genet.* 48, 705–709. doi: 10.1136/jmedgenet-2011-100166

Knust, J., Ochs, M., Gundersen, H. J., and Nyengaard, J. R. (2009). Stereological estimates of alveolar number and size and capillary length and surface area in mice lungs. *Anat. Rec.* 292, 113–122. doi: 10.1002/ar.20747

Li, J., Yu, K. H., Oehlert, J., Jeliffe-Pawlowski, L. L., Gould, J. B., Stevenson, D. K., et al. (2015). Exome sequencing of neonatal blood spots and the identification of genes implicated in bronchopulmonary dysplasia. *Am. J. Respir. Crit. Care Med.* 192, 589–596. doi: 10.1164/rccm.201501-0168OC

Makarenkova, H. P., Hoffman, M. P., Beenken, A., Eliseenkova, A. V., Meech, R., Tsau, C., et al. (2009). Differential interactions of FGFs with heparan sulfate control gradient formation and branching morphogenesis. *Sci. Signal.* 2:ra55. doi: 10.1126/scisignal.2000304

Meyerholz, D. K., Stoltz, D. A., Gansemer, N. D., Ernst, S. E., Cook, D. P., Strub, M. D., et al. (2018). Lack of cystic fibrosis transmembrane conductance regulator disrupts fetal airway development in pigs. *Lab. Investig.* 98, 825–838. doi: 10.1038/s41374-018-0026-7

Miller, A. J., Dye, B. R., Ferrer-Torres, D., Hill, D. R., Overeem, A. W., Shea, L. D., et al. (2019). Generation of lung organoids from human pluripotent stem cells in vitro. *Nat. Protoc.* 14, 518–540. doi: 10.1038/s41596-018-0104-8

Miller, A. J., Hill, D. R., Nagy, M. S., Aoki, Y., Dye, B. R., Chin, A. M., et al. (2018). In vitro induction and in vivo engraftment of lung bud tip progenitor cells derived from human pluripotent stem cells. *Stem Cell Reports* 10, 101–119. doi: 10.1016/j.stemcr.2017.11.012

Milunsky, J. M., Zhao, G., Maher, T. A., Colby, R., and Everman, D. B. (2006). LADD syndrome is caused by FGF10 mutations. *Clin. Genet.* 69, 349–354. doi: 10.1111/j.1399-0004.2006.00597.x

Nikolic, M. Z., Caritg, O., Jeng, Q., Johnson, J. A., Sun, D., Howell, K. J., et al. (2017). Human embryonic lung epithelial tips are multipotent progenitors that can be expanded in vitro as long-term self-renewing organoids. *elife* 6. doi: 10.7554/eLife.26575

Nikolic, M. Z., Sun, D., and Rawlins, E. L. (2018). Human lung development: recent progress and new challenges. *Development* 145. doi: 10.1242/dev.163485

Ochs, M., Nyengaard, J. R., Jung, A., Knudsen, L., Voigt, M., Wahlers, T., et al. (2004). The number of alveoli in the human lung. *Am. J. Respir. Crit. Care Med.* 169, 120–124. doi: 10.1164/rccm.200308-1107OC

Olsen, S. K., Garbi, M., Zampieri, N., Eliseenkova, A. V., Ornitz, D. M., Goldfarb, M., et al. (2003). Fibroblast growth factor (FGF) homologous factors share structural but not functional homology with FGFs. *J. Biol. Chem.* 278, 34226–34236. doi: 10.1074/jbc.M303183200

Ornitz, D. M., and Itoh, N. (2015). The Fibroblast Growth Factor signaling pathway. *Wiley Interdiscip. Rev. Dev. Biol.* 4, 215–266. doi: 10.1002/wdev.176

Prince, L. S. (2018). FGF10 and human lung disease across the life spectrum. *Front. Genet.* 9:517. doi: 10.3389/fgene.2018.00517

Ren, J. T., Feng, K., Wang, P., Peng, W. H., Jia, H. Y., Liu, K., et al. (2013). Relationship between the gene polymorphism in fibroblast growth factor-10 and susceptibility to chronic obstructive pulmonary disease 220 cases. *Zhonghua Jie He He Hu Xi Za Zhi* 36, 935–939.

Rezvani, M., Wilde, J., Vitt, P., Mailaparambil, B., Grychtol, R., Krueger, M., et al. (2013). Association of a FGFR-4 gene polymorphism with bronchopulmonary dysplasia and neonatal respiratory distress. *Dis. Markers* 35, 633–640. doi: 10.1155/2013/932356

Robertson, S. C., Meyer, A. N., Hart, K. C., Galvin, B. D., Webster, M. K., and Donoghue, D. J. (1998). Activating mutations in the extracellular domain of the fibroblast growth factor receptor 2 function by disruption of the disulfide bond in the third immunoglobulin-like domain. *Proc. Natl. Acad. Sci. U. S. A.* 95, 4567–4572.

Rohmann, E., Brunner, H. G., Kayserili, H., Uyguner, O., Nurnberg, G., Lew, E. D., et al. (2006). Mutations in different components of FGF signaling in LADD syndrome. *Nat. Genet.* 38, 414–417. doi: 10.1038/ng1757

Sekine, K., Ohuchi, H., Fujiwara, M., Yamasaki, M., Yoshizawa, T., Sato, T., et al. (1999). Fgf10 is essential for limb and lung formation. *Nat. Genet.* 21, 138–141. doi: 10.1038/5096

Seymen, F., Koruyucu, M., Toptanci, I. R., Balsak, S., Dedeoglu, S., Celepkolu, T., et al. (2017). Novel FGF10 mutation in autosomal dominant aplasia of lacrimal and salivary glands. *Clin. Oral Investig.* 21, 167–172. doi: 10.1007/s00784-016-1771-x

Smith, B. M., Traboulsi, H., Austin, J. H. M., Manichaikul, A., Hoffman, E. A., Bleecker, E. R., et al. (2018). Human airway branch variation and chronic obstructive pulmonary disease. *Proc. Natl. Acad. Sci. U. S. A.* 115, E974–E981. doi: 10.1073/pnas.1715564115

Teramoto, H., Yoneda, A., and Puri, P. (2003). Gene expression of fibroblast growth factors 10 and 7 is downregulated in the lung of nitrofen-induced diaphragmatic hernia in rats. *J. Pediatr. Surg.* 38, 1021–1024. doi: 10.1016/S0022-3468(03)00183-0

Volckaert, T., Campbell, A., Dill, E., Li, C., Minoo, P., and De Langhe, S. (2013). Localized Fgf10 expression is not required for lung branching morphogenesis but prevents differentiation of epithelial progenitors. *Development* 140, 3731–3742. doi: 10.1242/dev.096560

Wang, J., Liu, H., Gao, L., and Liu, X. (2018). Impaired FGF10 signaling and epithelial development in experimental lung hypoplasia with esophageal atresia. *Front. Pediatr.* 6:109. doi: 10.3389/fped.2018.00109

Wansleeben, C., Barkauskas, C. E., Rock, J. R., and Hogan, B. L. (2013). Stem cells of the adult lung: their development and role in homeostasis, regeneration, and disease. *Wiley Interdiscip. Rev. Dev. Biol.* 2, 131–148. doi: 10.1002/wdev.58

Wong, C. H., Siah, K. W., and Lo, A. W. (2018). Estimation of clinical trial success rates and related parameters. *Biostatistics* doi: 10.1093/biostatistics/kxx069

Wright, T. J., Ladher, R., McWhirter, J., Murre, C., Schoenwolf, G. C., and Mansour, S. L. (2004). Mouse FGF15 is the ortholog of human and chick FGF19, but is not uniquely required for otic induction. *Dev. Biol.* 269, 264–275. doi: 10.1016/j.ydbio.2004.02.003

Yuan, T., Volckaert, T., Chanda, D., Thannickal, V. J., and De Langhe, S. P. (2018). Fgf10 signaling in lung development, homeostasis, disease, and repair after injury. *Front. Genet.* 9:418. doi: 10.3389/fgene.2018.00418

16

An *In Vitro* Microfluidic Alveolus Model to Study Lung Biomechanics

*Vardhman Kumar[1], Sajeesh Kumar Madhurakkat Perikamana[2], Aleksandra Tata[3], Jiaul Hoque[2], Anna Gilpin[1], Purushothama Rao Tata[3,4] and Shyni Varghese[1,2,5]**

[1]Department of Biomedical Engineering, Duke University, Durham, NC, United States, [2]Department of Orthopaedic Surgery, Duke University School of Medicine, Durham, NC, United States, [3]Department of Cell Biology, Duke University School of Medicine, Durham, NC, United States, [4]Regeneration Next, Duke University, Durham, NC, United States, [5]Department of Mechanical Engineering and Material Science, Duke University, Durham, NC, United States

***Correspondence:**
Shyni Varghese
shyni.varghese@duke.edu

The gas exchange units of the lung, the alveoli, are mechanically active and undergo cyclic deformation during breathing. The epithelial cells that line the alveoli contribute to lung function by reducing surface tension *via* surfactant secretion, which is highly influenced by the breathing-associated mechanical cues. These spatially heterogeneous mechanical cues have been linked to several physiological and pathophysiological states. Here, we describe the development of a microfluidically assisted lung cell culture model that incorporates heterogeneous cyclic stretching to mimic alveolar respiratory motions. Employing this device, we have examined the effects of respiratory biomechanics (associated with breathing-like movements) and strain heterogeneity on alveolar epithelial cell functions. Furthermore, we have assessed the potential application of this platform to model altered matrix compliance associated with lung pathogenesis and ventilator-induced lung injury. Lung microphysiological platforms incorporating human cells and dynamic biomechanics could serve as an important tool to delineate the role of alveolar micromechanics in physiological and pathological outcomes in the lung.

Keywords: microfluidics, organ-on-a-chip, lung, microphysiological system, *in vitro* system

INTRODUCTION

The lung is a key organ that ensures blood oxygenation by means of respiration. Mechanical cues arising from cyclic expansion and contraction of alveoli during breathing have an important role in maintaining tissue homeostasis (Ingenito et al., 2005; Faffe and Zin, 2009; Perlman et al., 2011; Chen et al., 2014; Hsia et al., 2016; Knudsen and Ochs, 2018; Plantier et al., 2018). Conventional *in vitro* models of lung tissues frequently neglect the dynamic tissue biomechanics associated with respiration. Development of microfluidic organ-on-a-chip technology enables recapitulation of mechanical and structural aspects of the organ microenvironment, thus potentially narrowing the gap between *in vitro* and *in vivo* models (Bhatia and Ingber, 2014; Aung et al., 2016, 2020; Agrawal et al., 2017; Kumar and Varghese, 2019; Low et al., 2021). Toward this, various microphysiological platforms such as lung-on-a-chip, airway-on-a-chip, and alveolus-on-chip have been developed to model lung functions such as barrier properties, immune responses to infections, and lung pathologies such as asthma, edema, thrombosis, and lung cancer progression (Huh et al., 2010, 2012; Stucki et al., 2015, 2018; Benam et al., 2016a, 2016b, 2017; Jain et al., 2018; Park et al., 2018; Felder et al., 2019; Elias-Kirma et al., 2020; Ishahak et al., 2020; Jimenez-Valdes et al., 2020; Khalid et al.,

2020; Mejías et al., 2020; Nawroth et al., 2020; Shrestha et al., 2020, 2021; Zamprogno et al., 2021).

Lung distention occurs in three dimensions (3D) as a result of not only the alveolar air pressure but also the difference between the alveolar air pressure and the pleural fluid pressure, the transpulmonary pressure. Model systems incorporate such dynamic mechanical movements associated with breathing using deformable membranes subjected to dynamic pressure (Guenat and Berthiaume, 2018). While most *in vitro* studies and microphysiological systems incorporating dynamic stretch have been limited to generating in-plane strain or uniaxial strain in the 5–12% range reported *in vivo* (Birukov et al., 2003; Guenat and Berthiaume, 2018; Nossa et al., 2021; Sznitman, 2021), recent studies have delved into incorporating out-of-plane stretching to mimic the 3D movements of the alveoli during respiration (Stucki et al., 2018; Doryab et al., 2021a; Huang et al., 2021; Zamprogno et al., 2021). These advances offer unique *in vitro* tools to study the micromechanical changes such as the strain heterogeneity that develops as a result of the out-of-plane stretch and its subsequent role in lung physiology and pathology. Although the precise strain profile that develops in the lung during respiration is yet to be accurately mapped, it is well established that not just different regions of the lung but even a single alveolus experiences varying strains during respiration (Roan and Waters, 2011). These spatially varying mechanical cues have been shown to be associated with several lung conditions and vulnerabilities. For example, regions with intrinsically high strains—such as in aerated alveoli next to fluid-filled alveoli—are prone to experiencing increased strains during mechanical ventilation, thus predisposing them to ventilator-induced lung injury (VILI) (Perlman et al., 2011; Smith, 2016). Apart from such spatial variations in strain during breathing, progressive changes in local tissue mechanics (e.g., changes in compliance) are key characteristics of various respiratory disorders such as pulmonary fibrosis and emphysema (Ingenito et al., 2005; Faffe and Zin, 2009; Plantier et al., 2018; Hurtado et al., 2020).

In this study, we report a microfluidic alveolar tissue model that mimics dynamic out-of-plane stretching akin to alveolar inflation and deflation associated with breathing. The device consists of a fluidic and pneumatic layer separated by a thin polydimethylsiloxane (PDMS) membrane, which was functionalized by covalent conjugation of collagen-I to enable cell culture. We characterized the heterogeneous strain experienced by the membrane as a result of breathing-like movements by using computational analyses and examined the effect of spatial heterogeneity on cell alignment. Employing this platform, we also examined the effect of biomechanics on the function of alveolar epithelial cells. Specifically, we studied the effect of breathing-like movements on surfactant production by alveolar epithelial cells and how it is affected by heterogeneous strain and altered matrix compliance. Furthermore, we incorporated transpulmonary pressure into the device to have the membrane deform in response to a combination of pneumatic and hydrostatic pressure. Using this approach, we determined the applicability of this platform to model ventilator-induced lung injury (VILI). Finally, we also examined the potential of the platform to support the culture of human primary alveolar epithelial type 2 (AT2) cells and AT2 cells derived from human induced pluripotent stem cells (hiPSC).

METHODS

Photolithography of the Master Mold

Silicon wafers (UniversityWafers) were used for patterning arrays of 200-µm-wide and 100-µm-high channels by using SU-8 photolithography. Briefly, 4 ml of SU-8 100 photoresist was spin-coated on a cleaned wafer at 3,000 rpm/s for 30 s. The wafer was baked at 65°C for 10 min, followed by 95°C for 30 min. The wafer was then exposed to 365 nm wavelength light through a custom photomask designed in AutoCAD and baked at 65°C for 1 min and 95°C for 10 min. The wafer was then rinsed with SU-8 developer to remove the undeveloped photoresist. The resulting master mold was cleaned with isopropanol followed by water and stored until use.

Device Fabrication, Assembly, and Operation

To fabricate the device, a 10:1 (base:crosslinker) polydimethylsiloxane (PDMS) (Sylgard 184, Dow Inc.) precursor solution containing the crosslinker was poured onto the master mold and allowed to cure for 2 h at 60°C. Post curing, PDMS was cut around the channels and 8 mm diameter holes were punched in the top fluidic layer and bottom pneumatic layer to create cell culture chambers and pneumatic chambers, respectively (**Figure 1A**). The same channel dimensions were used for both fluidic and pneumatic channels. One-mm-diameter inlet and outlet were punched in the fluidic layer, and a 1-mm-diameter inlet was punched in the pneumatic layer of the device (**Figure 1A**). PDMS membranes were prepared by curing the precursor solution between two glass slides separated using stainless steel spacers with a thickness of 250 µm. The cell culture chamber was capped on the top by a glass coverslip using either double-sided tape (for reversible adhesion) or plasma bonding (for irreversible adhesion). The fluidic microchannels were capped at the base by plasma bonding the PDMS membrane to the fluidic layer. Separately, the pneumatic chamber and the pneumatic channels were capped at the bottom by plasma bonding a rectangular coverslip to the pneumatic layer (**Figure 1B**). The fluidic and pneumatic layers were assembled using double-sided tape to get a reversible adhesion between the two layers. This enabled easy disassembly of the device for imaging. The PTFE tubing from the programmable air pump (Elveflow) was connected to the inlet of the pneumatic layer, while the inlets of the fluidic layer were fed through syringes loaded onto a syringe pump (Harvard Apparatus) at a rate of 50 µl/h unless stated otherwise. For all experiments involving breathing-like motions, sinusoidal pressure waveforms with a minimum and maximum at 0 and 50 mbar, respectively, at a frequency of 0.5 Hz were used unless stated otherwise.

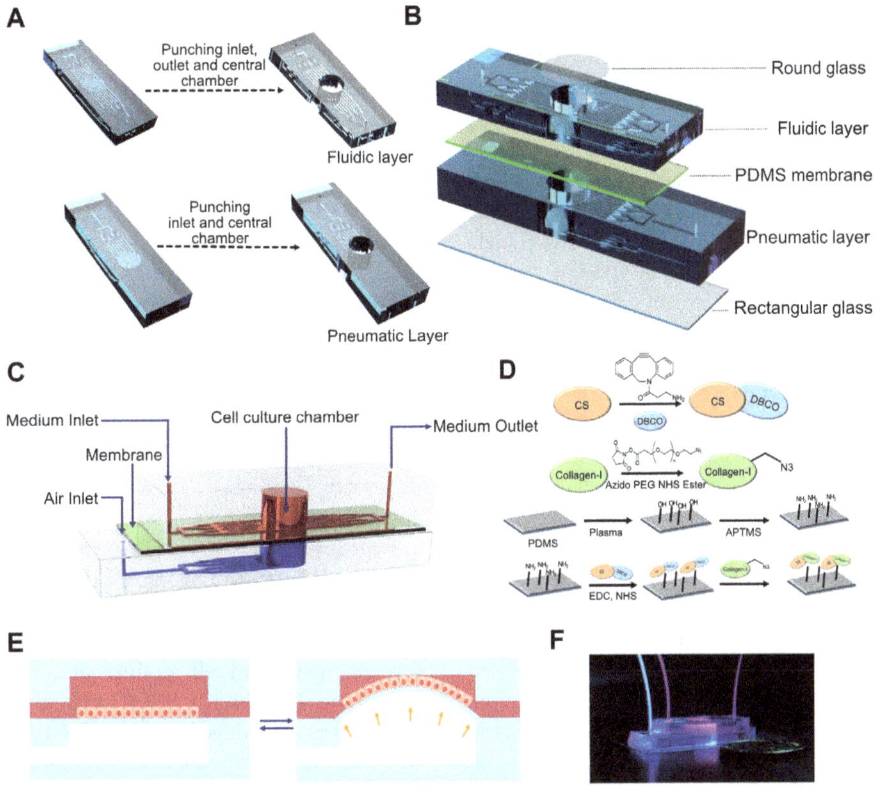

FIGURE 1 | (A) Computer-aided design (CAD) of the fabrication process of fluidic and pneumatic layers with microchannels. **(B)** Schematic of device assembly showing the different layers of the device in an exploded view. **(C)** Schematic depicting the assembled device. **(D)** Reaction scheme used for collagen functionalization of the PDMS membrane. **(E)** Schematic of breathing-like movements within the device. **(F)** Digital photograph of the device showing the media/cell chamber (red) and air chamber (blue).

Computational Modeling to Determine Strain Fields

The breathing movements of the membrane were modeled in COMSOL. The membrane was modeled as a cylindrical disc made from PDMS. A Mooney-Rivlin hyperelastic model (Rivlin, 1948) was used to describe the membrane:

$$W_s = \sum_{i,j=0}^{n} C_{i,j}(I_1 - 3)^i (I_2 - 3)^j + \frac{1}{2} K (J_{el} - 1)^2, \qquad (1)$$

where I_1 and I_2 are the first and second invariant of the left isochoric Cauchy-Green deformation tensor, K is the bulk modulus, J_{el} is the elastic Jacobian, and $C_{i,j}$ are material parameters.

Two-parameter Mooney–Rivlin material parameters for the PDMS membrane of 10:1 base to crosslinker were approximated from Yoon et al. (2010). The values used are listed in **Supplementary Table S1**. Zero displacement boundary condition was applied at the curved surface of the cylindrical membrane, while load (resulting from air pressure) was applied at the base of the membrane. Displacement field was used to calculate the resulting radial and circumferential strain as a function of radial distance from the center of the membrane (Winkler et al., 2014).

$$Radial\ Strain = \frac{\left|(x_2^s - x_1^s) + (y_2^s - y_1^s) + (z_2^s - z_1^s)\right| - \left|(x_2 - x_1) + (y_2 - y_1) + (z_2 - z_1)\right|}{\left|(x_2 - x_1) + (y_2 - y_1) + (z_2 - z_1)\right|} \qquad (2)$$

$$Circumferential\ Strain = \frac{2\pi r^s - 2\pi r}{2\pi r}, \qquad (3)$$

where (x_1, y_1, z_1) and (x_2, y_2, z_2) are coordinates of two arbitrary points on the membrane before stretching and (x_1^s, y_1^s, z_1^s) and (x_2^s, y_2^s, z_2^s) are the coordinates of the points after stretching. Similarly, r and r^s are the radial distance of a point from the center of the membrane before and after stretching, respectively.

Synthesis of Chondroitin Sulfate–Dibenzocyclooctyne and Collagen Azide

Five hundred milligrams of chondroitin sulfate (CS) (Alfa Aesar, J60341) was dissolved into 60 ml DI water. To this, 35 ml of dimethyl sulfoxide (DMSO) was added, followed by 287.5 mg of 1-ethyl-3-(3-dimethylaminopropyl) carbodiimide hydrochloride (EDC.HCl) (TCI Chemical, D1601). Then 172.6 mg of *N*-hydroxy succinimide (NHS) (Sigma, 130672) and 138.15 mg of dibenzocyclooctyne–amine (DBCO-amine) (Click Chemistry Tools, A103) were dissolved in 5 ml of DMSO and were added to the reaction mixture at 15-min intervals. The reaction was continued for 24 h under constant stirring. The reaction mixture was then dialyzed against water for 4 days and freeze-dried to obtain DBCO-conjugated chondroitin sulfate (CS-DBCO). The product was stored at −20°C until use. The product was characterized by a combination of Fourier transform infrared spectroscopy (FTIR) and proton nuclear magnetic resonance (^{1}HNMR) spectroscopy. The peaks in attenuated total reflection (ATR) FTIR spectra at 1,612 cm^{-1} due to C=O stretching and 1,559 cm^{-1} due to N–H deformation in the CS spectrum were shown to be shifted to 1,648 and 1,569 cm^{-1} in the CS-DBCO spectrum, respectively, indicating the presence of new amide bonds formed via the reaction between the carboxylic acid group of CS and the amine group of DBCO. In addition, peaks were observed at 1,480 and 1,441 cm^{-1}, which represented the aromatic C=C stretching in the rings of DBCO (**Supplementary Figure S1**). The successful conjugation of DBCO to CS was further confirmed by ^{1}HNMR where the spectrum showed the appearance of aromatic protons from DBCO at 7.34–7.44 ppm. The degree of DBCO conjugation was calculated by taking the ratio of area under the curve for the aromatic protons of DBCO at 7.34–7.44 ppm to the $-CH_3$ protons of the $-NHCOCH_3$ groups of CS at 1.9 ppm and found to be 39 ± 2% with respect to the dimeric sugar unit of CS (**Supplementary Figure S2**).

For collagen azide, 1 mg of collagen type I (Corning, 354236) and 500 µl of azide-polyethylene glycol-NHS) (Click Chemistry Tools, AZ103) were dissolved in 10 ml PBS each. The reaction was performed by mixing the solutions under constant stirring for 3 h at 0–4°C. The reaction mixture was then dialyzed against water at 4°C for 3 days. The product was freeze-dried and stored at -20°C until use. The product was characterized via FTIR spectroscopy where the spectra revealed a sharp peak at 2,141 cm^{-1} characteristic to the N≡N stretching frequency of the azide functional group (**Supplementary Figure S3**).

Collagen Functionalization of the Membrane

The PDMS membrane in the bonded devices was treated with corona treater (ETP, BD-20AC) for 1 min to plasma-activate the surface. Approximately 100 µl of 2% (v/v) (3-aminopropyl)-trimethoxysilane (APTMS) (Sigma, 281778) in 100% ethanol was introduced into the cell culture chamber, and the devices were incubated for 60 min at room temp and washed with distilled water. Meanwhile, 5 mg of CS-DBCO was dissolved in 1 ml of PBS and reacted with 5 mg of EDC for 15 min, followed by 2.1 mg of NHS to convert CS-DBCO into CS-DBCO-NHS ester. The devices were incubated with this activated CS-DBCO-NHS ester at 37°C for overnight to covalently immobilize CS-DBCO on the PDMS surface. The next day, the devices were washed 2–3 times with distilled water, and 10 µg/ml of collagen-azide solution in PBS was introduced into the devices. The devices were incubated overnight to immobilize collagen onto the PDMS surface via a strain-promoted azide–alkyne cycloaddition (SPAAC) reaction between the azide group of collagen zide and the DBCO group of surface-bound CS-DBCO. The devices were washed with PBS before culturing cells.

Isolation and Culture of Human Primary AT2 Cells

Healthy human lungs were procured through the BioRepository and Precision Pathology Center at Duke University in accordance with institutional procedures (Duke University Pro00082379—"Human Lung Stem Cells"; exempt research as described in 45 CFR 46.102(f), 21 CFR 56.102(e) and 21 CFR 812.3(p) which satisfies the Privacy Rule as described in 45CFR164.514). Human lung dissociation was performed as described previously (Zacharias et al., 2018). Briefly, approximately 2 g human lung tissue was cut into small pieces and incubated with 30 ml of enzyme mixture (collagenase type I (Gibco, 17100–017): 1.68 mg/ml, dispase (Corning, 354235): 5 U/ml, DNase (Thermo Fisher Scientific, 10104159001): 10 U/ml) at 37°C for 1 h with continuous rotation. The cells were filtered through a 100-µm cell strainer and rinsed with DMEM/F12 containing 10% FBS and anti-anti through the strainer. The sample was centrifuged at 450 g for 10 min, and the cell pellet was resuspended in red blood cell lysis buffer for 10 min, washed with DMEM/F12 containing 10% FBS, and filtered through a 40-µm strainer. Total cells were centrifuged at 450 g for 5 min at 4°C and the cell pellet was processed for alveolar type 2 cell (AT2s) purification. AT2s were isolated by magnetic-activated cell sorting (MACS) or fluorescence-activated cell sorting (FACS)-based protocols as described previously (Katsura et al., 2020). Approximately 2–10 million total human lung cells were resuspended in MACS buffer and incubated with Human TruStain FcX (Biolegend, 422032) for 15 min at 4°C, followed by incubation with HTII-280 (Terrace Biotech, TB-27AHT2-280) (1:60 dilution) antibody for 1 h at 4°C. The cells were washed twice with MACS buffer and incubated with anti-mouse IgM microbeads for 15 min at 4°C. The sample was loaded into the LS column (Miltenyi Biotec), and cells were collected magnetically. For FACS based purification of human AT2s, the total lung cell pellets were resuspended in MACS buffer and the EpCAM-positive population was purified using microbeads according to the manufacturer's instructions (Miltenyi Biotec, 130-061-101). CD326-positive cells were stained with HTII-280 and LysoTracker (Thermo Fisher Scientific, L7526) at 37°C for 25 min, followed by incubation with secondary antibody Alexa anti-mouse IgM-488 (Thermo Fisher Scientific, 10680) for 10 min at 37°C, washed twice and sorted using a FACS Vantage SE and SONY SH800 S. The cells were expanded as alveolospheres in growth factor reduced Matrigel (Corning, 354230) as described previously (Katsura et al., 2020), using Advanced DMEM/F12 medium containing 10 µM SB431542 (Abcam, 120163), 3 µM CHIR99021 (Tocris, 4423), 1 µM BIRB796 (Tocris, 5989), 10 µM Y27632 (Selleckchem, S1049) (for first 4 days of culture), 50 ng/ml Human EGF (Gibco, PHG0313), 10 ng/ml Human FGF10 (Biolegend, 559304),

5 μg/ml Heparin (Sigma, H3149), 1X B27 supplement (Thermo Fisher Scientific, 17504044), 1X Antibiotic-Antimycotic (Thermo Fisher Scientific, A5955), 15 mM HEPES, 1X Glutamax (Thermo Fisher Scientific, 35050061), and 1.25 mM N-Acetyl-L-Cysteine (Sigma, A9165).

Culture of Human Induced Pluripotent Stem Cell (hiPSC)-Derived AT2 Cells (iAT2 Cells)

IPSCs-derived human alveolar type 2 cells (iAT2s) (differentiated from the SPC2-ST-B2 iPSC line) were expanded as alveolospheres in growth factor reduced Matrigel (Corning, 354230) as described elsewhere (Jacob et al., 2019). The iAT2s were maintained in IMDM medium containing 25% Ham's F12 (Cellgro, 10–080-CV), 1% B27 supplement, 0.5% N2 supplement, 0.05% BSA (Invitrogen, 15260037), 200 ng/ml Primocin (Invivogen, NC9141851), 1X GlutaMAX, 50 μg/ml ascorbic acid (Sigma, A4544), 0.45 mM monothioglycerol (Sigma, M6145), 3 μM CHIR99021, 10 ng/ml rhKGF (R&D, 251-KG-010), 50 nM Dexamethasone (Sigma, D4902), 10 μM Y27632 (for first 3 days of culture), 0.1 mM 8-bromoadenosine 3′,5′-cyclic monophosphate sodium salt (Sigma, B7880), and 0.1 mM 3-isobutyl-1-methylxanthine (Sigma, I5879).

Culture of MLE-12 and H441 Cell Lines

MLE-12 cells were maintained in HITES medium consisting of DMEM/F12 (ATCC, 30-2006), 2% fetal bovine serum (FBS), 0.005 mg/ml insulin, 0.01 mg/ml transferrin (Fitzgerald, 31C-CH1026), 30 nM sodium selenite (Santa Cruz, 253595), 10 nM hydrocortisone (Sigma, H0888), 10 nM β-estradiol, 10 mM HEPES (Gibco, 15630106), 2 mM L-glutamine (Gibco, 25030081), and 1% Pen-Step (Gibco, 15140122). H441 cells were maintained in RPMI-1640 (ATCC, 30-2001) medium supplemented with 10% FBS and 1% Pen-Strep.

Cell Seeding Within the Device

For seeding hAT2s and iAT2s into the devices, alveolosphere dissociation was carried out by incubating the cultures in 2 mg/ml dispase for 30 min to release the alveolospheres from the Matrigel matrix. This was followed by centrifugation at 200 g for 4 min and resuspension of the alveolospheres in 0.05% Trypsin-EDTA for 5 min. The cell suspension was centrifuged at 300 g for 5 min and the cells were resuspended in their medium before counting. For cell lines, the cells were detached from the culture plate using 0.25% trypsin–EDTA, centrifuged, and resuspended in medium before counting.

Single cells were suspended in their corresponding medium at a concentration of 2×10^5 cells/ml; 100 μl of the cell suspension was perfused into the fluidic chamber of the device. The cell-loaded devices were left undisturbed (2 h for cell lines and 6 h for hAT2s and iAT2 cells) to allow the cells to adhere to the membrane before they were connected to the syringe pump to start the perfusion. The cells were cultured in a submerged condition within the device. A tubing was connected from the fluidic outlet into an Eppendorf tube to collect the perfusate. Twenty-four hours after cell seeding, the air pump was connected to the pneumatic inlet of the devices to induce breathing-like motion.

Immunofluorescence Staining and Quantification

The fluidic layer was separated from the pneumatic layer, and the cover slip was removed from the top. The cells were washed three times with PBS and fixed with 4% PFA for 15 min. The cells were washed again with PBS and treated with a permeabilization solution for 15–20 min (PBS/0.1% Triton-X). After permeabilization, the cells were blocked using 5% normal donkey serum in 1% BSA. Cells were then treated with anti-prosurfactant protein C primary antibody (Sigma, AB3786) for overnight at 4°C (1:150). The next day, the cells were washed 3 times with PBS and incubated with the secondary antibody (anti-rabbit Alexa Flour 647, 1:200) for 1 h. The staining solution was then removed, Hochest (1:1,000) was added, and the mixture was incubated for 4 min. Finally, cells were washed and imaged using a Keyence BZ microscope. Mean fluorescence intensity was quantified using ImageJ. Another set of cultures were stained with phalloidin (1:200) for 1 h and with Hochest (1:1,000) for 4 min. The cells were washed, and images of various locations within the membrane were acquired. OrientationJ plugin (Püspöki et al., 2016) within ImageJ was used to analyze the images.

Surfactant Protein-A ELISA

For Surfactant Protein-A (SP-A) ELISA experiments, devices were seeded with H441 cells, which were allowed to grow to confluence for 3 days before exposing them to breathing-like motions. Just before the start of the experiments, the outlet reservoir was emptied, and the flow rate was reduced to 5 μl/h to concentrate the secreted surfactant. After 24 h of breathing, it was visually confirmed under a microscope that the cell layer had not detached during the experiment. Perfusate collected in the outlet reservoir was used for surfactant protein-A ELISA using the SP-A kit (Biovender, RD191139200R) according to the manufacturer's instructions.

Determining Concave Volume and Compliance Curves

The concave volume of the membrane in response to applied air pressure (0–50 mbar) was calculated using COMSOL. The side view of the computational model of the membrane in stretched position was projected onto a 2D plane. The boundary of the membrane was traced to obtain the spatial points. A 6-order polynomial curve was fitted onto the points to obtain the equation for the curve. The volume encompassed was calculated by integrating the equation in three dimensions using Wolfram Alpha. This was done for membranes of different thicknesses 250 μm and 1,000 μm subjected to different pressures. The obtained volumes were plotted against the corresponding applied pressure to obtain the compliance plot.

Transpulmonary Pressure Setup

To introduce hydrostatic pressure, the outlet of the fluidic microchannels was blocked using knotted PTFE tubing. A 10-ml syringe was filled with cell culture medium and its plunger was removed to expose the media to the atmosphere. A lid was placed at the end of the syringe to reduce the chances of contamination.

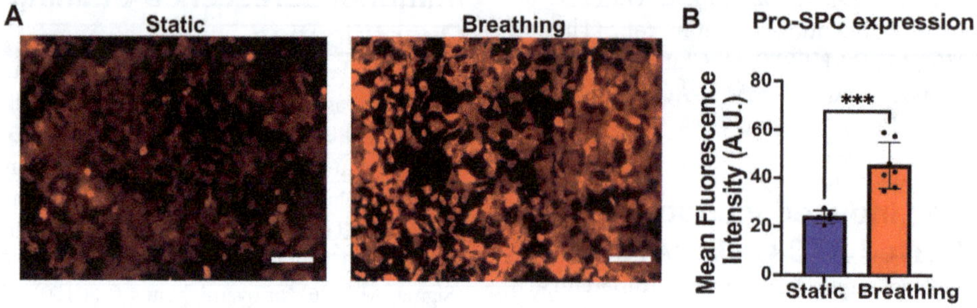

FIGURE 2 | (A) Immunofluorescent staining of Pro-SPC (red) of MLE-12 cells cultured under static and breathing conditions. **(B)** Quantification of the fluorescent intensity reveals that cells exposed to breathing-like motions express significantly higher pro-SPC. Each data point is an average of fluorescence intensity measurement from 6 to 11 images per independent device (N = 5 for static and N = 7 for breathing). Scale: 100 μm.

Tubing was connected from the syringe to the inlet of the fluid microchannels of the device. To generate positive hydrostatic pressure of 50 mbar, the syringe was placed 50 cm above the height of the device throughout the experiment.

Live-Dead Analysis

A viability/cytotoxicity kit (Thermo Fisher Scientific, L3224) was used to determine cell viability. Briefly, media was aspirated from the fluidic layer of the device, and the cells were washed with PBS. Then 100 μl of solution containing 0.05% calcein AM and 0.2% ethidium homodimer-1 was introduced into the device. The cells were incubated in the solution for 30 min before washing them with PBS and imaging them.

Statistics

Statistical analysis was performed on GraphPad Prism 9. An unpaired *t*-test was used to compare the mean fluorescent intensity in **Figure 2** and **Figure 6**; the cell shape in **Figure 6** and the SP-A levels in **Supplementary Figure S5**. For comparison of mean fluorescence intensity of cells cultured on 250- and 1,000-μm-thick membranes across center and edge, respectively, 2-way repeated measures ANOVA followed by multiple comparisons was used, with "center" and "edge" values being the repeated measures for each device. $N \geq 3$ independent devices per experimental group were used across all experiments. p-values < 0.05 were considered statistically significant.

RESULTS AND DISCUSSION

Device Fabrication and Cell Culture

The device consists of a bottom pneumatic layer and a top fluidic layer separated by a thin PDMS membrane (**Figure 1C**). The top layer consists of an inlet that diverges into an array of microchannels leading to a cylindrical cell culture chamber. This chamber is lined with a thin membrane at the base. Another array of microchannels connects the cell culture chamber to the device outlet. These channels are used for cell seeding and medium perfusion. In the bottom layer, the inlet diverges into an array of microchannels that lead to a cylindrical chamber whose ceiling is formed by the thin membrane and whose base is capped by a cover glass. The bottom layer is devoid of any outlets so that the device can be subjected to a pressure waveform to induce breathing-like movements. The PDMS membrane facing the fluid side was functionalized with collagen type I to promote cell attachment (**Figure 1D**). When subjected to a positive pressure in the bottom layer, the membrane concaves downward, which induces stretching of the membrane (**Figure 1E**). Applying a pressure waveform *via* the air pump facilitates cyclic stretching of the membrane, thus mimicking the breathing movements of alveoli (**Supplementary Movie S1**). Digital images of the device and of the setup are shown in **Figure 1F** and **Supplementary Figure S4**, respectively. Cells were perfused into the device *via* the inlet channel and allowed to adhere before introducing continuous perfusion of medium. The cells were cultured for 24 h before subjecting them to breathing-like movements. The device supported culture of alveolar epithelial cell lines, human primary alveolar epithelial cells (hAT2s) and human induced pluripotent (hiPSC)-derived alveolar epithelial cells (iAT2s).

Effect of Breathing-Like Motion on Surfactant Production

To study the effect of breathing-like motion-mediated active mechanical cues on alveolar cell functions, the epithelial cells within the device were subjected to cyclic stretching. The MLE-12 cells were subjected to breathing-like motions for 24 h, following which they were fixed and stained for surfactant protein-C (pro-SPC). Cells that were exposed to breathing-like motion expressed significantly higher levels of pro-SPC than cells cultured in static conditions (**Figures 2A, B**). Higher surfactant production in breathing cultures was further confirmed by H441 cells. As shown in **Supplementary Figure S5**, the cells subjected to dynamic breathing showed more secreted surfactant protein-A (SP-A). These results are in line with previous reports which showed increased surfactant production in response to cells subjected to stretching (Sanchez-Esteban et al., 1998; Torday and Rehan, 2002). The effect of mechanical cues on surfactant production has also been established in *in vivo* studies where mechanical ventilation-induced stretch has been reported to increase surfactant production in rat lungs (Martinez et al., 2004).

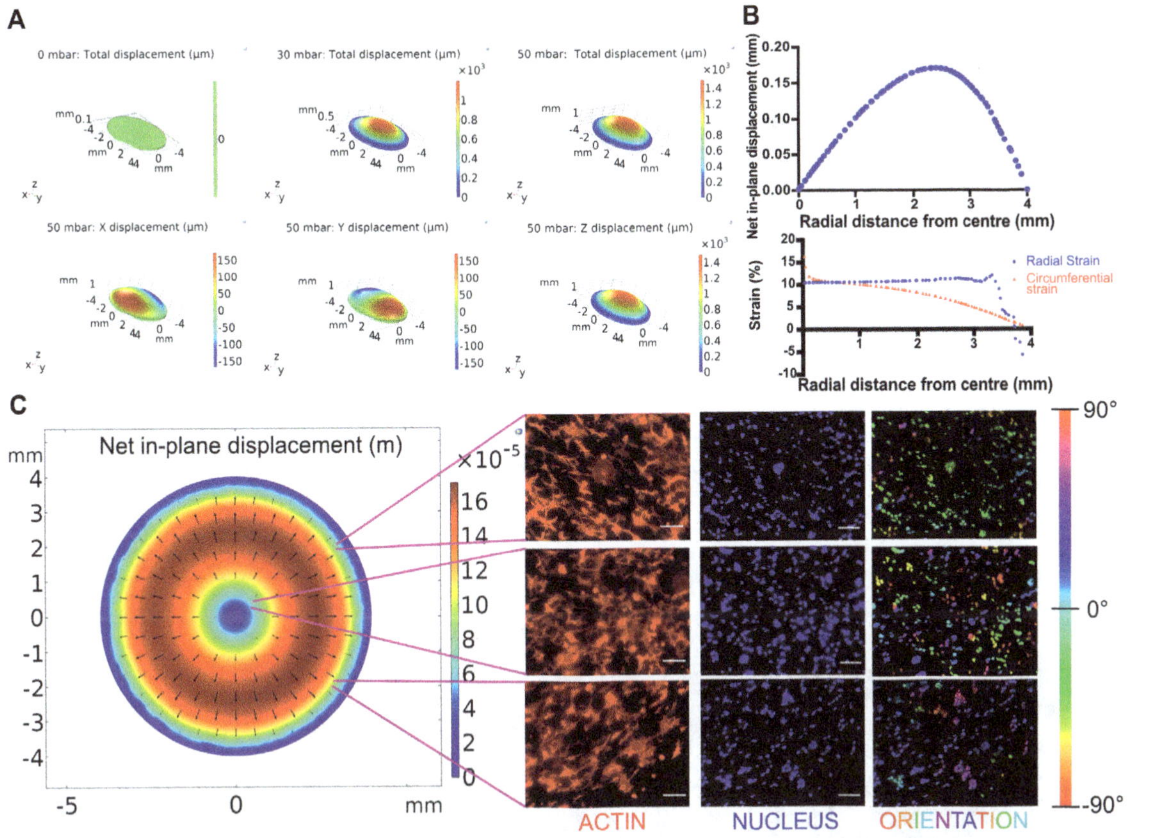

FIGURE 3 | (A) Displacement profiles of the breathing membrane subjected to various peak pressures. **(B)** In-plane displacement, radial strain and circumferential strain profile of the cell culture membrane at 50 mbar. **(C)** Effect of spatial strain heterogeneity of the cell culture substrate on cell alignment. Left: COMSOL computed in-plane displacement of the cell culture membrane. Right: Cellular alignment of MLE-12 cells was visualized by phalloidin (first column), and nucleus (second column) staining and cellular alignment at different locations in breathing devices was quantified using nuclear orientation (third column) where color of the nuclei in the third column represents their angle of alignment. Cells at the center of the membrane align randomly while those away from center align perpendicular to the radius. Scale: 100 μm.

Breathing-Induced Heterogeneous Strain Profile and Its Effect on Cell Shape

While dynamic stretching was found to promote surfactant production overall, we next analyzed the out-of-plane stretching-induced heterogeneous strain profile and its effect on the cells. Toward this, the membrane deformation during cyclic stretch was modeled in COMSOL as detailed in the experimental section. The effect of applied pressure on the membrane displacement field was determined by mapping the strain profile (**Figure 3A**). Using the displacement field, radial and circumferential strains were calculated at a peak pressure of 50 mbar. This pressure was chosen as it falls within the range of air pressure in the human lung during breathing and also results in physiological levels of strain (Roan and Waters, 2011). At this pressure, the in-plane displacement increases with increasing radial distance from the center (r) and gradually decreases, peaking at around r = 2.5 mm (**Figure 3B**). The circumferential strain was found to gradually decrease from 17 to 0% with increasing radial distance from the center. The radial strain largely remains constant at around 10% until a sharp decline after r > 3 mm due to the membrane being constricted at the edges (**Figure 3B**). MLE-12 cells on the membrane responded to the radial strain heterogeneity and exhibited a differential alignment. Specifically, at the center of the membrane, the cells were aligned randomly, while away from the center, they were aligned perpendicular to the direction of the major strain (i.e., the direction of radial displacement) (**Figure 3C**). In addition to epithelial cells, we have also examined the effect of strain heterogeneity on NIH 3T3 cells as fibroblasts are known to be highly sensitive to mechanical cues, including cyclic strain (Neidlinger-Wilke et al., 2002). Akin to epithelial cells, the fibroblasts displayed strain profile-dependent cell alignment, where cells away from the center aligned perpendicular to the direction of major strain, while those at the center were randomly aligned (**Supplementary Figure S6**). The strain-dependent alignment was more pronounced in the case of fibroblasts than in the epithelial cells, which is most likely attributed to the propensity of fibroblasts to polarize in cultures and acquire elongated morphology.

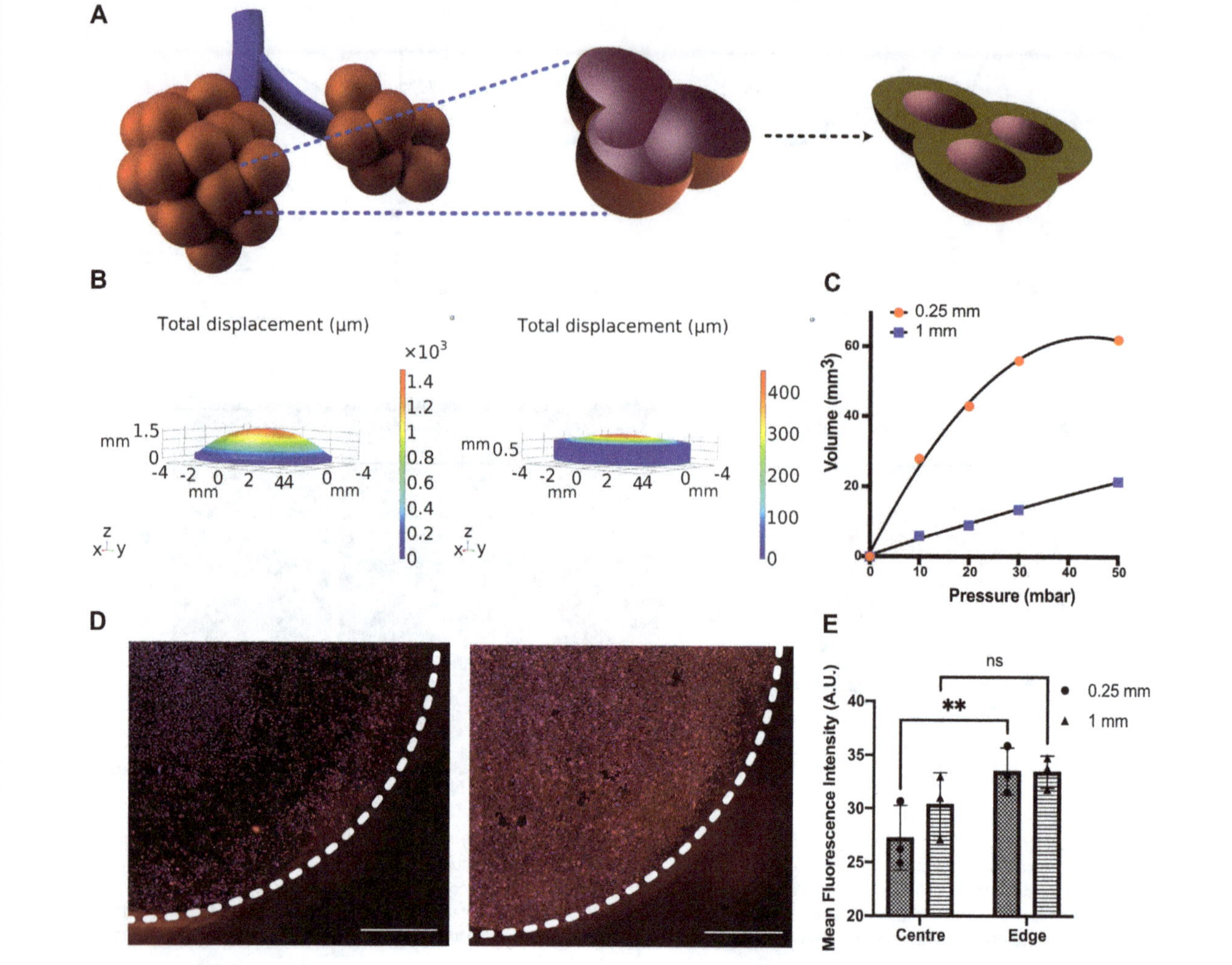

FIGURE 4 | (A) Schematic depicting the change in alveolar wall thickness as a result of interstitial wall thickening. **(B)** Displacement profiles of membranes with 250 and 1,000 µm thickness subjected to 50 mbar pressure **(C)** Pressure–volume compliance curves for membranes with 250 and 1,000 µm thickness when subjected to a breathing-like motion **(D)** Immunofluorescent staining for Pro-SPC (red) and nucleus (blue) in MLE-12 cells cultured on 250-µm (left) and 1,000-µm (right)-thick membranes and **(E)** its quantification at center (r < 3 mm) and edge (3 mm < r < 4 mm) of the device. N = 3 where each data point is an average of fluorescence intensity measurement from 7 to 12 images per independent device. White-dotted line represents the boundary of the membrane Scale: 1 mm.

Modeling Matrix Compliance

Changes in tissue compliance are a key characteristic of various lung diseases. For example, diseases like pulmonary fibrosis are characterized by alveolar wall thickening due to excessive accumulation of extracellular matrix and an increase in tissue stiffness, resulting in lowered compliance (**Figure 4A**). We have modeled the lowered tissue compliance by increasing the thickness of the membrane from 250 to 1,000 µm. With increasing thickness, the membrane will offer higher resistance to the same pressure profile than a 250-µm membrane, which results in less expansion/contraction and thereby a different breathing pattern (**Supplementary Movie S2**). The pulmonary compliance, which is expressed as the change in lung volume in response to a change in pressure ($\frac{\Delta V}{\Delta P}$), was calculated by computationally measuring the changes in the concave volume of the membrane as a function of pressure during breathing-like movements (**Figures 4B,C**). We chose a membrane thickness of 250 and 1,000 µm as they offer ~2.8 fold difference in volume at peak pressure, which is in the range of volume differences observed between healthy and fibrotic human lungs (Harris, 2005).

We examined the membrane compliance-mediated strain profile for an applied peak pressure of 50 mbar. As expected, the high compliance membrane (i.e., 250-µm membrane) encountered a significantly higher strain heterogeneity than the low compliance membrane (1,000 µm membrane). This is attributed to the lower resistance imposed by the 250 µm membrane, permitting higher deformation (**Figure 4B**). To examine the effect of cell response to the altered matrix compliance, MLE-12 cells were cultured in the device with membranes of thickness 250 µm and 1,000 µm and analyzed after subjecting them to 24 h of breathing-like motion. A significant difference in cell number was observed between the two, with the 1,000-µm membrane that experiences lower strains

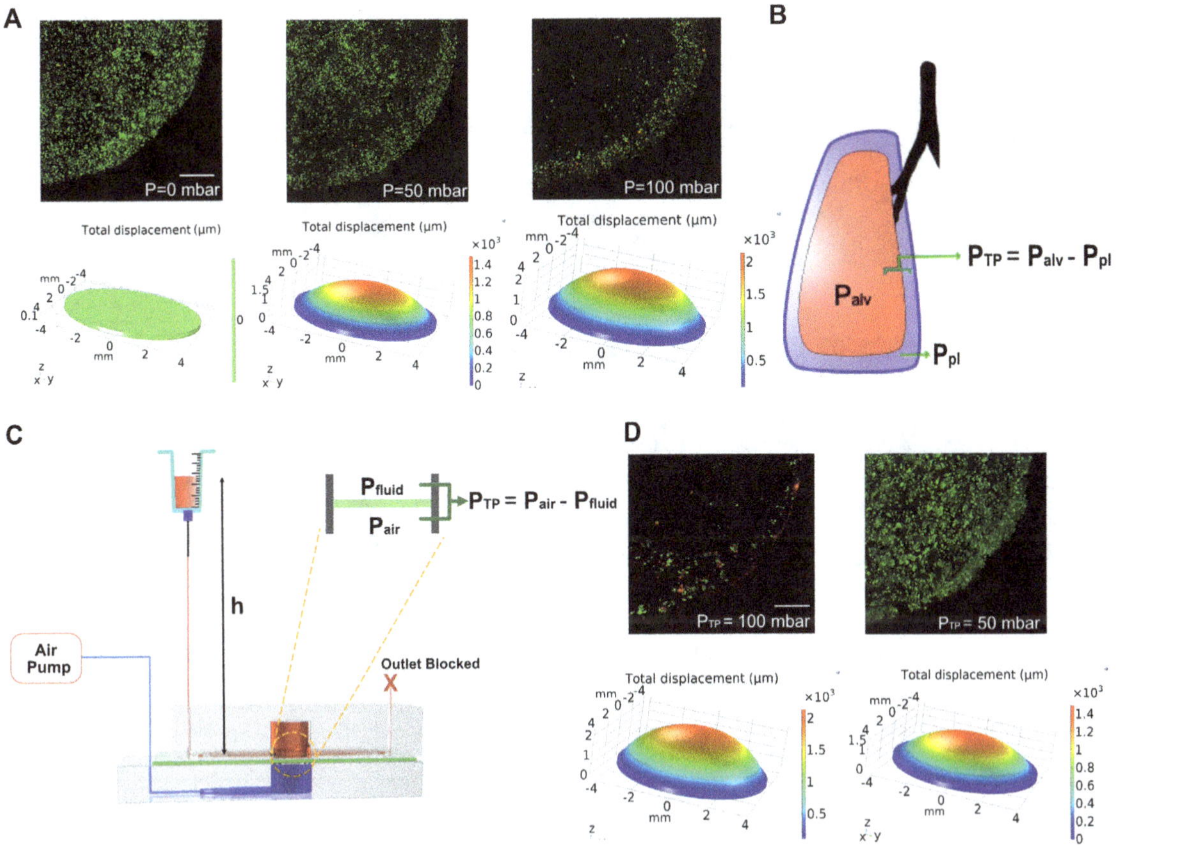

FIGURE 5 | (A) COMSOL modeling and corresponding cell experiments for studying the effect of volutrauma as a result of applied air pressure of 0 mbar, 50, and 100 mbar. Higher air pressure leads to higher concave volume. Viability of MLE-12 cells was determined using live-dead assay. Live cells are stained green while the dead cells are stained red. **(B)** Schematic depicting transpulmonary pressure in a lung. P_{TP}, P_{alv}, and P_{pl} are transpulmonary pressure, air pressure in the alveoli and pleural pressure, respectively. **(C)** Schematic showing the modeling of transpulmonary pressure in the device. P_{air} and P_{fluid} represent the air pressure and hydrostatic pressure in the device. **(D)** COMSOL modeling and corresponding cell experiment for studying barotrauma as a result of applied transpulmonary pressure of 50 and 100 mbar. Scale: 1 mm.

showing the presence of more cells (**Figure 4D**). Furthermore, the strain-dependent spatial variation in cell number was prominently observed on the 250-μm membrane, where the strain varies spatially over a wider range. Specifically, areas with high displacement exhibited lower cell numbers. On the contrary, such regional differences in cell number were not observed in the 1,000-μm membrane. Concomitant with these findings, spatial differences in surfactant production were also observed between the two conditions, as evident from the quantification of pro-SPC immunofluorescence intensity (**Figure 4D**).

Modeling Transpulmonary Pressure and Ventilator-Induced Lung Injury

Ventilator-induced lung injury (VILI) is thought to be closely related to strain heterogeneity in the lung, such that the injury occurs at high-strain regions (Beitler et al., 2016). The described fluidic-pneumatic platform is thus an ideal platform to model VILI. The two most commonly observed ventilator-induced lung injuries are volutrauma and barotrauma, which are closely related and result from alveolar overdistension caused by high tidal volumes and high transpulmonary pressure, respectively. To model volutrauma, the peak pressure of the air pressure waveform was increased from 50 to 100 mbar to generate increased concave volume and overdistension of the membrane. The concave volume for 50 and 100 mbar was 62.46 and 101.926 mm^3, respectively. As evident from the live/dead assay for MLE-12 cell cultures under these conditions, the increased pressure and the associated overdistention caused cell death and/or detachment of the cells (**Figure 5A**). At higher pressures/volumes, the effect of spatial strain heterogeneity on cell number was amplified, as seen in the case of 100 mbar, where more cells were found to be at the edges (3 mm < r < 4 mm) than in the center (r < 3 mm). Among the two pressures imposed, the devices exposed to 50 mbar air pressure had higher cell numbers at the edges than those exposed to 100 mbar. Comparing the experimental observations with the corresponding strain derived from COMSOL simulation suggests that strains above ~18% could be detrimental to the cells.

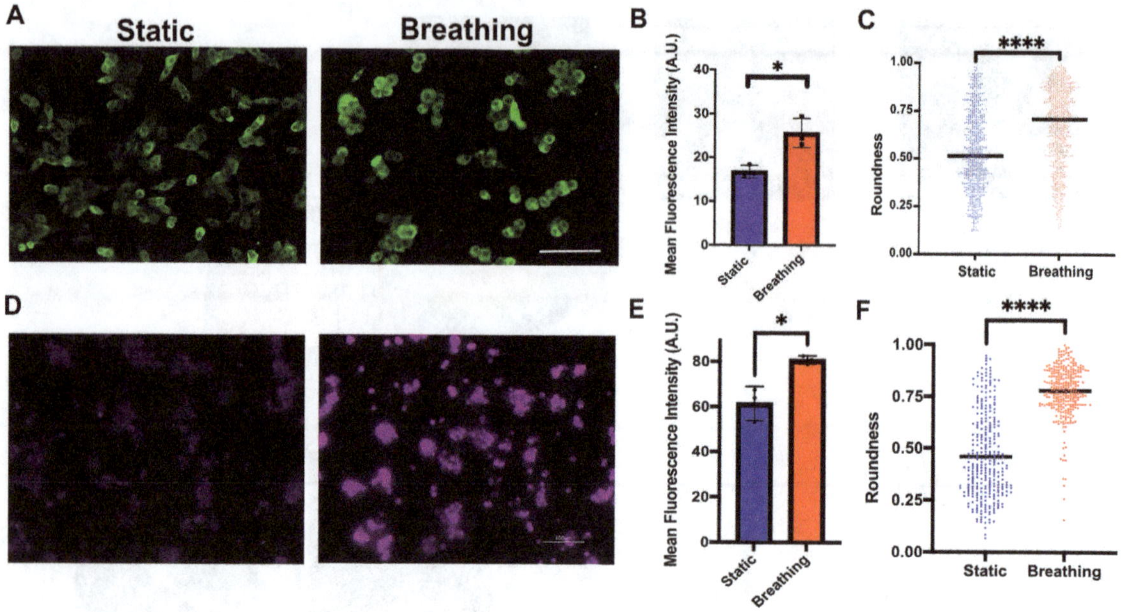

FIGURE 6 | (A) Immunofluorescence staining of Pro-SPC (green) in primary human AT2 cells cultured under static and breathing conditions and **(B)** its quantification. N = 3 where each data point is an average of fluorescence intensity measurement from 8 to 15 images per independent device. **(C)** Quantification of cell morphology in static and breathing conditions. **(D)** Immunofluorescent staining of Pro-SPC (magenta) in iAT2 cells cultured under static and breathing conditions and **(E)** its quantification. N = 3 where each data point is an average of fluorescence intensity measurement from 9 to 13 images per independent device. **(F)** Quantification of cell morphology in static and breathing conditions. Scale: 100 μm.

To model the lung transpulmonary pressure (alveolar air pressure—pleural fluid pressure) (**Figure 5B**), we have made a slight modification to the device to incorporate pleural fluid pressure. This was achieved by blocking the outlet of the media channels and replacing the syringe pump at the inlet with an open-ended syringe whose height can be easily varied (**Figure 5C**). The hydrostatic pressure developed in the chip by increasing the height of the syringe was used to mimic the pleural pressure, which applies a force on the membrane opposite to that of the air pressure, thus allowing us to define the transpulmonary pressure of the device as follows:

$$P_{TP} = P_{air} - P_{fluid} = P_{air} - \rho g h, \quad (4)$$

where P_{TP} is the transpulmonary pressure of the device, P_{air} is the applied peak pressure through the air pump, P_{fluid} is the hydrostatic pressure on the fluid side of the device, ρ is the density of the medium, g is the gravitational constant, and h is the height of the syringe above the device.

Leveraging this approach, we tested two conditions of varying transpulmonary pressure (50 and 100 mbar). To generate transpulmonary pressures of 50 mbar and 100 mbar, the syringe height was raised to 50 cm above the device height or kept at device height, respectively, while maintaining the applied air pressure at 100 mbar in both conditions. After 24 h of breathing, devices that were subjected to a transpulmonary pressure of 50 mbar showed minimal cell loss, despite the high air pressure encountered (**Figure 5D**). This is due to the hydrostatic pressure from the medium in the syringe opposing the high air pressure supplied from the air pump, which is akin to pleural fluid pressure opposing the high air pressure in the lung. Together these data highlight the ability of this biomechanically active platform to model VILI and its associated components and how such systems can be used as a predictive tool for determining regions that are predisposed to injury when subjected to mechanical ventilation.

Device Supports Human Alveolar Cell Cultures

Finally, we examined the potential of the platform to support human primary alveolar epithelial type 2 (hAT2) cells and human iPSC-derived alveolar type 2 (iAT2) cells. These cells were grown as alveolospheres in 3D cultures before dissociating them and seeding them onto the devices. Although the device can support long-term cultures of the cells (**Supplementary Figure S7**), hAT2 cells readily differentiate into alveolar type 1 (AT1) cells in 2D cultures and cease surfactant production. Therefore, the studies reported here were performed within 48 h of seeding the cells. The primary hAT2 cells were seeded at a density of 60,000 cells/cm^2 and cultured on collagen type 1-coated membranes. The cells were exposed to breathing-like motion for 24 h and compared against the corresponding static cultures. We observed significantly higher levels of pro SP-C in cells that encountered breathing-like motions (**Figures 6A, B**). Additionally, we also observed distinct differences in cell morphology between the two conditions, wherein the cells that were exposed to breathing-like motions were significantly more rounded than cells in static conditions (**Figure 6C**). The roundness of the cell, which is defined as $\frac{4*area}{\pi*major\ axis^2}$, was uniform across the device cultured in the static condition and no difference was observed between the center and edge of the membrane. On the contrary, the cells that were exposed to breathing-like motions displayed a significant difference between the edge and the center of the membrane. The cells at the center of the membrane were significantly more rounded than those at the edges, likely due to the spatially heterogeneous strain profile in the two regions (**Supplementary Figure S8**). We observed similar results with iAT2 cells, where cells cultured under breathing-like movements displayed significantly higher expression of pro-SPC as than static cultures (**Figures 6D, E**). As observed with primary hAT2 cells, iAT2 displayed more rounded morphologies in breathing-like conditions as than cells in static conditions (**Figure 6F**), although spatial differences in morphology were not observed in these cells. These results highlight the ability of culturing human alveolar epithelial cells within the device, a more clinically relevant cell source to model tissue-specific functions.

CONCLUSION

This study describes the development of a microfluidic-pneumatic platform consisting of pneumatic and fluidic chambers separated by a thin membrane that supports alveolar epithelial cell culture. The device utilizes out-of-plane stretching of the membrane *via* cyclic air pressurization to mimic strain heterogeneity experienced during alveolar expansion due to breathing, thus allowing us to study the effect of strain heterogeneity within a single device.

Our results show that breathing-like motions and micromechanics in the local environment had a significant effect on cell morphology and critical functions of alveolar epithelial cells, such as surfactant production. We also utilized this platform to model VILI by incorporating transpulmonary pressure. One of the limitations of the current study is that the dimensions of the membrane used are much greater than alveolar size, which can prevent the cells from feeling curvature at a cellular level during stretch (Nossa et al., 2021). The length scale of the alveolar architecture will have a significant effect on the strain heterogeneity generated from breathing-like motions. Recent studies have recapitulated alveolar size and curvature within lung-on-chip systems (Huang et al., 2021; Zamprogno et al., 2021), although further studies are needed to characterize heterogeneous strain and its effect on cells within such systems mimicking the alveolar architecture. While our device incorporates only the epithelial cells in its current configuration, our approach provides a framework for developing more complex systems that capture alveolar micromechanics and spatial strain heterogeneity. The incorporation of other distal lung cells such as fibroblasts within these devices will facilitate the study of progressive changes in lung biomechanics in diseases involving heterotypic cell–cell interactions such as pulmonary fibrosis. Replacing the non-porous PDMS membrane used in this study with porous membranes would allow cell–cell interactions, while also enabling air–liquid interface culture (Huh et al., 2010; Stucki et al., 2018; Doryab et al., 2021a, Doryab et al., 2021b; Huang et al., 2021; Zamprogno et al., 2021). Finally, although we have only modeled positive pleural pressure by raising the height of the syringe, negative pleural pressure can be similarly modeled by lowering the syringe height below the device height and dynamic pleural pressure changes by using an automated system that adjusts the height of the syringe in concert with the air pressure. Apart from providing insights into the role of biomechanics on lung function, these platforms can also potentially serve as important predictive tools to prevent lung injuries or for drug screening (Artzy-Schnirman et al., 2021).

AUTHOR CONTRIBUTIONS

SV and VK conceived the idea. VK, SP, and AG performed the experiments and collected the data. JH helped with the synthesis of chemicals. AT helped with human lung cell isolation. All authors wrote and edited the manuscript.

ACKNOWLEDGMENTS

We acknowledge the BioRepository and Precision Pathology Center (BRPC), a shared resource of the Duke University School of Medicine and Duke Cancer Institute, for supporting this project under Institutional Review Board oversight. The infrastructure receives support from P30 CA014236 and UM1 CA239755. We would also like to thank Dr. Darrell N. Kotton at Boston University and his laboratory members for providing the iAT2 cells.

REFERENCES

Agrawal, G., Aung, A., and Varghese, S. (2017). Skeletal Muscle-On-A-Chip: an *In Vitro* Model to Evaluate Tissue Formation and Injury. *Lab. Chip* 17, 3447–3461. doi:10.1039/C7LC00512A

Artzy-Schnirman, A., Arber Raviv, S., Doppelt Flikshtain, O., Shklover, J., Korin, N., Gross, A., et al. (2021). Advanced Human-Relevant *In Vitro* Pulmonary Platforms for Respiratory Therapeutics. *Adv. Drug Deliv. Rev.* 176, 113901. doi:10.1016/j.addr.2021.113901

Aung, A., Bhullar, I. S., Theprungsirikul, J., Davey, S. K., Lim, H. L., Chiu, Y.-J., et al. (2016). 3D Cardiac μtissues within a Microfluidic Device with Real-Time Contractile Stress Readout. *Lab. Chip* 16, 153–162. doi:10.1039/C5LC00820D

Aung, A., Kumar, V., Theprungsirikul, J., Davey, S. K., and Varghese, S. (2020). An

Engineered Tumor-On-A-Chip Device with Breast Cancer-Immune Cell Interactions for Assessing T-Cell Recruitment. *Cancer Res.* 80, 263–275. doi:10.1158/0008-5472.CAN-19-0342

Beitler, J. R., Malhotra, A., and Thompson, B. T. (2016). Ventilator-induced Lung Injury. *Clin. Chest Med.* 37, 633–646. doi:10.1016/j.ccm.2016.07.004

Benam, K. H., Mazur, M., Choe, Y., Ferrante, T. C., Novak, R., and Ingber, D. E. (2017). Human Lung Small Airway-On-A-Chip Protocol. *Methods Mol. Biol.* 1612, 345–365. doi:10.1007/978-1-4939-7021-6_25

Benam, K. H., Novak, R., Nawroth, J., Hirano-Kobayashi, M., Ferrante, T. C., Choe, Y., et al. (2016a). Matched-Comparative Modeling of Normal and Diseased Human Airway Responses Using a Microengineered Breathing Lung Chip. *Cel Syst.* 3, 456–466. e4. doi:10.1016/j.cels.2016.10.003

Benam, K. H., Villenave, R., Lucchesi, C., Varone, A., Hubeau, C., Lee, H.-H., et al. (2016b). Small Airway-On-A-Chip Enables Analysis of Human Lung Inflammation and Drug Responses *In Vitro*. *Nat. Methods* 13, 151–157. doi:10.1038/nmeth.3697

Bhatia, S. N., and Ingber, D. E. (2014). Microfluidic Organs-On-Chips. *Nat. Biotechnol.* 32, 760–772. doi:10.1038/nbt.2989

Birukov, K. G., Jacobson, J. R., Flores, A. A., Ye, S. Q., Birukova, A. A., Verin, A. D., et al. (2003). Magnitude-dependent Regulation of Pulmonary Endothelial Cell Barrier Function by Cyclic Stretch. *Am. J. Physiology-Lung Cell Mol. Physiol.* 285, L785–L797. doi:10.1152/ajplung.00336.2002

Chen, Z.-l., Chen, Y.-z., and Hu, Z.-y. (2014). A Micromechanical Model for Estimating Alveolar wall Strain in Mechanically Ventilated Edematous Lungs. *J. Appl. Physiol.* 117, 586–592. doi:10.1152/japplphysiol.00072.2014

Doryab, A., Taskin, M. B., Stahlhut, P., Schröppel, A., Orak, S., Voss, C., et al. (2021a). A Bioinspired *In Vitro* Lung Model to Study Particokinetics of Nano-/ Microparticles under Cyclic Stretch and Air-Liquid Interface Conditions. *Front. Bioeng. Biotechnol.* 9, 616830. doi:10.3389/fbioe.2021.616830

Doryab, A., Taskin, M. B., Stahlhut, P., Schröppel, A., Wagner, D. E., Groll, J., et al. (2021b). A Biomimetic, Copolymeric Membrane for Cell-Stretch Experiments with Pulmonary Epithelial Cells at the Air-Liquid Interface. *Adv. Funct. Mater.* 31, 2004707. doi:10.1002/adfm.202004707

Elias-Kirma, S., Artzy-Schnirman, A., Das, P., Heller-Algazi, M., Korin, N., and Sznitman, J. (2020). In Situ-Like Aerosol Inhalation Exposure for Cytotoxicity Assessment Using Airway-On-Chips Platforms. *Front. Bioeng. Biotechnol.* 8, 91. doi:10.3389/fbioe.2020.00091

Faffe, D. S., and Zin, W. A. (2009). Lung Parenchymal Mechanics in Health and Disease. *Physiol. Rev.* 89, 759–775. doi:10.1152/physrev.00019.2007

Felder, M., Trueeb, B., Stucki, A. O., Borcard, S., Stucki, J. D., Schnyder, B., et al. (2019). Impaired Wound Healing of Alveolar Lung Epithelial Cells in a Breathing Lung-On-A-Chip. *Front. Bioeng. Biotechnol.* 7, 3. doi:10.3389/fbioe.2019.00003

Guenat, O. T., and Berthiaume, F. (2018). Incorporating Mechanical Strain in Organs-On-A-Chip: Lung and Skin. *Biomicrofluidics* 12, 042207. doi:10.1063/1.5024895

Harris, R. S. (2005). Pressure-volume Curves of the Respiratory System. *Respir. Care* 50 (1), 78–79.

Hsia, C. C. W., Hyde, D. M., and Weibel, E. R. (2016). Lung Structure and the Intrinsic Challenges of Gas Exchange. *Compr. Physiol.* 6, 827–895. doi:10.1002/cphy.c150028

Huang, D., Liu, T., Liao, J., Maharjan, S., Xie, X., Pérez, M., et al. (2021). Reversed-engineered Human Alveolar Lung-On-A-Chip Model. *Proc. Natl. Acad. Sci. USA* 118, e2016146118. doi:10.1073/pnas.2016146118

Huh, D., Leslie, D. C., Matthews, B. D., Fraser, J. P., Jurek, S., Hamilton, G. A., et al. (2012). A Human Disease Model of Drug Toxicity-Induced Pulmonary Edema in a Lung-On-A-Chip Microdevice. *Sci. Transl. Med.* 4, 159ra147 LP. doi:10.1126/scitranslmed.3004249

Huh, D., Matthews, B. D., Mammoto, A., Montoya-Zavala, M., Hsin, H. Y., and Ingber, D. E. (2010). Reconstituting Organ-Level Lung Functions on a Chip. *Science* 328, 1662 LP–1668. doi:10.1126/science.1188302

Hurtado, D. E., Erranz, B., Lillo, F., Sarabia-Vallejos, M., Iturrieta, P., Morales, F., et al. (2020). Progression of Regional Lung Strain and Heterogeneity in Lung Injury: Assessing the Evolution under Spontaneous Breathing and Mechanical Ventilation. *Ann. Intensive Care* 10, 107. doi:10.1186/s13613-020-00725-0

Ingenito, E. P., Tsai, L. W., Majumdar, A., and Suki, B. (2005). On the Role of Surface Tension in the Pathophysiology of Emphysema. *Am. J. Respir. Crit. Care Med.* 171, 300–304. doi:10.1164/rccm.200406-770PP

Ishahak, M., Hill, J., Amin, Q., Wubker, L., Hernandez, A., Mitrofanova, A., et al. (2020). Modular Microphysiological System for Modeling of Biologic Barrier Function. *Front. Bioeng. Biotechnol.* 8, 581163. doi:10.3389/fbioe.2020.581163

Jacob, A., Vedaie, M., Roberts, D. A., Thomas, D. C., Villacorta-Martin, C., Alysandratos, K.-D., et al. (2019). Derivation of Self-Renewing Lung Alveolar Epithelial Type II Cells from Human Pluripotent Stem Cells. *Nat. Protoc.* 14, 3303–3332. doi:10.1038/s41596-019-0220-0

Jain, A., Barrile, R., van der Meer, A., Mammoto, A., Mammoto, T., De Ceunynck, K., et al. (2018). Primary Human Lung Alveolus-On-A-Chip Model of Intravascular Thrombosis for Assessment of Therapeutics. *Clin. Pharmacol. Ther.* 103, 332–340. doi:10.1002/cpt.742

Jimenez-Valdes, R. J., Can, U. I., Niemeyer, B. F., and Benam, K. H. (2020). Where We Stand: Lung Organotypic Living Systems that Emulate Human-Relevant Host-Environment/Pathogen Interactions. *Front. Bioeng. Biotechnol.* 8, 989. doi:10.3389/fbioe.2020.00989

Katsura, H., Sontake, V., Tata, A., Kobayashi, Y., Edwards, C. E., Heaton, B. E., et al. (2020). Human Lung Stem Cell-Based Alveolospheres Provide Insights into SARS-CoV-2-Mediated Interferon Responses and Pneumocyte Dysfunction. *Cell Stem Cell* 27, 890–904. e8. doi:10.1016/j.stem.2020.10.005

Khalid, M. A. U., Kim, Y. S., Ali, M., Lee, B. G., Cho, Y.-J., and Choi, K. H. (2020). A Lung Cancer-On-Chip Platform with Integrated Biosensors for Physiological Monitoring and Toxicity Assessment. *Biochem. Eng. J.* 155, 107469. doi:10.1016/j.bej.2019.107469

Knudsen, L., and Ochs, M. (2018). The Micromechanics of Lung Alveoli: Structure and Function of Surfactant and Tissue Components. *Histochem. Cel Biol.* 150, 661–676. doi:10.1007/s00418-018-1747-9

Kumar, V., and Varghese, S. (2019). *Ex Vivo* Tumor-on-a-Chip Platforms to Study Intercellular Interactions within the Tumor Microenvironment. *Adv. Healthc. Mater.* 8, 1801198. doi:10.1002/adhm.201801198

Low, L. A., Mummery, C., Berridge, B. R., Austin, C. P., and Tagle, D. A. (2021). Organs-on-chips: into the Next Decade. *Nat. Rev. Drug Discov.* 20, 345–361. doi:10.1038/s41573-020-0079-3

Martinez, F., Lewis, J., Copland, I., Engelberts, D., Kavanagh, B. P., Post, M., et al. (2004). Mechanical Ventilation Effect on Surfactant Content, Function, and Lung Compliance in the Newborn Rat. *Pediatr. Res.* 56, 19–25. doi:10.1203/01.PDR.0000128980.82797.29

Mejías, J. C., Nelson, M. R., Liseth, O., and Roy, K. (2020). A 96-well Format Microvascularized Human Lung-On-A-Chip Platform for Microphysiological Modeling of Fibrotic Diseases. *Lab. Chip* 20, 3601–3611. doi:10.1039/D0LC00644K

Nawroth, J. C., Lucchesi, C., Cheng, D., Shukla, A., Ngyuen, J., Shroff, T., et al. (2020). A Microengineered Airway Lung Chip Models Key Features of Viral-Induced Exacerbation of Asthma. *Am. J. Respir. Cel Mol. Biol.* 63, 591–600. doi:10.1165/rcmb.2020-0010MA

Neidlinger-Wilke, C., Grood, E., Claes, L., and Brand, R. (2002). Fibroblast Orientation to Stretch Begins within Three Hours. *J. Orthop. Res.* 20, 953–956. doi:10.1016/S0736-0266(02)00024-4

Nossa, R., Costa, J., Cacopardo, L., and Ahluwalia, A. (2021). Breathing *In Vitro*: Designs and Applications of Engineered Lung Models. *J. Tissue Eng.* 12, 204173142110086. doi:10.1177/20417314211008696

Park, J. Y., Ryu, H., Lee, B., Ha, D.-H., Ahn, M., Kim, S., et al. (2018). Development of a Functional Airway-On-A-Chip by 3D Cell Printing. *Biofabrication* 11, 015002. doi:10.1088/1758-5090/aae545

Perlman, C. E., Lederer, D. J., and Bhattacharya, J. (2011). Micromechanics of Alveolar Edema. *Am. J. Respir. Cel Mol. Biol.* 44, 34–39. doi:10.1165/rcmb.2009-0005OC

Plantier, L., Cazes, A., Dinh-Xuan, A.-T., Bancal, C., Marchand-Adam, S., and Crestani, B. (2018). Physiology of the Lung in Idiopathic Pulmonary Fibrosis. *Eur. Respir. Rev.* 27, 170062. doi:10.1183/16000617.0062-2017

Püspöki, Z., Storath, M., Sage, D., and Unser, M. (2016). Transforms and Operators for Directional Bioimage Analysis: A Survey. *Adv. Anat. Embryol. Cel Biol.* 219, 69–93. doi:10.1007/978-3-319-28549-8_3

Rivlin, R. S. (1948). Large Elastic Deformations of Isotropic Materials IV. Further Developments of the General Theory. *Phil. Trans. R. Soc. Lond. A.* 241, 379–397. doi:10.1098/rsta.1948.0024

Roan, E., and Waters, C. M. (2011). What Do We Know about Mechanical Strain in Lung Alveoli? *Am. J. Physiology-Lung Cell Mol. Physiol.* 301, L625–L635. doi:10.1152/ajplung.00105.2011

Sanchez-Esteban, J., Tsai, S.-W., Sang, J., Qin, J., Torday, J. S., and Rubin, L. P. (1998). Effects of Mechanical Forces on Lung-specific Gene Expression. *Am. J. Med. Sci.* 316, 200–204. doi:10.1097/00000441-199809000-00009

Shrestha, J., Razavi Bazaz, S., Aboulkheyr Es, H., Yaghobian Azari, D., Thierry, B., Ebrahimi Warkiani, M., et al. (2020). Lung-on-a-chip: the Future of Respiratory Disease Models and Pharmacological Studies. *Crit. Rev. Biotechnol.* 40, 213–230. doi:10.1080/07388551.2019.1710458

Shrestha, J., Ryan, S. T., Mills, O., Zhand, S., Razavi Bazaz, S., Hansbro, P. M., et al. (2021). A 3D-Printed Microfluidic Platform for Simulating the Effects of CPAP on the Nasal Epithelium. *Biofabrication* 13, 035028. doi:10.1088/1758-5090/abe4c1

Smith, B. J. (2016). Strain Heterogeneity in the Injured Lung: Cause or Consequence? *J. Appl. Physiol.* 121, 1363–1364. doi:10.1152/japplphysiol.00818.2016

Stucki, A. O., Stucki, J. D., Hall, S. R. R., Felder, M., Mermoud, Y., Schmid, R. A., et al. (2015). A Lung-On-A-Chip Array with an Integrated Bio-Inspired Respiration Mechanism. *Lab. Chip* 15, 1302–1310. doi:10.1039/C4LC01252F

Stucki, J. D., Hobi, N., Galimov, A., Stucki, A. O., Schneider-Daum, N., Lehr, C.-M., et al. (2018). Medium Throughput Breathing Human Primary Cell Alveolus-On-Chip Model. *Sci. Rep.* 8, 14359. doi:10.1038/s41598-018-32523-x

Sznitman, J. (2021). Revisiting Airflow and Aerosol Transport Phenomena in the Deep Lungs with Microfluidics. *Chem. Rev.* doi:10.1021/acs.chemrev.1c00621

Torday, J. S., and Rehan, V. K. (2002). Stretch-stimulated Surfactant Synthesis Is Coordinated by the Paracrine Actions of PTHrP and Leptin. *Am. J. Physiology-Lung Cell Mol. Physiol.* 283, L130–L135. doi:10.1152/ajplung.00380.2001

Winkler, M., Simon, M. G., Vu, T., Gartner, T. L., Jester, J. V., Lee, A. P., et al. (2014). A Microfabricated, Optically Accessible Device to Study the Effects of Mechanical Cues on Collagen Fiber Organization. *Biomed. Microdevices* 16, 255–267. doi:10.1007/s10544-013-9829-x

Yoon, S.-H., Reyes-Ortiz, V., Kim, K.-H., Seo, Y. H., and Mofrad, M. R. K. (2010). Analysis of Circular PDMS Microballoons with Ultralarge Deflection for MEMS Design. *J. Microelectromech. Syst.* 19, 854–864. doi:10.1109/JMEMS.2010.2049984

Zacharias, W. J., Frank, D. B., Zepp, J. A., Morley, M. P., Alkhaleel, F. A., Kong, J., et al. (2018). Regeneration of the Lung Alveolus by an Evolutionarily Conserved Epithelial Progenitor. *Nature* 555, 251–255. doi:10.1038/nature25786

Zamprogno, P., Wüthrich, S., Achenbach, S., Thoma, G., Stucki, J. D., Hobi, N., et al. (2021). Second-generation Lung-On-A-Chip with an Array of Stretchable Alveoli Made with a Biological Membrane. *Commun. Biol.* 4, 168. doi:10.1038/s42003-021-01695-0

17

A Volatile and Dynamic Longitudinal Microbiome is Associated with Less Reduction in Lung Function in Adolescents with Cystic Fibrosis

*Marisa I. Metzger[1,2], Simon Y. Graeber[3,4,5], Mirjam Stahl[3,4,5], Olaf Sommerburg[2,6,7], Marcus A. Mall[3,4,5], Alexander H. Dalpke[8] and Sébastien Boutin[1,2]**

[1] Department of Infectious Diseases, Medical Microbiology and Hygiene, University of Heidelberg, Heidelberg, Germany, [2] Translational Lung Research Center Heidelberg (TLRC), German Center for Lung Research (DZL), University of Heidelberg, Heidelberg, Germany, [3] German Centre for Lung Research (DZL), Associated Partner Site, Berlin, Germany, [4] Department of Pediatric Respiratory Medicine, Immunology and Critical Care Medicine and Cystic Fibrosis Center, Charité - Universitätsmedizin Berlin, Berlin, Germany, [5] Berlin Institute of Health (BIH), Berlin, Germany, [6] Division of Pediatric Pulmonology & Allergy and Cystic Fibrosis Center, Department of Pediatrics, University of Heidelberg, Heidelberg, Germany, [7] Department of Translational Pulmonology, University of Heidelberg, Heidelberg, Germany, [8] Institute of Medical Microbiology and Virology, Technische Universität Dresden, Dresden, Germany

***Correspondence:**
Sébastien Boutin
sebastien.boutin@med.uni-heidelberg.de

Progressive impairment in lung function caused by chronic polymicrobial airway infection remains the major cause of death in patients with cystic fibrosis (CF). Cross-sectional studies suggest an association between lung function decline and specific lung microbiome ecotypes. However, longitudinal studies on the stability of the airway microbiome are missing for adolescents with CF constituting the age group showing the highest rate of decline in lung function. In this study, we analyzed longitudinal lung function data and sputum samples collected over a period of 3 to 5 years from 12 adolescents with CF. The sputum microbiome was analyzed using 16S rRNA gene sequencing. Our results indicate that the individual course of the lung microbiome is associated with longitudinal lung function. In our cohort, patients with a dynamic, diverse microbiome showed a slower decline of lung function measured by $FEV_{1\%}$ predicted, whereas a more stable and less diverse lung microbiome was related to worse outcomes. Specifically, a higher abundance of the phyla Bacteroidetes and Firmicutes was linked to a better clinical outcome, while Proteobacteria were correlated with a decline in $FEV_{1\%}$ predicted. Our study indicates that the stability and diversity of the lung microbiome and the abundance of Bacteroidetes and Firmicutes are associated with the lung function decline and are one of the contributing factors to the disease severity.

Keywords: lung microbiome, cystic fibrosis, longitudinal study, volatility analysis, *Pseudomonas aeruginosa*, adolescent

INTRODUCTION

Patients with the autosomal recessive disorder cystic fibrosis (CF) suffer progressive impairment of lung function, which is the most common reason for reduced quality of life and mortality (Bell et al., 2020; Mall et al., 2020). Infections with potential respiratory pathogens (PRP) increase mortality (Sherrard et al., 2014). PRP such as *Pseudomonas aeruginosa* or *Staphylococcus aureus* may overgrow the commensal microbiota of the airways causing a decreased microbial diversity in the lung, which is associated with a decrease in lung function and an increase of pulmonary exacerbations in adult CF patients (Boutin et al., 2015; Coburn et al., 2015; O'Neill et al., 2015; Boutin et al., 2017).

Analysis of the lung microbiome in cross-sectional studies revealed variable microbial compositions among patients with CF (Coburn et al., 2015). Of note, the lung microbiome of pediatric patients with CF was shown to be more diverse as compared to adult patients with more advanced lung disease states (Cox et al., 2010; Zemanick et al., 2017). Furthermore, it was demonstrated that patients harbor an individual lung microbiome; thus, longitudinal instead of cross-sectional studies are required to reveal the functional role of microbiome alterations (Whelan et al., 2017).

A few longitudinal studies in CF patients have already been performed (Carmody et al., 2015; Cuthbertson et al., 2016; Whelan et al., 2017; Ahmed et al., 2019) confirming a patient-specific microbiome. No overall community change in the microbiome could be detected upon the first exacerbation in infants (Ahmed et al., 2019), as well as in adults with CF (Whelan et al., 2017). The PRP *P. aeruginosa* was reported to occur in a high relative amount during an exacerbation but also in phases of stable lung function. Cuthbertson et al. reported no change in the microbiome community upon exacerbation and antibiotic treatment indicating a high resistance and resilience of the lung microbiome (Cuthbertson et al., 2016).

We focused on the adolescent age group when the microbiome often shifts from a diverse microbiome to a stable microbiome with a higher load of PRPs, which goes along with a fast decline in lung function and an increase of the CF disease's burden (Szczesniak et al., 2017). The aim of our study was to evaluate the long-term evolution of the microbiome over a period of more than 3 years. We hypothesized that the personalized lung microbiome of each patient is related to lung disease progression and that patients with a better lung function show a more diverse, volatile lung microbiome.

MATERIAL AND METHODS

Study Subjects and Design

Adolescent patients, diagnosed with CF based on established diagnostic criteria (De Boeck et al., 2011), provided sputum samples *via* spontaneous expectorations during clinical visits. These included routine visits every 3 months and unforeseen visits due to pulmonary exacerbations and elective treatments. The study was approved by the Ethics Committee of the University of Heidelberg (S-370/2011), and all patients, their parents, and/or legal guardians gave written informed consent. Only patients having expectorated sputum at least during three routine visits per year during the full course of 3 to 5 years were included, resulting in 12 patients included in the study. Clinical data including demographics, lung function, and information on antibiotic therapy are provided in **Table 1**. Lung function was determined by the forced expiratory volume in one second expressed as percent predicted (FEV_1%pred) according to the global lung function initiative reference values (Cooper et al., 2017). Infections with *P. aeruginosa* were classified as negative, intermittent, or chronic based on culture results and *P. aeruginosa* antibody titers as previously described (Stahl et al., 2017). None of the patients were under CFTR modulator therapy during the course of the study.

Sputum Microbiome Analysis

Details are provided in the online supplement. After sample preparation, DNA was extracted with the QIAamp Mini Kit (Qiagen, Hilden, Germany) according to the manufacturer's protocol. DNA amplification *via* PCR was done using universal barcoded bacterial primers flanking the V4 region of the 16S

TABLE 1 | Clinical characteristics of patients with cystic fibrosis.

	Stable	Decliner
Number of subjects	4	8
Age in years (sd) NS	17.1 (1.18)	17.3 (1.4)
Sex males/females	2/2	3/5
BMI [kg/m^2] (sd)***	20.5 (1.41)	18.4 (2.04)
$FEV_{1\%}$ predicted (sd)***	86.8 (16.3)	58.2 (22.5)
CFTR genotype		
F508del/F508del	1	3
F508del/other	3	4
other/other		1
Number if i.v. treatment per year (sd)**	1.1 (0.5)	3.5 (1.77)
Pancreatic insufficiency	4	8

*Data are expressed as mean with the standard deviation. The difference in age, BMI, and $FEV_{1\%}$ predicted between the two groups was evaluated by a t-test. **$p < 0.05$), ***$p < 0.001$, NS, not significant.*

BMI, body mass index, FEV_1, forced expiratory volume in 1 s.

rRNA gene (515F: GTGCCAGCMGCCGCGGTAA and 806R: GGACTACHVGGGTWTCTAAT). A mock community (HM-782D, BEI Resources, Manassas, USA) was used in the PCR as a positive control. Next-generation paired-end sequencing was performed on an Illumina MiSeq system (2 × 250 cycles) by Eurofins Genomics. Processing the raw sequences was done using DADA2 as previously described to amplicon sequence variants (ASV) (Schmitt et al., 2020). Shortly, raw sequences were processed through quality control (no ambiguities (N), less than one error per reads, truncation of the reads after quality score < 2) merged as contigs and checked for chimera with the default parameters of DADA2. Taxonomy was defined based on the Silva database (Version 132). Negative control from DNA extraction and PCR reaction were performed to evaluate contamination. However, none of the blanks produced a visible amplicon (QIAxcel DNA screen) or showed enough DNA to be quantified with PicoGreen (<2.5 ng/ml), indicating no contamination. A quantitative PCR was performed with a universal 16S rRNA primer to evaluate the number of 16S rRNA gene copies as previously published (Boutin et al., 2017; Schoilew et al., 2019).

Statistics

A time index (t_i) was created starting at the 14th year for each patient to align all patients accordingly to their age. The time range of this study is monthly to obtain rational numbers needed for the volatility analysis. Descriptive indices and statistics were calculated using the R packages *phyloseq* (McMurdie and Holmes, 2013) and *microbiome* (Leo Lahti et al., 2017). Statistical variation of the β-diversity and clinical values was investigated by permutational analysis of variance (PERMANOVA) with the *vegan* R package (Jari Oksanen et al., 2019). Variation of descriptive values and clinical values between groups was tested with a Wilcoxon rank-sum test. The R packages *stats* (Team RC, 2019) and *cluster* (Maechler et al., 2019) were used to perform hierarchical cluster analysis on the samples. The hierarchical cluster tree based on *Ward's minimum variance* was used to calculate the cluster groups of all microbiome samples. A phylogenetic tree of all ASVs was constructed by multiple-sequence alignment with the *DECIPHER* R package (Wright, 2016), and the constructed neighbor-joining tree served as a template for a maximum likelihood tree calculated by the *phangorn* R package (Schliep, 2011). The *longitudinal* plugin for Qiime2 (Bokulich et al., 2018) was used to perform metadata Volatility Analysis and Feature Volatility Analysis at the ASV level and phylum level. In the "feature volatility analysis," the machine learning algorithm uses the structure of the data as a learning input to identify features (ASV or phyla) that are the most important ones in the prediction of the different states (= time points). The n_estimators input value was set to 1,000, and Random Forest Regression was used as an estimator. The details are provided in the online supplement. Raw data and scripts are available in the GitHub repository https://github.com/MarisaIsabell/CF-lung-microbiome-longitudinal-development. All analysis in R was done with R 3.6.0 and RStudio 1.1.463.

RESULTS

Patient With a Declining Lung Function Showed a Higher Number of Intravenous Therapies per Year

We were able to collect 286 sputum samples from 12 patients with at least three samples per year over a 3–5-year period (**Supplementary Figure 1**). To group patients for different functional outcomes, we calculated the change of the mean FEV_1%pred per year with a linear regression and used the slope as the rate of decline per year. By using a grouping threshold of 0%, we defined "stable" patients (n = 4) showing a stable FEV_1%pred over the years with the change ranging from 0.34% to 1.84% per year. The "decliner" patients (n = 8) had a decline of the FEV_1%pred values between -0.08% and -9.14% per year.

We then analyzed this dynamic, functional parameter in comparison to different demographic and clinical variables. We observed that the number of intravenous (i.v.) antibiotic therapies per year correlated with the change of FEV_1%pred per year: Patients showing a decline in lung function experienced more i.v. antibiotic therapies (**Supplementary Figure 1**). Antibiotic therapy is a known to have a high influence of the microbiome. Therefore, we compared the impact of the number of i.v. antibiotic therapies per year on the median values of each patient's microbiome alpha diversity (Shannon index), dominance (relative), and evenness (Simpson index) and on the microbial burden (copies/μl). We observed no significant relationship between the numbers of i.v. antibiotic therapies per year on either alpha-diversity parameter.

The Temporal Evolution of the Lung Microbiome Is Driven by a Personalized Microbial Fingerprint

When analyzing the airway microbiome, we identified the individual patient as a factor in the PERMANOVA explaining 49% (Morisita-Horn distance) or 33% (weighted UniFrac distance) of the variance. The β-diversity calculated between two samples from the same patient at different time points was significantly lower ($p < 0.001$) than the β-diversity between two samples from different patients. Thus, the microbiomes of individual patients in this cohort stayed more similar over time compared to the microbiome of different patients. These results show that each patient harbors a dynamic but individual microbiome evolution.

Patients With Stable Lung Function Have a More Diverse Microbiome With Less Dominance

We found 137 distinct ASVs and 38 genera, which were present in at least one sample with a relative abundance ≥5%. All samples were clustered based on their microbiome composition in 24 hierarchical clusters (**Figure 1**). Cluster A consists mostly of samples with high abundance of *Pseudomonas* (relative abundance > 60%) and was characteristic for samples from patients with a chronic infection of the mentioned bacteria.

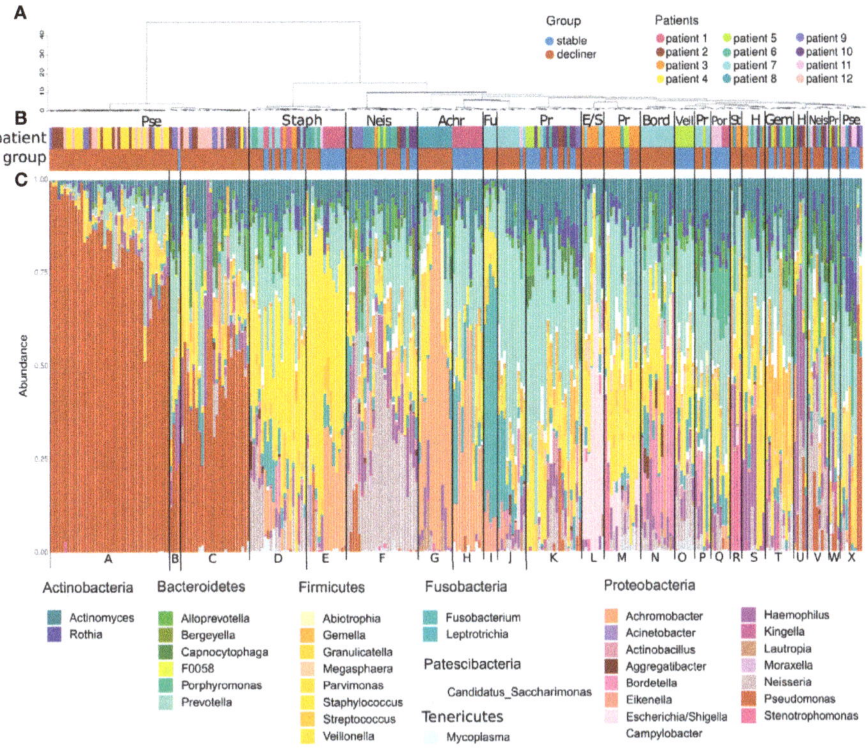

FIGURE 1 | Microbiome composition of each sample grouped by hierarchical clustering. **(A)** Dendrogram representing the hierarchical clustering of the samples. **(B)** Colored bars showing the affiliation of the samples to a patient (pat) and the patient FEV-group (group; stable or decliner). The most abundant genera are written above the colored bars to name the clusters. Pse, *Pseudomonas*; Staph, *Staphylococcus*; Neis, *Neisseria*; Achr, *Achromobacter*; Fu, *Fusobacteria*; Pr, *Prevotella*; E/S, *Escherichia/Shigella*; Bord, *Bordetella*; Veil, *Veillonella*; Por, *Porphyromonas*; St, *Stenotrophomonas*; H, *Haemophilus*; Gem, *Gemella*. **(C)** Relative abundance of the genera, which occurs in at least one sample with a relative abundance ≥5%. All other genera are cumulated as "Others." The letter at the bottom indicates the cluster groups.

Related clusters were cluster C with a mid-level *Pseudomonas* infection (relative abundance primary > 25%) and cluster B with samples harboring a low-level infection (relative abundance primary < 25%). Indeed, the clinical data reported chronic infection with *Pseudomonas aeruginosa* (**Supplementary Figure 1**) for patients 2, 4, 9, and 12, whose samples mostly build up these clusters.

The genus *Pseudomonas* was almost exclusively present in the "decliner" population, suggesting a worsening of the lung function associated with the infection with the pathogen (**Figure 1B**). The β-diversity from samples from the same patient affiliated to the *Pseudomonas* clusters was much lower than the β-diversity within the commensal clusters (**Supplementary Figure 2**), indicating a less diverse and more stable microbiome for *Pseudomonas*-infected samples. Other reported pathogens in CF like *Staphylococcus* and *Haemophilus* dominated clusters, which are composed of samples from both decliner and stable patients (cluster M, D, and S). Clusters dominated by commensals like *Porphyromonas* or *Veillonella* were composed of samples from stable patients.

We next intended to probe whether differences in individual fluctuations of the microbiome instead of the analysis of a static assignment into a microbial cluster would be more appropriate to link microbiome to clinical changes in individual patients. We used a volatility analysis in which the temporal development of each patient's microbiome parameters (alpha diversity, dominance, evenness) was used to visualize the fluctuation of the corresponding descriptive parameter in two patient groups (**Figure 2A**). The α-diversity was higher in patients from the "stable" groups compared to the "decliner" group over the whole time period. When calculating the mean of the alpha diversity for each patient, the trend stayed the same (**Figure 2A**, boxplot; $p < 0.05$). Accordingly, the relative dominance, as analyzed in a longitudinal manner, was higher for the patients with a decline in FEV_1%pred than for the "stable" patients (**Figure 2B**) with a significant p-value of 0.03 when comparing the patient means for relative dominance. Thus, patients with a decline in lung function had a less diverse and more dominated microbiome. Furthermore, the volatility analysis also clearly revealed the high variation of single-point measurements as revealed by the high variation of the microbial parameters, most pronounced in the decliner group.

The evenness of the microbiome did not reveal a large difference between the two patient groups in the longitudinal volatility analysis as well as in the boxplot comparing the mean evenness for each patient with a p-value of 0.57 (**Figure 2C**).

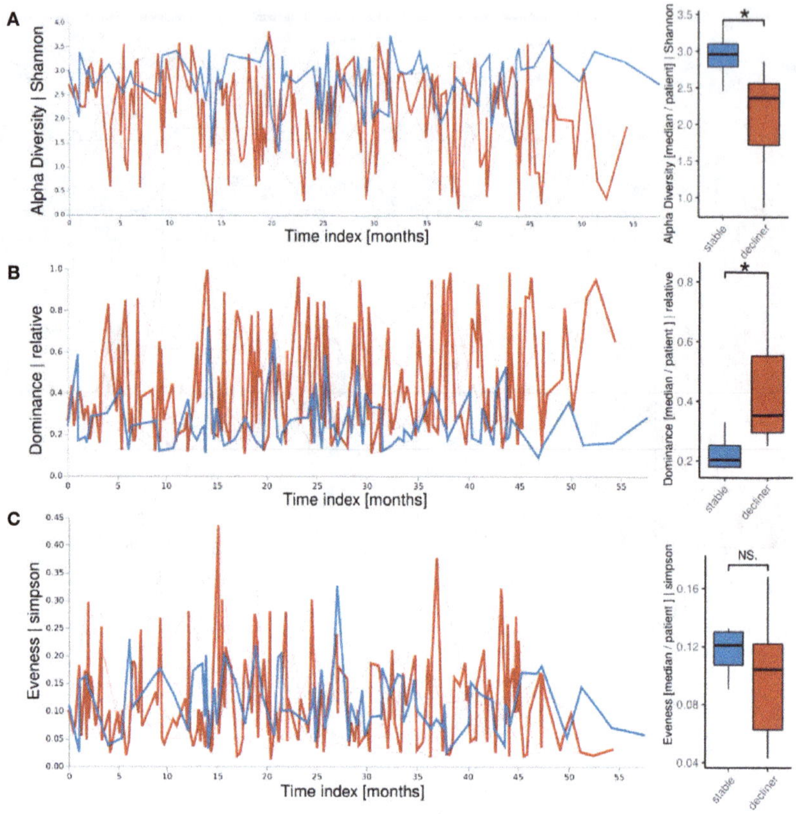

FIGURE 2 | Longitudinal volatility analysis and boxplot visualization of descriptive microbiome statistics grouped by the patient groups: Alpha diversity **(A)**, relative dominance **(B)**, and the evenness **(C)**. The thick lines represent how the variable changes over time in the patient group while the thin lines represent each patient. *$p < 0.05$, NS, not significant.

The microbiome of the "decliner" population was indeed dominated by mostly one pathogen.

The "Decliner" Group Is Dominated by Pseudomonas ASV While the "Stable" Group Showed Higher Abundance of Commensal Bacteria

We performed a "Feature Volatility Analysis" on the ASV level which can identify ASVs that are most discriminatory between the patient groups. The first seven ASVs reported by the Feature Volatility Analysis, which hold the highest importance for the random forest classifier to discriminate between the states, belonged to commensal bacteria (**Figure 3A**). Among those, *Prevotella melaninogenica* and *Veillonella* sp. had a high global median (referring to the relative abundance of the taxa in all samples) indicating the frequent presence in the samples. Together, high global median and identification by feature volatility analysis indicated the ubiquitous abundance of those commensals in the microbiome and importance for the ecology of the lung microbiome. Calculating the statistical difference between the relative abundances of the respective genera reported a decrease in the "decliner" group, which was significant for *Prevotella* ($p = 0.03$), but not for *Veillonella* ($p = 0.15$) (**Figure 3B**).

The first ASV with a very high global variance in the microbiome, indicating a great difference in relative abundance between the groups, was a *Pseudomonas* sp. The high variance and high global mean (not shown), but low global median, suggest that this ASV was not frequently found in the samples but dominated the microbiome if present. Indeed, the prevalence of *Pseudomonas* in our cohort (including all samples) was 54.2% with relative individual abundances up to almost 100% (**Figure 1C**). In the boxplot analysis based on the *Pseudomonas* mean abundance per patient, the decliner group revealed a higher relative abundance of the genus *Pseudomonas* ($p = 0.3$). We also observed a slightly higher bacterial burden in the sputum of patients from the decliner group (**Supplementary Figure 3**).

The Phylum Proteobacteria Is the Main Driver for the "Decliner" Patient Group

At the phylum level, the Feature Volatility Analysis reported Proteobacteria as the most important phylum to distinguish the longitudinal microbiome development between the two patient groups, which also comprises *Pseudomonas* (**Figure 4A**). In the volatility plot, the "stable" patients had a lower amount of Proteobacteria in their microbiome, whereas the "decliner"

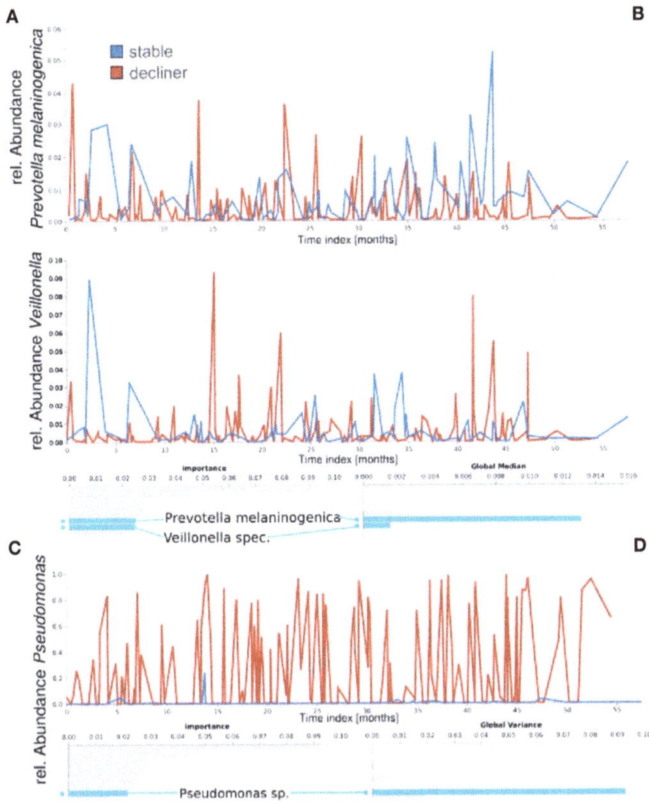

FIGURE 3 | Longitudinal feature volatility analysis on ASV level **(A, C)** and boxplot visualization **(B, D)** grouped by patient groups. The feature volatility analysis was done on ASV levels, and the boxplots are median values for each patient for all species with the respective genus name. **(A, B)** Shown are two examples of important commensals (*Prevotella* and *Veillonella*), which do also reveal a high global median in the feature volatility analysis. **(C, D)** A *Pseudomonas* ASV is the eighth important feature (ASV), but the first with a very high global variance indicates a high impact on the microbiome development, and it is important for distinguishing between patient groups. *$p < 0.05$), NS, not significant.

patients harbored more Proteobacteria. For the Proteobacteria phylum volatility as well as the *Pseudomonas* volatility, the graph for the "decliner" group is more variable than for the "stable" group. We observed an enrichment of the Proteobacteria ($p = 0.03$) but a decrease of the next following important phyla Firmicutes ($p = 0.07$), Fusobacteria ($p = 0.05$), Actinobacteria ($p = 0.15$), and Bacteroides ($p = 0.05$) in the "decliner" compared to the "stable" patients (**Figure 4B**). The non-significance for the differences observed in Firmicutes, Fusobacteria, and Actinobacteria when comparing the mean per patient for those values is not surprising due to the low number of patients and thus data points for this comparison.

DISCUSSION

This study with 12 patients and the continuous sampling for up to 5 years is to our knowledge the first long-term longitudinal study in adolescents with CF. Other studies have focused on infants (Frayman et al., 2017; Ahmed et al., 2019) or adults (Whelan et al., 2017). Compared to other studies that have been focusing on the impact of clinical state or age on microbiome data from infant to adulthood (Cox et al., 2010; Carmody et al., 2018), we focused on the use of volatility and machine learning to establish the important factors that are associated with the decline in lung function during the period of the life when a fast decline in lung function and an increase of the CF disease's burden are observed (Szczesniak et al., 2017). Our data show that the temporal dynamics of the patient's lung microbiome in a period of 3–5 years are linked with the individual microbiome composition and the dominance by Proteobacteria as well as the decline in the lung function. Patients with a diverse microbiome showed a high variability of the microbiome over time while patients carrying a monospecific and less diverse microbiome showed high stability that was associated with decrease in lung function. These results agree with a study of a cohort of adults showing a relatively stable microbiome dominated by Proteobacteria while patients with a more diverse microbiome had also a more variable microbiome composition (Whelan et al., 2017). Furthermore, our group-wise analysis comparing patients with lung function decline to stable patients showed that a milder disease progression in CF is linked to a volatile, dynamic, and diverse microbiome in the lower airways (**Figures 2, 3**). Using a new analysis of the volatility of the lung microbiome, the

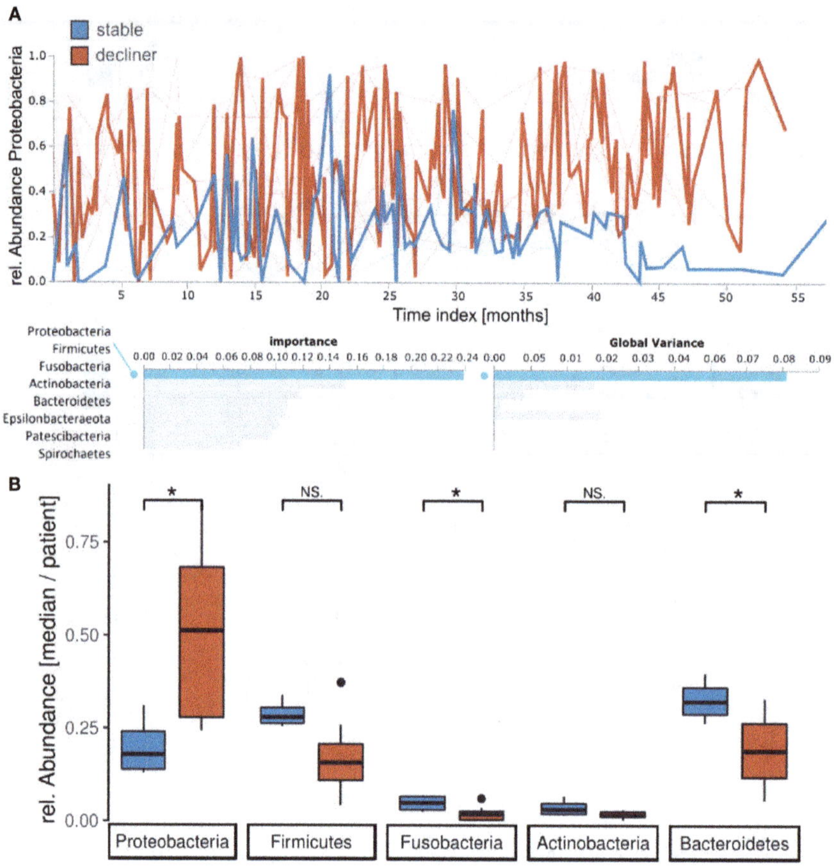

FIGURE 4 | Proteobacteria are enriched for patients in the decliner group. **(A)** Longitudinal feature volatility analysis at the phylum level reveals the Proteobacteria as the most important feature for the microbiome progression in this study. **(B)** Median relative abundance for each patient of the five most important phyla grouped by the patient groups. *$p < 0.05$, NS, not significant.

necessity of multiple sampling becomes very obvious, since single data from just one time-point might be misleading (e.g., see the large variation in the volatility analysis) (**Figures 2, 3**). Our findings highlight that analysis of single time-points holds the problem of high variance. Therefore, considerable changes in the lung microbiome can only be studied by longitudinal means combined with a volatility analysis.

High variability might indicate a cycle of bacterial immigration and removal due to a functional lung clearance system (Dickson et al., 2015). A stable microbiome in contrast is more probably linked to a pathogen-infected lung with local bacterial replication and worse outcome of the disease. In most of the patients presenting a higher diversity and higher temporal variability, the decline in lung function is reduced compare to patients with a high dominance of Proteobacteria. Yet, the question of which factors trigger the transition from an unstable but diverse microbiome to a microbiome dominated by chronic infection with a high abundant pathogen remains open. We propose to use the observed difference in the phylum abundances between the two patient groups identified here as a hint to an answer. Proteobacteria were the most responsible phylum for a chronically infected lung. Moreover, the phyla Bacteroidetes and Firmicutes were decreased and imbalanced for the "decliner." Other studies have also reported associations between the reduction of *Prevotella* or in general anaerobic bacteria and the worsening of the lung function (Zemanick et al., 2013; O'Neill et al., 2015). Our data also demonstrate that the microbiome composition at a single time-point alone does not explain the classification of the patients in "stable" and "decliner" (**Figure 1**). The individual course and development are important, which can be analyzed in a longitudinal study. To our knowledge, this is the first analysis of the CF lung microbiome using the volatility analysis. The advantage of this approach is the use of machine learning (Random Forest) to highlight how microbial communities change over time. This method is useful to identify the influence of relative abundance and alpha-diversity associated not only with the overall temporal evolution but also with specific time points across individual courses. In our study, we run the model to find predictors of stability and decline in the lung function. The results emphasize the urgency to monitor the microbiome over time with a proper method. It becomes obvious that a single time-point analysis or comparison between two time-points can only give a snapshot and may lead to false impressions since the two curves in the volatility plot usually overlap strongly (**Figure 2**). Only the multiple and longitudinal analyses identify the average development and highlight the differences between the patient groups.

The role of Bacteroidetes and Firmicutes in a microbial community is a highly discussed topic in microbiome research (Fabbrizzi et al., 2019). A higher amount of short-chain fatty acids like acetate and butyrate were reported in individuals with increased Firmicutes abundance in the gut (Turnbaugh et al., 2006). Butyrate was shown in animal models to decrease oxidative stress in the gut and inhibit inflammation (Hamer et al., 2008). The lower abundance of Firmicutes in the "decliner" leads to the speculation that the level of butyrate could as well be decreased in this patient group. Assuming the butyrate amount in the lung also affects oxidative stress and inflammation, as it does in the gut microbiome; this could be a functional factor explaining our findings. Further analysis of metabolome products is necessary.

One of the main Proteobacteria found in our cohort was *Pseudomonas aeruginosa*. The lungs of four patients in this study cohort were chronically infected with *Pseudomonas*. Those patients showed a higher decrease in lung function as well as a microbiome which was more dominated by one ASV and thus less diverse but more stable. Chronic infections with the pathogen *Pseudomonas aeruginosa* were previously associated with lower diversity, higher dominance, increase in bacterial biomass of the lung microbiome (Boutin et al., 2017), and lower FEV_1 values (Zemanick et al., 2013). In this longitudinal study, we confirm these observations partially, although there were also three patients with a moderate decrease of FEV_1%pred per year and one patient with the highest worsening of the lung function without *Pseudomonas* infection. The microbiome of the latter patient revealed the occurrence of genera like *Aggregatibacter*, *Escherichia/Shigella*, *Eikenella*, *Bordetella*, *Stenotrophomonas*, and *Actinobacillus*, which are not characteristic for a healthy lung microbiome, and *Staphylococcus* which was already reported as a pathogen in CF (Akil and Muhlebach, 2018). Taken together, the infection with *Pseudomonas* correlates with the clinical data from the patients, but it cannot be the only reason for the decline in lung function of the CF patients.

Environmental factors are also affecting the lung function of CF patients by triggering exacerbation. I.v. antibiotic treatment was reported to increase lung function after an acute pulmonary exacerbation temporarily (Carmody et al., 2018). The higher frequency of antibiotic usage was linked to a worsening of lung function in the analyzed period in our study. However, this is a typical causality-consequence paradox and could be just a confounding factor because antibiotics have been the major improvement to treat pulmonary exacerbations in patients with CF. Whether the more frequent antibiotic therapies or the high frequency of clinical worsening led to a higher decline of FEV1%pred cannot be answered yet. Most likely, it is an interplay between both and other factors.

This study must be interpreted considering some limitations, which need to be addressed in future studies, like the relatively small cohort. Unfortunately, we also did not observe patients who started with a healthy-like microbiome and ended with a dominated microbiome to analyze the cause/consequence relationship between Proteobacteria and lung decline. The longitudinal analysis requires a repeated long-term sampling of the same patients; thus, we have a high number of samples with a low number of patients with the use of 16S rRNA gene-targeted sequencing. Further, we were limited in the depth of taxonomic analysis and were not capable to report virus or fungus abundances in the microbiome as well as information about existing genes, expression patterns, and biochemical pathways. Furthermore, we used spontaneous sputum expectoration as a proxy for the lower-airway state of health, limiting this study to patients who naturally expectorate sputum and therefore to patients with more severe lung diseases.

In summary, our data demonstrate that adolescents with CF showed an individual course of their lung microbiome over a 3–5-year period. The decrease in the variability of the microbiome was associated with the worsening of lung function mostly linked to a decline in the lung clearance and accumulation of PRPs. Furthermore, our data show that decliners present a disturbed microbiome dominated by a single species and a higher prevalence of i.v. antibiotic usage. While the benefit of antibiotics is undeniable, this makes one think about antibiotic stewardship and especially a shift toward more targeted therapy and alternative strategies.

ETHICS STATEMENT

The studies involving human participants were reviewed and approved by the ethics committee of the University of Heidelberg (S 370/2011). Written informed consent to participate in this study was provided by the participants' legal guardian/next of kin.

AUTHOR CONTRIBUTIONS

MAM, AD, and SB contributed to the conception and design of the study. SG, MS, and OS organized the clinical database. MIM and SB performed the bioinformatic and statistical analysis. MIM and SB wrote the first draft of the manuscript. All authors contributed to manuscript revision, read, and approved the submitted version.

ACKNOWLEDGMENTS

We acknowledge the excellent technical support by Selina Hassel. The authors thank all patients with CF for their participation in this study.

REFERENCES

Ahmed, B., Cox, M. J., Cuthbertson, L., James, P., Cookson, W. O. C., Davies, J. C., et al. (2019). Longitudinal Development of the Airway Microbiota in Infants With Cystic Fibrosis. *Sci. Rep.* 9, 5143. doi: 10.1038/s41598-019-41597-0

Akil, N., and Muhlebach, M. S. (2018). Biology and Management of Methicillin Resistant Staphylococcus Aureus in Cystic Fibrosis. *Pediatric Pulmonology* 53, S64–S74. doi: 10.1002/ppul.24139

Bell, S. C., Mall, M. A., Gutierrez, H., Macek, M., Madge, S., Davies, J. C., et al. (2020). The Future of Cystic Fibrosis Care: A Global Perspective. *Lancet Respir. Med.* 8, 65–124. doi: 10.1016/S2213-2600(19)30337-6

Bokulich, N. A., Dillon, M. R., Zhang, Y., Rideout, J. R., Bolyen, E., Li, H., et al. (2018). Q2-Longitudinal: Longitudinal and Paired-Sample Analyses of Microbiome Data. *mSystems* 3, e00219–e00218. doi: 10.1128/mSystems.00219-18

Boutin, S., Graeber, S. Y., Stahl, M., Dittrich, A. S., Mall, M. A., and Dalpke, A. H. (2017). Chronic But Not Intermittent Infection With Pseudomonas Aeruginosa is Associated With Global Changes of the Lung Microbiome in Cystic Fibrosis. *Eur. Respir. J.* 50, 1701086. doi: 10.1183/13993003.01086-2017

Boutin, S., Graeber, S. Y., Weitnauer, M., Panitz, J., Stahl, M., Clausznitzer, D., et al. (2015). Comparison of Microbiomes From Different Niches of Upper and Lower Airways in Children and Adolescents With Cystic Fibrosis. *PLoS One* 10, e0116029. doi: 10.1371/journal.pone.0116029

Carmody, L. A., Caverly, L. J., Foster, B. K., Rogers, M. A. M., Kalikin, L. M., Simon, R. H., et al. (2018). Fluctuations in Airway Bacterial Communities Associated With Clinical States and Disease Stages in Cystic Fibrosis. *PLoS One* 13, e0194060. doi: 10.1371/journal.pone.0194060

Carmody, L. A., Zhao, J., Kalikin, L. M., LeBar, W., Simon, R. H., Venkataraman, A., et al. (2015). The Daily Dynamics of Cystic Fibrosis Airway Microbiota During Clinical Stability and at Exacerbation. *Microbiome* 3, 12. doi: 10.1186/s40168-015-0074-9

Coburn, B., Wang, P. W., Diaz Caballero, J., Clark, S. T., Brahma, V., Donaldson, S., et al. (2015). Lung Microbiota Across Age and Disease Stage in Cystic Fibrosis. *Sci. Rep.* 5, 10241. doi: 10.1038/srep10241

Cooper, B. G., Stocks, J., Hall, G. L., Culver, B., Steenbruggen, I., Carter, K. W., et al. (2017). The Global Lung Function Initiative (GLI) Network: Bringing the World's Respiratory Reference Values Together. *Breathe (Sheff)* 13, e56–e64. doi: 10.1183/20734735.012717

Cox, M. J., Allgaier, M., Taylor, B., Baek, M. S., Huang, Y. J., Daly, R. A., et al. (2010). Airway Microbiota and Pathogen Abundance in Age-Stratified Cystic Fibrosis Patients. *PLoS One* 5, e11044. doi: 10.1371/journal.pone.0011044

Cuthbertson, L., Rogers, G. B., Walker, A. W., Oliver, A., Green, L. E., Daniels, T. W., et al. (2016). Respiratory Microbiota Resistance and Resilience to Pulmonary Exacerbation and Subsequent Antimicrobial Intervention. *Isme J.* 10, 1081–1091. doi: 10.1038/ismej.2015.198

De Boeck, K., Derichs, N., Fajac, I., de Jonge, H. R., Bronsveld, I., Sermet, I., et al. (2011). New Clinical Diagnostic Procedures for Cystic Fibrosis in Europe. *J. Cyst Fibros* 10 Suppl 2, S53–S66. doi: 10.1016/S1569-1993(11)60009-X

Dickson, R. P., Erb-Downward, J. R., Freeman, C. M., McCloskey, L., Beck, J. M., Huffnagle, G. B., et al. (2015). Spatial Variation in the Healthy Human Lung Microbiome and the Adapted Island Model of Lung Biogeography. *Ann. Am. Thorac. Soc.* 12, 821–830. doi: 10.1513/AnnalsATS.201501-029OC

Fabbrizzi, A., Amedei, A., Lavorini, F., Renda, T., and Fontana, G. (2019). The Lung Microbiome: Clinical and Therapeutic Implications. *Internal Emergency Med.* 14, 1241–1250. doi: 10.1007/s11739-019-02208-y

Frayman, K. B., Armstrong, D. S., Carzino, R., Ferkol, T. W., Grimwood, K., Storch, G. A., et al. (2017). The Lower Airway Microbiota in Early Cystic Fibrosis Lung Disease: A Longitudinal Analysis. *Thorax* 72, 1104–1112. doi: 10.1136/thoraxjnl-2016-209279

Hamer, H. M., Jonkers, D., Venema, K., Vanhoutvin, S., Troost, F. J., and Brummer, R. J. (2008). Review Article: The Role of Butyrate on Colonic Function. *Aliment Pharmacol. Ther.* 27, 104–119. doi: 10.1111/j.1365-2036.2007.03562.x

Jari Oksanen, F. G. B., Friendly, M., Kindt, R., Legendre, P., McGlinn, D., Minchin, P. R., et al. (2019) *Vegan: Community Ecology Package. R Package Version 2.5-4.* Available at: https://CRAN.R-project.org/package=vegan.

Leo Lahti, S. S., Tineka, B., and Jarkko, S. (2017). *Microbiome R Package. 2012.*

Maechler, M., Rousseeuw, P., Struyf, A., Hubert, M., and Hornik, K. (2019). *Cluster: Cluster Analysis Basics and Extensions. R Package Version 2.0.9.*

Mall, M. A., Mayer-Hamblett, N., and Rowe, S. M. (2020). Cystic Fibrosis: Emergence of Highly Effective Targeted Therapeutics and Potential Clinical Implications. *Am. J. Respir. Crit. Care Med.* 201, 1193–1208. doi: 10.1164/rccm.201910-1943SO

McMurdie, P. J., and Holmes, S. (2013). Phyloseq: An R Package for Reproducible Interactive Analysis and Graphics of Microbiome Census Data. *PLoS One* 8, e61217. doi: 10.1371/journal.pone.0061217

O'Neill, K., Bradley, J. M., Johnston, E., McGrath, S., McIlreavey, L., Rowan, S., et al. (2015). Reduced Bacterial Colony Count of Anaerobic Bacteria is Associated With a Worsening in Lung Clearance Index and Inflammation in Cystic Fibrosis. *PLoS One* 10, e0126980. doi: 10.1371/journal.pone.0126980

Schliep, K. P. (2011). Phangorn: Phylogenetic Analysis in R. *Bioinformatics* 27, 592–593. doi: 10.1093/bioinformatics/btq706

Schmitt, F. C. F., Lipinski, A., Hofer, S., Uhle, F., Nusshag, C., Hackert, T., et al. (2020). Pulmonary Microbiome Patterns Correlate With the Course of the Disease in Patients With Sepsis-Induced ARDS Following Major Abdominal Surgery. *J. Hosp Infect.* S0195-6701(20)30203-6. doi: 10.1016/j.jhin.2020.04.028

Schoilew, K., Ueffing, H., Dalpke, A., Wolff, B., Frese, C., Wolff, D., et al. (2019). Bacterial Biofilm Composition in Healthy Subjects With and Without Caries Experience. *J. Oral. Microbiol.* 11, 1633194. doi: 10.1080/20002297.2019.1633194

Sherrard, L. J., Tunney, M. M., and Elborn, J. S. (2014). Antimicrobial Resistance in the Respiratory Microbiota of People With Cystic Fibrosis. *Lancet* 384, 703–713. doi: 10.1016/S0140-6736(14)61137-5

Stahl, M., Wielputz, M. O., Graeber, S. Y., Joachim, C., Sommerburg, O., Kauczor, H. U., et al. (2017). Comparison of Lung Clearance Index and Magnetic Resonance Imaging for Assessment of Lung Disease in Children With Cystic Fibrosis. *Am. J. Respir. Crit. Care Med.* 195, 349–359. doi: 10.1164/rccm.201604-0893OC

Szczesniak, R. D., Li, D., Su, W., Brokamp, C., Pestian, J., Seid, M., et al. (2017). Phenotypes of Rapid Cystic Fibrosis Lung Disease Progression During Adolescence and Young Adulthood. *Am. J. Respir. Crit. Care Med.* 196, 471–478. doi: 10.1164/rccm.201612-2574OC

Team RC (2019). *R: A Language and Environment for Statistical Computing* (Vienna, Austria: R Foundation for Statistical Computing). Available at: https://www.R-project.org/.

Turnbaugh, P. J., Ley, R. E., Mahowald, M. A., Magrini, V., Mardis, E. R., and Gordon, J. I. (2006). An Obesity-Associated Gut Microbiome With Increased Capacity for Energy Harvest. *nature* 444, 1027. doi: 10.1038/nature05414

Whelan, F. J., Heirali, A. A., Rossi, L., Rabin, H. R., Parkins, M. D., and Surette, M. G. (2017). Longitudinal Sampling of the Lung Microbiota in Individuals With Cystic Fibrosis. *PLoS One* 12, e0172811. doi: 10.1371/journal.pone.0172811

Wright, E. S. (2016). Using DECIPHER V2.0 to Analyze Big Biological Sequence Data in R. *R J.* 8, 352–359. doi: 10.32614/RJ-2016-025

Zemanick, E. T., Harris, J. K., Wagner, B. D., Robertson, C. E., Sagel, S. D., Stevens, M. J., et al. (2013). Inflammation and Airway Microbiota During Cystic Fibrosis Pulmonary Exacerbations. *PLoS One* 8, e62917. doi: 10.1371/journal.pone.0062917

Zemanick, E. T., Wagner, B. D., Robertson, C. E., Ahrens, R. C., Chmiel, J. F., Clancy, J. P., et al. (2017). Airway Microbiota Across Age and Disease Spectrum in Cystic Fibrosis. *Eur. Respir. J.* 50 (5), 1700832. doi: 10.1183/13993003.00832-2017

Permissions

All chapters in this book were first published by Frontiers; hereby published with permission under the Creative Commons Attribution License or equivalent. Every chapter published in this book has been scrutinized by our experts. Their significance has been extensively debated. The topics covered herein carry significant findings which will fuel the growth of the discipline. They may even be implemented as practical applications or may be referred to as a beginning point for another development.

The contributors of this book come from diverse backgrounds, making this book a truly international effort. This book will bring forth new frontiers with its revolutionizing research information and detailed analysis of the nascent developments around the world.

We would like to thank all the contributing authors for lending their expertise to make the book truly unique. They have played a crucial role in the development of this book. Without their invaluable contributions this book wouldn't have been possible. They have made vital efforts to compile up to date information on the varied aspects of this subject to make this book a valuable addition to the collection of many professionals and students.

This book was conceptualized with the vision of imparting up-to-date information and advanced data in this field. To ensure the same, a matchless editorial board was set up. Every individual on the board went through rigorous rounds of assessment to prove their worth. After which they invested a large part of their time researching and compiling the most relevant data for our readers.

The editorial board has been involved in producing this book since its inception. They have spent rigorous hours researching and exploring the diverse topics which have resulted in the successful publishing of this book. They have passed on their knowledge of decades through this book. To expedite this challenging task, the publisher supported the team at every step. A small team of assistant editors was also appointed to further simplify the editing procedure and attain best results for the readers.

Apart from the editorial board, the designing team has also invested a significant amount of their time in understanding the subject and creating the most relevant covers. They scrutinized every image to scout for the most suitable representation of the subject and create an appropriate cover for the book.

The publishing team has been an ardent support to the editorial, designing and production team. Their endless efforts to recruit the best for this project, has resulted in the accomplishment of this book. They are a veteran in the field of academics and their pool of knowledge is as vast as their experience in printing. Their expertise and guidance has proved useful at every step. Their uncompromising quality standards have made this book an exceptional effort. Their encouragement from time to time has been an inspiration for everyone.

The publisher and the editorial board hope that this book will prove to be a valuable piece of knowledge for researchers, students, practitioners and scholars across the globe.

List of Contributors

Jasmin Matuszak
Institute of Physiology, Charité - Universitätsmedizin Berlin, Corporate Member of Freie Universität Berlin, Humboldt-Universität zu Berlin, and Berlin Institute of Health, Berlin, Germany

Arata Tabuchi
The Keenan Research Centre for Biomedical Science at St. Michael's, Toronto, ON, Canada

Wolfgang M. Kuebler
Institute of Physiology, Charité - Universitätsmedizin Berlin, Corporate Member of Freie Universität Berlin, Humboldt-Universität zu Berlin, and Berlin Institute of Health, Berlin, Germany
Departments of Surgery and Physiology, University of Toronto, Toronto, ON, Canada

Samer Bou Jawde, Ayuko Takahashi and Béla Suki
Biomedical Engineering, Boston University, Boston, MA, United States

Jason H. T. Bates
Department of Medicine, Larner College of Medicine, University of Vermont, Burlington, VT, United States

Bradford J. Smith
Department of Bioengineering, College of Engineering, Design & Computing, University of Colorado Denver | Anschutz Medical Campus, Aurora, CO, United States
Department of Pediatric Pulmonary and Sleep Medicine, School of Medicine, University of Colorado Anschutz Medical Campus, Aurora, CO, United States

Gregory S. Roy, Alyx Cleveland and Chantel M. Charlebois
Vermont Lung Center, Larner College of Medicine, The University of Vermont, Burlington, VT, United States

Courtney Mattson and Kayo Okamura
Department of Bioengineering, College of Engineering, Design & Computing, University of Colorado Denver | Anschutz Medical Campus, Aurora, CO, United States

Katharine L. Hamlington
Department of Pediatric Pulmonary and Sleep Medicine, School of Medicine, University of Colorado Anschutz Medical Campus, Aurora, CO, United States

Michael V. Novotny
Lerner Research Institute, Cleveland Clinic, Cleveland, OH, United States

Lars Knudsen
Institute of Functional and Applied Anatomy, Hannover Medical School, Hanover, Germany
Biomedical Research in Endstage and Obstructive Lung Disease Hannover (BREATH), Member of the German Center for Lung Research, Hanover, Germany

Matthias Ochs
Institute of Functional Anatomy, Charité Medical University of Berlin, Berlin, Germany

R. Duncan Hite
Lerner Research Institute, Cleveland Clinic, Cleveland, OH, United States
Division of Pulmonary, Critical Care and Sleep Medicine, Department of Internal Medicine, College of Medicine, University of Cincinnati, Cincinnati, OH, United States

Vitor Mori
Department of Medicine, Vermont Lung Center, Larner College of Medicine, The University of Vermont, Burlington, VT, United States
Department of Telecommunications and Control Engineering, University of São Paulo, São Paulo, Brazil

Bela Suki
Department of Biomedical Engineering, Boston University, Boston, MA, United States

Jason H. T. Bates
Department of Medicine, Vermont Lung Center, Larner College of Medicine, The University of Vermont, Burlington, VT, United States

Henri Schulte
Institute of Functional and Applied Anatomy, Hannover Medical School, Hanover, Germany

Christian Mühlfeld and Christina Brandenberger
Cluster of Excellence REBIRTH (From Regenerative Biology to Reconstructive Therapy), Hanover, Germany
Biomedical Research in Endstage and Obstructive Lung Disease Hannover (BREATH), Member of the German Center for Lung Research (DZL), Hanover, Germany

Kirsten Sehlmeyer and Jannik Ruwisch
Institute of Functional and Applied Anatomy, Hannover Medical School, Hanover, Germany
Biomedical Research in Endstage and Obstructive Lung Disease Hannover, Member of the German Centre for Lung Research, Hanover, Germany

Nuria Roldan
Alveolix AG and ARTORG Center, University of Bern, Bern, Switzerland

Elena Lopez-Rodriguez
Institute of Functional and Applied Anatomy, Hannover Medical School, Hanover, Germany
Biomedical Research in Endstage and Obstructive Lung Disease Hannover, Member of the German Centre for Lung Research, Hanover, Germany
Institute of Functional Anatomy, Charité - Universitätsmedizin Berlin, Berlin, Germany

Tiziana P. Cremona and Johannes C. Schittny
Institute of Anatomy, Department of Preclinical Medicine, Faculty of Medicine, University of Bern, Bern, Switzerland

Andrea Hartner
Department of Pediatrics and Adolescent Medicine, University Hospital of Erlangen-Nürnberg, Erlangen, Germany

Jacob Herrmann
Roy J. Carver Department of Biomedical Engineering, University of Iowa, Iowa City, IA, United States
Department of Anesthesia, University of Iowa, Iowa City, IA, United States
OscillaVent, Inc., Iowa City, IA, United States

Sarah E. Gerard
Roy J. Carver Department of Biomedical Engineering, University of Iowa, Iowa City, IA, United States

Wei Shao
Department of Electrical and Computer Engineering, University of Iowa, Iowa City, IA, United States

Monica L. Hawley
OscillaVent, Inc., Iowa City, IA, United States

Joseph M. Reinhardt
Roy J. Carver Department of Biomedical Engineering, University of Iowa, Iowa City, IA, United States
Department of Radiology, University of Iowa, Iowa City, IA, United States

Gary E. Christensen
Department of Electrical and Computer Engineering, University of Iowa, Iowa City, IA, United States
Department of Radiation Oncology, University of Iowa, Iowa City, IA, United States

Eric A. Hoffman
Roy J. Carver Department of Biomedical Engineering, University of Iowa, Iowa City, IA, United States
Department of Radiology, University of Iowa, Iowa City, IA, United States
Department of Internal Medicine, University of Iowa, Iowa City, IA, United States

David W. Kaczka
Roy J. Carver Department of Biomedical Engineering, University of Iowa, Iowa City, IA, United States
Department of Anesthesia, University of Iowa, Iowa City, IA, United States
OscillaVent, Inc., Iowa City, IA, United States
Department of Radiology, University of Iowa, Iowa City, IA, United States

Joshua Satalin, Sarah J. Blair and Gary F. Nieman
Department of Surgery, SUNY Upstate Medical University, Syracuse, NY, United States

Penny L. Andrews
Department of Critical Care, R Adams Cowley Shock Trauma Center, University of Maryland Medical Center, Baltimore, MD, United States

Louis A. Gatto
Department of Surgery, SUNY Upstate Medical University, Syracuse, NY, United States
Department of Biological Sciences, SUNY Cortland, Cortland, NY, United States

Karolin Albert, Jeanne-Marie Krischer and Alexander Pfaffenroth
Institute of Functional and Applied Anatomy, Hannover Medical School, Hanover, Germany

Sabrina Wilde and Armin Braun
Fraunhofer Institute for Toxicology and Experimental Medicine, Hanover, Germany
Biomedical Research in Endstage and Obstructive Lung Disease Hannover (BREATH), German Center for Lung Research, Hanover, Germany

Carrie E. Perlman
Department of Biomedical Engineering, Stevens Institute of Technology, Hoboken, NJ, United States

Gary F. Nieman, Joshua Satalin and Sarah Blair
Department of Surgery, SUNY Upstate Medical University, Syracuse, NY, United States

Hassan Al-Khalisy and Girish Trikha
Department of Surgery, SUNY Upstate Medical University, Syracuse, NY, United States
Department of Medicine, SUNY Upstate Medical University, Syracuse, NY, United States

Michaela Kollisch-Singule
Department of Pediatric Surgery, Arkansas Children's Hospital, Little Rock, AR, United States

Penny Andrews, Maria Madden and Nader M. Habashi
Department of Trauma Critical Care Medicine, R Adams Cowley Shock Trauma Center, University of Maryland School of Medicine, Baltimore, MD, United States

Haoran Ma and Donald P. Gaver III
Department of Biomedical Engineering, Tulane University, New Orleans, LA, United States

Hideki Fujioka
Center for Computational Science, Tulane University, New Orleans, LA, United States

David Halpern
Department of Mathematics, University of Alabama, Tuscaloosa, AL, United States

Paolo Jose Cesare Biselli
Intensive Care Unit, University Hospital, University of Sao Paulo, Sao Paulo, Brazil

Fernanda Degobbi Tenorio Quirino Dos Santos Lopes, Iolanda Fátima Lopes Calvo Tibério and Milton Arruda Martins
Laboratory of Experimental Therapeutics, Department of Clinical Medicine, School of Medicine, University of Sao Paulo, Sao Paulo, Brazil

Renato Fraga Righetti
Laboratory of Experimental Therapeutics, Department of Clinical Medicine, School of Medicine, University of Sao Paulo, Sao Paulo, Brazil
Hospital Sírio-Libanês, Serviço de Reabilitação, São Paulo, Brazil

Henrique Takachi Moriya
Biomedical Engineering Laboratory, Escola Politecnica, University of Sao Paulo, Sao Paulo, Brazil

Soula Danopoulos, Jessica Shiosaki and Denise Al Alam
Saban Research Institute, Children's Hospital Los Angeles, Los Angeles, CA, United States

Vardhman Kumar and Anna Gilpin
Department of Biomedical Engineering, Duke University, Durham, NC, United States

Sajeesh Kumar Madhurakkat Perikamana and Jiaul Hoque
Department of Orthopaedic Surgery, Duke University School of Medicine, Durham, NC, United States

Aleksandra Tata
Department of Cell Biology, Duke University School of Medicine, Durham, NC, United States

Purushothama Rao Tata
Department of Cell Biology, Duke University School of Medicine, Durham, NC, United States
Regeneration Next, Duke University, Durham, NC, United States

Shyni Varghese
Department of Biomedical Engineering, Duke University, Durham, NC, United States
Department of Orthopaedic Surgery, Duke University School of Medicine, Durham, NC, United States
Department of Mechanical Engineering and Material Science, Duke University, Durham, NC, United States

Marisa I. Metzger and Sébastien Boutin
Department of Infectious Diseases, Medical Microbiology and Hygiene, University of Heidelberg, Heidelberg, Germany
Translational Lung Research Center Heidelberg (TLRC), German Center for Lung Research (DZL), University of Heidelberg, Heidelberg, Germany

Simon Y. Graeber and Mirjam Stahl and Marcus A. Mall
German Centre for Lung Research (DZL), Associated Partner Site, Berlin, Germany
Department of Pediatric Respiratory Medicine, Immunology and Critical Care Medicine and Cystic Fibrosis Center, Charité-Universitätsmedizin Berlin, Berlin, Germany
Berlin Institute of Health (BIH), Berlin, Germany

Olaf Sommerburg
Translational Lung Research Center Heidelberg (TLRC), German Center for Lung Research (DZL), University of Heidelberg, Heidelberg, Germany
Division of Pediatric Pulmonology & Allergy and Cystic Fibrosis Center, Department of Pediatrics, University of Heidelberg, Heidelberg, Germany
Department of Translational Pulmonology, University of Heidelberg, Heidelberg, Germany

Alexander H. Dalpke
Institute of Medical Microbiology and Virology, Technische Universität Dresden, Dresden, Germany

Index